Contemporary Cardiology

Series Editor

For more than a decade, cardiologists have relied on the Contemporary Cardiology series to provide them with forefront medical references on all aspects of cardiology. Each title is carefully crafted by world-renown cardiologists who comprehensively cover the most important topics in this rapidly advancing field. With more than 75 titles in print covering everything from diabetes and cardiovascular disease to the management of acute coronary syndromes, the Contemporary Cardiology series has become the leading reference source for the practice of cardiac care.

George J. Arnaoutakis • Ibrahim Sultan
Gilbert R. Upchurch Jr.
Editors

Aortic Aneurysms

Pathogenesis and Treatment

Second Edition

Humana Press

Editors
George J. Arnaoutakis
University of Texas at Austin Dell Medical School
Austin, TX, USA

Ibrahim Sultan
University of Pittsburgh
Pittsburgh, PA, USA

Gilbert R. Upchurch Jr.
University of Florida
Gainesville, FL, USA

ISSN 2196-8969 ISSN 2196-8977 (electronic)
Contemporary Cardiology
ISBN 978-3-032-13133-1 ISBN 978-3-032-13134-8 (eBook)
https://doi.org/10.1007/978-3-032-13134-8

This Humana imprint is published by the registered company Springer Nature Switzerland AG
The registered company address is: Gewerbestrasse 11, 6330 Cham, Switzerland

To my beloved family—thank you for your support and encouragement, which inspires me to pursue meaningful advances in the care of patients living with aortic disease.

George J. Arnaoutakis, MD

Thanks to all of the students, residents, and fellows I have mentored for all your selfless care as you became educated about aortic disease.

Gilbert R. Upchurch Jr. MD, DHA

Preface to the Second Edition

Aortic disease remains a frequently undetected and highly lethal condition, often asymptomatic until rupture has occurred. Yet, since the publication of the first edition of *Aortic Aneurysms: Pathogenesis and Treatment*, the understanding and treatment of aortic disease has undergone significant transformation. Innovations in imaging, genetics, endovascular therapy, and surgical technique have expanded our understanding of aortic pathology and broadened the spectrum of available treatments. With this second edition, we have significantly expanded the scope of the textbook to comprehensively address not only abdominal but also thoracic aortic disease—including ascending aorta, arch, and descending thoracic aorta pathology. This evolution reflects advances in multidisciplinary care and the increasing complexity of managing patients with aortic disease across the entire aortic continuum, emphasizing the need for a collaborative approach.

This edition brings together contributions from world-renowned experts in vascular and cardiac surgery, cardiology, radiology, and genetics, ensuring that each chapter reflects the most current evidence and clinical practice. We are grateful to them for contributing their time and expertise. In this edition, we have emphasized clarity, clinical relevance, and scholarly rigor, integrating updated guidelines, surgical strategies, and endovascular techniques while also highlighting emerging frontiers such as connective tissue disorders, and new branched endovascular technology. Whether you are a trainee seeking foundational knowledge or a seasoned clinician looking for nuanced insight into advanced care, we hope this expanded volume serves as a valuable and enduring resource in your practice.

Austin, TX, USA — George J. Arnaoutakis
Pittsburgh, PA, USA — Ibrahim Sultan
Gainesville, FL, USA — Gilbert R. Upchurch Jr.

Contents

Chapter 1
Genetics of Aortic Aneurysm

Karen Kim and Courtney Bromberek

Thoracic Aortic Aneurysm

Thoracic aortic aneurysm (TAA) is a dilation of the thoracic aorta involving all three layers (intima, media, and adventitia) of at least 50% increase in diameter compared to the expected normal diameter. The 2022 ACC/AHA aortic guidelines defined a thoracic aorta measuring 4.0 cm as "dilated" and 4.5 cm or greater as an "aneurysm" [8]. Due to disruption and loss of elastic fibers and increased deposition of proteoglycans in an aneurysmal aortic wall, as well as forces of Laplace's Law, aneurysms are at risk for rupture or dissection. In a 2022 systematic review of population-based studies, Gouveia et al. found that the prevalence of TAAs is 5–10 per 100,000 individuals per year, while the incidence of rupture within this population was 1.6 per 100,000 individuals per year [5]. Most TAA are asymptomatic and are undiagnosed until an emergent event occurs [10], making early detection and proactive screening essential to avoiding early mortality from acute aortic syndrome [13]. While risk factors for thoracic aortic aneurysm include older age, gender, hypertension, atherosclerotic disease, tobacco use, lifestyle, and environment, it has become more and more evident that genetics is a major factor in developing aortic disease. It is currently estimated that about 20% of TAA have a hereditary or genetic component [1].

K. Kim
Department of Cardiovascular and Thoracic Surgery, Dell Medical School, University of Texas, Austin, TX, USA
e-mail: karen.kim@austin.utexas.edu

C. Bromberek (✉)
Department of Cardiovascular and Thoracic Surgery, Dell Medical School, University of Texas, Austin, TX, USA

Institute for Cardiovascular Health, Austin, TX, USA
e-mail: courtney.bromberek@austin.utexas.edu

G. J. Arnaoutakis et al. (eds.), *Aortic Aneurysms*, Contemporary Cardiology,
https://doi.org/10.1007/978-3-032-13134-8_1

Heritable thoracic aortic disease (HTAD) occurs in approximately 1 in 5000 individuals and is divided into syndromic and non-syndromic conditions. The genes identified to date that contribute to HTAD can be broadly categorized based on the cellular components they affect:

- *Extracellular Matrix (ECM) Genes:* These genes encode proteins crucial for the structural integrity of the aortic wall. Examples include *FBN1*, *MFAP5*, *LOX*, and *COL3A1*.
- *TGFβ Pathway Genes:* These genes are involved in the transforming growth factor-beta signaling pathway, which regulates cell growth, differentiation, and extracellular matrix production. Examples include *TGFBR1*, *TGFBR2*, *SMAD2*, *SMAD3*, *TGFB2*, and *TGFB3*.
- *Smooth Muscle Cell (SMC) Contractile Mechanism Genes:* These genes affect the function of smooth muscle cells in the aortic wall, which are vital for maintaining vessel tone and integrity. Examples include *ACTA2*, *MYH11*, *MYLK*, and *PRKG1*.

Syndromic HTAD includes multisystem disorders such as Marfan syndrome, Loeys-Dietz syndrome, and vascular Ehlers-Danlos syndrome (vEDS) [13]. In addition to risk for acute aortic syndrome, these conditions often exhibit additional physical traits such as joint hyper-flexibility, skin extensibility, scoliosis, myopia, and distinct facial features. Non-syndromic HTAD, or familial thoracic aortic aneurysm and dissection (FTAAD), is associated with isolated symptoms of aortic disease. Currently, there are approximately 30 genes that have been identified to be associated with TAA (Table 1.1) [2]. The familial nature of TAA and dissections is significant, with up to 20% of affected individuals having at least one affected first-degree relative [11]. Familial cases are associated with a significantly increased risk of TAA and aortic dissection compared to sporadic cases. Due to the overlapping expression and phenotypes of aortic disease, initial gene panel testing via next-generation sequencing [13], rather than individual gene testing, is recommended [3].

Table 1.1 HTAD genes

Condition	Gene
Syndromic HTAD	
Marfan syndrome	FBN1
Vascular Ehlers-Danlos syndrome (vEDS)	COL3A1
Loey-Dietz syndrome	TGFBR1, TGFBR2, SMAD3, TGFB2, TGFB3
Classical Ehlers-Danlos syndrome	COL5A1, COL5A2
Congenital contractual arachnodactyly	FBN2
Ehlers-Danlos syndrome with periventricular nodular heterotopia	FLNA
Osteogenesis Imperfecta and Ehlers-Danlos syndrome	COL1A1, COL1A2
Arterial tortuosity syndrome	SLC2A10
Shprintzen-Goldberg syndrome	SKI
Meester-Loeys syndrome (MRLS)	BGN
Multisystemic Smooth Muscle Dysfunction Syndrome (MSMDS)	ACTA2
LOX-related TAA	LOX
Autosomal recessive cutis laxa type 1B	EFEMP2
Non-syndromic HTAD (Familial TAAD)	
FTAAD/BAV	NOTCH1
FTAAD	ACTA2
FTAAD	FOXE3
FTAAD	MAT2A
FTAAD	MFAP5
FTAAD	MYLK
FTAAD	MYH11
FTAAD	PRKG1
FTAAD	THSD4

BAV bicuspid aortic valve, *FTAAD* familial thoracic aortic aneurysm and dissection, *HTAD* heritable thoracic aortic disease

Abdominal Aortic Aneurysm

In addition to TAA, abdominal aortic aneurysms (AAA) contribute significantly to the likelihood of a cardiovascular event or mortality. According to the Society for Vascular Surgery, ruptured AAA is ranked the 15th leading cause of death overall in individuals and the tenth leading cause of death in men over the age of 55 [15]. However, a 2024 cross-sectional analysis observed that there has been a significant reduction in AAA-related deaths in older individuals, specifically, a 59.6% decrease from 1999 to 2020. This decrease in mortality may be due to factors such as primary prevention, healthcare advancements, and better screening practices [6]. One emerging area of screening for AAA risk is through the use of genetic testing.

Like TAA, there are many factors that can contribute to AAA, such as lifestyle (e.g., smoking), atherosclerosis, age, and hypertension. However, AAA is a multifactorial disease that is known to have a significant genetic component, with studies indicating a heritability of 70% [14]. However, the genetic basis of AAA is not as well-known as TAA. Nevertheless, pathogenic variants in multiple genes have been linked to various aortic aneurysms, including AAA. Specifically, genes such as *FBN1, LOX, PRKG1, SMAD2, SMAD3, TGFB3, TGFBR1,* and *TGFBR2* have been implicated in predisposing individuals to other arteriopathies, including AAA, though some experimental evidence is weaker for certain genes. Therefore, ongoing research is important in fully understanding the genetic causes of AAA. Through genome-wide association studies (GWAS), 24 loci have been identified to be linked to AAA [9]. However, this leaves much of the hereditary aspects of AAA unknown. This highlights the importance of continuing GWAS studies and genetic studies as there is much to still be learned about the genetics of AAA.

Genetic Counseling

Genetic testing has become increasingly accessible and available to patients within the past two decades due to the advancements in technology, increased understanding and awareness of the role of genetics in disease, and clinic laboratories offering cost-effective genetic testing options for patients. Genetic testing can be ordered by any healthcare provider such as genetic counselors, primary care providers, cardiologists, and cardiovascular surgeons [1]. Additionally, genetic testing can be facilitated in both an inpatient and an outpatient setting. Collecting a sample for genetic testing is a simple process in which a blood, saliva, or buccal sample suffices for most situations. These sample collection kits can be ordered and mailed to the clinician from the laboratory by simply placing a request on the laboratory's website. These genetic testing samples can be collected at the time of a patient's visit, or a sample collection kit can be mailed to a patient's home address for at-home collection. Billing for genetic testing typically begins with authorizations through insurance. However, if insurance denies coverage for the genetic test, most laboratories offer patient assistance programs or self-pay options ranging from $249 to $1000 [4, 7]. Due to the better understanding of TAA genetics, most genetic aortopathy panels are tailored to genes associated with TAA rather than AAA. However, some syndromic HTAD that are included on genetic panels, such as vEDS, also have risk for AAA along with the risk for TAA.

Most of the genetic conditions associated with TAD are inherited in an autosomal dominant pattern and are caused by a single causative gene; therefore, first-degree relatives have up to a 50% chance of also inheriting the genetic variant [4]. Although it is not as common, some genetic conditions associated with TAD are inherited in an autosomal recessive pattern; Therefore, a child of two carrier parents has a 25% risk to inherit both pathogenic variants. When performing genetic testing, there are three possible results: positive, negative, and uncertain [4]. The return and discussion of genetic testing results should be performed using post-testing genetic counseling to ensure that the individual has a complete understanding of the results and receives clear guidance on next steps for their own health, as well as their family members' [12].

A positive result indicates that a known likely pathogenic or pathogenic variant (commonly known as a mutation) was identified. This positive result would confirm that an individual has an increased hereditary risk or predisposition to develop thoracic aortic aneurysms, dissections, or ruptures. More frequent screening, earlier surgical intervention, and lifestyle modifications may be recommended. Additionally, depending on the result, there may be implications to surveil other body systems. For example, if the patient were to test positive for syndromic HTAD, such as Marfan syndrome, then a multidisciplinary approach focused on monitoring and addressing the various manifestations of the disorder is essential. Early and ongoing management by a multidisciplinary team of specialists—cardiologists, cardiovascular surgeons, genetic counselors, orthopedists, physical therapists, ophthalmologists, and others—is recommended and crucial for optimizing outcomes and preventing complications for individuals with syndromic HTAD. When an individual tests positive for a known pathogenic variant, predictive testing should be utilized for all first-degree relatives. Most genetic testing laboratories offer free targeted familial cascade testing within 150 days of the positive result. Knowing a family member's genetic status can also help understand their future risk for an aortic aneurysm, dissection, or rupture. Many of the causative genes associated with aortic disease have variable expressivity and reduced penetrance. Therefore, if a family member tests positive for a familial variant but is asymptomatic, it is still crucial to recommend aortic screening and management due to the variation of disease onset that can be seen among individuals with the same genetic mutation [11]. If a family member does not have the known familial variant, then no additional imaging surveillance or management is typically required.

A negative genetic test, which is indicated by the classification of likely benign or benign, means that no known pathogenic variants were identified. This result does not entirely rule out the possibility for there to be a genetic explanation for a personal or family history of aortic aneurysms. This negative result may be due to inadequate technologies to identify the genetic variant, as we do not currently understand all genetic causes for aortic aneurysms at this time, or there may not be a variant in the family. Based on a negative result, no management modifications are necessary for the individual. Genetic testing for the biological children of an individual who has a negative genetic test is not recommended. However, this does not eliminate the possibility of children inheriting a genetic change from their other parent's side of the family. Siblings might consider their own genetic testing, as a negative result does not provide definitive information about their risk given, and they still have a 50% chance of inheriting different alleles from their parents. In the absence of an identifiable genetic cause and based on an individual's personal or family history, first-degree relatives may consider beginning follow-up cardiovascular screening, including cardiac imaging every 2–5 years [8]. Additionally, new genes are continuing to be discovered. Therefore, patients with negative results are encouraged to consider repeat testing and meeting with a genetic counselor every 3–5 years [4].

Finally, an uncertain result, or a variant of uncertain significance (VUS), indicates there is a genetic change that is not currently understood or that the laboratory does not have enough information to know if the VUS is disease-causing or non-disease-causing. In these cases, the result is typically treated as a negative and no management modifications or early surgical intervention are recommended based on this result. Family member testing for the VUS is not recommended. However, some laboratories do offer complimentary VUS family member testing for select genetic variants. In these cases, family members can complete free genetic testing for the VUS, and this will contribute to the information needed to reclassify the variant from uncertain. If in the future the laboratory does gather enough information about the variant and upgrades or downgrades it, the ordering provider will be contacted, and the patient will be updated at that point in time. It is important to note that a VUS result can be frustrating and stressful news for a patient to receive. Therefore, supportive and compassionate counseling is necessary [4].

Current Clinical Guidelines and Management

With the uptake of genetic testing in the cardiac clinical setting, guidelines for management and screening have also been developed. The 2022 ACC/AHA Guideline for the Diagnosis and Management of Aortic Disease provides recommendations to guide clinicians in the process of diagnosing, managing, and surgically treating thoracic aortic aneurysms. For example, aortic dissections account for 22% of all deaths in patients with vEDS, with these dissections being fatal 68% of the time [13]. Therefore, prophylactic aortic surgery for vEDS patients at aortic diameters less than the typical aortic diameter of 5.0–5.5 cm is critical in preventing these fatal aortic dissections. For patients identified to have a pathogenic mutation in causative gene associated with vEDS, surgical intervention is recommended at an aortic diameter of 4.5–5.0 cm [13]. Additionally, these guidelines aid in understanding when genetic testing is warranted in an individual and when genetic testing should be extended to family members (Table 1.2). Examples of instances in which a referral to a genetic specialist or genetic testing should be considered include an aortic aneurysm or dissection diagnosed in an individual before the age of 60, the presence of syndromic features of connective tissue disorders such as Marfan syndrome, Loeys-Dietz syndrome, or vEDS, a positive family history of thoracic aortic or intracranial aneurysms, or a family history of unexplained sudden death before the age of 50 [8]. Currently, there are no guidelines for genetic testing for AAA. However, many of the syndromic HTAD, such as vEDS, include risks for AAA in addition to the risk for a TAA.

Table 1.2 Guidelines for genetic testing in patients with TAD

Indication	Genetic testing?	Family members
TAD diagnosed before the age of 60	Yes—aortopathy panel	If positive, cascade testing offered to family members. If negative or VUS, imaging for aortic imaging recommended for at-risk family members
TAD with the presence of features of MFS, LDS, or vEDS	Yes—aortopathy panel or CTD panel	If positive, cascade testing offered to family members. If negative or VUS, imaging for aortic imaging recommended for at-risk family members
TAD with a family history of thoracic aortic disease or peripheral/intracranial aneurysm	Yes—aortopathy panel	If positive, cascade testing offered to family members. If negative or VUS, imaging for aortic imaging recommended for at-risk family members
TAD with a family history of unexplained/cardiac sudden death <50 yo	Yes—aortopathy panel	If positive, cascade testing offered to family members. If negative or VUS, imaging for aortic imaging recommended for at-risk family members
A family history of a known disease-causing variant associated with thoracic aortic disease	Yes—targeted cascade testing for the known genetic variant	If positive for family variant, cascade testing for offspring. If negative, offspring at general population risk for TAD
"Sporadic" TAD (diagnosed after the age of 60 yo)	Dependent on family history and presence of syndromic features	Aortic imaging recommended for at-risk family members

TAD indicates thoracic aortic disease, *CTD* connective tissue disorder, *MFS* Marfan syndrome, *LDS* Loey-Dietz syndrome, *vEDS* vascular Ehler-Danlos syndrome

Conclusion: The Future of Aneurysm Genetics

TAA and AAA are complex, multifactorial disorders that are known to have a hereditary component. The use of genetic information plays an essential role in personalizing management plans, early detection, and timely surveillance and surgical interventions. Although there have been advancements and increase in knowledge about the genetics of aortic aneurysms, there is still much that is unknown. Additionally, it is important to increase the awareness and availability of genetic testing for individuals with a personal or family history of aortic aneurysms or connective tissue disorders as this will allow for better treatment and screening.

References

1. Acharya M, Maselli D, Mariscalco G. Genetic screening in heritable thoracic aortic disease-rationale, potentials and pitfalls. Indian J Thorac Cardiovasc Surg. 2022;38(Suppl 1):24–35. https://doi.org/10.1007/s12055-020-01124-7.
2. Brownstein AJ, Kostiuk V, Ziganshin BA, Zafar MA, Kuivaniemi H, Body SC, Bale AE, Elefteriades JA. Genes associated with thoracic aortic aneurysm and dissection: 2018 update and clinical implications. Aorta (Stamford). 2018;6(1):13–20. https://doi.org/10.1055/s-0038-1639612. Epub 2018 Jul 27. PMID: 30079932; PMCID: PMC6136681.
3. Demo E, Rigelsky C, Rideout AL, Graf M, Pariani M, Regalado E, MacCarrick G. Genetics and precision medicine: heritable thoracic aortic disease. Med Clin North Am. 2019;103(6):1005–19. https://doi.org/10.1016/j.mcna.2019.08.001. Epub 2019 Aug 31. PMID: 31582001.
4. Elefteriades JA, Zafar MA, Ziganshin BA. Genetics of aortic aneurysm disease: 10 key points for the practitioner. JTCVS Open. 2024;21:58–63.
5. Gouveia E, Melo R, Silva Duarte G, Lopes A, Alves M, Caldeira D, Fernandes E, Fernandes R, Mendes Pedro L. Incidence and prevalence of thoracic aortic aneurysms: a systematic review and meta-analysis of population-based studies. Semin Thorac Cardiovasc Surg. 2022;34(1):1–16. https://doi.org/10.1053/j.semtcvs.2021.02.029. Epub 2021 Mar 8. PMID: 33705940.
6. Goyal A, Saeed H, Shahnoor S, Arshad MK, Wasay A, Abdullah N, et al. Mortality trends, gender, and racial disparities in older adults due to abdominal aortic aneurysm: a nationwide cross-sectional analysis. Int J Surg. 2024;110(12):8241–5.
7. Halbisen AL, Lu CY. Trends in availability of genetic tests in the United States, 2012-2022. J Pers Med. 2023;13(4):638. https://doi.org/10.3390/jpm13040638. PMID: 37109024; PMCID: PMC10142561.
8. Isselbacher EM, et al. 2022 ACC/AHA Guideline for the Diagnosis and Management of Aortic Disease: a report of the American Heart Association/American College of Cardiology Joint Committee on Clinical Practice Guidelines. Circulation. 2022;146(24):e334–482.
9. Klarin D, Verma SS, Judy R, Dikilitas O, Wolford BN, Paranjpe I, et al. Genetic architecture of abdominal aortic aneurysm in the million veteran program. Circulation. 2020;142(17):1633–46.
10. Milewicz DM, Carlson AA, Regalado ES. Genetic testing in aortic aneurysm disease: PRO. Cardiol Clin. 2010;28(2):191–7. https://doi.org/10.1016/j.ccl.2010.01.017. PMID: 20452526; PMCID: PMC3615454.
11. Milewicz DM, Regalado ES. Use of genetics for personalized management of heritable thoracic aortic disease: how do we get there? J Thorac Cardiovasc Surg. 2015;149:S3–5.
12. Musunuru K, et al. Genetic testing for inherited cardiovascular diseases: a scientific statement from the American Heart Association. Circ Genome Precis Med. 2020;13(4):e000067.
13. Ostberg NP, Zafar MA, Ziganshin BA, Elefteriades JA. The genetics of thoracic aortic aneurysms and dissection: a clinical perspective. Biomolecules. 2020;10:182. https://doi.org/10.3390/biom10020182.
14. Wahlgren CM, Larsson E, Magnusson PKE, Hultgren R, Swedenborg J. Genetic and environmental contributions to abdominal aortic aneurysm development in a twin population. J Vasc Surg. 2010 [cited 2022 Mar 27];51(1):3–7.
15. Yamanouchi D. Unpacking the complexities of a silent killer. Int J Mol Sci. 2023;24(8):7125.

Chapter 2
Inflammatory Pathogenesis and Pathophysiology of Thoracic and Abdominal Aortic Aneurysms

Lee M. Fuentes and George J. Arnaoutakis

Introduction

The aorta is a complex structure in which form follows function. The aorta is a high-pressure conduit that also conserves the energy output of the heart (elastic recoil). The main structural proteins of the aorta—collagen (strength) and elastin—serve these functions. In addition to these proteins, there are thousands of other proteins that make up the extracellular matrix (ECM) of the aorta. Together, these structures are organized into lamellae or plates [1]. The ECM is not a passive structure but contains growth factors and encrypted protein fragments. The packaging of growth factors and the dysregulation of transforming growth factor-beta (TGF-β) play a central role in the pathogenesis of Marfan's disease [2, 3]. The ECM, therefore, may also play a central role in healing and disease.

Aortic Heterogeneity

Aortic architecture is heterogenous and varies from the thoracic aorta to the abdominal aorta [4]. This variation in aortic structure may be explained in part by differences in embryology, anatomy, and mechanics. Embryologically, the second heart field leads to the formation of the aortic root, neural crest cells to the ascending aorta and aortic arch, and mesoderm to the descending and abdominal aorta [5]. Anatomically, the three aortic layers—intima, media, and adventitia—grow in

L. M. Fuentes · G. J. Arnaoutakis (✉)
Division of Cardiovascular and Thoracic Surgery, Department of Cardiovascular and Thoracic Surgery, University of Texas at Austin Dell Medical School, Austin, TX, USA
e-mail: lee.m.fuentes@austin.utexas.edu; george.arnaoutakis@austin.utexas.edu

G. J. Arnaoutakis et al. (eds.), *Aortic Aneurysms*, Contemporary Cardiology,
https://doi.org/10.1007/978-3-032-13134-8_2

different patterns above and below the diaphragm. With particular focus on the media, the thoracic aorta contains between 55 and 60 lamellar units compared to the 28–32 lamellar units of the abdominal aorta. This difference accounts for the increased adventitial vasa vasorum of the thoracic aorta because trans-intimal diffusion of oxygen can only support 28–30 lamellar units [6]. Mechanically, the abdominal aorta is subjected to more wall stress and is stiffer, relative to the thoracic aorta. Aging leads to medial thickening, but the mechanism for thickening differs based on aortic region. The thoracic aorta media thickens by lamellar unit synthesis, increasing the quantity. The abdominal aorta media thickens by medial widening of lamellar units, changing the quality [7]. This leads to more stress per lamellar unit in the abdominal aorta because there are relatively fewer lamellar units to share the intraluminal pressure. The synthesis of lamellar units may explain the increased elastin in the thoracic aorta and relatively increased stiffness of the abdominal aorta due to less elastin [8].

Epidemiologically, the aortic heterogeneity results in abdominal aortic aneurysm (AAA) being more prevalent than thoracic aortic aneurysm (TAA), 0.92% vs 0.16% respectively [9, 10]. Regardless, both are largely asymptomatic until dissection or rupture, with the latter carrying a sobering mortality of >90% [11, 12]. Environmental, lifestyle, and genetic factors influence aortic aneurysms and have differing effects throughout the aorta. However, the scope of this chapter is to review the inflammatory processes contributing to thoracic and abdominal aortic aneurysms (TAAA).

Inflammatory Pathogenesis of Aortic Aneurysms

With these basic understandings of the aortic structure and inflammatory pathways in mind, the role that inflammation plays in the pathogenesis of TAAA becomes more apparent. Before immune mediators—cytokines, growth factors, and chemoattractants—can act on the aortic organ, immune cells must infiltrate. Infiltration can occur for a variety of reasons—atherosclerosis, stenosis, thrombosis, and aneurysm formation [13]. In 1951, Dubost reported the first successful repair of an AAA using a human homograft and described this infiltration [14]: "The main feature, together with the destruction of the elastic tissue is the presence throughout the outer half of the aorta of masses of lymphocytic cells accompanying the vaso vasorum; these cells form concentric sheets but are also seen sometimes to follow the vessels at right angles to all layers of the wall. … In summary … this endarteritis and periarteritis would suggest an inflammatory process without any specific indication as to its nature." This observation was not studied in detail until the mid-1980s.

Immune Cell Infiltrates

Rizzo et al. described an inflammatory infiltrate in the outer walls of the aorta in biochemical studies of patients with aneurysms and occlusive disease [15]. This inflammatory infiltrate was later characterized by Koch who found that the majority of cells within the media and adventitia of AAA were CD3-positive T lymphocytes ranging from 67% to 80% [16]. In addition, CD19-positive B cells were also found within the arterial wall. This data suggested that aortic aneurysms may represent an immune-mediated event rather than simple degeneration of the arterial wall. Brophy et al. also described the presence of Russell bodies, which are the accumulation of large amounts of immunoglobulins in the arterial wall [17]. Tilson et al. purified these immunoglobulins and characterized a potential antigenic source, aneurysm-associated protein-40 [18]. Spinosa et al. explored B cell inhibition via B cell-activating factor (BAFF) in AAA formation [19]. Both the innate and adaptive roles of B cells in vitro were identified.

The histological and cytokine profiles of the inflammatory infiltrate suggest both an adaptive and an innate immune response. Eliason et al. explored innate involvement by studying neutropenic animal models exposed to pro-aneurysmal conditions. The control group experienced an increase in aortic diameter of 104 ± 14% compared to 42 ± 33% in the neutropenic group [20]. Platsoucas et al. examined adaptive responses whether the infiltrate represented a monoclonal or a polyclonal T-cell amplification [21]. The β-chain T-cell receptor transcripts from patients with AAA were amplified and characterized. In nine of the ten patients studied, there was an oligoclonal population of T cells. In addition, they found that many of the mononuclear cells found in AAA expressed early, intermediate, and late activation antigens. They concluded that AAA are a specific antigen-driven Th2-predominant cell disease with evidence of ongoing inflammation [22].

Tang et al. examined thoracic aortas and determined that normal aortas, non-infiltrated, and infiltrated—referring to transmural lymphocyte presence—TAA have varying levels of lymphocyte infiltration. TAA were associated with increased levels of CD45-positive lymphocytes throughout the aortic wall compared to non-aneurysmal aortas, as expected. Contrary to previous understanding, TAA are associated with higher levels of CD4 vs CD8-positive T lymphocytes in the media and adventitia. This means that TAA inflammation is a predominantly Th1-driven process while AAA inflammation is a mix of both Th1 and Th2 [23].

Cytokines and Inflammatory Mediators

The relationship between inflammatory infiltrate and the subsequent damage to the arterial wall has been evaluated in many animal models [24]. Using an elastase-induced aneurysm model, Thompson et al. studied the progression of disease [25].

Three days following an acute response, a transitional inflammatory state exists. By days 10–14, the inflammation becomes chronic (Fig. 2.1). During this period, there are alterations in the cytokine proteins as well as the expression of metalloproteinases and their inhibitors—tissue inhibitors of metalloproteinases (TIMP) [13]. However, experimental aneurysms may occur without an initial injury. APO E knockout mice when exposed to angiotensin II spontaneously develop aortic aneurysms without the sequence of events described above [26]. Thus, the role that inflammation plays in the initiation of AAA is uncertain.

Matrix metalloproteinases (MMPs) appear to play a critical role in the pathogenesis of aneurysms. Busuttil et al. first described collagenase-like activity in the wall of patients with AAA in 1980 [27]. Since then many investigators have described the role that MMPs play in aneurysm formation. The metalloproteinases are a subfamily of the metazincin superfamily of proteinases [28]. The majority of these proteins are secreted as a proenzyme, requiring extracellular activation. However, several MMPs are membrane-bound. Aortic aneurysms have been associated with a variety of MMPs, including 2, 9, and 13 [29]. The substrate specificity of each MMP is variable and, while at first it was thought to be only ECM proteins, other substrates have been identified. Enzyme substrates include both non-collagenase ECM proteins, such as fibronectin and laminin, as well as non-structural components. The non-structural components may be even more important to the pathogenesis of AAA. Non-structural substrates of the MMPs include interleukin-1 alpha (IL-1α), active MMP-9, chemokine (C-X-C motif) ligand 5 (CXCL-5), IL-1β, IL-2 receptor, TGF-β, and many of the pro-MMPs [30]. Thus, MMPs may regulate the inflammatory response.

The immune response is highly regulated to prevent injury to the host. Usually, the inflammatory process leads to a healing process and tissue repair. However, in some instances, this process becomes pathologic, leading to continued tissue damage secondary to the immune response. An infectious etiology is clear in many cases; however, the initiating event may be unknown. The key intersection of MMPs in the regulations of inflammation may be the central process in the pathogenesis of TAAA. The modification of proinflammatory cytokines, chemokines, and the shedding of the membrane receptors by the MMPs are critical. CXCL-7, CXCL-12, CXCL-5 (chemokine), and TGF-β are substrates of MMP-2, MMP-3, and MMP-9 [31]. The lack of critical control of the immune response at multiple layers may, therefore, lead to the same phenotype—aortic aneurysm. The specific route for thoracic and abdominal aortic aneurysms is different. MMP-9 is essential for AAA formation. In animal models, the abdominal aorta demonstrates higher MMP-9 expression compared to the aortic arch. Ailawadi et al. demonstrated the regional, rather than structural, impact of MMP-9 expression by translocating the thoracic and abdominal aorta [32]. Freestone et al. harvested 64 aortic tissue samples from patients undergoing AAA repair. MMP-2 was more concentrated in smaller aneurysms, suggesting MMP-2′s role in early AAA formation [33]. In contrast, TAA formation is driven by MMP-2. Several murine models have shown an increase in MMP-9 during early TAA formation [34, 35]. While MMP-9 expression increases in early TAA formation, Schomaker et al. demonstrated the increasing MMP-2 to

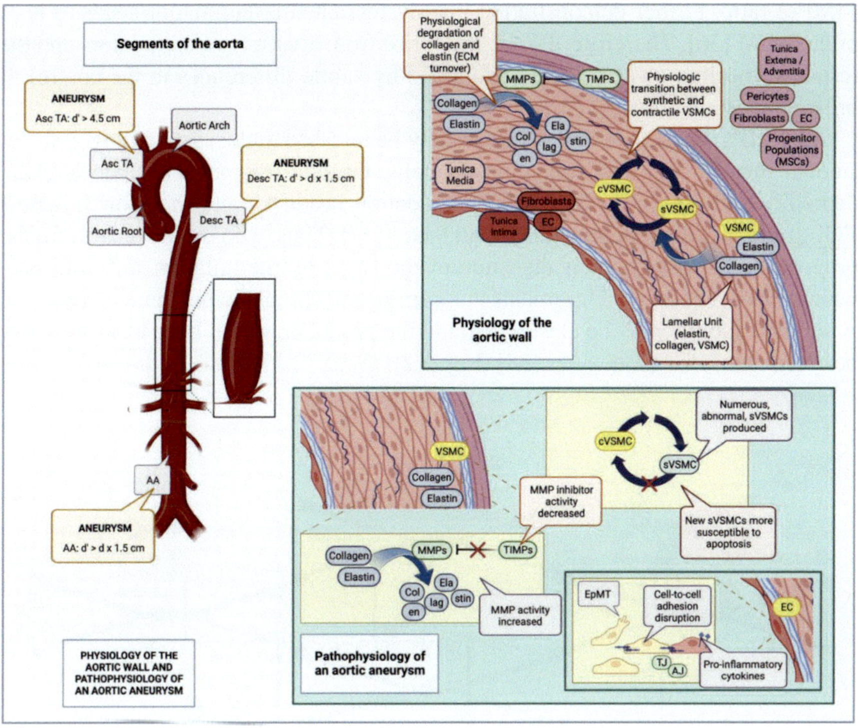

Fig. 2.1 Physiology of the aortic wall and pathophysiology of an aortic aneurysm (Created with BioRender.com): The aorta is composed of three layers, the tunica intima containing ECs along with fibroblasts in the subendothelial layer, the tunica media, composed of elastin interlaced with collagen, and VSMCs (lamellar units), and the tunica externa (adventitia), composed of pericytes, fibroblasts, ECs, and various progenitor cell populations, such as MSCs. Normally, there is a constant turnover of collagen and elastin fibers in the tunica media, carried out by MMPs and inhibited by TIMPs; there is also an equilibrium between synthetic (sVSMC) and contractile VSMC (cVSMC) populations. Aneurysm definitions may vary according to location; thus, for the Asc TA, it is defined as a diameter (d') exceeding 4.5 cm, while for the Desc TA, AA, as well as many visceral vessels, it is defined as an increase in diameter greater than the product of the initial vessel diameter multiplied by 1.5 ($d' > d \times 1.5$). During aneurysm development, many of these normal physiological processes are disrupted. Abnormal sVSMCs, more susceptible to apoptosis, accumulate, there is increased MMP activity along with associated decreased TIMP activity, leading to augmented fragmentation of collagen and elastin fibers. In addition, EC intercellular adhesion is interrupted, due to AJ and TJ derangements, as well as switching of the EC phenotype, from an epithelial to a mesenchymal type; pro-inflammatory cytokines are also expressed on the EC surface, facilitating leukocyte entry into the aortic wall. *MSC* mesenchymal stem cells, *TIMP* tissue inhibitors of metalloproteinase, *MMP* matrix metalloproteinase, *EC* endothelial cell, *VSMC* vascular smooth muscle cell, *TJ* tight junctions, *AJ* adherens junctions, *EpMT* epithelial-to-mesenchymal transition, *Asc TA* ascending thoracic aorta, *Desc TA* descending thoracic aorta, *AA* abdominal aorta, *d* initial aortic diameter, *d'* aneurysmal aortic diameter. (Stougiannou TM, Christodoulou KC, Georgakarakos E, Mikroulis D, Karangelis D. Promising Novel Therapies in the Treatment of Aortic and Visceral Aneurysms. Journal of Clinical Medicine. 2023 Jan;12(18):5878)

TIMP-2 ratio, further demonstrating that dysregulated inflammation leads to lysis of the ECM [36]. Therefore, TAAA may arise from a variety of stimulators and the response (healing or destruction) is guided by subtle differences in the control of inflammation.

As MMPs digest the matrix, signals may be released to the surrounding vascular smooth muscle cells and inflammatory cells. Cryptic fragments include arrestin, deprellin, endostatin, restin, elastin degradation products, and the growth factors TGF-β and vascular endothelial growth factor [37]. Thus, a possible scenario for the progression of aneurysms is digestion of the ECM by the inflammatory infiltrate, which exposes encrypted fragments that continue to stimulate the immune response. A simple example may be elastin degradation products, which have been shown to be chemotactic for monocytes [38] (Fig. 2.2).

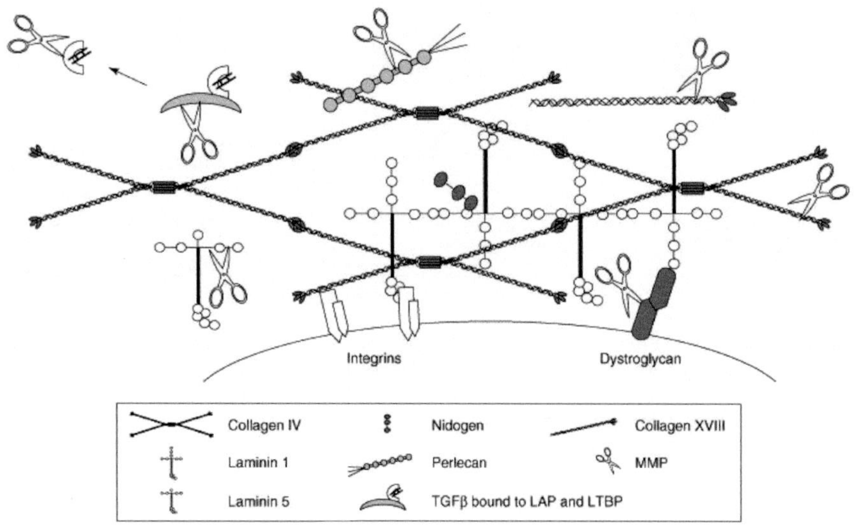

Fig. 2.2 A schematic diagram of some of the proteins that comprise the extracellular matrix (*ECM*) and the potential for matrix metalloproteinase (*MMP*) cleavage. The ECM is composed of both laminin and collagen networks. Within ECM network, many laminins and collagens are present as well as proteins such as nidogen, perlecan (i.e., heparin sulfate proteoglycans), and fibronectin (not shown). Cell surface receptors such as integrins and dystroglycan interact with proteins of the basement membrane network. Cleavage of ECM molecules releases bioactive fragments that have been referred to as matricryptins or matrikines. Furthermore, growth factors, such as latent transforming growth factor-beta (*TGF-β*), are embedded with ECM, and proteolysis of binding proteins that keep the growth factors in a latent state is a major activation pathway. In addition, some of the cell surface receptors such as dystroglycan are targets for proteolysis. Cleavage of these types of molecules breaks cell–ECM contact. (Reprinted from Mott and Werb [34]. Reproduced with permission from Elsevier)

The Genetic Basis of the Inflammatory Response in Thoracic and Abdominal Aortic Aneurysms

The differential expression of genes involved in immune function in AAA versus control aortic tissue was described by Lenk et al. [39]. They used Illumina and Affymetrix microarray platforms to obtain gene expression profiles, and Gene Ontology and Kyoto Encyclopedia of Genes and Genomes database tools to analyze biological pathways. The AAA tissues showed significantly more expression of genes involved in immune function, most notably in pathways regulating cell adhesion molecules, natural killer cell-mediated cytotoxicity, and leukocyte transendothelial migration. The authors acknowledged that a limitation of their study was sampling of AAA tissue from late-stage disease. However, their gene expression data provides valuable insight into the future development of immune-based treatment strategies, as well as direction to the search for underlying genetic factors in AAA.

Family history, or genetics, and sex are significant and independent risk factor for AAA [40, 41]. Which genes predispose to AAA is yet to be determined, but several candidate gene polymorphism studies have shown an association between AAA and genes mediating inflammation. A review by Sandford et al. includes a comprehensive evaluation of genetic research in AAA, based on familial, segregation, and candidate gene studies [42]. In a case-control study of 100 AAA patients and age- and gender-matched controls, Bown et al. reported cytokine gene polymorphism data for the proinflammatory IL−1p + 3953, IL−6 − 174, and tumor necrosis factor-alpha (TNF−α) − 308, and the anti-inflammatory IL−10 promoter polymorphisms at positions 81082 and −592. The A allele for IL−10 R̂ 1082 was found in association with AAA, while the others failed to reach statistical significance [43]. This allele is associated with low IL−10 secretion, and may contribute to the chronic inflammation that is characteristic of AAA. In another study, Ghilardi et al. reported the association of chemokine receptor CCR5 Δ32 deletion and AAA when compared to patients with peripheral arterial occlusive disease, carotid artery disease, and controls. Within the AAA subjects, CCR5 Δ32 was also more commonly found in patients with ruptured aneurysms [44]. The deletion results in the production of fewer receptors and, in theory, less cytokine activation through this receptor pathway. This would appear contrary to increased cytokine levels found in AAA tissue, although the mechanism of this receptor has not been fully described.

TAA contrasts AAA by having a significant genetic association, accounting for 20% of all TAA [45]. Klarin et al. conducted genome-wide association study (GWAS) of 8626 veterans with TAA and dissection and identified 4 known pathologic loci and 17 novel loci [46]. The genetic syndromes—Marfan, Loeys-Dietz, and Heritable Thoracic Aortic Disease—are associated with aberrant signaling pathways—such as upregulation of TGF-β—but outside the scope of this chapter. Recommendations for testing and management are reflected in the 2022 ACC/AHA and 2024 EACTS/STS guidelines [47, 48]. Polymorphisms of IL-6 and IL-1B are associated with TAA formation and are possibly prognostic with severity of systemic and tissue inflammation [49]. After testing both blood-based DNA and aortic tissue samples from 144 patients with TAA and 150 age and gender matched healthy subjects, Scola et al. identified the IL-6 and IL-1B polymorphisms, -174G > C and -511C > T, respectively. Patients expressing both recessive polymorphisms were found to have statistically significant increases of CD-3,4,8,20, and 68+ lymphocytes in the aortic samples.

Evidence of Inflammation in the Circulation of Thoracic and Abdominal Aortic Aneurysm Patients

The presence of inflammatory cells and a number of cytokines within TAAA tissue has been well-documented through histology, immunohistochemistry, and in situ hybridization, although reports of elevated circulating levels of cytokines have been fewer. One exception is IL-6. Dawson et al. reported elevated levels of plasma IL-6 in TAAA patients, and a positive correlation between aneurysm surface area and mean plasma IL-6 concentration [50].

As our understanding of inflammation moves beyond proinflammatory cytokines, a number of interesting studies have emerged. Duftner et al. reviewed serological markers, CRP and ESR, of inflammation in AAA [51]. Duftner also described data from her own studies that showed an increased prevalence of circulating CD4+, CD8+, and CD28- T cells in AAA patients free of preexisting immune-mediated disease, cancer, or acute infection. This subgroup of T cells is known to produce large amounts of interferon-γ, and has been previously seen in patients with a variety of autoimmune diseases.

Plasma samples from 100 of AAA patients and 109 normal controls were analyzed for the soluble forms of the following T-cell costimulatory factors: sCD28, sCTLA-4, sCD86, and sCD80, as well as MMP-9. Compared to controls, plasma from AAA patients showed elevated levels of the T-cell-activating sCD28 and sCD86 ($p = 0.0001$), and a decrease in an inhibitor of T-cell activation, sCTLA-4 ($p = 0.0018$). We also found a significant inverse relationship between concentrations of sCTLA-4 and sCD80 with MMP-9 [52]. Soluble costimulatory molecules of T-cell activation may provide a new set of markers of immune activation in AAA and possible therapeutic targets for future therapies.

Koprulu et al. analyzed the inflammatory markers of 135 patients with TAA, and identified possible association of high sensitivity CRP (hsCRP) and a monocyte to HDL ratio (MHR) to TAA. Granted, the sensitivity and specificity of the hsCRP were 68% and 60%, respectively [53].

Differences in Thoracic and Abdominal Aortic Aneurysm Inflammation

The aorta is a heterogeneous organ from its embryology, structure, mechanics, and inflammatory processes. The various differences are illustrated in Fig. 2.3 created by Ruddy et al. [54] (Fig. 2.3). While both TAA and AAA exhibit immune activation, their inflammatory profiles differ: TAA is predominantly a Th1-driven process with elevated CD4+ lymphocyte infiltration, whereas AAA features a mixed Th1/

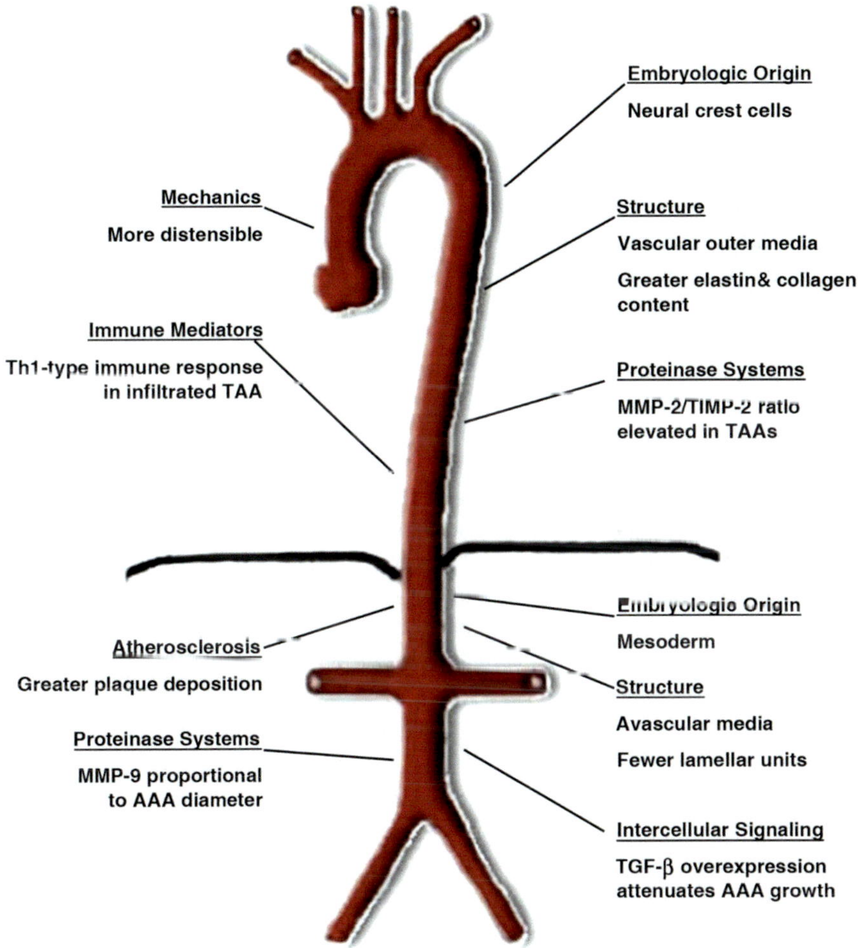

Fig. 2.3 Pertinent disparities between the thoracic and abdominal aorta. *TAA* thoracic aortic aneurysm, *MMP* matrix metalloproteinase, *TIMP* tissue inhibitor of metalloproteinase, *AAA* abdominal aortic aneurysm, *TGF-β* transforming growth factor β. (Reprinted from Ruddy et al. [54]. Reproduced with permission from Elsevier)

Th2 response with significant macrophage and B-cell involvement. MMPs also contribute differentially, with MMP-9 playing a dominant role in TAA and MMP-2 driving AAA progression. Genetic polymorphisms further modulate the inflammatory response, with IL-6 and IL-1B variants influencing TAA severity, while AAA is associated with IL-10, CCR5, and CTLA-4 polymorphisms. Elevated systemic inflammatory markers, such as plasma IL-6 and high-sensitivity CRP, further highlight the immune dysregulation underlying aneurysm progression. Understanding these inflammatory mechanisms and their genetic underpinnings is crucial for developing targeted immune-modulating therapies aimed at preventing aneurysm expansion and rupture.

Conclusions

Inflammatory pathogenesis of TAAA is a complex interplay of immune cell infiltration, cytokine signaling, and ECM remodeling that is influenced by the distinct embryologic, anatomic, and mechanical properties of the thoracic and abdominal aorta. While inflammation appears to play a central role in the formation of both TAA and AAA, the nature of the response differs. The initiating factors that begin the inflammatory cascade are unknown. It is certainly possible that atherosclerosis may be the initiating event. However, smoking is an essential component to the progression of the disease. Once the inflammatory response has been initiated, it appears to be self-perpetuating. A possible explanation for this perpetuation of the inflammation is repeated exposures of cryptic protein fragments. However, once these patients are treated with endovascular grafts, the aneurysm sac regresses, and continued destruction of the aneurysm ceases. If it were true that the inflammatory process was self-sustained, then it is unclear how to explain that the aneurysm sac shrinks when an endograft is placed. Thus, mechanical forces must also play a role in sustaining the process. From the endovascular aneurysm repair experience, it is not pulsatility in as much as the continued pressure. Additional research is needed to further understand the relationship between mechanical forces, inflammatory disease, and genetics.

References

1. Wolinsky H, Glagov S. A lamellar unit of aortic medial structure and function in mammals. Circ Res. 1967;20(1):99–111.
2. Neptune ER, Frischmeyer PA, Arking DE, Myers L, Bunton TE, Gayraud B, et al. Dysregulation of TGF-β activation contributes to pathogenesis in Marfan syndrome. Nat Genet. 2003;33(3):407–11.
3. Boileau C, Guo DC, Hanna N, Regalado ES, Detaint D, Gong L, et al. TGFB2 loss of function mutations cause familial thoracic aortic aneurysms and acute aortic dissections associated with mild systemic features of the Marfan syndrome. Nat Genet. 2012;44(8):916–21.

4. Jauhiainen S, Kiema M, Hedman M, Laakkonen JP. Large vessel cell heterogeneity and plasticity: focus in aortic aneurysms. Arterioscler Thromb Vasc Biol. 2022;42(7):811–8.
5. Maleszewski JJ. Inflammatory ascending aortic disease: perspectives from pathology. J Thorac Cardiovasc Surg. 2015;149(2):S176–83.
6. Wolinsky H, Glagov S. Comparison of abdominal and thoracic aortic medial structure in mammals. Circ Res. 1969;25(6):677–86.
7. Wolinsky H. Comparison of medial growth of human thoracic and abdominal aortas. Circ Res. 1970;27(4):531–8.
8. Halloran BG, Davis VA, McManus BM, Lynch TG, Baxter BT. Localization of aortic disease is associated with intrinsic differences in aortic structure. J Surg Res. 1995;59(1):17–22.
9. Song P, He Y, Adeloye D, Zhu Y, Ye X, Yi Q, et al. The global and regional prevalence of abdominal aortic aneurysms: a systematic review and modeling analysis. Ann Surg. 2023;277(6):912–9.
10. Gouveia E, Melo R, Silva Duarte G, Lopes A, Alves M, Caldeira D, Fernandes E, Fernandes R, et al. Incidence and prevalence of thoracic aortic aneurysms: a systematic review and meta-analysis of population-based studies. Semin Thorac Cardiovasc Surg. 2022;34(1):1–16.
11. Robinson WP, Schanzer A, Li Y, Goodney PP, Nolan BW, Eslami MH, et al. Derivation and validation of a practical risk score for prediction of mortality after open repair of ruptured abdominal aortic aneurysms in a U.S. regional cohort and comparison to existing scoring systems. J Vasc Surg. 2013;57(2):354–61.
12. Johansson G, Markström U, Swedenborg J. Ruptured thoracic aortic aneurysms: a study of incidence and mortality rates. J Vasc Surg. 1995;21(6):985–8.
13. Galis ZS, Khatri JJ. Matrix metalloproteinases in vascular remodeling and atherogenesis: the good, the bad, and the ugly. Circ Res. 2002;90(3):251–62.
14. Dubost C, Allary M, Oeconomos N. Resection of an aneurysm of the abdominal aorta: reestablishment of the continuity by a preserved human arterial graft, with result after five months. AMA Arch Surg. 1952;64(3):405–8.
15. Rizzo RJ, McCarthy WJ, Dixit SN, Lilly MP, Shively VP, Flinn WR, et al. Collagen types and matrix protein content in human abdominal aortic aneurysms. J Vasc Surg. 1989;10(4):0365–73.
16. Koch AE, Haines GK, Rizzo RJ, Radosevich JA, Pope RM, Robinson PG, et al. Human abdominal aortic aneurysms. Immunophenotypic analysis suggesting an immune-mediated response. Am J Pathol. 1990;137(5):1199–213.
17. Brophy CM, Reilly JM, Smith GJW, Tilson MD. The role of inflammation in nonspecific abdominal aortic aneurysm disease. Ann Vasc Surg. 1991;5(3):229–33.
18. Tilson MD, editor. The abdominal aortic aneurysm: genetics, pathophysiology, and molecular biology. Boston: Blackwell; 2006. 411 p. (Annals of the New York Academy of Sciences).
19. Spinosa MD, Montgomery WG, Lempicki M, Srikakulapu P, Johnsrude MJ, McNamara CA, et al. B cell activating factor antagonism attenuates the growth of experimental abdominal aortic aneurysm. Am J Pathol. 2021;191(12):2231–44.
20. Eliason JL, Hannawa KK, Ailawadi G, Sinha I, Ford JW, Deogracias MP, et al. Neutrophil depletion inhibits experimental abdominal aortic aneurysm formation. Circulation. 2005;112(2):232–40.
21. Platsoucas CD, Lu S, Nwaneshiudu I, Solomides C, Agelan A, Ntaoula N, et al. Abdominal aortic aneurysm is a specific antigen-driven T cell disease. Ann N Y Acad Sci. 2006;1085(1):224–35.
22. Schönbeck U, Sukhova GK, Gerdes N, Libby P. TH2 predominant immune responses prevail in human abdominal aortic aneurysm. Am J Pathol. 2002;161(2):499–506.
23. Tang PCY, Yakimov AO, Teesdale MA, Coady MA, Dardik A, Elefteriades JA, et al. Transmural inflammation by interferon-γ-producing T cells correlates with outward vascular remodeling and intimal expansion of ascending thoracic aortic aneurysms. FASEB J. 2005;19(11):1528–30.
24. Halpern VJ, Nackman GB, Gandhi RH, Irizarry E, Scholes JV, Ramey WG, et al. The elastase infusion model of experimental aortic aneurysms: synchrony of induction of endogenous proteinases with matrix destruction and inflammatory cell response. J Vasc Surg. 1994;20(1):51–60.

25. Thompson RW, Curci JA, Ennis TL, Mao D, Pagano MB, Pham CTN. Pathophysiology of abdominal aortic aneurysms: insights from the elastase-induced model in mice with different genetic backgrounds. Ann N Y Acad Sci. 2006;1085(1):59–73.
26. Daugherty A, Rateri DL, Cassis LA. Role of the renin-angiotensin system in the development of abdominal aortic aneurysms in animals and humans. Ann N Y Acad Sci. 2006;1085(1):82–91.
27. Busuttil RW. Collagenase activity of the human aorta: a comparison of patients with and without abdominal aortic aneurysms. Arch Surg. 1980;115(11):1373.
28. Lee MH, Murphy G. Matrix metalloproteinases at a glance. J Cell Sci. 2004;117(18):4015–6.
29. Pearce WH, Shively VP. Abdominal aortic aneurysm as a complex multifactorial disease: interactions of polymorphisms of inflammatory genes, features of autoimmunity, and current status of MMPs. Ann N Y Acad Sci. 2006;1085(1):117–32.
30. Somerville RP, Oblander SA, Apte SS. Matrix metalloproteinases: old dogs with new tricks. Genome Biol. 2003;4(6):216.
31. Parks WC, Wilson CL, López-Boado YS. Matrix metalloproteinases as modulators of inflammation and innate immunity. Nat Rev Immunol. 2004;4(8):617–29.
32. Ailawadi G, Knipp BS, Lu G, Roelofs KJ, Ford JW, Hannawa KK, et al. A nonintrinsic regional basis for increased infrarenal aortic MMP-9 expression and activity. J Vasc Surg. 2003;37(5):1059–66.
33. Freestone T, Turner RJ, Coady A, Higman DJ, Greenhalgh RM, Powell JT. Inflammation and matrix metalloproteinases in the enlarging abdominal aortic aneurysm. Arterioscler Thromb Vasc Biol. 1995;15(8):1145–51.
34. Jones JA, Barbour JR, Lowry AS, Bouges S, Beck C, McClister DM, et al. Spatiotemporal expression and localization of matrix metalloproteinas-9 in a murine model of thoracic aortic aneurysm. J Vasc Surg. 2006;44(6):1314–21.
35. Barbour JR, Stroud RE, Lowry AS, Clark LL, Leone AM, Jones JA, et al. Temporal disparity in the induction of matrix metalloproteinases and tissue inhibitors of metalloproteinases after thoracic aortic aneurysm formation. J Thorac Cardiovasc Surg. 2006;132(4):788–95.
36. Schmoker JD, McPartland KJ, Fellinger EK, Boyum J, Trombley L, Ittleman FP, et al. Matrix metalloproteinase and tissue inhibitor expression in atherosclerotic and nonatherosclerotic thoracic aortic aneurysms. J Thorac Cardiovasc Surg. 2007;133(1):155–61.
37. Mott JD, Werb Z. Regulation of matrix biology by matrix metalloproteinases. Curr Opin Cell Biol. 2004;16(5):558–64.
38. Senior RM, Griffin GL, Mecham RP. Chemotactic activity of elastin-derived peptides. J Clin Invest. 1980;66(4):859–62.
39. Lenk GM, Tromp G, Weinsheimer S, Gatalica Z, Berguer R, Kuivaniemi H. Whole genome expression profiling reveals a significant role for immune function in human abdominal aortic aneurysms. BMC Genomics. 2007;8(1):237.
40. Blanchard JF, Armenian HK, Friesen PP. Risk factors for abdominal aortic aneurysm: results of a case-control study. Am J Epidemiol. 2000;151(6):575–83.
41. Ailawadi G, Eliason JL, Roelofs KJ, Sinha I, Hannawa KK, Kaldjian EP, et al. Gender differences in experimental aortic aneurysm formation. Arterioscler Thromb Vasc Biol. 2004;24(11):2116–22.
42. Sandford RM, Bown MJ, London NJ, Sayers RD. The genetic basis of abdominal aortic aneurysms: a review. Eur J Vasc Endovasc Surg. 2007;33(4):381–90.
43. Bown MJ, Burton PR, Horsburgh T, Nicholson ML, Bell PRF, Sayers RD. The role of cytokine gene polymorphisms in the pathogenesis of abdominal aortic aneurysms: a case-control study. J Vasc Surg. 2003;37(5):999–1005.
44. Ghilardi G, Biondi ML, Battaglioli L, Zambon A, Guagnellini E, Scorza R. Genetic risk factor characterizes abdominal aortic aneurysm from arterial occlusive disease in human beings: CCR5 Delta 32 deletion. J Vasc Surg. 2004;40(5):995–1000.
45. Pinard A, Jones GT, Milewicz DM. Genetics of thoracic and abdominal aortic diseases. Circ Res. 2019;124(4):588–606.

46. Klarin D, Devineni P, Sendamarai AK, Angueira AR, Graham SE, Shen YH, et al. Genome-wide association study of thoracic aortic aneurysm and dissection in the Million Veteran Program. Nat Genet. 2023;55(7):1106–15.
47. Isselbacher EM, Preventza O, Hamilton Black J, Augoustides JG, Beck AW, Bolen MA, et al. 2022 ACC/AHA Guideline for the diagnosis and management of aortic disease: a report of the American Heart Association/American College of Cardiology Joint Committee on Clinical Practice Guidelines. Circulation [Internet]. 2022 [cited 2024 Aug 19];146(24). Available from: https://www.ahajournals.org/doi/10.1161/CIR.0000000000001106
48. Czerny M, Grabenwöger M, Berger T, Aboyans V, Corte AD, Chen EP, et al. EACTS/STS guidelines for diagnosing and treating acute and chronic syndromes of the aortic organ. Ann Thorac Surg. 2024;118(1):5–115.
49. Scola L, Giarratana RM, Marinello V, Cancila V, Pisano C, Ruvolo G, et al. Polymorphisms of pro-inflammatory IL-6 and IL-1β cytokines in ascending aortic aneurysms as genetic modifiers and predictive and prognostic biomarkers. Biomolecules. 2021;11(7):943.
50. Dawson J, Cockerill GW, Choke E, Belli AM, Loftus I, Thompson MM. Aortic aneurysms secrete interleukin-6 into the circulation. J Vasc Surg. 2007;45(2):350–6.
51. Duftner C, Seiler R, Dejaco C, Fraedrich G, Schirmer M. Increasing evidence for immune-mediated processes and new therapeutic approaches in abdominal aortic aneurysms—a review. Ann N Y Acad Sci. 2006;1085:331–8.
52. Sakthivel P, Shively V, Kakoulidou M, Pearce W, Lefvert AK. The soluble forms of CD28, CD86 and CTLA-4 constitute possible immunological markers in patients with abdominal aortic aneurysm. J Intern Med. 2007;261(4):399–407.
53. Köprülü D, Hassan MO, Atmaca H, Albayrak S, Işcanlı E. Inflammatory markers and aortic aneurysms: exploring the role of Hs-CRP and MHR in ascending aortic aneurysm development. Int J Gen Med. 2024;17:2899–905.
54. Ruddy JM, Jones JA, Spinale FG, Ikonomidis JS. Regional heterogeneity within the aorta: relevance to aneurysm disease. J Thorac Cardiovasc Surg. 2008;136(5):1123.

Chapter 3
Contemporary Imaging of Aortic Disease

Brennan A. Lanier, Lakshya Trivedi, and Sneha Vakamudi

Introduction

In the modern era, computed tomography (CT) scans and magnetic resonance imaging (MRI) devices are the standard diagnostic tools for imaging of the vascular system. Contemporary CT and MR techniques have revolutionized the diagnosis of vascular pathology, without the procedural risks of transarterial catheterization. In the evaluation of aneurysmal disease, cross-sectional imaging is particularly important for depiction of the length of diseased vessel, total aortic and arterial diameters, true vascular diameter, including the patent lumen and the extent of mural thrombus formation [1] (Fig. 3.1), and distance of diseased wall from critical aortic branches. Cross-sectional techniques also provide valuable information on extravascular pathology (Fig. 3.2a–c). Noninvasive cross-sectional imaging is now frequently used as a single examination for both diagnosis and preprocedural planning of aortic interventions, with demonstrable decrease in operative morbidity and mortality [2]. Furthermore, noninvasive imaging is also an excellent method for monitoring the postoperative patient for complications, including both traditional open repairs and endovascular therapies [3, 4]. Three-dimensional reformatted and volume-rendered images can be made to aid in clinical diagnosis and easily depict pathology (Fig. 3.3a, b). The basic principles of computed tomography angiography (CTA) and magnetic resonance angiography (MRA) will be discussed, as will their specific relevance toward aneurysmal disease. Despite the advances in cross-sectional imaging, there remains a solid basis

B. A. Lanier · L. Trivedi · S. Vakamudi (✉)
Department of Cardiology, University of Texas at Austin Dell Medical School, Austin, TX, USA
e-mail: brennan.lanier@ascension.org; lakshya.trivedi@ascension.org; sneha.vakamudi@ascension.org

G. J. Arnaoutakis et al. (eds.), *Aortic Aneurysms*, Contemporary Cardiology,
https://doi.org/10.1007/978-3-032-13134-8_3

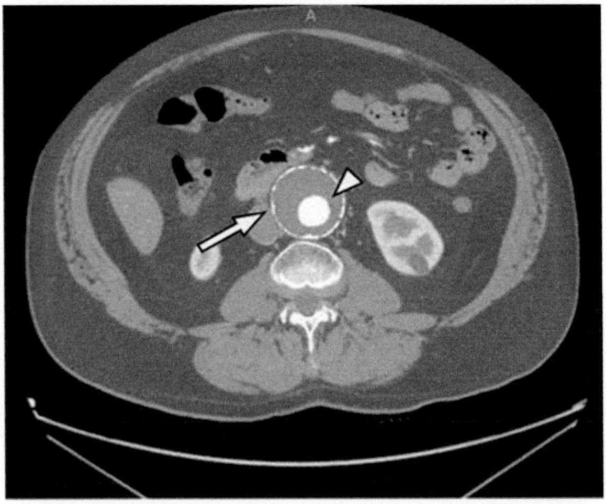

Fig. 3.1 Axial contrast-enhanced computed tomography (*CT*) image demonstrates a 5.4-cm infrarenal abdominal aortic aneurysm. Cross-sectional imaging nicely depicts how the patent vascular lumen (*arrowhead*) comprises only a portion of the total aortic diameter (*arrow*)

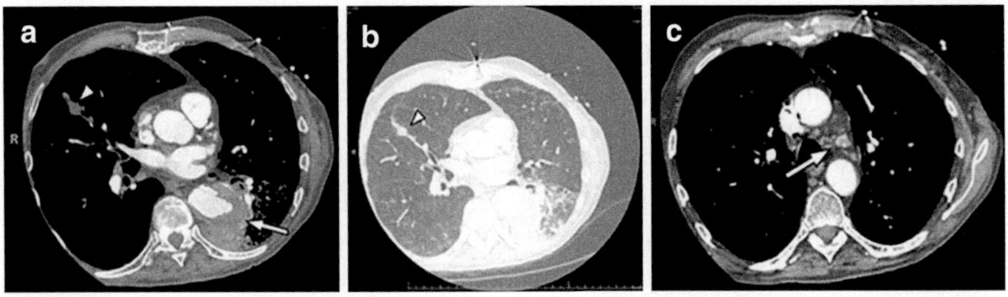

Fig. 3.2 (**a**) Axial contrast-enhanced computed tomography (*CT*) image (soft tissue windowing) demonstrates a focal saccular aneurysm involving the distal descending thoracic aorta (*arrow*). There is abnormal attenuation in the right middle lobe (arrowhead). (**b**) Axial contrast-enhanced CT image (lung windowing) reveals spiculation associated with the right middle lobe mass (*arrowhead*). Biopsy was positive for non-small cell lung carcinoma. (**c**) Axial contrast-enhanced CT image (soft tissue windowing) demonstrates mediastinal adenopathy (arrow) that was positive on subsequent PET scan

for catheter-based angiography. Although it has lost its primary importance as a diagnostic modality, catheter-based angiography must be discussed in the setting of its still irreplaceable role in the endovascular treatment of aortic disease. As it is currently integrated with contemporary cross-sectional imaging, catheter-based angiography entails the use of carbon dioxide angiography and intravascular ultrasound (IVUS). Transthoracic and transesophageal echocardiography are also useful modalities to evaluate for aortic disease noninvasively.

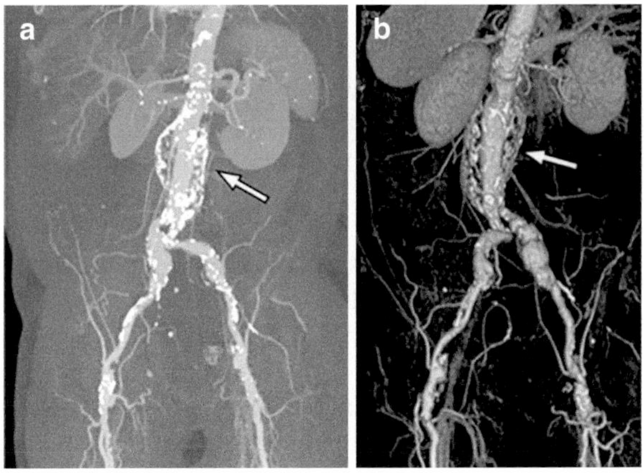

Fig. 3.3 (**a**) 3D Reformatted image demonstrates abdominal aortic aneurysm (*arrow*) with atherosclerotic calcification throughout the abdominal aorta and branch vessels. (**b**) Surface-shaded display of same data set redemonstrates the abdominal aortic aneurysm (*arrow*)

Computed Tomography

Computed tomography is an x-ray-based method of imaging which uses a rotating gantry including an x-ray tube and detector plate to generate tomographic images of the body. Early on, CT played only a minor role in clinical vascular imaging, as it was mostly used for stationary anatomic imaging due to slow acquisition speed. However, the development of helical scanning technique and multidetector row technology in the early 1990s revolutionized the role of CT in angiographic applications [3, 5]. Slip-ring technology allows continuous rotation of the gantry without the need to unwind power/electricity cables, allowing modern gantry rotation speeds of approximately 0.33 s per rotation. When combined with a moving table, the data acquisition changes from axial 2D imaging to volumetric 3D imaging. The overall scan time is reduced, and the acquired data can be reconstructed into traditional axial slices or other reformatted planes. In the early implementation of this technology, the anatomy recorded by detectors at the beginning of the gantry rotation was different than at the end of the gantry rotation (due to continuous table movement), leading to exaggerated volume-averaging effects and decreased through-plane resolution. The development of multiple detector rows on the circulating gantry addressed this problem, thereby allowing multiple rows of data to be acquired in a single rotation [6]. With advances in detector technology, thinner detector elements were developed with subsequent gains in through-plane resolution (individual detector size) as well as overall z-axis coverage (total number of rows on the gantry). Currently, detector element width is approximately 0.5–0.625 mm. The combination of helical scanning and multiple detector rows is the foundation for modern multidetector CT (MDCT) scanners, which can provide data sets with equal spatial and contrast resolution in all three planes and ultrafast imaging times (complete vascular interrogation from arch to toes in less than 30 s) [7].

Recent advances in scanners have improved temporal resolution even further, to 0.275–0.35 s/rotation, which helps greatly reduce motion artifacts. Furthermore, ECG gating techniques have enabled timing the scan for an appropriate cardiac phase, to reduce heartbeat-related motion artifacts, especially in cases of aortic dissection [8]. Unfortunately, ECG-gated techniques increase acquisition time and the breath hold required [9]. For cases of patients who cannot hold their breath for a long period of time, or who have urgent cardiovascular issues, high-pitch dual-source, or FLASH, CT is an option [10]. This technology does not use ECG gating and is able to scan the entire aorta in about 2 s [10]. Furthermore, in contrast to ECG gating, it allows for a heart rate above 70 beats per minute while obtaining images [10].

CT studies focused on vascular disease often involve MDCT scanners with protocols consisting of multiple imaging phases, including a precontrast image series and at least one contrast-enhanced image series. Although the contrast-enhanced images provide exquisite luminal imaging, it is important not to overlook the precontrast images. Precontrast images are critical for the detection of blood, as acute hemorrhage/hematoma is usually hyperdense on noncontrast images (Fig. 3.4a, b). Although CT attenuation values are absolute numbers related to the constituents that make up a given voxel, subtle areas of acute hemorrhage can be less conspicuous when dense intraluminal contrast is present (Fig. 3.5a, b). From the standpoint of clinical management, the presence of extraluminal high attenuation in a patient suspected of ruptured aneurysm should obviate the need for further imaging and decrease the delay time to definitive treatment [7]. Additionally, atherosclerotic calcifications, calcified old hematomas, surgical grafts, and felt pledgets/rings are

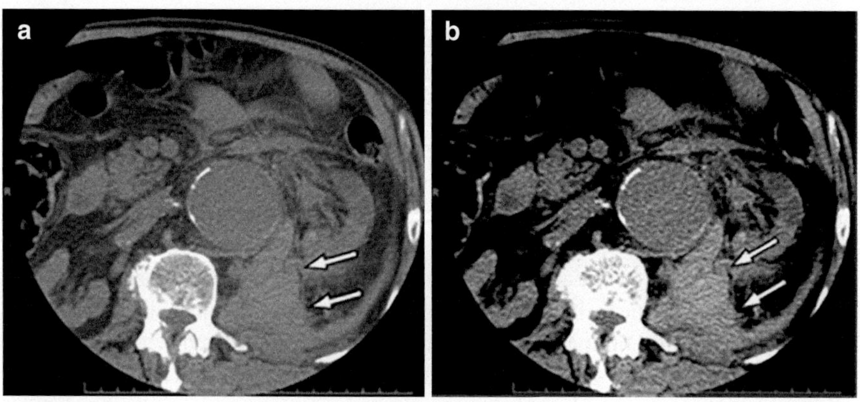

Fig. 3.4 (**a**) Axial noncontrast computed tomography (*CT*) image through the abdomen in standard abdominal soft tissue windowing (window = 400, level = 40) demonstrates retroperitoneal high attenuation (*arrows*) with concomitant fascial thickening around the anterolaterally displaced left kidney, indicating retroperitoneal hemorrhage. (**b**) Axial noncontrast CT image with narrow window settings (window = 100, level = 30) demonstrates increased conspicuity of high attenuation related to suspected retroperitoneal hemorrhage (*arrows*). The patient expired during attempted open repair of abdominal aortic aneurysm rupture

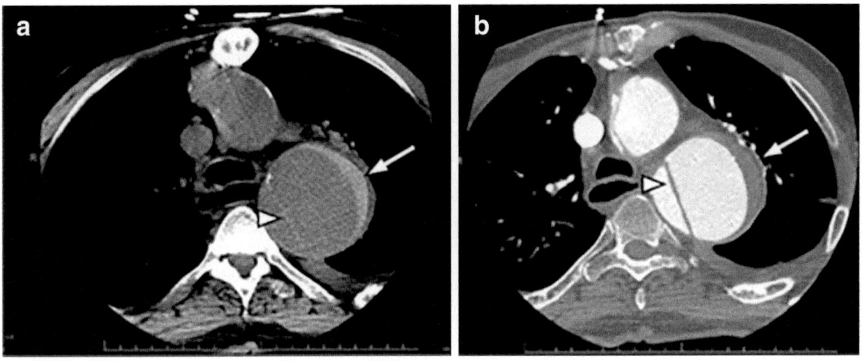

Fig. 3.5 (**a**) Axial noncontrast computed tomography (*CT*) image through the chest demonstrates crescentic high attenuation (*arrow*) associated with the left lateral aspect of the descending thoracic aorta, compatible with an intramural hematoma. There is also a suggestion of a dissection flap on the medial aspect of the aorta (*arrowhead*). (**b**) Axial contrast-enhanced CT image at the same level easily demonstrates the suspected dissection flap (*arrowhead*). However, the visual conspicuity of the intramural hematoma on the left-lateral aspect of the aorta is decreased (*arrow*) versus the dense contrast bolus in the aortic lumen

often more reliably seen on precontrast images than postcontrast images [11] (Fig. 3.6a, b). Identification of these components will aid in rendering a final opinion about the patient's disease status.

The contrast-enhanced portion of a CTA study is typically performed with mechanical dual-chamber power injectors. Given the potential coverage speed of MDCT, contrast bolus geometry and injection protocols have become areas of considerable research with the rapid evolution of MDCT technology; a detailed discussion of this research is beyond the scope of this chapter and includes consideration of physiological and anatomical factors, injection rate, total volume, and iodine concentration [13]. Generally, CTA studies utilize contrast media with iodine concentrations of 300–400 mmol iodine/ml, injection rates of 3–5 ml/s, and a total volume of 70–150 ml. However, the fundamental challenge in CTA is optimal delivery of the appropriate amount of contrast to the volume of interest. This often requires some degree of protocol specificity particular to the scanner being used. The scan time to cover a certain distance can vary considerably depending on the number of detectors available on a given MDCT system, and therefore the contrast injection protocol must vary to meet the ability of the scanner. As an example, a 4-detector scanner may take 21 s to cover a 25 cm length with standard parameters, whereas a 64-detector scanner could achieve similar or better imaging parameters in 4 s [14]. In contrast, FLASH CT is able to image the entire chest in less than 1 s [12]. Additionally, delayed postcontrast images can be valuable portions of a complete aortic protocol, especially in patients who have had prior endovascular therapy for aneurysms [15]. Therefore, it is critical to tailor scan protocols for the specific task toward the actual device being used for acquisition.

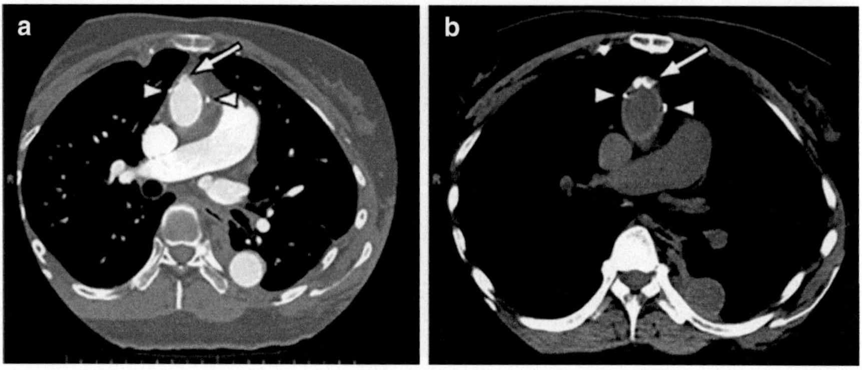

Fig. 3.6 (**a**) Axial contrast-enhanced computed tomography (*CT*) image of the chest demonstrates irregularity of the anterior aspect of the ascending aorta (*arrow*). The patient had prior surgical graft repair of the ascending aorta for aneurysm. Tiny clips are present (arrowheads) around the ascending aorta as well. (**b**) Axial noncontrast CT image at the same level demonstrates very high attenuation in the area of questioned abnormality on the contrast-enhanced CT image (*arrow*). This area was stable for over 5 years and had been present on every postoperative scan, probably representing felt pledgets buttressing closure of an aortotomy wound. Surgical clips are again demonstrated (*arrowheads*)

There are specific advantages and disadvantages of CTA when compared to other cross-sectional techniques such as MRA. In general, CTA requires less technical sophistication to achieve a diagnostic quality examination than does MRA, which leads to more generalized reproducibility among studies obtained at different institutions [16]. CTA is also superior to MRA in terms of spatial resolution and temporal acquisition, making it the test of choice for trauma or clinically unstable patients (Fig. 3.7). As opposed to the high degree of background suppression obtained in MRA, the extraluminal detail is retained during the angiographic/contrast-enhanced portion of the CTA, which offers a single comprehensive evaluation of the vascular system [7] (Fig. 3.8). Moreover, CTA is more time-efficient than MRA, an important aspect to consider in the management of a potentially hemodynamically unstable patient. The major clinical disadvantages associated with CTA include the use of ionizing radiation (which limits dynamic or real-time imaging of contrast bolus propagation) and a nephrotoxic contrast agent, while other technical disadvantages include artifacts related to the injected contrast material, indwelling metallic prostheses, or adjacent osseous structures [17].

Given the risks of radiation, episodic and cumulative ionizing radiation doses should be kept as low as possible while still obtaining quality images. On a technical note, when performing MRI or CT imaging, the root and ascending aorta should be measured from inner edge to inner edge [19]. In cases of asymmetric or oval contour, the longest diameter and its perpendicular diameter should be reported [19].

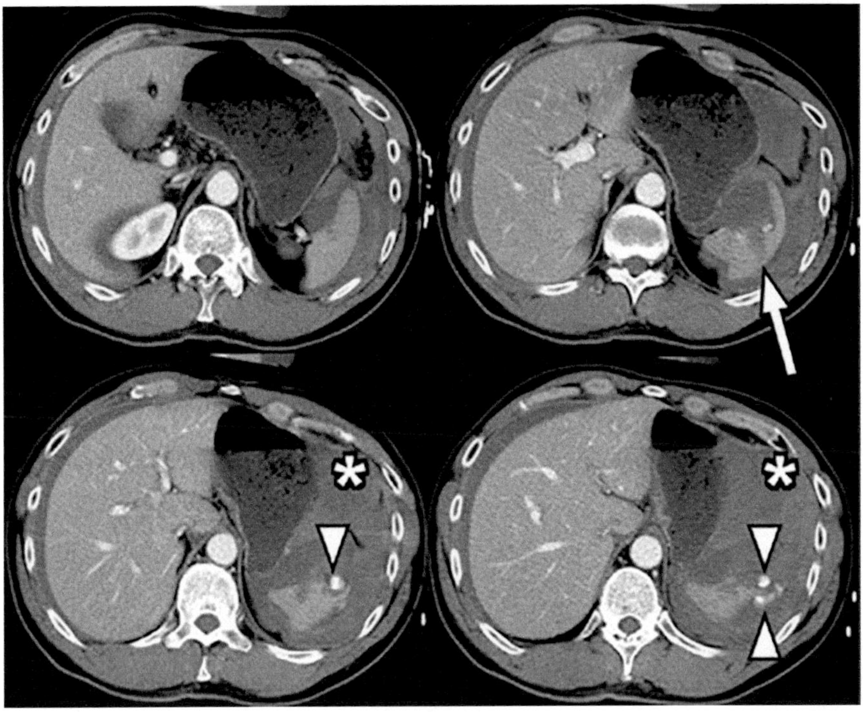

Fig. 3.7 Four contiguous axial contrast-enhanced computed tomography (*CT*) images through the upper abdomen in a patient after motor vehicle collision demonstrate a hypodense linear tract through the spleen (*arrow*), compatible with a splenic laceration. There are scattered foci of very high attenuation within the laceration bed (*arrowheads*) that represent active extravasation of iodinated contrast material into left upper quadrant, or hemoperitoneum (*). The patient was taken for emergent embolization of active hemorrhage in order to maintain splenic function. Because of its short scan times, CT is ideally suited for the initial imaging of trauma patients

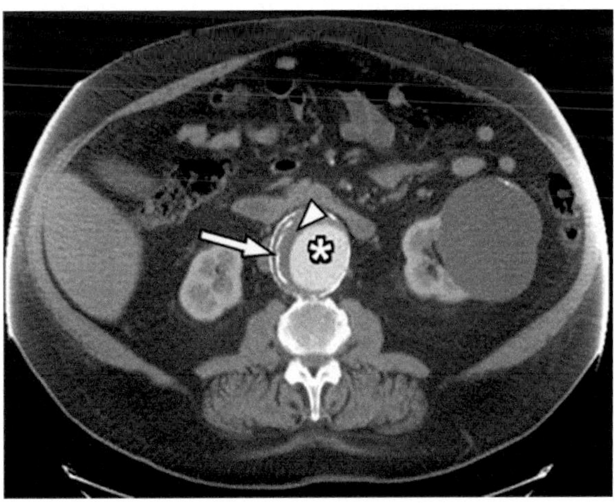

Fig. 3.8 Axial contrast-enhanced computed tomography (*CT*) image demonstrates a 6.8-cm abdominal aortic aneurysm. Note how CT demonstrates the luminal and extraluminal components of the vessel wall, including the patent lumen (*), incorporated mural thrombus (*arrowhead,*), and intimal calcifications (*arrow*). The patient underwent subsequent successful endovascular repair

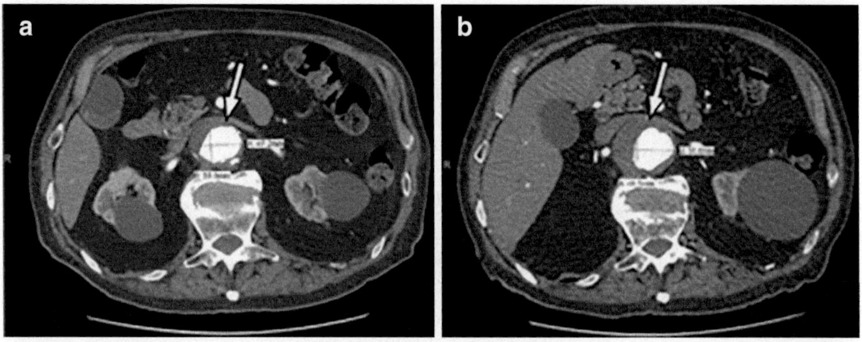

Fig. 3.9 (**a**) Axial contrast-enhanced computed tomography (*CT*) image demonstrates an abdominal aortic aneurysm (*arrow*) with maximal axial dimensions of 3.88 × 4.72 cm. (**b**) Axial contrast-enhanced CT image of the same patient in a similar location approximately 1 year later demonstrates interval growth of the aneurysm, now measuring 4.85 × 5.56 cm

With respect to aneurysmal disease, CTA provides a fast, reproducible study that yields important clinical information. CTA is frequently the first-line tool for the emergent evaluation of patients with suspected aortic aneurysm rupture; noncontrast studies can be performed rapidly and can render a diagnosis that expedites definitive surgical treatment [18]. CTA can be used to follow patients with known aneurysms for rate of interval growth, to facilitate the preoperative management of such patients when their aneurysm reaches critical dimensions, and to follow up patients in the postoperative period for complication development [17] (Fig. 3.9a, b). In the era of endovascular repair, CTA has become even more valuable as the acquired data set from MDCT scanners can be loaded into postprocessing software to generate the salient preoperative parameters for stent-graft deployment (Fig. 3.10a–d). Additionally, CTA is a robust modality for following endograft patients in the postoperative period, as CT can directly visualize the intraluminal graft and look for stent graft complications such as endoleaks [20] (Fig. 3.11a, b). With the increasing use of endovascular systems for the aortic aneurysmal disease, CTA has become the definitive imaging modality used for both planning and follow-up of surgery.

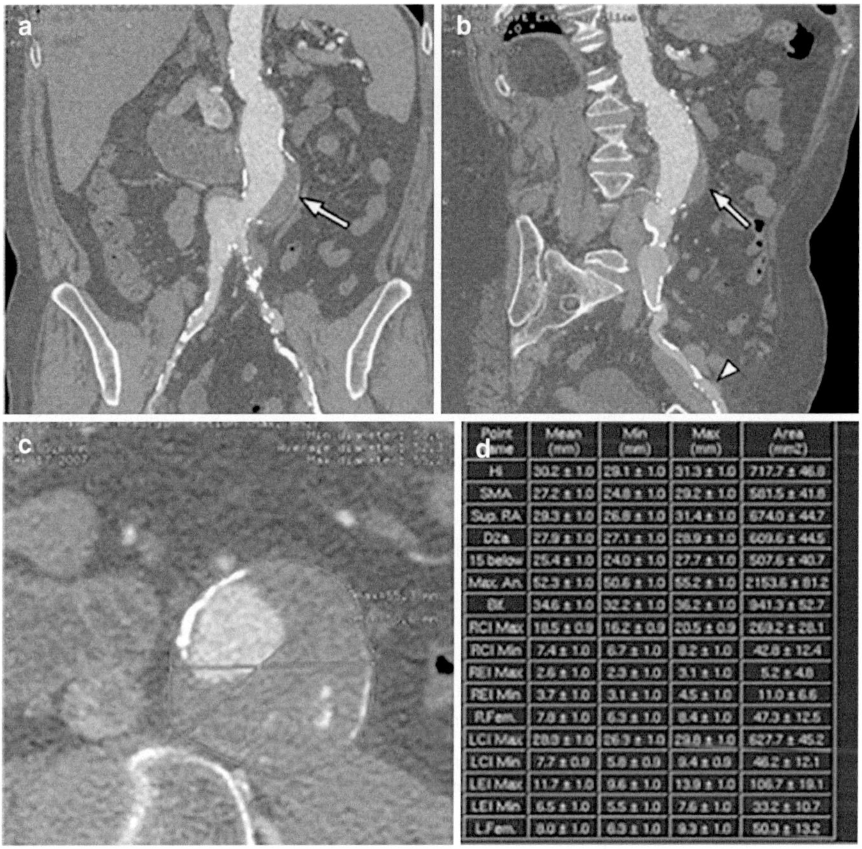

Point name	Mean (mm)	Min (mm)	Max (mm)	Area (mm2)
HI	30.2 ± 1.0	29.1 ± 1.0	31.3 ± 1.0	717.7 ± 46.8
SMA	27.2 ± 1.0	24.8 ± 1.0	29.2 ± 1.0	581.5 ± 41.8
Sup. RA	29.3 ± 1.0	26.8 ± 1.0	31.4 ± 1.0	674.0 ± 44.7
D2a	27.9 ± 1.0	27.1 ± 1.0	28.9 ± 1.0	609.6 ± 44.5
15 below	25.4 ± 1.0	24.0 ± 1.0	27.7 ± 1.0	507.6 ± 40.7
Max. An.	52.3 ± 1.0	50.6 ± 1.0	55.2 ± 1.0	2153.6 ± 81.2
Bif.	34.6 ± 1.0	32.2 ± 1.0	36.2 ± 1.0	941.3 ± 52.7
RCI Max	18.5 ± 0.9	16.2 ± 0.9	20.5 ± 0.9	269.2 ± 28.1
RCI Min	7.4 ± 1.0	6.7 ± 1.0	8.2 ± 1.0	42.8 ± 12.4
REI Max	2.6 ± 1.0	2.3 ± 1.0	3.1 ± 1.0	5.2 ± 4.8
REI Min	3.7 ± 1.0	3.1 ± 1.0	4.5 ± 1.0	11.0 ± 6.6
RFem.	7.8 ± 1.0	6.3 ± 1.0	8.4 ± 1.0	47.3 ± 12.5
LCI Max	28.9 ± 1.0	26.3 ± 1.0	29.8 ± 1.0	627.7 ± 45.2
LCI Min	7.7 ± 0.9	5.8 ± 0.9	9.4 ± 0.9	46.2 ± 12.1
LEI Max	11.7 ± 1.0	9.6 ± 1.0	13.9 ± 1.0	106.7 ± 19.1
LEI Min	6.5 ± 1.0	5.5 ± 1.0	7.6 ± 1.0	33.2 ± 10.7
LFem.	8.0 ± 1.0	6.3 ± 1.0	9.3 ± 1.0	50.3 ± 13.2

Fig. 3.10 (**a**) Coronal maximum intensity projection from contrast-enhanced computed tomography angiography (*CTA*) study demonstrates a 5.5-cm abdominal aortic aneurysm (*arrow*). (**b**) Curved reformatted image from the same CTA data set using a center-line automated approach allows continuous visualization of the arterial anatomy through the left external iliac artery (*arrowhead*) for endovascular treatment planning. Abdominal aortic aneurysm is again seen (*arrow*). (**c**) Single oblique image from postprocessing software package demonstrates how the vessel is sized at this specific level. The user may modify the included area based on visual inspection. (**d**) Final vessel analysis provides maximal and minimal luminal diameter at various levels to assist in planning the endovascular operative approach

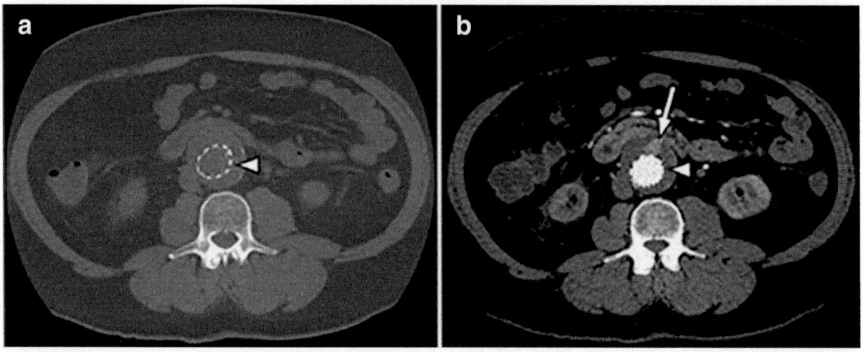

Fig. 3.11 (**a**) Axial noncontrast computed tomography (*CT*) image of the abdomen demonstrates an abdominal aortic aneurysm with indwelling endovascular stent graft (*arrowhead*). There is no abnormal high attenuation in the excluded aneurysm sac on these noncontrast images. (**b**) Axial contrast-enhanced CT image at the same level demonstrates a blush of contrast within the aneurysm sac (*arrow*), which is outside the stent graft itself (*arrow*). Since this was not present on the precontrast images, this area fills through an endoleak. Contrast angiography confirmed a type II endoleak from retrograde flow through the inferior mesenteric artery (*IMA*)

Magnetic Resonance Imaging

Magnetic resonance imaging allows imaging of the body utilizing a magnetic field and radiofrequency pulses. The patient is placed within a strong magnetic field (modern clinical scanners function at 1.5–3.0 T) that aligns the net magnetic field of the protons within a patient's body along the bore of the main magnetic field [21]. When a radiofrequency pulse is sent out from a transmitter, the net magnetization is deflected from its resting axis along the main magnetic field. As the protons relax back to their original state in the main magnetic field, a detectable signal—called an echo—is generated and localized by a receiver coil [22]. The frequency data ("k-space data") received by the coil is converted into an image via the Fourier transform [23]. Magnetic recovery after a radiofrequency pulse has been sent out by the transmitter has two discrete components: a longitudinal relaxation (parallel to the main magnetic field) and a transverse relaxation (perpendicular to the main magnetic field) [21]. Tissue-specific parameters related to longitudinal and transverse recovery are called T1 and T2 relaxation times, respectively. Depending on the parameters of the imaging sequence, the acquired data set (and subsequent generated images) can demonstrate T1- or T2-weighting to highlight these characteristics [23]. Additionally, the imaging contrast can be altered either by changing the intrinsic contrast of an organ (the addition of Gadolinium-based intravenous contrast) or by selectively nullifying certain tissues based on known T1/T2 values (fat saturation techniques), particularly in evaluation of the vascular tree [24]. In general, the more specific lesion characterization that is offered by MRI relies on the integrated spectrum of tissue appearances on various types of T1- and T2-weighted sequences.

The use of magnetic resonance imaging in noninvasive vascular imaging has been termed magnetic resonance angiography (MRA). Similar to other applications in MRI, angiographic applications require more than one sequence to generate a complete diagnosis. Precontrast T1-weighted images can be used to obtain information about anatomy, including delineation of the aortic wall and adjacent mediastinal or retroperitoneal pathology [25] (Fig. 3.12a). Fat-saturated T1-weighted images often increase the conspicuity of extracellular methemoglobin in hematomas, which is particularly important in angiographic applications (Fig. 3.13a, b). T2-weighted images are used less in angiographic applications than in other anatomic regions, mainly due to their lengthy time of acquisition, though these sequences remain useful in cases of vasculitis or suspected vascular malformation [25, 26] (Fig. 3.14a, b). Black-blood vascular imaging technique is a technique based on fast spin-echo imaging that uses a set of two inversion pulses to "prepare" the imaging slice, ultimately leading to nullification of blood protons within the slice and yielding excellent depiction of intraluminal and mural abnormalities [27]. Contrast-enhanced MRA has become the predominant method of evaluating the vascular tree, as the injection of Gadolinium-based contrast agents allows accurate depiction of the luminal appearance on fast T1-weighted imaging [25, 28] (Fig. 3.12b, c). Because MR techniques do not have ionizing radiation, similar images at multiple time points can be acquired without harm to the patient. Therefore, imaging techniques are frequently used in MRA which will demonstrate multiple phases of vascular contrast, including arterial, venous, and delayed phases of imaging. Contrast-enhanced MRA is particularly useful for aneurysmal disease of the aorta and iliac arteries, as the slow swirling flow in such aneurysms can degrade other MR sequences [29]. For aneurysm evaluation, both arterial and delayed images are critical to evaluate (Fig. 3.12b, c); the arterial images will accurately demonstrate the luminal contour while delayed images are useful for looking at the vascular wall and extent of mural thrombus formation [25].

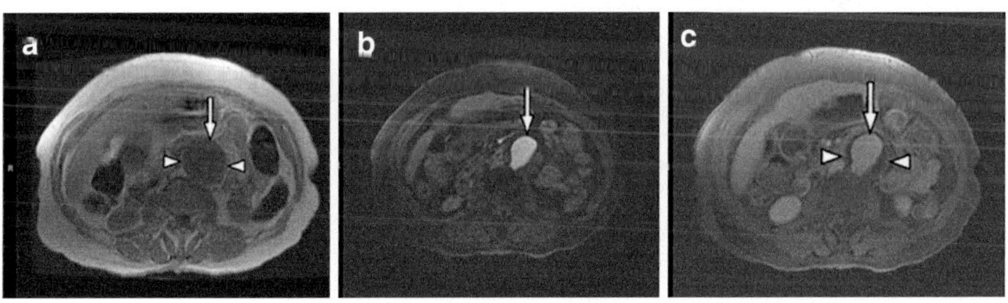

Fig. 3.12 (**a**) Axial precontrast T1-weighted in-phase gradient echo image of the abdomen demonstrates a 4.9-cm abdominal aortic aneurysm (*arrow*). Note that the complete/full diameter of the aneurysm (*arrowheads*) is depicted on this sequence. (**b**) Axial fat-suppressed postcontrast T1-weighted spoiled gradient echo image at the same level as panel a during the arterial phase of enhancement demonstrates that the aneurysm lumen (*arrow*) is most conspicuous with relative paucity of signal in the wall and background tissues. (**c**) Axial fat-suppressed postcontrast T1-weighted spoiled gradient echo image at same level as panel a, obtained 5 min after injection, demonstrates aneurysm (*arrow*) with increased conspicuity of the vascular wall (*arrowheads*). There is higher signal in the background tissues as well

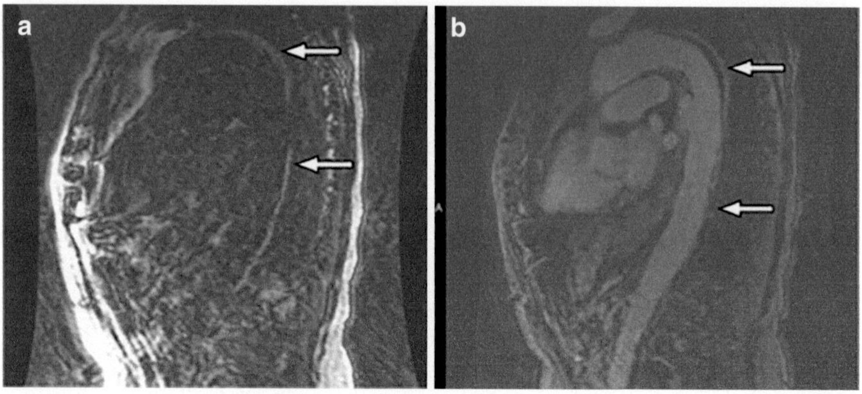

Fig. 3.13 (**a**) Oblique sagittal fat-suppressed precontrast T1-weighted spoiled gradient echo image of the thoracic aorta demonstrates curvilinear foci of high attenuation (arrows) which parallel the expected aortic channel, suspect for a thrombosed false lumen in a thoracic aortic dissection. The use of fat-suppression techniques allows greater conspicuity of the blood products versus the background tissues, as the mediastinal fat is nullified. (**b**) Oblique sagittal fat-suppressed postcontrast T1-weighted spoiled gradient echo image at the same location as panel a confirms suspected false lumen in aortic dissection. Note that the high signal intensity on the precontrast image is less conspicuous on this postcontrast image, which validates the need to look carefully at the precontrast image

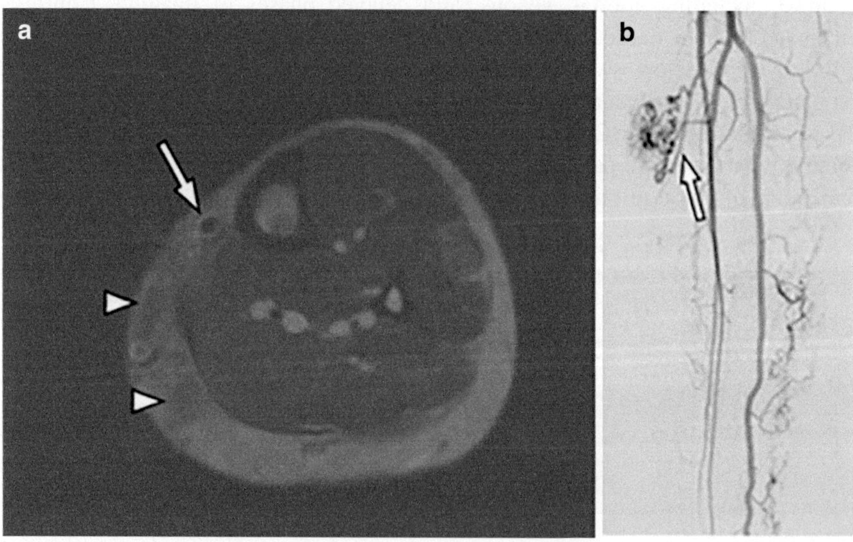

Fig. 3.14 (**a**) Axial T2-weighted *fast spin echo* image of the lower leg in a patient with suspected vascular malformation. There is infiltration of the subcutaneous fat (*arrowheads*) with numerous small curvilinear foci of signal, likely representing small vessels. Larger area of flow-void (*arrow*) likely represents a high-flow channel. (**b**) Digital subtraction angiography on the same patient reveals high-flow within numerous subcutaneous vascular malformations in the lower leg, supplied by discrete arterial feeding vessels. Note high arterial flow in matched lesion (*arrow*) to magnetic resonance imaging (*MRI*) image in panel a

Prior to the use of contrast-enhanced MRA sequences, luminal flow information could be obtained on MRI from noncontrast techniques. With previously used Gadolinium-based contrast agents being linked to nephrogenic systemic fibrosis (NSF) in patients with impaired renal function, certain noncontrast MRA techniques became valuable in these at-risk patients [30, 31]. Principal among these techniques is a variant T1-weighted gradient echo sequence called "time-of-flight" (TOF) imaging. TOF MRA relies on the difference in longitudinal magnetization of flowing protons in a bloodstream that enters into a slice of interest versus static protons within that slice of interest [27, 32]. This signal difference can be manipulated by imaging parameters to provide luminal contrast. In fact, by using selective saturation bands adjacent to the slice of interest, isolated arterial or venous flow can be displayed [27, 32] (Fig. 3.15a–c). Other techniques such as phase-contrast MRA and bright-blood steady-state free procession provide high signal intensity within vascular lumen without the addition of intravenous contrast [23, 25, 32] (Fig. 3.16). With the development of newer Gadolinium-containing contrast agents, guidelines highlight these agents to have very low, if any, risk of NSF development including those patients with advanced chronic renal insufficiencies. Given that many patients with aortic aneurysmal disease often have coexistent other medical comorbidities, including chronic renal insufficiency, contrast-enhanced MRI with newer Gadolinium-containing contrast agents should be considered for evaluation of aortopathies [33–35].

MRA has numerous benefits compared to other imaging modalities including native/direct multiplanar imaging, high soft tissue contrast, flow quantification, and the ability to evaluate both the vascular lumen and its wall [25]. As opposed to the rotating machinery involved in CT, MRI localizes signal in the body via the sophisticated interplay of magnetic gradients and radiofrequency pulses [27]. Therefore, it is not dependent on particular geometric constraints for acquiring images, and can

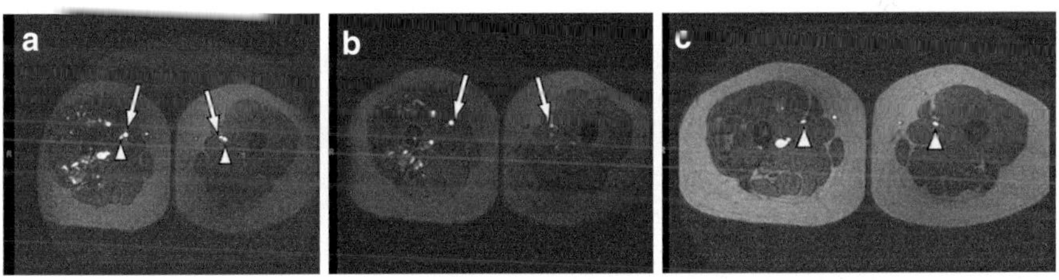

Fig. 3.15 (**a**) Axial time-of-flight magnetic resonance angiography (*MRA*) image in the upper leg without any flow selection (*saturation band*) demonstrates flow in both arterial (*arrow*) and venous (*arrowheads*) directions with the superficial femoral arteries (*SFA*) and superficial femoral veins (*SFV*), respectively. No intravenous contrast was given. (**b**) Axial time-of-flight MRA image in the upper leg with inferior saturation band (arterial flow selection) demonstrates near complete nullification of venous signal and only flow-related enhancement in the arterial structures. Arrows = arterial flow in bilateral SFAs. (**c**) Axial time-of-flight MRA image in the upper leg with superior saturation band (venous flow selection) demonstrates reversal of panel b, with near complete nullification of arterial signal and only venous flow-related enhancement. Arrowheads = venous flow in bilateral SFVs

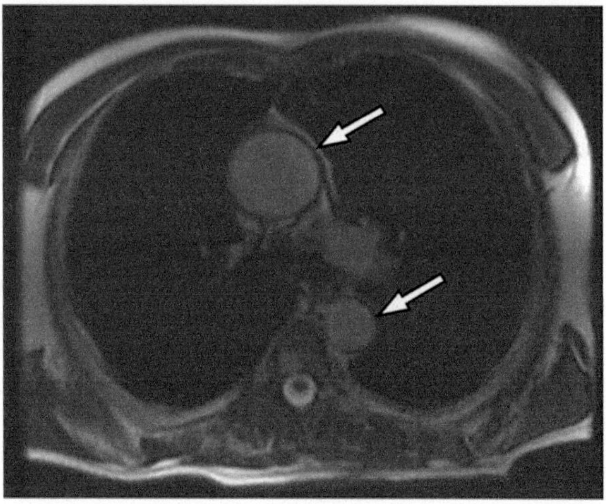

Fig. 3.16 Axial balanced steady-state free procession image through the chest demonstrates high signal intensity within the aortic lumen (*arrows*). No intravenous contrast was administered

image the body in any plane prescribed by the user. This is particularly useful in the thoracic aorta, where images can be obtained in the oblique sagittal plane to anatomically follow the oblique course of the thoracic aorta. The intrinsic difficulty in MRI of visualizing calcification can actually be useful for MRA applications—cortical bone structures are relatively inconspicuous on MRI versus CT where such structures can be quite confounding due to their high attenuation [7, 25] (Fig. 3.17). MRI is also recommended and considered advantageous over CT in the guidelines for surveillance of conditions including Turner Syndrome, aortic diseases in pregnancy, and Takayau arteritis [35].

With respect to CTA, there are some recognized disadvantages of MRA that must be considered, including decreased spatial resolution, increased examination length, contraindication with implantable electronically active hardware (such as pacemakers or defibrillator devices), interference with imaging by ferromagnetic components of vascular prostheses, and decreased equipment availability [17]. Additionally, the technical variability of MRA is higher than in CTA due to fluctuations in technologist skill level and inconsistency in available pulse sequences or gating techniques on different machines. Despite those limitations, MRA remains a useful vascular imaging tool whose future utility, particularly in stable patients, may continue to increase, given the recent increased concern about radiation doses in medical imaging and nephrotoxic effects of iodinated contrast material [36].

MRA can be used effectively in the management of aneurysmal disease, particularly in detection and surveillance. MRA is indicated as a screening technique in patients with high risk of developing aneurysms, such as those with connective tissue disease or vasculitis [17]. A patient with known aneurysmal disease is well suited for noncontrast MRA surveillance, given that this technique has no ionizing radiation and does not use potentially nephrotoxic contrast agents (Fig. 3.18a, b). MRA provides excellent detail about the status of disease, including assessment of

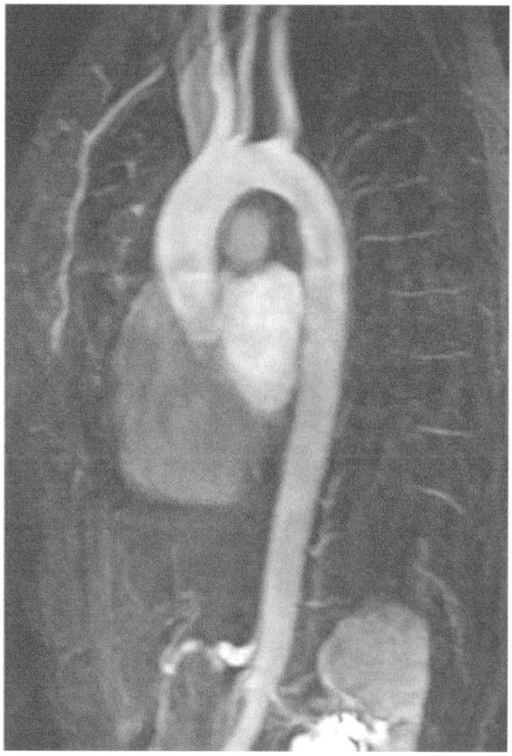

Fig. 3.17 Thick slab maximum intensity projection (*MIP*) from postgadolinium fat-suppressed T1-weighted oblique sagittal spoiled gradient echo data set demonstrates normal thoracic aorta. Note the lack of artifact related to osseous structures incorporated into the *MIP* image, as cortical bone is dark on magnetic resonance imaging (*MRI*)

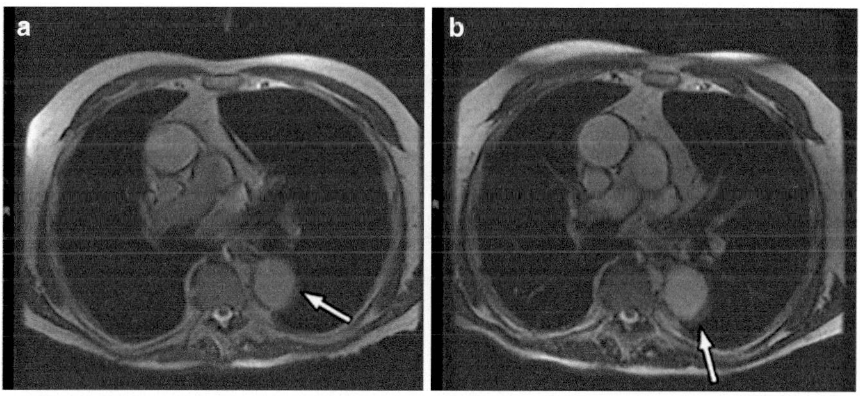

Fig. 3.18 (**a**) Axial balanced steady-state free procession image through the chest demonstrates a 4.2-cm thoracic aortic aneurysm of the descending thoracic aorta. (**b**) Axial balanced steady-state free procession image through a similar level 9 months later redemonstrates a 4.2-cm aortic aneurysm without interval change. This set of noncontrast images highlights how magnetic resonance angiography (*MRA*) can excel in following known aneurysmal disease without ionizing radiation or nephrotoxic iodinated contrast

the true aneurysm diameter [17, 27]. MRI is not frequently used in the emergent evaluation of patients with suspected aortic rupture due to examination time and generalized equipment availability. Because of slice thickness considerations, MRA has not been used as frequently as CTA for preoperative stent-graft measurements; nevertheless, studies have demonstrated that high spatial-resolution MRA can in fact be used as a sole preoperative test for endovascular planning, including integration with automated vessel analysis programs [37–39]. MRA can also be used in the postoperative period to follow patients with both open and endovascular repairs of aortic aneurysms. In patients with prior endovascular repair of aneurysm, the ability to visualize the stent graft itself is highly dependent on the graft material composition [16]. Nitinol-based devices cause only minor distortions on acquired images, while stainless steel devices create substantial artifact that often precludes any detailed evaluation [40]. As opposed to CTA, the device itself is usually seen in negative contrast versus the blood pool on T1-weighted gradient echo images. Endoleaks following endovascular repair with nonferromagnetic materials are also well delineated by MRA, with published studies demonstrating at least similar efficacy to CTA and perhaps superior detection of subtle type II endoleaks [41–43] (Fig. 3.19a, b). Newer techniques in MRA that allow blood pool and dynamic imaging may in fact improve endoleak detection even further and are an area of active investigation [44, 45]. MRA is a robust tool for imaging both preoperative and postoperative patients with aneurysmal disease.

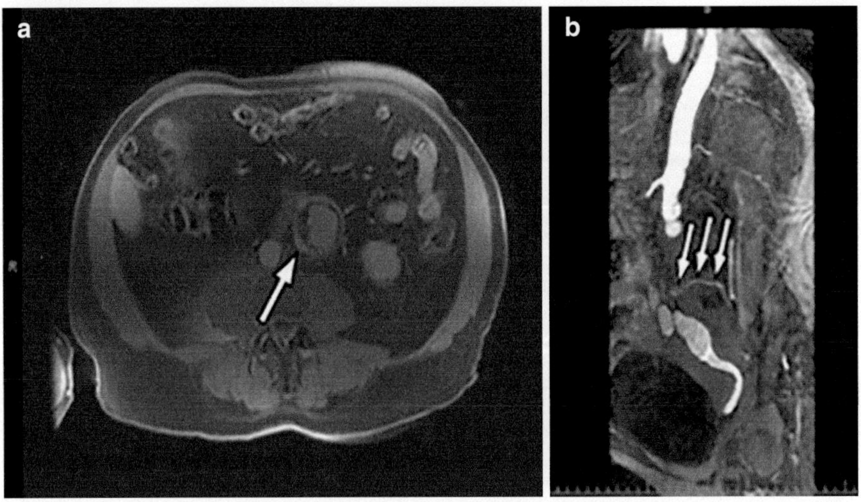

Fig. 3.19 (**a**) Axial fat-suppressed postcontrast T1-weighted spoiled gradient echo image of the abdomen demonstrates a 4.8-cm abdominal aortic aneurysm. There is also an indwelling stent graft. Along the right posterior aspect of the aorta, there is a small area of high signal intensity (*arrow*), outside the stent graft itself, suspect for an endoleak. (**b**) Reformatted maximum intensity projection image using arterial data set from an axial fat-suppressed postcontrast T1-weighted spoiled gradient echo sequence, demonstrating an enlarged lumbar artery leading into the aneurysm sac (*arrows*), thought to be responsible for the type II endoleak

In addition to traditional MRI & MRA imaging techniques, the addition of four-dimensional flow magnetic resonance imaging (4D flow MRI) provides additional utility in aortic imaging. Compared to conventional two- or three-dimensional phase contrast MR imaging, 4D flow MRI includes time as an additional dimension to generate time-constructed images [46]. 4D flow MRI evaluates average velocities across multiple heart cycles for every pixel obtained through 3D imaging to visualize various blood patterns including abnormal helical and vortical flow [47]. In regard to aortic imaging, the utility of 4D flow MRI continues to be established. For instance, 4D flow MRI can assist in evaluating aortic wall stiffness [47]. 4D flow MRI can also be useful to evaluate the development of aortic aneurysm and better assess risk for dissections by combining aortic diameter measurements with aortic hemodynamics and wall shear stress [48]. Additionally, in patients with bicuspid aortic valves, wall shear stress measurements due to eccentric blood flow can better identify aortopathies. 4D flow MRI can also serve as an alternative to catheterization to evaluate hemodynamics and wall parameters in aortic coarctation [49]. 4D flow MRI imaging can also be obtained without contrast with the addition of contrast improving imaging quality/resolution even further [50]. Limitations of 4D flow MRI include longer study time and postprocessing time, unreliable accuracy of blood flow with irregular heart cycles, lower spatial resolution compared to traditional 2D MRI, and lack of consensus on the optimal locations for flow parameter measurements. Further studies will be required to better evaluate the role of 4D flow MRI in aortic imaging [48].

Catheter-Based Vascular Imaging

The technical improvements in CTA and MRA have almost completely eliminated the role of catheter-based angiography from diagnostic imaging of the aorta and its first-order branches. Limited roles for catheter-based angiography using vascular contrast agents remain in fine-adjusting final endograft placement with respect to renal or other critical branch artery origins, in monitoring branch artery interventions such as embolization of renal or internal iliac arteries, or in demonstrating and/or treating endoleaks. These are straightforward and fairly routine, and will not be discussed further.

Renal impairment has always been a relative contraindication to the use of iodinated contrast materials. The use of renal-protective strategies such as oral *N*-acetylcysteine or intravenous bicarbonate infusions appears to mitigate the renotoxicity of iodinated contrast agents, although unequivocal demonstration of their benefit has not yet been documented. Nevertheless, the safety margin of these agents is so broad that preimaging administration of one or both has won wide acceptance. Gadolinium-based contrast agents, the mainstay of contrast-enhanced MRI, were championed as renal-friendly contrast agents used in off-label applications as an x-ray contrast material, until the discovery of nephrogenic systemic sclerosis specifically affecting patients in renal failure. In contrast, the use of intravascular carbon dioxide contrast, long championed by pioneers in the interventional radiology community, is gaining wide acceptance by all peripheral interventionalists. Safe use requires unflagging attention to numerous safety precautions and clinical rules of thumb, which have to be adopted in total by the entire angiographic team [51]. For example, intra-arterial carbon dioxide cannot be considered safe if injected above the diaphragm. This and other precautions are based on the physical properties of carbon dioxide gas and idiosyncrasies of delivering a high-volume arterial bolus in a clinically tolerable fashion. For example, a patient with a previous right radical nephrectomy needed endograft treatment of an abdominal aortic aneurysm. This is an ideal application of carbon dioxide angiography. The goal is to display the renal and internal iliac artery origins, in order to guide endograft deployment; in this well-defined clinical scenario, carbon dioxide can reliably substitute for iodinated contrast agents. Subtraction angiography with carbon dioxide injections unequivocally localizes the solitary left renal artery and internal iliac arteries (Fig. 3.20a, b). The inferior mesenteric artery

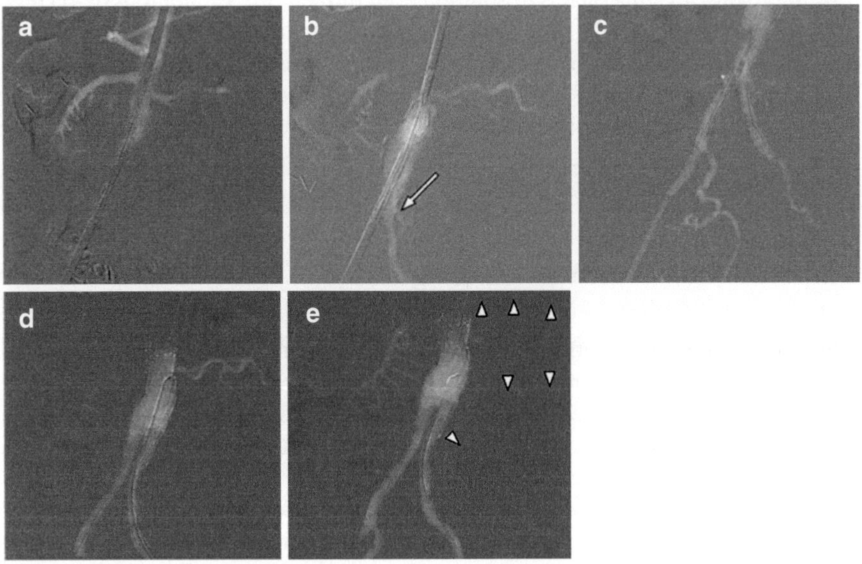

Fig. 3.20 Five images from carbon dioxide angiography during deployment of a Zenith endograft in a patient with prior right nephrectomy. Initial bolus injection (**a**) localizes the left renal artery origin, confirmed after deployment of the first two covered segments (**b**). Note expected filling of the patent inferior mesenteric artery (*IMA*) (**b**, *arrow*). After deployment of the iliac limbs, carbon dioxide gas injected into the right iliac artery (**c**) continues to fill the IMA, indicating a subtle junctional endoleak. It would be unusual to see such a leak after injection of iodinated contrast material. Final aortography with carbon dioxide confirms sparing of the left renal and internal iliac arteries (**d**). However, there is continued filling of the IMA (**e**), but this finding is inconclusive because, due to its low viscosity, the carbon dioxide quickly fills the superior mesenteric artery, middle colic artery, and arc of Riolan (**e**, *arrowheads*). Further research is needed to determine the clinical significance of endoleaks demonstrated by carbon dioxide angiography

(IMA) is also filled because of its anterior origin off the aneurysm sac and preferential filling of nondependent structures by the buoyant gas (Fig. 3.20b, arrow). The IMA continues to fill after endograft deployment, both from iliac artery injection and from suprarenal aortic injection (Fig. 3.20c–e). This case illustrates a limit in our current understanding of carbon dioxide angiography, which has been encountered in the context of TIPS construction, diagnosis of gastrointestinal or traumatic hemorrhage, or arteriovenous shunting, namely, that carbon dioxide angiography may be too sensitive. The reliability of carbon dioxide in demonstrating clinically significant endoleaks requires further systematic study.

IVUS imaging of the aorta is based on 8–9 Fr catheter systems; imaging of arteries such as the superior mesenteric or renal arteries is best accomplished with 5–6 Fr systems. The former allows visualization of a 60-mm-diameter field of view, the latter an 8- to 20-mm-diameter field of view. IVUS is best for high-resolution clarification of specific localized anatomical questions. For example, in treating aortic aneurysmal disease, it is sometimes useful to place an IVUS catheter at the celiac or left common carotid origin, to allow absolute localization of the vessel origin independent of beam divergence, center of the fluoroscopic field, magnification, or other confounding geometrical distortion. IVUS imaging is even more generally useful during interventions to treat aortic dissection. IVUS allows unequivocal distinction between true and false lumens at any given level and permits immediate localization of a catheter or guidewire with respect to the aortic true and false lumens, without contrast injection. As such, it can guide interventions in the dissected aorta as well as the superior mesenteric or other branch artery. Passing the IVUS over a guidewire allows positive identification of the entire course of the wire, which can inconspicuously traverse from one lumen across the flap into another. Lack of appreciation of an errant guidewire pathway, when implanting an aortic stent or endograft, can lead to anatomical blunders which can be disastrous at worst and time-consuming to correct at best. IVUS may be used to guide creation of fenestration tears and assess the response of the true lumen to creation of a fenestration tear or implantation of an endograft IVUS catheters. The guidewire lumen of the IVUS catheter can be attached to an electronic manometer for direct correlation of pressure drops with anatomical features of the aortic lumen. These and other applications make IVUS an indispensable tool in any high-volume aortic practice.

Echocardiography

Due to its widespread availability and usefulness in emergent situations to identify a broad range of cardiovascular pathologies, echocardiography is frequently used in cases of undifferentiated chest pain. Transthoracic echocardiography (TTE) can be used to identify acute aortic pathology involving the aortic root or proximal ascending aorta, with a 70–85% sensitivity in diagnosing ascending aortic dissection (Fig. 3.21) [52, 53]. Additionally, TTE is useful to evaluate the functional consequences of dissection, such as potential aortic insufficiency and myocardial

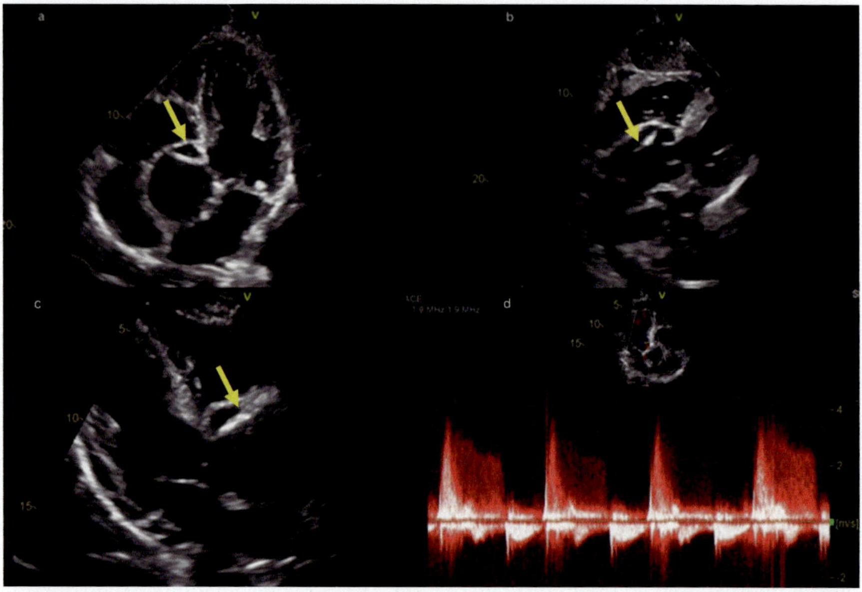

Fig. 3.21 Four images from transthoracic echocardiogram demonstrating a type A aortic dissection (yellow arrow). (**a**) shows an apical five-chamber view with perhaps the best view of the dissection flap and dilated root. (**b, c**) offer subcostal and parasternal long views of the dissection flap at the level of the sinotubular junction and proximal aorta. (**d**) demonstrates the moderate aortic regurgitation that is present as a result of this proximal type A aortic dissection

ischemia when the dissection extends into a coronary [53]. Finally, TTE allows for assessment for a bicuspid aortic valve, which is frequently present in cases of congenital aortopathy. Assessment of the aortic root is best carried out in a parasternal long-axis view, while suprasternal views allow for evaluation of the supra-aortic vessels and a portion of the descending aorta. The aortic valve should be examined for regurgitation from a parasternal short-axis view, directed toward the base of the heart and great vessels [53]. Five- and three-chamber views can also evaluate aortic regurgitation.

Transesophageal echocardiography (TEE) permits high-resolution images of the aorta from the root to the descending section. The one portion it cannot evaluate is a small portion of the distal ascending aorta near the innominate artery [53]. It is certainly useful in cases of acute dissection, especially if a patient is too hemodynamically unstable to go to the CT scanner or has renal disease preventing administration of contrast (Fig. 3.22). TEE is portable and has a sensitivity of over 80% with specificity over 90% for aortic dissection [53]. Classical aortic dissection is diagnosed when seeing an intimal flap that divides the aorta into true and false lumina [54]. Color Doppler generally shows false lumen flow but may not in cases of retrograde or thrombosed dissection [54].

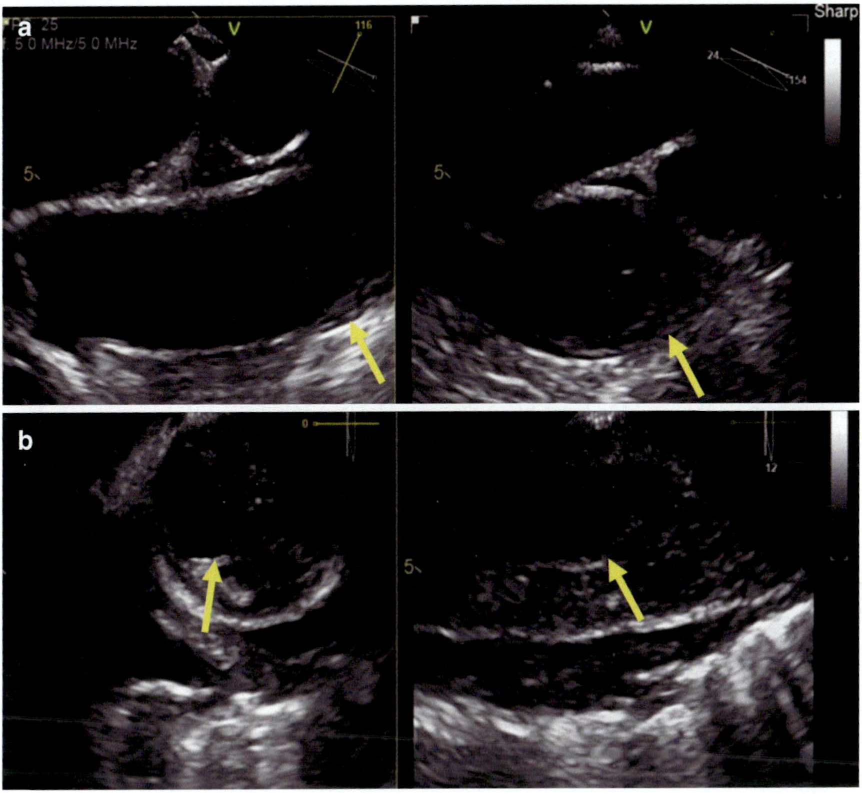

Fig. 3.22 Demonstrates transesophageal echocardiographic windows of a type A intramural hematoma (**a**) with a type B aortic dissection (**b**) at yellow arrows. We use the biplane technique to evaluate the area of interest from multiple angles at once

Acknowledgements Peter S. Liu and David M. Williams, who wrote the previous version of this chapter.

References

1. Costello P, Ecker CP, Tello R, Hartnell GG. Assessment of the thoracic aorta by spiral CT. Am J Roentgenol. 1992;158(5):1127–30.
2. Shapira OM, Aldea GS, Cutter SM, Fitzgerald CA, Lazar HL, Shemin RJ. Improved clinical outcomes after operation of the proximal aorta: a 10-year experience. Ann Thorac Surg. 1999;67(4):1030–7.
3. Tatli S, Yucel EK, Lipton MJ. CT and MR imaging of the thoracic aorta: current techniques and clinical applications. Radiol Clin North Am. 2004;42(3):565–85.
4. Armerding MD, et al. Aortic aneurysmal disease: assessment of stent-graft treat-ment-CT versus conventional angiography. Radiology. 2000;215:138–46.

5. Dillon EH, van Leeuwen MS, Fernandez MA, Mali WP. Spiral CT angiography. Am J Roentgenol. 1993;160(6):1273–8.
6. Weg N, Scheer MR, Gabor MP. Liver lesions: improved detection with dual-detector-array CT and routine 2.5-mm thin collimation. Radiology. 1998;209(2):417–26.
7. Kaufman JA. Noninvasive vascular imaging. In: Vascular and interventional radiology: the requisites. 1st ed. Philadelphia: Mosby; 2004. p. 71–82.
8. Tanaka R, Yoshioka K, Abiko A. Updates on computed tomography imaging in aortic aneurysms and dissection. Ann Vasc Dis. 2020;13(1):23–7.
9. Di Cesare E, Splendiani A, Barile A, Squillaci E, Di Cesare A, Brunese L, Masciocchi C. CT and MR imaging of the thoracic aorta. Open Med. 2016;11(1):143–51.
10. Liu Y, Xu J, Li J, Ren J, Liu H, Xu J, Wei M, Hao Y, Zheng M. The ascending aortic image quality and the whole aortic radiation dose of high-pitch dual-source CT angiography. J Cardiothorac Surg. 2013;8(1):1–5.
11. Sundaram B, Quint LE, Patel HJ, Deeb GM. CT findings following thoracic aortic surgery. Radiographics. 2007;27(6):1583–94.
12. Sandfort V, Ahlman MA, Jones EC, Selwaness M, Chen MY, Folio LR, Bluemke DA. High pitch third generation dual-source CT: coronary and cardiac visualization on routine chest CT. J Cardiovasc Comput Tomogr. 2016;10(4):282–8.
13. Napoli A, et al. Computed tomography angiography: state-of-the-art imaging using multidetector-row technology. J Comput Assist Tomogr. 2004;28:S32–45.
14. Lell MM, et al. New techniques in CT angiography. Radiographics. 2006;26:S45–62.
15. Rozenblit AM, et al. Detection of endoleaks after endovascular repair of abdominal aortic aneurysm: value of unenhanced and delayed helical CT acquisitions. Radiology. 2003;227(2):426–33.
16. Stavropoulos SW, Charagundla SR. Imaging techniques for detection and management of endoleaks after endovascular aortic aneurysm repair. Radiology. 2007;243(3):641–55.
17. Olin JW, et-al. Atherosclerotic vascular disease conference: writing group IV: imaging. Circulation. 2004;109(21):2626–33.
18. Federle MP, Pan KT, Pealer KM. CT criteria for differentiating abdominal hemorrhage: anticoagulation or aortic aneurysm rupture ? Am J Roentgenol. 2007;188(5):1324–30.
19. Isselbacher EM, Preventza O, Hamilton Black J III, et al. 2022 ACC/AHA guideline for the diagnosis and Management of Aortic Disease: a report of the American Heart Association/American College of Cardiology Joint Committee on clinical practice guidelines. J Am Coll Cardiol. 2022;80(24):e223–393.
20. Rozenblit A, Marin ML, Veith FJ, Cynamon J, Wahl SI, Bakal CW. Endovascular repair of abdominal aortic aneurysm: value of postoperative follow-up with helical CT. Am J Roentgenol. 1995;165(6):1473–9.
21. Pooley RA. AAPM/RSNA physics tutorial for residents: fundamental physics of MR imaging. Radiographics. 2005;25(4):1087–99.
22. Jacobs MA, Ibrahim TS, Ouwerkerk R. AAPM/RSNA physics tutorials for residents: MR imaging: brief overview and emerging applications. Radiographics. 2007;27(4):1213–29.
23. Bitar R, et-al. MR pulse sequences: what every radiologist wants to know but is afraid to ask. Radiographics. 2006;26(2):513–37.
24. Creasy JL, Price RR, Presbrey T, Goins D, Partain CL, Kessler RM. Gadolinium-enhanced MR angiography. Radiology. 1990;175:280–3.
25. Roberts D, Siegelman ES. Imaging and MR arteriography of the aorta. In: Body MRI. 1st ed. Philadelphia: Elsevier; 2005. p. 481–507.
26. Dobson MJ, Hartley RW, Ashleigh R, Watson Y, Hawnaur JM. MR angiography and MR imaging of symptomatic vascular malformations. Clin Radiol. 1997;52(8):595–602.
27. Tatli S, Lipton MJ, Davison BD, Skorstad RB, Yucel EK. From the RSNA refresher courses: MR imaging of aortic and peripheral vascular disease. Radiographics. 2003;23 Spec No:S59–78.
28. Zhang H, Maki JH, Prince MR. 3D contrast-enhanced MR angiography. J Magn Reson Imaging. 2007;25(1):13–25.

29. Prince MR. Gadolinium-enhanced MR aortography. Radiology. 1994;191(1):155–64.
30. Marckmann P, et al. Nephrogenic systemic fibrosis: suspected causative role of gadodiamide used for contrast-enhanced magnetic resonance imaging. J Am Soc Nephrol. 2006;17:2359–62.
31. Stafford RB, Sabati M, Mahallati H, Frayne R. 3D non-contrast-enhanced MR angiography with balanced steady-state free precession dixon method. Magn Reson Med. 2008;59(2):430–3.
32. Saloner D. The AAPM/RSNA physics tutorial for residents. An introduction to MR angiography. Radiographics. 1995;15(2):453–65.
33. ACR Committee on Drugs and Contrast Media. ACR manual on contrast media, version 10.3. https://www.acr.org/-/media/ACR/Files/Clinical-Resources/Contrast_Media.pdf. Published June 2018. Accessed 9 May 2019.
34. European Society of Urogenital Radiology. ESUR guidelines on contrast agents, version 10.0. http://www.esur-cm.org/index.php/a-general-adverse-reactions-2. Published March 2018. Accessed 9 May 2019.
35. Woolen SA, Shankar PR, Gagnier JJ, MacEachern MP, Singer L, Davenport MS. Risk of nephrogenic systemic fibrosis in patients with stage 4 or 5 chronic kidney disease receiving a group II gadolinium-based contrast agent: a systematic review and meta-analysis. JAMA Intern Med. 2020;180(2):223–30. https://doi.org/10.1001/jamainternmed.2019.5284.
36. Brenner DJ, Hall EJ. Computed tomography—an increasing source of radiation exposure. N Engl J Med. 2007;357(22):2277–84.
37. Thurnher SA, et al. Evaluation of abdominal aortic aneurysm for stent-graft placement: comparison of gadolinium-enhanced MR angiography versus helical CT angiography and digital subtraction angiography. Radiology. 1997;205(2):341–52.
38. Lutz AM, et al. Evaluation of aortoiliac aneurysm before endovascular repair: comparison of contrast-enhanced magnetic resonance angiography with multidetector row computed tomographic angiography with an automated analysis software tool. J Vasc Surg. 2003;37(3):619–27.
39. Ludman CN, et al. Feasibility of using dynamic contrast-enhanced magnetic resonance angiography as the sole imaging modality prior to endovascu-Lar repair of abdominal aortic aneurysms. Eur J Vasc Endovasc Surg. 2000;19(5):524–30.
40. Thurnher S, Cejna M. Imaging of aortic stent-grafts and endoleaks. Radiol Clin North Am. 2002;40(4):799–833.
41. Cejna M, et al. MR angiography vs CT angiography in the follow-up of niti-nol stent grafts in endoluminally treated aortic aneurysms. Eur Radiol. 2002;12(10):2443–50.
42. Engellau L, et al. Magnetic resonance imaging and MR angiography of endo-luminally treated abdominal aortic aneurysms. Eur J Vasc Endovasc Surg. 1998;15(3):212–9.
43. Haulon S, et al. Prospective evaluation of magnetic resonance imaging after endovascular treatment of infrarenal aortic aneurysms. Eur J Vasc Endovasc Surg. 2001;22(1):62–9.
44. Stavropoulos SW, Baum RA. Imaging modalities for the detection and management of endoleaks. Semin Vasc Surg. 2004;17(2):154–60.
45. Cohen EI, et al. Time-resolved MR angiography for the classification of endoleaks after endovascular aneurysm repair. J Magn Reson Imaging. 2008;27(3):500–3.
46. Ramaekers MJFG, Westenberg JJM, Adriaans BP, et al. A clinician's guide to understanding aortic 4D flow MRI. Insights Imaging. 2023;14:114. https://doi.org/10.1186/s13244-023-01458-x.
47. Burris NS, Hope MD. 4D flow MRI applications for aortic disease. Magn Reson Imaging Clin N Am. 2015;23(1):15–23. https://doi.org/10.1016/j.mric.2014.08.006. Epub 2014 Oct 5. PMID: 25476670; PMCID: PMC5127263.
48. Takahashi K, Sekine T, Ando T, Ishii Y, Kumita S. Utility of 4D flow MRI in thoracic aortic diseases: a literature review of clinical applications and current evidence. Magn Reson Med Sci. 2022;21(2):327–39. https://doi.org/10.2463/mrms.rev.2021-0046. Epub 2021 Sep 8. PMID: 34497166; PMCID: PMC9680552.

49. Saitta S, Pirola S, Piatti F, Votta E, Lucherini F, Pluchinotta F, Carminati M, Lombardi M, Geppert C, Cuomo F, Figueroa CA, Xu XY, Redaelli A. Evaluation of 4D flow MRI-based non-invasive pressure assessment in aortic coarctations. J Biomech. 2019;94:13–21. https://doi.org/10.1016/j.jbiomech.2019.07.004. Epub 2019 Jul 9.
50. Dyverfeldt P, Bissell M, Barker AJ, et al. 4D flow cardiovascular magnetic resonance consensus statement. J Cardiovasc Magn Reson. 2015;17:72. https://doi.org/10.1186/s12968-015-0174-5.
51. Cho KJ, Hawkins IR, editors. Carbon dioxide angiography: principles, techniques, and practice. New York: Informa Healthcare USA, Inc; 2007.
52. Bhave NM, Nienaber CA, Clough RE, Eagle KA. Multimodality imaging of thoracic aortic diseases in adults. JACC Cardiovasc Imaging. 2018;11(6):902–19.
53. Evangelista A, Flachskampf FA, Erbel R, Antonini-Canterin F, Vlachopoulos C, Rocchi G, Sicari R, Nihoyannopoulos P, Zamorano J, Document Reviewers, Pepi M. Echocardiography in aortic diseases: EAE recommendations for clinical practice. Eur J Echocardiogr. 2010;11(8):645–58.
54. Upadhyaya K, Ugonabo I, Satam K, Hull SC. Echocardiographic evaluation of the thoracic aorta: tips and pitfalls. AORTA. 2021;9(01):001–8.

Chapter 4
Best Medical Management of AAA

Jason R. Cook, Jonathan R. Thompson, and B. Timothy Baxter

Introduction and Approach

Following identification of an abdominal aortic aneurysm (AAA), patients will routinely be referred for or seek out a vascular specialist with expertise in treating aortic aneurysms. Anyone with acute symptoms related to their AAA should be evaluated urgently, usually in the emergency department. However, most AAAs are not symptomatic when discovered, having been found at screening or incidentally during imaging for other concerns [1]. These patients are seen in the clinic and typically present with some degree of alarm and apprehension. For the majority of these patients, the AAA will be below the standard repair threshold and many will be followed for some years before intervention is warranted, if ever, as some will die of other causes. Reassurance, education, and surveillance become the plan for initial management. Because of the disease onset in later life and the strong association between AAA and tobacco use, many of these patients are receiving medical treatment for other health problems including atherosclerotic occlusive disease and obstructive lung disease [2]. In fact, one meta-analysis identified that COPD is associated with increased risk of rupture for AAA patients [3]. While a specific pharmacologic therapy to inhibit expansion of AAA does not yet exist, AAA progression, rupture rates, and long-term outcomes are significantly impacted by a host of factors. Optimal management of these patients requires a thorough understanding of factors that may influence the future behavior and progression of AAA. Using the highest level of available evidence, systematic reviews and prospective trial, we will provide an update on best management practices for AAA patients undergoing surveillance.

J. R. Cook · J. R. Thompson · B. T. Baxter (✉)
Department of Surgery, University of Nebraska Medical Center, Omaha, NE, USA
e-mail: jason.cook@unmc.edu; jonathan.thompson@unmc.edu; btbaxter@unmc.edu

G. J. Arnaoutakis et al. (eds.), *Aortic Aneurysms*, Contemporary Cardiology,
https://doi.org/10.1007/978-3-032-13134-8_4

Tobacco Use and AAA

The association between tobacco use and AAA is certain and was the topic of a systematic review and meta-analysis by Aune et al. [4]. The relative risk (RR) of developing an AAA for current or past smokers compared to nonsmokers was 4.9 and 2.1, respectively. The RR was dose dependent up to a threshold of 20 cigarettes per day or 20 pkg years; there was no further increase above these levels. The precise mechanism through which this occurs is not entirely clear. The etiology for AAA has been elusive, in part, because it is multifactorial. This is illustrated by two features concerning the relationship between tobacco use and AAA: (1) the majority of the patients seen and treated for peripheral or carotid artery disease with a significant smoking history have no abdominal aortic dilation; (2) some patients with AAA have no history of tobacco exposure [5]. Thus, tobacco use promotes AAA development when a permissive genetic background is present [6]. When AAA is present, continued tobacco use is associated with more rapid AAA expansion and increased risk of rupture (Fig. 4.1).

Given this clear association between tobacco exposure and AAA development, progression, and rupture, smoking cessation is the single, most effective strategy for reducing risk associated with AAA [7]. Providers should be aware that this is difficult and the percentage of smokers who quit in any given year is in the single digits. Factors proven in meta-analysis to increase quit rates include counseling and medication [8, 9]. Nicotine replacement therapy (NRT) during quitting, especially when a patch is used in combination with gum or lozenges, can significantly increase smoking cessation rates [10, 11]. The relative risk of abstinence

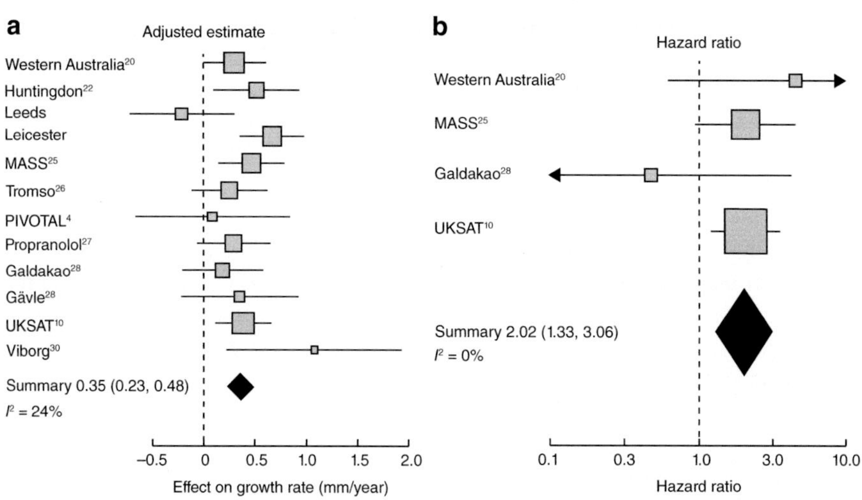

Fig. 4.1 Effect of smoking on aortic aneurysm growth rate (**a**, left panel) and aortic aneurysm rupture rate (**b**, right panel) in individual studies and meta-analysis. Adjusted estimates are shown with 95% confidence intervals [6]

for any form of NRT relative to control was 1.55 (95% confidence interval (CI) 1.49–1.61). Adverse and serious adverse events from NRT are rare. Aside from NRT, Varenicline is the only other medication proven to increase success. It was temporarily taken off the market by the FDA because of its high nitrosamine concentration. This has been addressed and it is now available [12]. Smoking cessation rates are highest when these aids are used in combination. Finally, a key factor that influences success is the number of attempts at quitting [13]. This is the reason it is important to have a discussion about risks of continued smoking, the benefits of cessation, and to encourage attempts at quitting during each patient encounter.

Antiplatelet and Antithrombotic Therapy

The effects of antiplatelet and antithrombotic therapy have been systematically assessed in retrospective reviews. When the impacts of all types of antiplatelet therapy are taken together, AAA growth rate is not affected (Fig. 4.2) [14]. However, analysis of the four observational studies (882 patients) that looked only at aspirin, rather than any type of antiplatelet therapy, found aspirin (vs. no aspirin) to be associated with slower AAA growth. The strength of the evidence for this finding was considered "low" and the magnitude of the difference small. The role of Ticagrelor, a potent antiplatelet therapy that blocks the P2Y12 receptor, was tested in a randomized trial in ASA-naïve patients testing the hypothesis that it would reduce growth by limiting intraluminal thrombus and inflammation [15]. Compared to placebo, ticagrelor did not decrease AAA progression determined by MRI measurements of both volume and diameter. Similarly, intraluminal thrombus volume was not affected at 12 months. When the potential role of anticoagulation on AAA growth was evaluated, no effect was found.

	Antithrombotic			Control			Mean difference in aneurysm growth	
Study or subgroup	Mean - mm/y	SD - mm/y	Total	Mean - mm/y	SD - mm/y	Total	IV, random, 95% CI - mm/y	Weight
Aspirin								
Lindholt 2008 (diameter > 40 mm)[53]	2.92	2.6154	14	5.18	2.6154	17	−2.26 [−4.11, −0.41]	3.7%
Karlsson 2008[83]	1.8	1.77	101	2.6	2	100	−0.80 [−1.32, −0.28]	16.4%
Behr-Rasmussen 2014[70]	2.42	2.46	209	3.01	2.67	207	−0.59 [−1.08, −0.10]	16.9%
Ahmad 2017[91]	2	2.2	40	2.4	2.2	77	−0.40 [−1.24, −0.44]	11.1%
Lindholt 2008 (diameter < 40 mm)[53]	2.23	1.683	48	2.52	1.683	69	−0.29 [−0.91, −0.33]	14.6%
Subtotal (95% CI)			**412**			**470**	**−0.61 [−0.94, −0.28]**	**62.6%**
Heterogeneity: Tau² = 0.02; *Chi²* = 4.83, df = 4 (*p* = .30); *I*² = 17%								
Test for overall effect: Z = 3.65 (*p* < .001)								
Other Antiplatelets								
Thompson 2010[74]	1.35	17.4695	443	1.54	4.127	757	−0.19 [−1.84, 1.46]	4.4%
Wanhainen 2020[21]	2.3	2.5533	72	2.2	2.1278	72	0.10 [−0.67, 0.87]	12.1%
Sweeting 2010[90]	2.91	2.632	501	2.76	2.632	1200	0.15 [−0.12, 0.42]	20.9%
Subtotal (95% CI)			**1 016**			**2 029**	**0.14 [−0.12, 0.39]**	**37.4%**
Heterogeneity: Tau² = 0.00; *Chi²* = 0.17, df = 2 (*p* = .92); *I*² = 0%								
Test for overall effect: Z = 1.05 (*p* = .30)								
Total (95% CI)			**1 428**			**2 499**	**−0.36 [−0.75, 0.02]**	**100.0%**
Heterogeneity: Tau² = 0.17; *Chi²* = 19.36, df = 7 (*p* = .007); *I*² = 64%								
Test for overall effect: Z = 1.85 (*p* = 0.60)								
Test for subgroup differences: *Chi²* = 12.39, df = 1 (*p* < .001); *I*² = 91.9%								

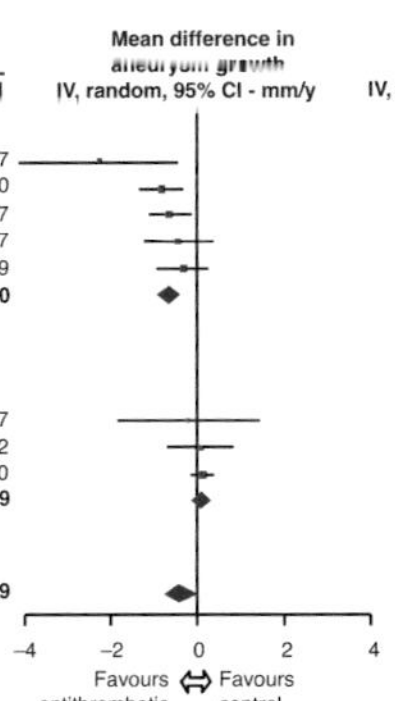

Fig. 4.2 Summary forest plot of aneurysm growth rate for patients with aneurysms treated with aspirin or other antiplatelets vs. no antiplatelet agent. *CI* confidence interval; inverse variance, *SD* standard deviation, *mm/y* mm growth per year [14]

ASA use was associated with a reduction in all-cause mortality after AAA intervention compared to those not taking ASA [14]. The strength of the evidence for this finding is considered to be "high". While ASA was used in the past for primary prevention of cardiovascular disease, the United States Preventive Service Task Force no longer recommends low-dose aspirin therapy for primary prevention of cardiovascular disease for those over 60 years of age [16]. Considering this recommendation along with (1) the relatively weak evidence of AAA growth inhibition and (2) the negative results of the ticagrelor randomized trial, the decision for low-dose ASA during surveillance should be individualized. It should not be used in patients with increased bleeding risk. After AAA repair, however, the evidence strongly favors ASA as a means of reducing all-cause mortality. Anticoagulation, on the other hand, is associated with increased all-cause mortality after AAA intervention.

Blood Pressure Control

Based simply on physiology and geometry, the pressure at the wall of the aneurysm is greater than in the remainder of the smaller diameter aorta, and this difference is inversely proportional to the radius. As such, one might assume that elevated blood pressure would have a detrimental impact on AAA growth rate. Meta-analysis of this subject included 21 cohort studies (20 publications) with data on 28,162 cases and 5,440,588 participants [17]. The RR for the presence of AAA in hypertensive patients is 1.66 (95% CI: 1.49–1.85, I^2 = 79.3%, n = 13) compared to non-hypertensive patients. In addition, there was a 14% (95% CI: 6–23%, I^2 = 30.5%, n = 6) and a 28% (95% CI: 12–46%, I^2 = 80.1%, n = 6) increase in the RR of AAA for every 20 mmHg and 10 mmHg increase in systolic blood pressure (SBP) and diastolic blood pressure (DBP), respectively. The analysis of DBP showed evidence of a strong and highly significant nonlinear dose-response relationship ($p < 0.001$) when the diastolic pressure was above 80 mmHg.

Perhaps somewhat surprisingly, three separate analyses, using different models, did not find a relationship between blood pressure and expansion rate of small AAA (Figs. 4.3 and 4.4) [6, 18, 19]. Additionally, two of these studies found no selective benefit to any particular antihypertensive medication. This is consistent with the results of randomized trials that tested the effects of four different classes of antihypertensive medications against placebo. Propranolol was tested in two separate randomized trials, neither of which showed slower growth with propranolol [20, 21]. Both studies were compromised by poor patient compliance secondary to side effects. Amlodipine, a calcium channel blocker, and perindopril, an angiotensin-converting enzyme inhibitor, were compared against placebo using 1:1:1 randomization [22, 23]. Amlodipine and perindopril both reduced blood pressure compared to baseline values but neither reduced AAA growth rates. Although blood pressure control did not directly contribute to decreasing the growth rate of abdominal aortic aneurysms, there was a statistically significant reduction in aortic rupture in patients

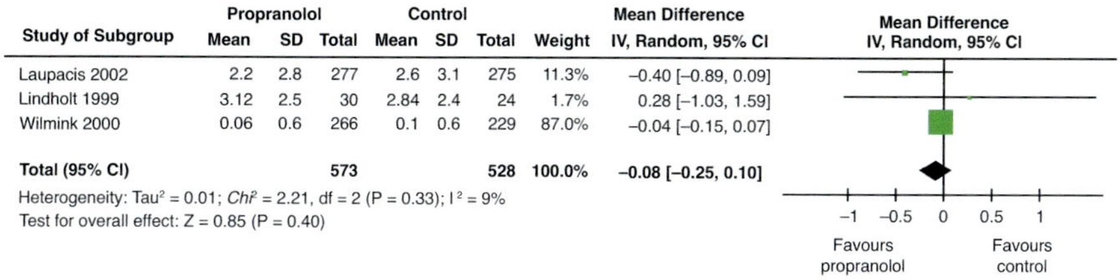

Fig. 4.3 Forest plot summarizing multiple trials regarding the effect of propranolol on abdominal aortic aneurysm growth rate shown in mean difference (MD) in mm/year growth rate and 95 confidence intervals (CI) [37]

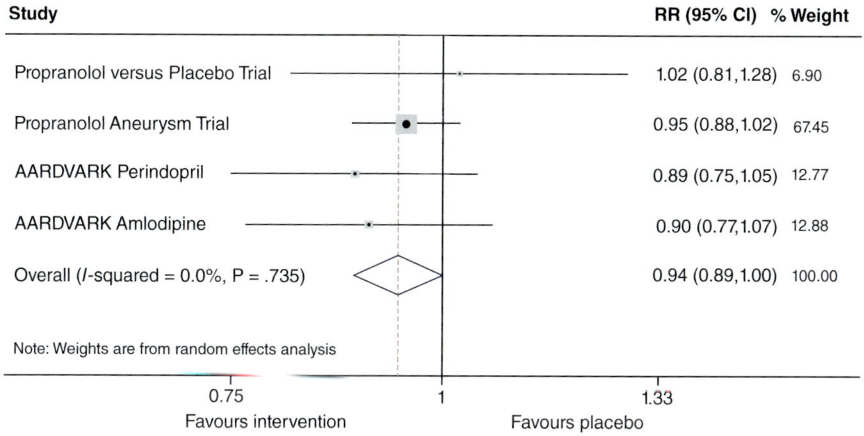

Fig. 4.4 Forest plot of antihypertensive regimens on aortic rupture in patients with abdominal aortic aneurysms [24]

treated with antihypertensive medications [24]. Blood pressure control in accordance with the Adult Treatment Protocols from the American Heart Association is critical to the well-being of all patients. The class of antihypertensive medication should not be influenced by the presence of AAA.

Statins

The effects of statin therapy on AAA has been the focus of two meta-analyses covering the range from impact on growth, rupture rates, and effect on long-term health outcomes [25, 26]. The data regarding impact on growth demonstrates an inhibitory effect on expansion rate (Fig. 4.5). This effect size is less in more recent studies and minimal among the studies with the largest number of patients [19] (Figs. 4.5 and 4.6). The data also suggest the effect may be greater in larger AAA (>4 cm) [25]. Statin therapy has been found to reduce AAA rupture and perioperative morbidity

Study or Subgroup	Statins Mean	Statins SD	Statins Total	Control Mean	Control SD	Control Total	Weight	Mean Difference IV. Fixed, 95% CI
Karrowni 2011	0.9	0.27	136	3.2	3.38	75	40.1%	−2.30 [−3.07, −1.53]
Kim 2016	−7.9	8.3	64	−4.9	5.9	45	3.3%	−3.00 [−6.67, −0.33]
Mosorin 2008	1.9	1.8	34	2.6	2.4	87	38.0%	−0.70 [−1.49, 0.09]
Schouten 2006	1.79	3.789	59	2.95	2.8	91	18.6%	−1.16 [−2.29, −0.03]
Total (95% CI)			**293**			**298**	**100.0%**	**−1.50 [−1.99, −1.02]**

Heterogeneity: Chi² = 9.72, df = 3 (P = 0.02); I² = 69%
Test for overall effect: Z = 6.07 (P < 0.00001)

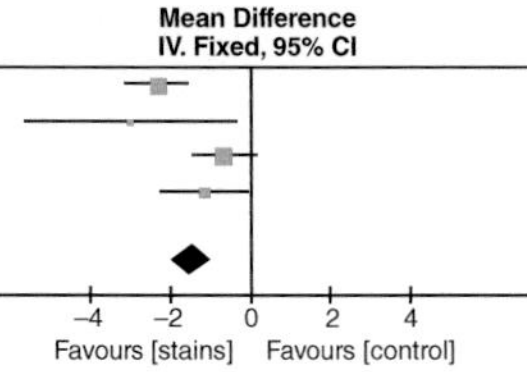

Fig. 4.5 The effect of statin therapy on mean difference of abdominal aortic aneurysm growth rate in mm/year [26]

Study or Subgroup	log[Odds Ratio]	SE	Weight	Odds Ratio IV, Fixed, 95% CI
Alshaikh 2018	−0.9284	0.1325	16.7%	0.40 [0.30, 0.51]
Feeney 2009	−1.195	0.5161	1.1%	0.30 [0.11, 0.83]
Galinanes 2014	−0.2337	0.0868	39.0%	0.79 [0.67, 0.94]
Leurs 2006	−0.557	0.316	2.9%	0.57 [0.31, 1.06]
Mathisen 2017	−1.455	0.376	2.1%	0.23 [0.11, 0.49]
Mcnally 2010	−2.992	1.4482	0.1%	0.05 [0.00, 0.86]
Tyerman 2018	0.1595	0.4002	1.8%	1.17 [0.54, 2.57]
Wemmelund 2014	−0.4403	0.0901	36.2%	0.64 [0.54, 0.77]
Total (95% CI)			**100.0%**	**0.63 [0.56, 0.70]**

Heterogeneity: Chi² = 33.90, df = 7 (P < 0.0001); I² = 79%
Test for overall effect: Z = 8.61 (P < 0.00001)

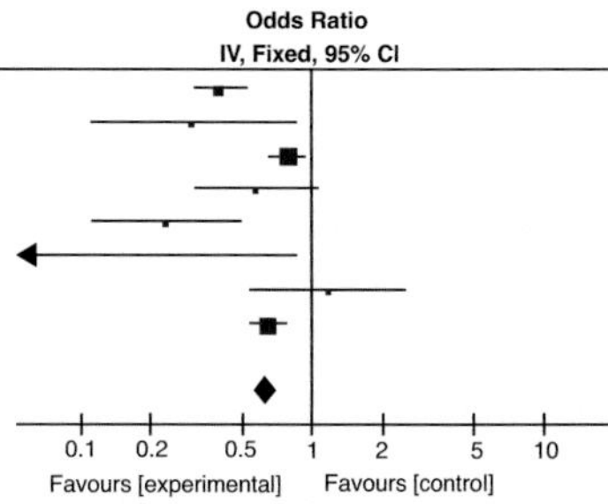

Fig. 4.6 Forest plot summarizing the effect of statin therapy on abdominal aortic aneurysm-related clinical events including rupture, repair, and/or death [26]

and mortality after open or endovascular repair [19, 25, 27, 28]. Long-term all-cause mortality is improved with statin therapy [28].

Metformin

It is well-known that AAAs grow more slowly in patients with type II diabetes. Of all the factors found to impact AAA progression, the presence of diabetes has the largest effect size (Figs. 4.7 and 4.8). While the mechanism for this association is unclear, a number of hypotheses have been proposed [29]. Hyperglycemia has an impact on protein structure through glycosylation of proteins. This effect is in fact the basis for the laboratory studies used clinically to determine average glucose levels, the percentage of glycated hemoglobin or hemoglobin 1Ac. Glycation occurs normally but is greatly enhanced in a high glucose milieu. Hemoglobin has a known half-life so its glycation reflects the glucose levels over its half-life (90 days). For proteins with very low turnover, such as fibrillar collagens and elastin, glycation is cumulative. This process leads to increasing crosslinking in these proteins, which makes them less susceptible to protease degradation. This is one potential mechanism for growth inhibition in diabetic patients. An alternative hypothesis, currently under investigation in an NIH-funded trial, is that metformin, a drug commonly used to treat type II DM, has pleotropic effects that may impact AAA growth in addition to its effects on

Study or Subgroup	Prescribe Metformin Mean	SD	Total	Not Prescribe Metformin Mean	SD	Total	Weight	Mean Difference IV, Random, 95% CI
Fujimura 2016	0.4	0.6	15	1.7	0.5	43	15.4%	−1.30 [−1.64, −0.96]
Golledge 2017 Cohort 1	1.03	2.68	118	1.62	2.45	1239	13.1%	−0.59 [−1.09, −0.09]
Golledge 2017 Cohort 2	1.4	2.99	39	2.55	3.04	248	7.3%	−1.15 [−2.16, −0.14]
Golledge 2017 Cohort 3	0.37	1.28	16	1.46	1.52	37	9.4%	−1.09 [−1.89, −0.29]
Golledge 2019 Cohort 1	0.63	1.42	129	1.15	1.99	105	13.8%	−0.52 [−0.97, −0.07]
Golledge 2019 Cohort 1	0.48	1.58	106	1.16	2.72	75	10.7%	−0.68 [−1.37, 0.01]
Itoga 2019	1.2	1.9	5496	1.5	2.2	8347	17.8%	−0.30 [−0.37, −0.23]
Unosson 2021	1.1	1.1	65	1.6	1.4	33	12.5%	−0.50 [−1.05, 0.05]
Total (95% CI)			**5984**			**10127**	**100.0%**	**−0.72 [−1.08, −0.37]**

Heterogeneity: Tau² = 0.18; Chi² = 40.49, df = 7 (P < 0.00001); I² = 83%
Test for overall effect: Z = 4.01 (P < 0.0001)

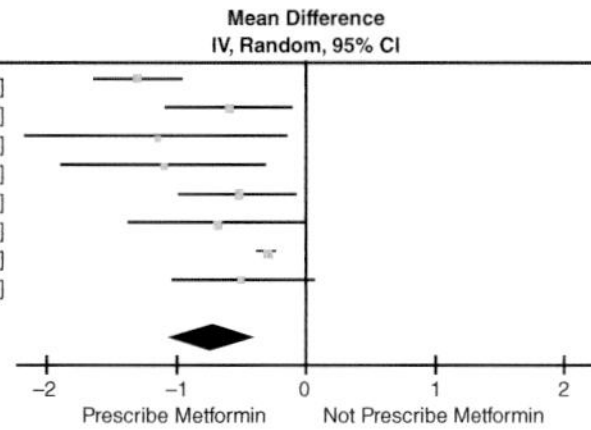

Fig. 4.7 Forest plot summarizing the effect of metformin on abdominal aortic aneurysm growth rate plotted as mean difference mm/year [38]

Study of Subgroup	Prescribe Metformin Events	Total	Not Prescribe Metformin Events	Total	Weight	Odds Ratio M-H, Random, 95% CI
Golledge 2019 Cohort 1	32	129	44	105	8.8%	0.46 [0.26, 0.80]
Golledge 2019 Cohort 2	14	106	19	75	5.1%	0.45 [0.21, 0.96]
Sutton 2020 Cohort 1	11749	24361	22185	43073	45.1%	0.88 [0.85, 0.91]
Sutton 2020 Cohort 2	698	2373	1633	5294	39.7%	0.93 [0.84, 1.04]
Turowicz 2021	2	54	7	23	1.2%	0.09 [0.02, 0.47]
Total (95% CI)		**27023**		**48570**	**100.0%**	**0.80 [0.66, 0.96]**
Total events	**12495**		**23888**			

Heterogeneity: Tau² = 0.02; Chi² = 16.86, df = 4 (P = 0.002); I² = 76%
Test for overall effect: Z = 2.40 (P = 0.02)

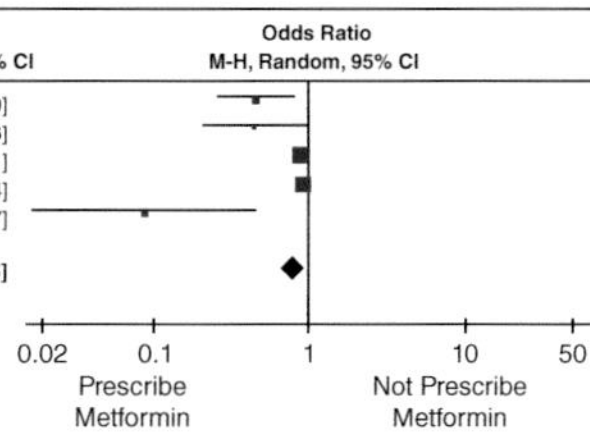

Fig. 4.8 Forest plot summarizing the effect of metformin on abdominal aortic aneurysm-related clinical events including rupture, repair, and/or related death [38]

blood sugar [30]. One meta-analysis suggests the growth rates of patients under treatment with metformin have a growth rate that is reduced by approximately 1 mm/year [19]. However, this decrease is consistent with the decreased growth seen in diabetics (not all of whom are on metformin), and one analysis comparing growth rates with prescription of various agents used to treat hyperglycemia found no difference in growth rates among the drugs [19]. Given these conflicting data and the well-documented detrimental effects of poorly controlled blood sugars, the selection of the medical regimen should be based on optimization of hemoglobin 1Ac.

Antibiotics

Antibiotics have been proposed to slow AAA expansion through different mechanisms. There was, at one time, a focus on the presence of Chlamydia in AAA tissue as having a causal role in AAA. This led to randomized trials of a number of anti-chlamydial antibiotic therapies [31]. The second potential mechanism through which antibiotics were considered to potentially impact AAA growth was their ability to inhibit the matrix-degrading enzymes, matrix metalloproteinases [32]. The role of antibiotics has been the focus of a recent meta-analysis [19]. When these study results are taken together, there is no evidence for the current use of antibiotics to suppress AAA growth or reduce untoward clinical events (Fig. 4.9).

Study of Subgroup	Antibiotic Mean	Antibiotic SD	Antibiotic Total	Placebo Mean	Placebo SD	Placebo Total	Weight	Mean Difference IV, Random, 95% CI
Hogh 2009	1.61	1.5	42	2.52	2.5	42	66.0%	−0.91 [−1.79, −0.03]
Vammen 2001	1.97	3	43	2.72	3	49	34.0%	−0.75 [−1.78, 0.48]
Total (95% CI)			**85**			**91**	**100.0%**	**−0.86 [−1.57, −0.14]**

Heterogeneity: Tau² = 0.00; Chi² = 0.04, df = 1 (P = 0.84); I² = 0%
Test for overall effect: Z = 2.34 (P = 0.02)

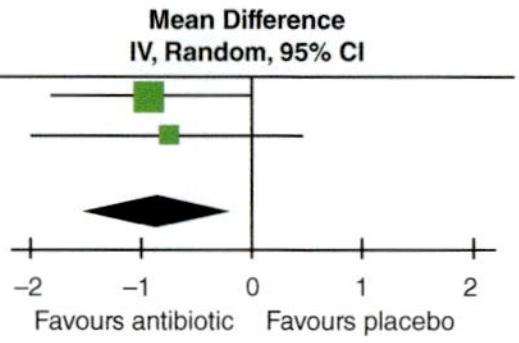

Fig. 4.9 Forest plot summarizing the effect of antibiotics on abdominal aortic aneurysm growth rate in mm/year [37]

Exercise Therapy

Aerobic exercise in patients with AAA has been the focus of a number of studies and these have been assessed in meta-analysis [33, 34]. Exercise appears to be safe. Patients enrolled in these studies had a cardiac event rate of 0.8% (95% CI 0.2–3.1%) and no ruptures were observed in study participants. Those in the exercise group had increases in anaerobic threshold and peak oxygen consumption. No change (increase or decrease) was seen in aortic diameter progression compared to control patients. In a previous NIH-funded randomized trial, AAA growth rate was not impacted by exercise. The studies of exercise therapy are important in reassuring AAA patients that, when approached with usual caution of all elderly patients with cardiovascular disease, they may safely perform aerobic exercise and achieve benefit without increased risk of cardiac events or AAA rupture.

Considerations for Evaluating Medical Therapies

There are three important features of AAA that lend themselves to prolonged medical treatment. Ultrasound evaluation provides a low-cost, safe, and accurate method for detection and serial surveillance imaging [35]. Patients with AAA have, on average, a life expectancy equal to the average population and opportunity for lifestyle modification and long periods of surveillance prior to intervention. With USPSTF recommendations, adult males with a history of smoking over the age of 65 should have at least one aortic ultrasound to evaluate for the presence of an AAA [36]. Increased public awareness and the ease of screening will continue to result in early AAA detection. In fact, 90% of aneurysms detected at screening are below the threshold for immediate repair resulting in a large population of patients who would benefit from long-term medical therapy [36]. AAA progression is relatively slow, therefore reducing the expansion rate of a 4.0 cm AAA by 50% potentially increases the time before surgical intervention is required to greater than 10 years, exceeding the life expectancy of many aneurysm patients. The current standard of care for small AAAs is "watchful waiting" after lifestyle modification including smoking cessation and blood pressure management is achieved. The provision of a relatively benign and efficacious medical therapy to these patients may reverse the diminished quality of life associated with detection of a potentially life-threatening condition for which no immediate treatment is offered.

Summary of Recommendations

1. Blood pressure should be controlled in accordance with ATPIII guidelines. There is no evidence that one class of antihypertensive medications is superior in slowing AAA growth. Selection of medication should be based on achieving blood pressure targets taking into account cogent patient factors such as demographics and comorbidities.
2. Statin therapy should be initiated in all patients with AAA and continued following any repair.
3. Low-dose aspirin should not be initiated routinely for the small AAA under surveillance. Unless bleeding risk is considered excessive, it should be started and continued after AAA intervention.
4. At each visit, patients with AAA should be educated regarding the increased rate of growth and rupture associated with smoking. All active smokers should be made aware of resources and programs available. Temporary nicotine replacement therapy is safe and can increase rates of quitting.
5. Anticoagulation has no primary role during surveillance or after treatment of AAA and is associated with worse long-term outcomes.
6. Patients should be educated regarding the safety and potential cardiovascular benefit of aerobic activity.

References

1. Sakalihasan N, Limet R, Defawe OD. Abdominal aortic aneurysm. Lancet. 2005;365:1577–89.
2. Takagi H, Umemoto T. A meta-analysis of the association of chronic obstructive pulmonary disease with abdominal aortic aneurysm presence. Ann Vasc Surg. 2016;34:84–94
3. Takagi H, Umemoto T. Association of chronic obstructive pulmonary, coronary artery, or peripheral artery disease with abdominal aortic aneurysm rupture. Int Angiol. 2017;36:322–31.
4. Aune D, Schlesinger S, Norat T, Riboli E. Tobacco smoking and the risk of abdominal aortic aneurysm: a systematic review and meta-analysis of prospective studies. Sci Rep. 2018;8:14786.
5. Wu AD, Lindson N, Hartmann-Boyce J, et al. Smoking cessation for secondary prevention of cardiovascular disease. Cochrane Database Syst Rev. 2022;8:Cd014936.
6. Sweeting MJ, Thompson SG, Brown LC, Powell JT. Meta-analysis of individual patient data to examine factors affecting growth and rupture of small abdominal aortic aneurysms. Br J Surg. 2012;99:655–65.
7. Lindson N, Klemperer E, Hong B, Ordóñez-Mena JM, Aveyard P. Smoking reduction interventions for smoking cessation. Cochrane Database Syst Rev. 2019;9:Cd013183.
8. Kalkhoran S, Glantz SA. E-cigarettes and smoking cessation in real-world and clinical settings: a systematic review and meta-analysis. Lancet Respir Med. 2016;4:116–28.

9. Lancaster T, Stead LF. Individual behavioural counselling for smoking cessation. Cochrane Database Syst Rev. 2017;3:Cd001292.
10. Wang RJ, Bhadriraju S, Glantz SA. E-cigarette use and adult cigarette smoking cessation: a meta-analysis. Am J Public Health. 2021;111:230–46.
11. Koegelenberg CF, Noor F, Bateman ED, et al. Efficacy of varenicline combined with nicotine replacement therapy vs varenicline alone for smoking cessation: a randomized clinical trial. JAMA. 2014;312:155–61.
12. FDA. FDA updates and press announcements on nitrosamine in varenicline (Chantix). 2022.
13. Chaiton M, Diemert L, Cohen JE, et al. Estimating the number of quit attempts it takes to quit smoking successfully in a longitudinal cohort of smokers. BMJ Open. 2016;6:e011045.
14. Wong KHF, Zlatanovic P, Bosanquet DC, et al. Antithrombotic therapy for aortic aneurysms: a systematic review and meta-analysis. Eur J Vasc Endovasc Surg. 2022;64:544–56.
15. Wanhainen A, Mani K, Kullberg J, et al. The effect of ticagrelor on growth of small abdominal aortic aneurysms—a randomized controlled trial. Cardiovasc Res. 2020;116:450–6.
16. Davidson KW, Barry MJ, Mangione CM, et al. Aspirin use to prevent cardiovascular disease: US preventive services task force recommendation statement. JAMA. 2022;327:1577–84.
17. Kobeissi E, Hibino M, Pan H, Aune D. Blood pressure, hypertension and the risk of abdominal aortic aneurysms: a systematic review and meta-analysis of cohort studies. Eur J Epidemiol. 2019;34:547–55.
18. Takagi H, Umemoto T. Association of hypertension with abdominal aortic aneurysm expansion. Ann Vasc Surg. 2017;39:74–89.
19. Su Z, Guo J, Gu Y. Pharmacotherapy in clinical trials for abdominal aortic aneurysms: a systematic review and meta-analysis. Clin Appl Thromb Hemost. 2022;28:10760296221120423.
20. Lindholt JS, Henneberg EW, Juul S, Fasting H. Impaired results of a randomised double blinded clinical trial of propranolol versus placebo on the expansion rate of small abdominal aortic aneurysms. Int Angiol. 1999;18:52–7.
21. Investigators TPAT. Propranolol for small abdominal aortic aneurysms: results of a randomized trial. J Vasc Surg. 2002;35:72–9.
22. Bicknell CD, Kiru G, Falaschetti E, Powell JT, Poulter NR. An evaluation of the effect of an angiotensin-converting enzyme inhibitor on the growth rate of small abdominal aortic aneurysms: a randomized placebo-controlled trial (AARDVARK). Eur Heart J. 2016;37:3213–21.
23. Golledge J, Singh TP. Effect of blood pressure lowering drugs and antibiotics on abdominal aortic aneurysm growth: a systematic review and meta-analysis. Heart. 2021;107:1465–71.
24. Golledge J, Moxon JV, Singh TP, Bown MJ, Mani K, Wanhainen A. Lack of an effective drug therapy for abdominal aortic aneurysm. J Intern Med. 2020;288:6–22.
25. Salata K, Syed M, Hussain MA, et al. Statins reduce abdominal aortic aneurysm growth, rupture, and perioperative mortality: a systematic review and meta-analysis. J Am Heart Assoc. 2018;7:e008657.
26. Pan Z, Cui H, Wu N, Zhang H. Effect of statin therapy on abdominal aortic aneurysm growth rate and mortality: a systematic review and meta-analysis. Ann Vasc Surg. 2020;67:503–10.
27. Xiong X, Wu Z, Qin X, et al. Meta-analysis suggests statins reduce mortality after abdominal aortic aneurysm repair. J Vasc Surg. 2022;75:356–362.e4.
28. Cheng W, Jia X, Li J, et al. Relationships of statin therapy and hyperlipidemia with the incidence, rupture, postrepair mortality, and all-cause mortality of abdominal aortic aneurysm and cerebral aneurysm: a meta-analysis and systematic review. J Cardiovasc Pharmacol. 2019;73:232–40.
29. Unosson J, Wågsäter D, Bjarnegård N, et al. Metformin prescription associated with reduced abdominal aortic aneurysm growth rate and reduced chemokine expression in a Swedish cohort. Ann Vasc Surg. 2021;70:425–33.
30. Wanhainen A, Unosson J, Mani K, Gottsäter A. The metformin for abdominal aortic aneurysm growth inhibition (MAAAGI) trial. Eur J Vasc Endovasc Surg. 2021;61:710–1.
31. Lindholt JS, Ashton HA, Scott RA. Indicators of infection with *Chlamydia pneumoniae* are associated with expansion of abdominal aortic aneurysms. J Vasc Surg. 2001;34:212–5.

32. Baxter BT, Matsumura J, Curci JA, et al. Effect of doxycycline on aneurysm growth among patients with small infrarenal abdominal aortic aneurysms: a randomized clinical trial. JAMA. 2020;323:2029–38.
33. Kato M, Kubo A, Green FN, Takagi H. Meta-analysis of randomized controlled trials on safety and efficacy of exercise training in patients with abdominal aortic aneurysm. J Vasc Surg. 2019;69:933–43.
34. Myers J, McElrath M, Jaffe A, et al. A randomized trial of exercise training in abdominal aortic aneurysm disease. Med Sci Sports Exerc. 2014;46:2–9.
35. Zucker EJ, Prabhakar AM. Abdominal aortic aneurysm screening: concepts and controversies. Cardiovasc Diagn Ther. 2018;8:S108–17.
36. Guirguis-Blake JM, Beil TL, Senger CA, Coppola EL. U.S. Preventive Services Task Force Evidence Syntheses, formerly Systematic Evidence Reviews. Primary care screening for abdominal aortic aneurysm: a systematic evidence review for the US Preventive Services Task Force. Rockville: Agency for Healthcare Research and Quality (US); 2019.
37. Rughani G, Robertson L, Clarke M. Medical treatment for small abdominal aortic aneurysms. Cochrane Database Syst Rev. 2012;2012(9):Cd009536.
38. Niu W, Shao J, Yu B, et al. Association between metformin and abdominal aortic aneurysm: a meta-analysis. Front Cardiovasc Med. 2022;9:908747.

Chapter 5
Surgery for Aortic Root Aneurysm

Lee M. Fuentes and George J. Arnaoutakis

Introduction

Structure and Function of the Aortic Root

The aortic root is the anatomic segment between the aortic annulus and the ascending aorta. The aortic root contains several elements: the aortic annulus, interleaflet triangles, sinuses of Valsalva, aortic cusps, and the sinotubular junction (Fig. 5.1) [2]. The aortic annulus attaches the aortic root to the left ventricle. Three interleaflet triangles are the "ventricular facing" extensions of the left ventricular outflow tract, named for their relation to the coronary arteries. Specifically, the noncoronary interleaflet triangle extends from the intervalvular fibrous body and the membranous septum. The right and left interleaflet triangles extend from the muscular interventricular septum. The sinuses of Valsalva are the "aortic facing" spaces bounded between the aortic cusps and the aortic wall. The right and left sinuses give rise to the respective coronary arteries. Three aortic cusps form the standard trileaflet aortic valve. The cusps have two edges, the base and free margin. The base anchors the cusps to the aortic root at the aortic annulus in a crescent shape. The free margins of the three cusps form the unidirectional valve mechanism through their coaptation. The junction of the free margins and the base form the aortic valve commissures. The sinotubular junction is the ridge of the aorta delineated by an imaginary circumferential line connecting the top of each of the aortic valve commissures (Figs. 5.2 and 5.3) [6].

Aortic valve function is dependent on a dynamic aortic root. The interrelated dimensions and geometry of the annulus, cusps, sinuses, and sinotubular junction

L. M. Fuentes · G. J. Arnaoutakis (✉)
Division of Cardiovascular and Thoracic Surgery, Department of Cardiovascular and Thoracic Surgery, University of Texas at Austin Dell Medical School, Austin, TX, USA
e-mail: george.arnaoutakis@austin.utexas.edu

G. J. Arnaoutakis et al. (eds.), *Aortic Aneurysms*, Contemporary Cardiology,
https://doi.org/10.1007/978-3-032-13134-8_5

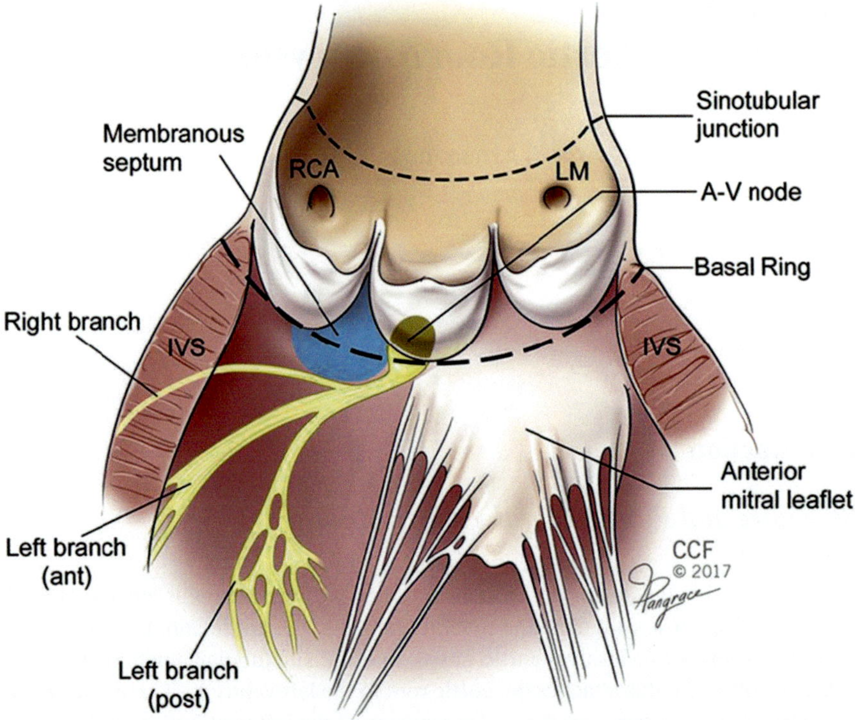

Fig. 5.1 Illustration of the aortic root displaying the sub-commissural triangles, aorto-ventricular junction, aortic cusps, aortic sinuses, coronary artery orifices, and sinotubular junction. Additionally, the relation of the AV node, membranous septum, and anterior mitral leaflet to the aortic root is depicted [1]

provide this dynamic nature. These relationships explain the form and function of the aortic root [7]. Proper coaptation of the aortic cusps is possible only if the sinotubular junction diameter is about 10–20% smaller than the aortic annulus diameter. This relationship renders the free margin length of the three aortic cusps to be about 1.5 times the diameter of the sinotubular junction. This size discrepancy allows the cusps to have sufficient coaptation to form a functional aortic valve [8]. The unique shape of the sinuses of Valsalva helps close the aortic cusps during diastole by inducing vortices and prevents occlusion of the coronary arteries during systole [9, 10]. To minimize stress on the aortic cusps, the root expands and contracts its diameter during the cardiac cycle by 16% [11]. As imaging modalities advance, computed tomography and magnetic resonance imaging demonstrate how the aortic root planar shape is not circular but ovoid and dynamically varies throughout the cardiac cycle [12, 13]. Pathologic disturbances of any of these relationships within the aortic root will eventually lead to valvular dysfunction and potentially adverse aortic events.

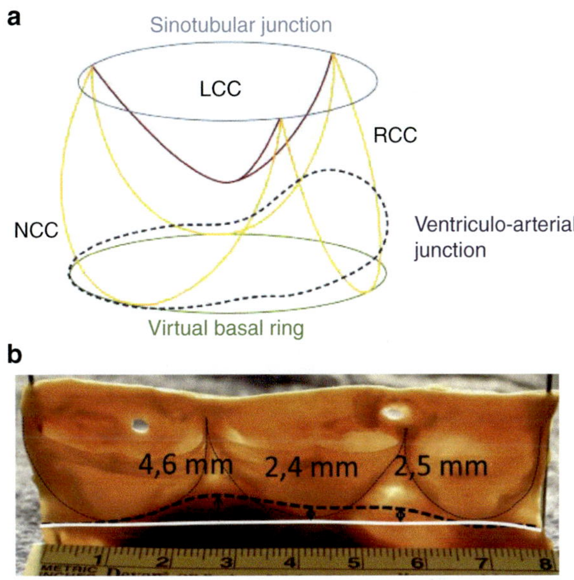

Fig. 5.2 Aortic root diagram. (**a**) Schematic of aortic root and the relationship between the virtual basal ring and the non-planar ventriculo-arterial junction [3]. (**b**) Longitudinal depiction of the aortic root with the white line depicting the virtual basal ring, located at the hinge points of the aortic cusps, and the non-planar ventriculo-arterial junction [4]

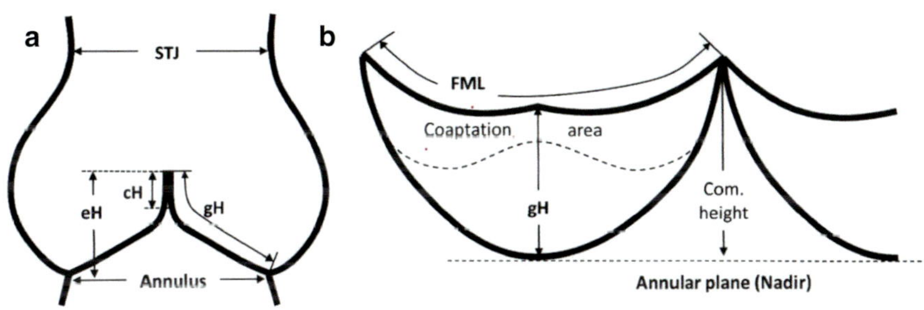

Fig. 5.3 (**a**) Profile of the aortic root. STJ sinotubular junction, GH geometric height of the cusp, eH effective height of the cusp, cH coaptation height of the cusp. (**b**) Diagram of the aortic cusp and pertinent measurements. *FML* free margin length, *gH* geometric height [5]

Epidemiology and Pathophysiology

Ascending aorta and root dilation is defined as a diameter ≥4.0 cm, and aneurysm is defined as ≥4.5 cm (Fig. 5.4). This is a departure from the usual definition of an aneurysm being 1.5× larger than a normal diameter employed throughout the rest of the aorta. The incidence of thoracic aortic aneurysms varies from 5.3 to 16.3 per 100,000 per year with 45.5% involving the ascending aorta and root [14, 15]. As the ascending aorta and root increase in size, the risk of dissection, rupture, and aortic valve insufficiency increases. Incidences of thoracic aortic dissection and rupture are 2.9–4.3 and 1.6 per 100,000 per year, respectively [14, 16].

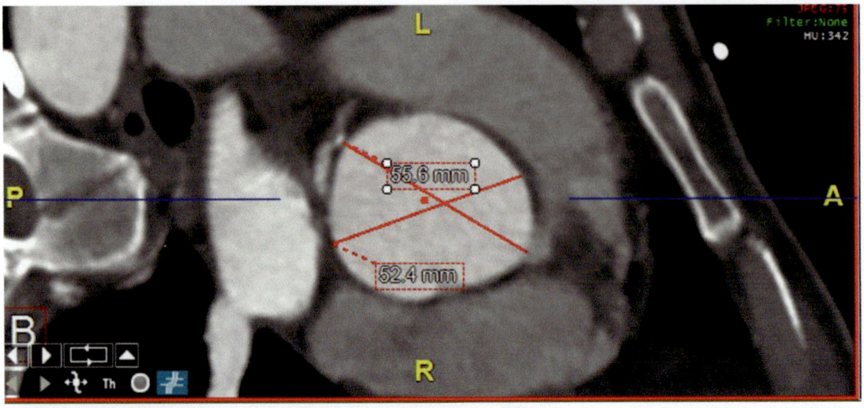

Fig. 5.4 Axial imaging of the aortic root demonstrating the non-uniform planar geometry and measurements of 55.6 mm and 52.4 mm, meeting criteria for an aortic root aneurysm. (Used with permission from Dr. George J. Arnaoutakis)

As the aortic root dilates, the dynamic relationships of its elements are disrupted. Aortic root dilation increases the sinotubular junction diameter. This alters the ability of the aortic cusps to coapt causing valvular insufficiency. The causes of aortic root dilatation are categorized as degenerative, heritable, congenital, inflammatory, and infectious etiologies. It is important to keep the embryologic origins of the aortic root, ascending aorta, aortic arch, and descending aorta in mind, as their different origins impact their predilection for pathologies and natural progression. The aortic root is derived from the second heart field or lateral plate mesoderm, the ascending aorta and arch from neural crest cells, and the descending aorta from paraxial mesoderm. Each of these origins produces different smooth muscle cells leading to different mechanical properties, suggesting regional discrepancies at their junctions (Fig. 5.5) [17, 18].

Degenerative Etiologies

The aortic wall has three layers (Fig. 5.6): intima, media, and adventitia. The intima is a layer of endothelium and connective tissue. The media contains about 50 layers of smooth muscle cells, elastic fibers, collagen, and structural proteins. The adventitia is composed of connective tissue, fibroblasts, nerves, and vasa vasorum [19]. Cystic medial necrosis results in the degradation of elastic fibers and smooth muscle cells within the aortic media, leading to the formation of a weakened aortic wall that is susceptible to aneurysmal dilatation. Risk factors include age, hypertension, hyperlipidemia, and smoking.

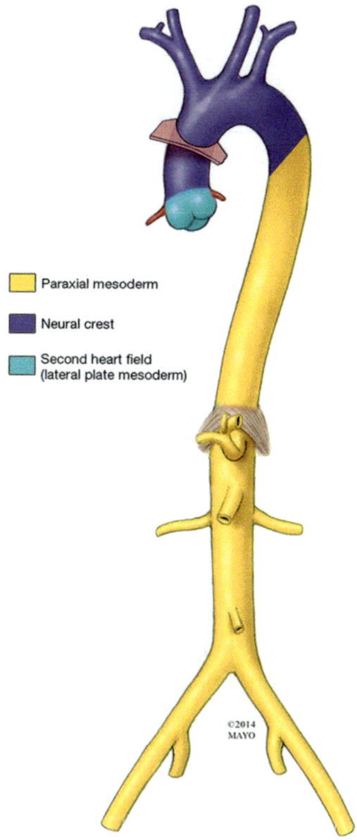

Fig. 5.5 Aortic schematic diagram. Regional differences in aortic pathology are probably explained, at least in part, by the varying embryologic origins. The aortic root is derived primarily from the second heart field (lateral plate mesoderm), whereas the ascending aorta and arch are of neural crest derivation. The remaining aorta is derived from the paraxial mesoderm [17]

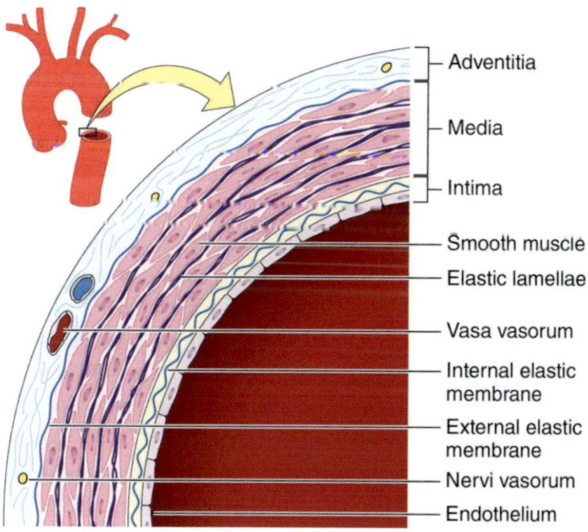

Fig. 5.6 The medial layer in human aortas contains >50 alternating layers of elastin and smooth muscle cells (whereas only 5 are shown in this simplified illustration). (Adapted (cropped) from "Illustration of tunics of the arteries vs veins" by Malgosia Wilk-Blaszczak, used under CC-BY 4.0. "Illustration of tunics of the arteries vs veins" is adapted (cropped) from fig. 20.3 in BC OpenStax Anatomy and Physiology used under CC-BY 4.0)

Heritable Etiologies

In contrast to the descending aorta, ascending aortopathies typically present at younger ages due to heritable associations [20]. These pathologies can present as either syndromic or non-syndromic. Syndromic presentations are associated with the extra-aortic manifestations of Marfan, Loeys-Dietz, and vascular Ehlers-Danlos phenotypes. Non-syndromic presentations are limited to the aorta and identified via family history and genetic testing. The cardiovascular presentation of Marfan syndrome (MFS) is associated with mitral valve prolapse and aortic root dilation. Excessive TGF-β activation and abnormal fibrillin production cause this abnormality [21]. The estimated prevalence of MFS is 1 in 5000 individuals. Loeys-Dietz syndrome (LDS) results from a mutation in TGF-β receptors. The presentation can range from a phenotype similar to Marfan syndrome to childhood aortic dissection or rupture [22]. The prevalence of LDS cannot be estimated. Vascular Ehlers-Danlos syndrome (vEDS) results from a mutation in *COL3A1* causing abnormal type III collagen synthesis. The abnormal collagen causes cardiovascular manifestations such as aortic root dilation and large-to-medium caliber arterial spontaneous rupture [23]. The prevalence of vEDS is between 1 in 50,000 and 1 in 200,000 individuals.

Heritable thoracic aortic disease (HTAD) represents the non-syndromic, autosomal dominant single gene disorders, currently comprised of 11 genes. These genes are identified to encode extracellular matrix proteins, TGF-β signaling, and smooth muscle cell contraction. All these genes significantly increase the patient's risk for aortic dissection and rupture [24]

Congenital Etiologies

Several congenital anomalies are associated with thoracic aortic aneurysm (TAA) with bicuspid aortic valve (BAV) being the most common. Other congenital heart defects that are associated with (TAA) include: Turner syndrome, aortic coarctation, tetralogy of Fallot, transposition of the great arteries, and truncus arteriosus. The abnormal flow through the bicuspid valve causes shear stresses that can lead to asymmetric aneurysmal dilatation. BAV occurs in 1–2% of the population, with a 4:1 female preponderance, making BAV aortopathy a common consultation for the modern surgeon. Michelena et al. described the modern consensus of the types and phenotypes of the BAV by adding imaging, surgical pathology, and clinical associations to the traditional Sievers classifications [25]. This classification describes the spectrum of phenotypes that are encountered. The most common of these phenotypes is the fused BAV, occurring in 90–95% of these patients. The surgical significance rests in the commissural angles of the non-fused cusp, ranging 180° to <130° because this impacts surgical repair techniques, which will be detailed in section "Surgical techniques for aortic root aneurysm". 20–30% of aortic dilation and aneurysms associated with BAV involve root or root with ascending phenotypes [26].

Inflammatory Etiologies

Aortitis is most associated with giant cell arteritis (GCA) and Takayasu arteritis (TA). GCA is a poorly understood pathology but leads to transmural panarteritis and adventitial perivasculitis. Aortic aneurysm and dissection can develop in up to 30% of GCA patients.

TA is not commonly diagnosed in the United States with an incidence of 2–3 per 1,000,000 per year. While usually diagnosed in women, men with this diagnosis have a higher frequency of aortic involvement. Between 5 and 55% of patients with aortic symptoms can present with aortic root dilation and subsequent aortic insufficiency. TA is also characterized with panarteritis, with the following differences when compared to GCA. TA is diagnosed in younger patients (20–30 s) compared to GCA (60–70 s). TA has a greater aortic wall thickness. TA has more severe adventitial scarring. GCA has more severe intimal inflammation. TA is associated with granulomas. Finally, GCA has a more varied "extra-vascular" phenotype, while all TA patients have large vessel pathology [27].

Infectious Etiologies

Syphilitic aortitis was the most common cause of infectious aortic aneurysm. Since the introduction of antibiotics as standard treatment, this has significantly decreased its prevalence to mainly historical note. The spirochete infiltrates the vasa vasorum of the aorta leading to adventitial fibrosis, initial atherosclerosis, and destruction of the medial elastic fibers. The relative increased density of vasa vasorum in the aortic arch explains this location of most syphilitic aortic aneurysms [28]. The aortic root and coronaries are also at risk of aneurysmal dilation [29].

Clinical Features and Diagnosis

95% of TAAs are asymptomatic until an acute event, making TAA silent and lethal [30]. Aortic root aneurysms are associated with signs and symptoms of aortic insufficiency and syndromic features of heritable pathologies. The chief complaint of patients with aortic insufficiency includes shortness of breath, cough, dyspnea on exertion, and chest pain. Transthoracic echocardiography (TTE), transesophageal echocardiography (TEE), computed tomography (CT), and magnetic resonance imaging (MRI) are all imaging modalities to diagnose aortic root aneurysms and their etiology. Selection of each modality should be based on the acuity of presentation, patient factors, and facility availability. TEE is best in detailing the cusp morphology, number of cusps, appearance of the free margins, coaptation, and presence of prolapse. CT and MRI are best for determining aortic root measurements. Dimensions taken from CT and MRI can correlate with TEE measurements [31].

Once a diagnosis of aortic root aneurysm is made, all patients with syndromic features, family history of TAA, or if less than 60 years of age should be counseled regarding genetic testing. The revised Ghent criteria for Marfan syndrome plus genetic testing help identify patients and at-risk family members for aortic root aneurysms. HTAD, MFS, LDS, and vEDS are all autosomal dominant hereditary disorders, with 50% of their offspring inheriting their condition. Some features classically associated with MFS are ectopia lentis, pectus carinatum, increased height, pes planus, and reduced upper segment to lower segment ratio [32]. LDS has similar features to MFS with the notable additions of hypertelorism, bifid uvula, and generalized arterial tortuosity [8]. vEDS has mainly cutaneous features of easy bruising, translucent skin, impaired wound healing, and hair loss [33].

Classification and Indications for Surgery

Compared to the normal ascending aorta, there are three types of aneurysmal dilatation: supracoronary, Marfanoid, and tubular [34]. Current indications recommend surgery for symptomatic and acute syndromes of the aortic root. For asymptomatic aortic root surgery, recommendations consider anatomy and etiology: tricuspid aortic valve, bicuspid aortic valve, and heritable. Table 5.1 is compiled from all current recommendations from the STS, EACTS, ACC, and AHA [19, 35]. In summary, the tricuspid aortic root should be replaced once greater than 55 mm. If the patient is low risk, then 50 mm is acceptable. For bicuspid aortic root aneurysms, the root should be replaced once greater than 50 mm. For both tricuspid and bicuspid aortic root aneurysms, the root can be replaced once greater than 45 mm if doing concomitant aortic valve surgery. Heritable aortic root aneurysms, recommendations are genetic and phenotype specific, should be replaced between 40 and 50 mm. While this review focuses on aortic root aneurysms, supracoronary aneurysms often have sinus of Valsalva dilation and introduce the question of whether to address a dilated aortic root.

Surgical Techniques for Aortic Root Aneurysm

Valve-Sparing Aortic Root Replacement

When aortic root aneurysmal disease has suitable aortic cusp tissue, a valve-sparing operation can be employed. Several methods have been developed since the 1980s, each with strengths and weaknesses.

Table 5.1 Recommended aortic root sizes for intervention based on STS/EACTS/ACC/AHA guidelines [19, 35]

Diagnosis	Indications for aortic root surgery	Class of recommendation
Tricuspid	≥55 mm ≥50 mm in low-risk patients ≥45 mm when undergoing aortic valve surgery	I–IIa
Bicuspid	≥50 mm ≥45 mm when undergoing aortic valve surgery	I–IIa
Heritable		
Marfan	≥50 mm ≥45 mm if high-risk features[a] ≥45 mm if no high-risk features + valve-sparing operation + low surgical risk	I–IIb
Loeys-Dietz	≥45 mm if TGFBR1/2 variant ≥40 mm if TGFBR1 + high-risk features[a] ≥40 mm if TGFBR2 + high-risk features[b] ≥50 mm if TGFBR3 ≥45 mm if SMAD3 ≥45 mm if TGFB2 or SMAD2	I–IIb
HTAD	≥45 mm if ACTA2 ≥42 mm if ACTA2 + high-risk features[c] ≥42 mm if PRKG1 ≥40 mm if PRKG1 + high-risk features[c] ≥45 mm if MYLK or MYH11	IIa–IIb

[a]Family history of aortic dissection; aortic growth >0.3 cm/year; diffuse aortic root and ascending aortic dilation, marked vertebral arterial tortuosity
[b]Certain specific pathogenic variants (R528H/C in TGFBR2); women with TGFBR2 and small body size; severe extra-aortic features (i.e., craniosynostosis, cleft palate, hypertelorism, bifid uvula, marked arterial tortuosity, widened scars, and translucent skin); family history of aortic dissection, especially at young age or aortic diameter <4.5 cm; aortic growth rate > 0.3 cm/year
[c]Family history of type A aortic dissection in the setting of no or minimal aortic dilation, aortic growth rate > 0.3 cm/year

Remodeling (Yacoub)

In 1992, Sir Magdi Yacoub published his experience with a novel technique for replacing the aortic root while preserving the aortic valve. The aorta is divided above the sinotubular junction. The aortic root is mobilized to the surgical aortic annulus. The aortic commissures are suspended. Coronary buttons are harvested with 3 mm cuffs. The sinuses of Valsalva are excised, leaving the aortic valve with 3–5 mm of surrounding aortic wall above the aortic annulus. Careful measurements of the aortic annulus are taken to make a calculation for the graft. The goal of the graft selection is to achieve a ratio of 0.9:1 sinotubular junction to annulus. The graft is cut at three points to fit the commissures, making the graft between the cuts the neo-sinuses (Fig. 5.7). The suspended aortic commissures are pulled inside the graft and attached to the apices of the previously made 3 cuts. A 3-0 or 4-0 polypropylene suture is then used to attach the neo-sinuses to the residual aortic wall. Openings are

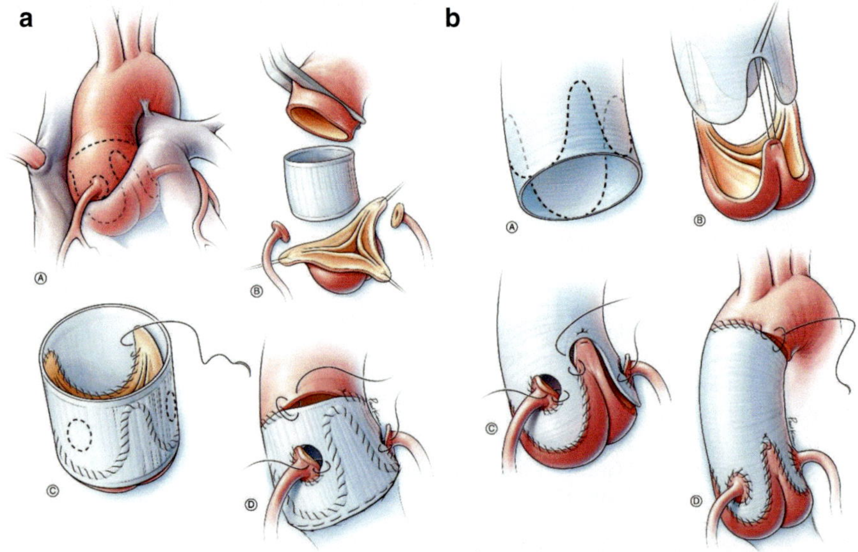

Fig. 5.7 Diagram of remodeling technique during the tailoring of the Dacron graft to create the neo-sinuses during this valve-sparing aortic root replacement [36]

created for the coronary buttons and attached with 5-0 polypropylene suture into the neo-sinuses. An end-to-end anastomosis of the graft to the distal aorta completes this technique [8, 36–38].

A benefit of the remodeling technique is restoration of the native aortic root shape by recreating the aortic sinuses allowing for conditions to closely mimic the native aortic root [39]. A critique of the remodeling technique was progressive aortic annular dilatation resulting in subsequent aortic insufficiency [40]. To combat this, ring and suture annuloplasties were added to the original remodeling procedure. Long-term outcomes are still pending [41].

Reimplantation (David)

In 1992, Dr. Tirone David published his experience with reimplantation of the aortic valve during aortic root replacement. The aorta is divided above the sinotubular junction. The aortic root is dissected to a few millimeters below the aortic annulus. Care is taken around the non-coronary cusp because the right atrial wall is adjacent. Extensive dissection is required because this is where the graft will sit. The aortic commissures are suspended with 4-0 or 5-0 polypropylene suture. Coronary buttons are harvested with 3mm cuffs. The sinuses of Valsava are excised, leaving 3–5 mm of surrounding aortic wall above the aortic annulus. Horizontal mattress sutures are placed below the aortic annulus for sub-annular stabilization and reduction annuloplasty using 2-0 or 3-0 polyester suture. Depending on the patient's anatomy, we prefer six to nine circumferential sutures to be placed. Care is taken to avoid the conduction system when placing these sutures near the membranous septum. There are various techniques to select graft size which are beyond the scope of this chapter, but a 32 mm or 34 mm Valsalva graft is usually selected in men and 32 mm or 30 mm is usually used in women. The commissure posts are pulled up into the graft and resuspended at the level of the sinotubular junction. A continuous hemostatic 3-0 or 4-0 polypropylene suture is used to attach the graft to the remnant cuff of the aortic wall. The aortic valve is tested with static saline. The coronary buttons are reimplanted into the graft. The graft is anastomosed to the distal aorta, completing this reconstruction (Figs. 5.8 and 5.9) [8, 36, 38, 41, 43]. The reimplantation technique has the benefit of more than two decades of experience and durability data with greater than 90% freedom from reintervention at 15–20 years in expert hands [44].

Florida Sleeve

To simplify the aortic root reconstruction another novel valve-sparing technique was developed known as the Florida Sleeve [45]. The aortic root is circumferentially dissected to the level of the aortic annulus, including subcoronary artery dissection. Next, care is taken to ensure an annulus measuring between 21 and 26 mm. Valsalva graft sizing is then based on the sinus of Valsalva measurements. If >36 mm, a 32 or 34-mm graft is used. Once a graft is selected, 2-0 polyester horizontal mattress sub-annular sutures are placed a few millimeters below the aortic annulus. Taking observation of the location of the coronary arteries respective to the sinuses, two vertical slit openings with coronary keyholes are created. The horizontal mattress sutures are placed into the base of the graft, the graft is lowered over the root and coronaries, and the horizontal mattress sutures are tied over a Hegar dilator. Sutures are passed under the coronary arteries to close the previously made slits. A hemostatic suture line is then made between the graft and the sinotubular junction with a 4-0 polypropylene suture (Fig. 5.10) [8, 45].

Strengths of the Florida Sleeve include its simplified suture lines and potential reduction in cusp stress. By maintaining the sinuses of Valsalva, this technique avoids coronary reimplantation and the associated complications of coronary button aneurysm. Additionally, this maintains the natural base margin of the aortic cusp which allows for distribution of stress during the cardiac cycle when compared to reimplantation [47].

Valve Replacing Aortic Root Replacement

When operations for aortic root aneurysms cannot salvage the aortic valve, complete root and valve replacement with composite grafts is performed.

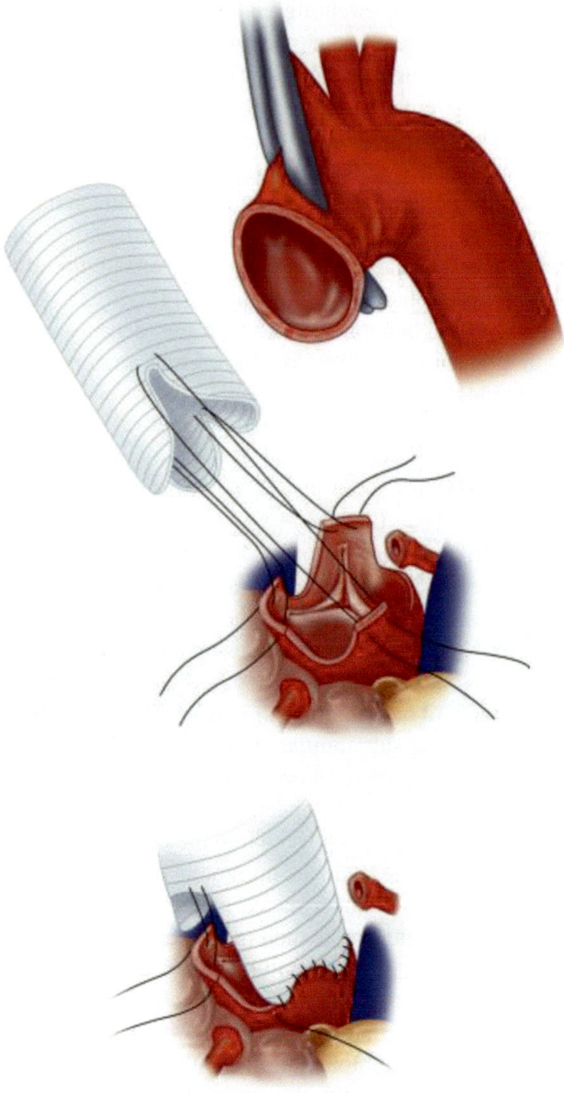

Fig. 5.8 Diagram of the completed reimplantation technique. The lower suture line representing the sub-annular annuloplasty. Coronary reimplantation is demonstration [36]

Composite Valve Graft (Bentall)

First described in 1968 by Bentall and De Bono, aortic root is prepared, and the aortic valve is excised. Coronary buttons with 3 mm cuffs are harvested. The remaining aortic sinuses and wall are circumferentially excised, leaving a 5–6 mm cuff of aortic wall. The aortic annulus is measured and appropriate composite graft, with biologic or mechanical valve, is selected. Circumferential 2-0 polyester sutures are passed from outside to inside on the aortic annulus when performing intra-annular replacement. The sutures are then placed through the graft. The sutures are tied once

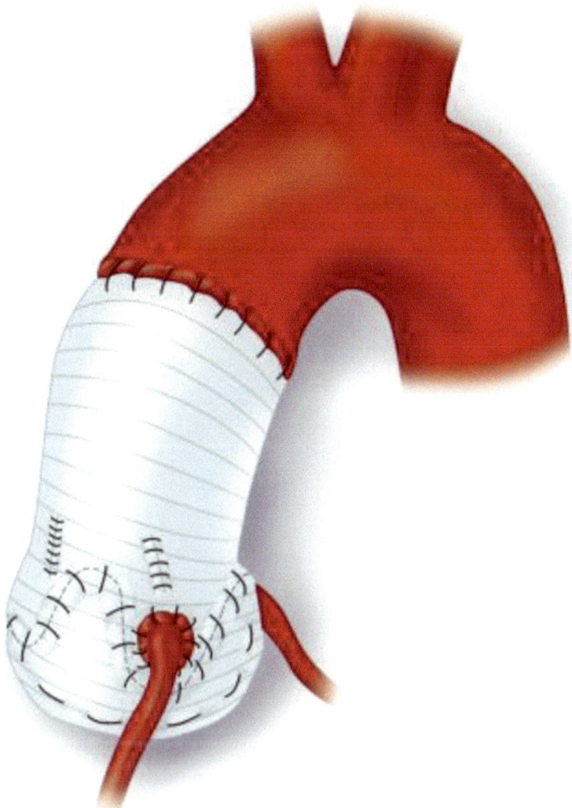

Fig. 5.9 Intraoperative depiction of the reimplantation operation during commissure resuspension. The sub-annular annuloplasty sutures are completed and depicted. The coronaries are suspended and not yet reimplanted. The sutures used to resuspend the commissures will be used to attach the remnant aortic root wall to the graft [42]

the valve is confirmed to be seated appropriately above the left ventricular outflow tract (Fig. 5.11). The coronary arteries are reimplanted using 5-0 polypropylene suture. The distal end-to-end anastomosis completes this reconstruction (Fig. 5.12) [8, 38, 49, 50].

Outcomes and Prognosis

Valve-Sparing Aortic Root Replacement Outcomes

With publication of valve-sparing root replacement (VSRR) techniques in the 1990s–2000s, these techniques were still being disseminated. Between 2004 and 2010, 13,743 aortic root replacements were performed, 1918 being VSRR and 11,825 being valved graft conduits. The trend for VSRR has increased over that period to between 15% and 17%. The concerning finding is that most centers perform ≤2 aortic root procedures per year with 5% of U.S. centers performing >16

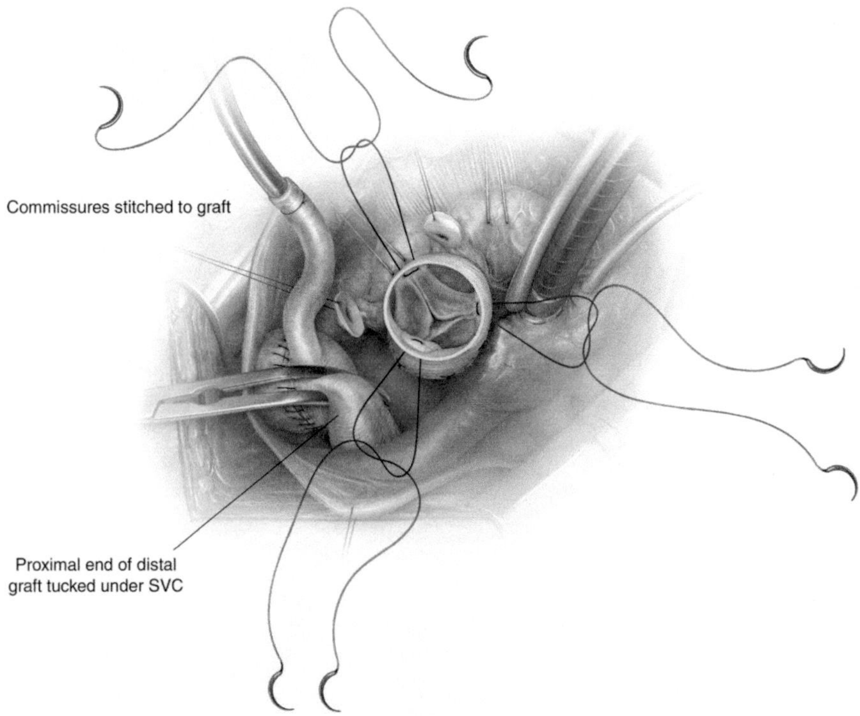

Fig. 5.10 Diagram of the Florida Sleeve technique. Note the spared sinuses that preclude coronary reimplantation as the graft fits over the coronary arteries via the previously constructed slit and keyhole incisions [46]

operations per year. However, the operative mortality for VSRR is 1.88% [51]. The technical nuances of these procedures can make generalizability difficult.

Remodeling

Schafers et al. conducted a meta-analysis for remodeling in the tricuspid aortic valve patient. The in-hospital and 30-day mortality rates ranged from 0% to 4.6%. The average 5-year survival was 93% and 86% at 10 years. Compared to Schafers et al.'s institutional findings of freedom from aortic insufficiency ≥2 at 10 years of 90% and at 15 years 77%, the pooled analysis showed a freedom of 53% to 87% at 5 years. Freedom from reoperation ranged from 84% to 96% at 10 years.

Schafers also detailed the 28-year experience of remodeling for non-tricuspid aortic valve patients and those with connective tissue disorder. 33 unicuspid, 472 bicuspid, and 684 tricuspid valve patients were included in the study. Bicuspid and unicuspid patients had less freedom from reoperation (84%) compared to tricuspid patients (94%). Patients with connective tissue disorder had similar freedom from reoperation at 15 years (97%) compared to those without (90%). Freedom from

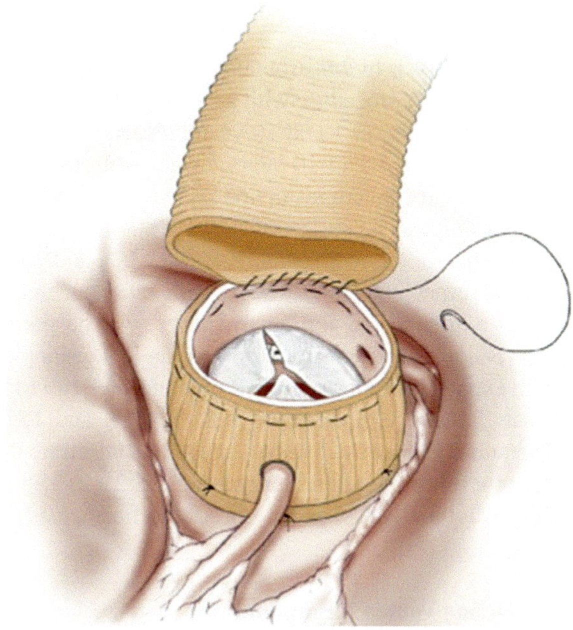

Fig. 5.11 Intraoperative photo during a Bio-Bentall operation. The aortic valve has been excised. The graft is being lowered onto the aortic annulus. The black silk sutures are retracting the coronary buttons that will be later reimplanted. (Used with permission from Dr. George J. Arnaoutakis [46])

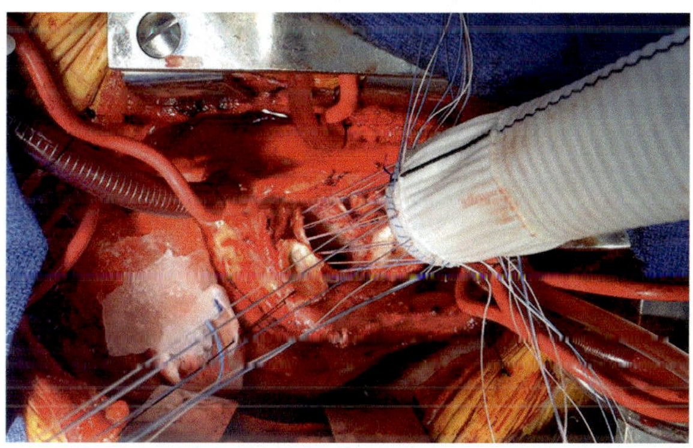

Fig. 5.12 The Bentall (composite valve graft) technique of valve replacing aortic root replacement [48]

recurrent aortic insufficiency ≥2 was lower for bicuspid and unicuspid patients at 10 years, 88% and 88% respectively, compared to tricuspid valve patients (90%). This is congruent with the Arnaoutakis et al. systematic review that showed a greater presence of ≥2 aortic insufficiency in remodeling for bicuspid aortic valve; however, this did not result in a greater need for reoperation [52].

Reimplantation

The meta-analysis by Mastrobuoni et al. included 7878 patients who had undergone a reimplantation procedure with an average follow-up of 4.8 years. Overall survival was 99% and 89% at 1 and 10 years, respectively. Freedom from reoperation was 99% and 91% at 1 and 10 years, respectively [53]. These findings are congruent with Dr. David's outcomes in 465 patients over 29 years with reoperation-free survival rates of 88.7%, 80.1%, and 69.1% at 10, 15, and 20 years respectively. Aortic insufficiency of ≥2 was found in 5.3%, 7.3%, and 10.2% of patients at 10, 15, and 20 years, respectively [44]. The reimplantation technique has comparable results for patients with bicuspid aortic valve. There was no statistically significant difference in survival and freedom from reoperation at 9 years [53].

Dr. David also reported VSRR outcomes for 149 Marfan patients, with 82.9% of patients having reimplantation. The 5-, 10-, and 15-year outcomes for survival, reoperation, and aortic insufficiency ≥2 demonstrate that reimplantation is a viable option for this population. Survival was 93.2% at 15 years, and freedom from reoperation was 95.1% at 15 years. Aortic insufficiency ≥2 was limited to 8% at 15 years.

Remodeling Versus Reimplantation

The Sá et al. meta-analysis examined 3044 patients who received either remodeling or reimplantation to examine 20 years of outcomes from 15 studies. The striking findings from this study were a significant difference in survival and aortic valve and/or aortic root reintervention with hazard ratios of 1.54 and 1.49, respectively, favoring reimplantation up to 4 years [54]. In regard to connective tissue disease patients, the difference between remodeling and reimplantation is less clear. The AVIATOR registry showed no difference in survival (92.3%), aortic insufficiency ≥2 (22.0%), and reintervention on the aortic valve (10.9%) at 10 years. Of note, remodeling without annuloplasty was associated with increased annulus size after 3 years, while reimplantation and remodeling with annuloplasty had similar diameters [55]. It is difficult to make conclusions from these large meta-analyses but with these techniques requiring highly technical surgeons, the ability to perform a randomized control trial is nearly impossible. When examining outcomes from leaders in the field, surgeon experience is a significant driver in the outcomes for VSRR patients. Centers with experienced surgeons and the means to follow these patients should continue to offer their preferred technique.

Florida Sleeve

The longer-term outcomes for the Florida Sleeve are promising. Aalaei-Andabili et al. report the 14-year outcomes from the Florida group. Survival was 93% at 8 years, with freedom from reoperation 98% at 8 years. There are not as many longer-term follow-up studies for the Florida Sleeve as compared to remodeling or reimplantation. Freedom from aortic insufficiency ≥2 was 93.6% at 5 years [56]. More data is needed before accurate conclusions can be made about the Florida Sleeve and patients with bicuspid aortic valves [57].

For Marfan patients, the Florida Sleeve is a viable option. Freedom from reoperation was 100% over 8 years. 1 out of 37 patients required a reoperation at year 9. There was 100% freedom from ≥2 aortic insufficiency at 5 years [46]. Of note, cusp repair was limited in this published series.

Valve Replacing Aortic Root Replacement Outcomes

Replacement of the aortic valve during root surgery is a durable and widely reproducible operation; however, aortic valve replacement introduces patients to inherent potential sequelae. In the United States from 2006 to 2010, 11,825 composite aortic root replacements (VRARR) were performed. Trends show a consistent use of mechanical valves with an increase in biological valves and a decrease in homograft usage [51]. The systematic review by Mookhoek et al. included 7629 patients over a 44-year period. Operative mortality was 5.6% without a decreasing trend. Survival was 79.8% at 10 years. Freedom from root reoperation was 95.4% at 10 years. The incidence of thromboembolism or bleeding was 14.1% at 10 years. Major adverse valve-related events had an incidence of 26.6% at 10 years [58].

Gott et al. describe their experience with VRARR for Marfan patients with excellent results. Operative mortality was 0.7% and only occurred in patients undergoing emergent or urgent operations. Survival was 89% and 67% at 5 and 20 years, respectively. Freedom from reoperation was 74% at 20 years. 5.6% of patients developed thromboembolic events due to inadequate therapeutic anticoagulation [59].

Future Directions in Surgical Management

Emerging Techniques and Innovations

Less invasive techniques are available to address aortic root aneurysms. Personalized external aortic root support (PEARS) was first published in 2004 to support the Marfan population [60]. A macroporous sleeve encapsulates the aortic root and ascending aorta with the attractive feature of not requiring to place the patient on cardiopulmonary bypass (Fig. 5.13). The premise behind this device is to restrict aortic dilatation thereby reducing risk of dissection or rupture. Early outcomes have shown that the largest change at 3 years has been a reduction in the root diameter [62]. While offering ease of placement, there have been no reported outcomes of dissection after implantation in these patients. Currently, the technique is slowly expanding as direct comparisons to VSRR or VRARR are difficult [61, 63].

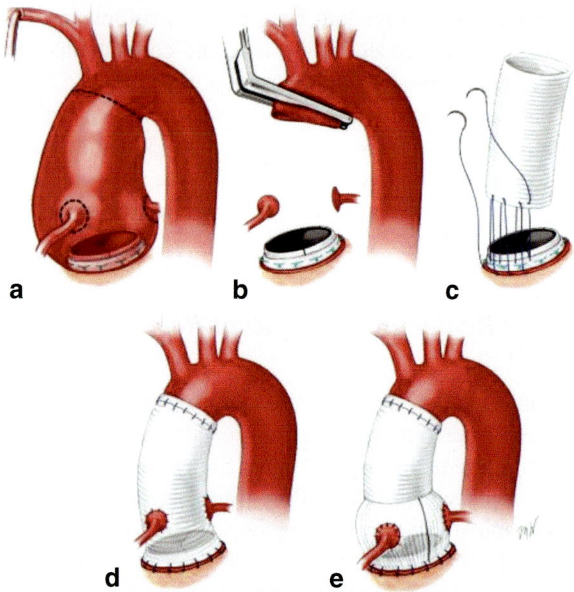

Fig. 5.13 The personalized external aortic root support (PEARS) is tailored to every patient's anatomy then wrapped around the aorta and secured to prevent further dilatation. The figure demonstrates how the PEARS device is secured around the coronaries through keyhole incisions and sutured in place [61]

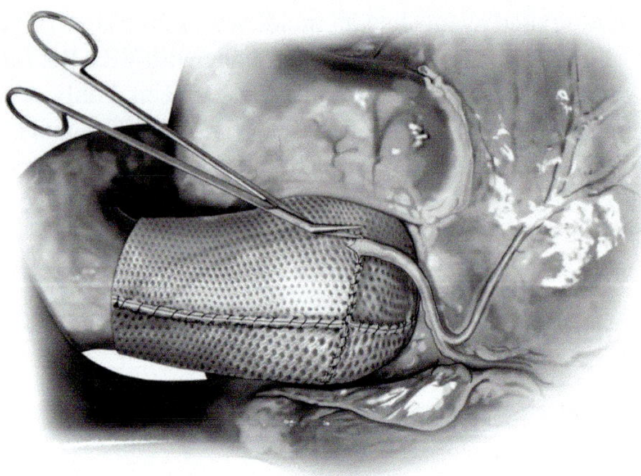

Fig. 5.14 Diagram showing a diagram for the "endo-bentall" demonstrating placement of the graft within the aortic root and coronary connecting stents to both the right and left coronary arteries [66]

The "endo-bentall" was described in 2020 as a compassionate use indication in patients where surgical risk was prohibitive [64]. While a viable solution for those unable to tolerate surgery, replacement of the dynamic aortic root under two-dimensional angiography is fraught with risk and needs further development until its use can be expanded [65]. The progress and modifications required to make such a feat possible are detailed in case series (Fig. 5.14) [66].

Research and Developments

VSRR has several areas of ongoing investigation. For example, it remains unknown how adding annuloplasty to remodeling impacts long-term outcomes. The central tenet of VSRR is to preserve the native aortic valve. To accomplish this, remodeling and reimplantation may require cusp repair techniques in upwards of 67% of patients. Adding any leaflet modification technique other than cusp plication significantly worsens long-term rates of recurrent aortic regurgitation [67]. In terms of fenestrations in the aortic cusps, David et al. report the "double layer suture" technique (Fig. 5.15) is associated with 4.8% aortic valve reoperation, 9.2% moderate/severe aortic insufficiency, and 5.1% thromboembolism rates at 15 years [68]. There is more to understand about the optimal implementation of VSRR in terms of managing cusp repair, especially in the setting of leaflet calcification or extensive fenestrations.

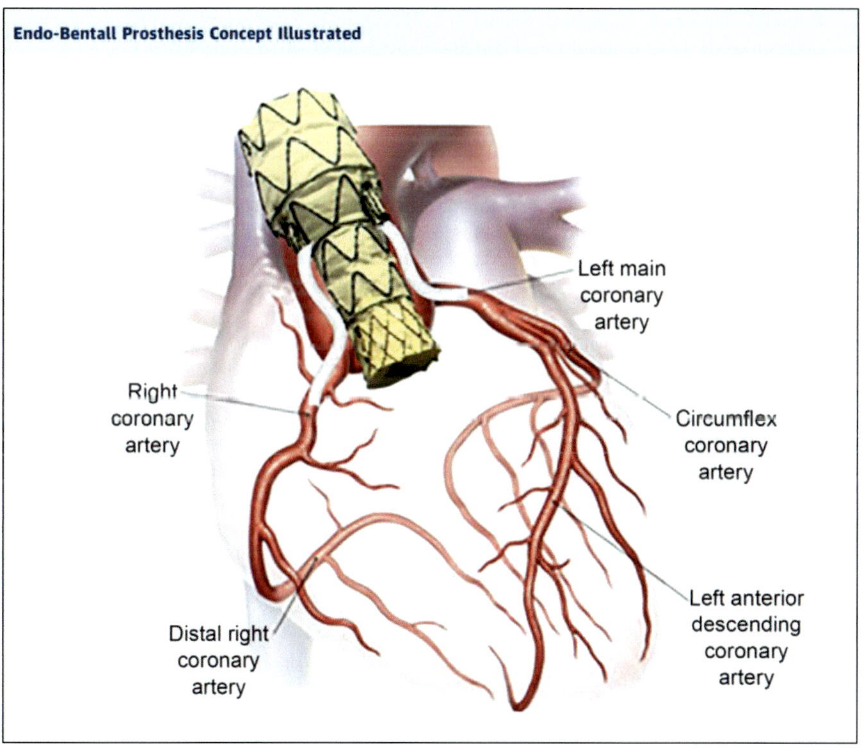

Fig. 5.15 The "double layer suture" technique described by Dr. David for repair of aortic cusp fenestrations. A fine Gore-Tex suture is weaved along the free margin of the cusp [68]

Conclusions

Aortic root aneurysms may pose significant consequences if not diagnosed and treated appropriately. Commonly associated with heritable disorders, patients with aortic root aneurysms should be counseled about genetic screening once diagnosed. Proper surgical planning relies on detailed imaging from TTE, TEE, CT, or MRI. Based on the presenting etiology, valve morphology, patient characteristics, and center experience, valve-sparing aortic root replacement techniques may be an attractive option. A composite root replacement, or modified Bentall operation, has been performed for many decades and remains a durable, excellent option in these patients. Valve-sparing operations, such as remodeling, reimplantation, and the Florida Sleeve, are technically nuanced operations that offer durable results. Newer technologies such as external aortic support and endovascular options are still in their infancy and not yet available for common application.

References

1. Hahn RT, Nicoara A, Kapadia S, Svensson L, Martin R. Echocardiographic imaging for transcatheter aortic valve replacement. J Am Soc Echocardiogr. 2018;31(4):405–33.
2. Sievers HH, Hemmer W, Beyersdorf F, Moritz A, Moosdorf R, Lichtenberg A, et al. The everyday used nomenclature of the aortic root components: the tower of Babel? Eur J Cardiothorac Surg. 2012;41(3):478–82.
3. Federspiel JM, Ehrlich T, Abeln K, Schäfers HJ. Aortic annuloplasty: subcommissural, intraannular suture techniques, external and internal rings. JTCVS Tech. 2021;7:98–102.
4. de Kerchove L, Jashari R, Boodhwani M, Duy KT, Lengelé B, Gianello P, et al. Surgical anatomy of the aortic root: implication for valve-sparing reimplantation and aortic valve annuloplasty. J Thorac Cardiovasc Surg. 2015;149(2):425–33.
5. Lansac E, de Kerchove L. Aortic valve repair techniques: state of the art. Eur J Cardiothorac Surg. 2018;53(6):1101–7.
6. Cook AC, Hlavacek AM, Backer CL, Spicer DE, Tretter JT, Anderson RH. Surgical anatomy of the valves of the heart. In: Wilcox's surgical anatomy of the heart. 5th ed. Cambridge: Cambridge University Press; 2024. p. 77–112.
7. Swanson WM, Clark RE. Dimensions and geometric relationships of the human aortic value as a function of pressure. Circ Res. 1974;35(6):871–82.
8. David TE. Chapter 70—surgery of the aortic root and ascending aorta. In: Sabiston and spencer surgery of the chest. 10th ed. Philadelphia: Elsevier Inc; 2024. p. 1291–312.
9. Bellhouse BJ, Bellhouse FH. Mechanism of closure of the aortic valve. Nature. 1968;217(5123):86–7.
10. Bissell MM, Dall'Armellina E, Choudhury RP. Flow vortices in the aortic root: in vivo 4D-MRI confirms predictions of Leonardo da Vinci. Eur Heart J. 2014;35(20):1344.
11. Brewer RJ, Deck JD, Capati B, Nolan SP. The dynamic aortic root. J Thorac Cardiovasc Surg. 1976;72(3):413–7.
12. de Heer LM, Budde RPJ, Mali WPTHM, de Vos AM, van Herwerden LA, Kluin J. Aortic root dimension changes during systole and diastole: evaluation with ECG-gated multidetector row computed tomography. Int J Card Imaging. 2011;27(8):1195–204.

13. Perinajová R, van de Ven T, Roelse E, Xu F, Juffermans J, Westenberg J, et al. A comprehensive MRI-based computational model of blood flow in compliant aorta using radial basis function interpolation. Biomed Eng Online. 2024;23:69.
14. Gouveia E, Melo R, Silva Duarte G, Lopes A, Alves M, Caldeira D, Fernandes E, Fernandes R, et al. Incidence and prevalence of thoracic aortic aneurysms: a systematic review and meta-analysis of population-based studies. Semin Thorac Cardiovasc Surg. 2022;34(1):1–16.
15. Olsson C, Thelin S, Ståhle E, Ekbom A, Granath F. Thoracic aortic aneurysm and dissection. Circulation. 2006;114(24):2611–8.
16. Lemaire SA, Russell L. Epidemiology of thoracic aortic dissection. Nat Rev Cardiol. 2011;8(2):103–13.
17. Maleszewski JJ. Inflammatory ascending aortic disease: perspectives from pathology. J Thorac Cardiovasc Surg. 2015;149(2):S176–83.
18. Cheung C, Bernardo AS, Trotter MWB, Pedersen RA, Sinha S. Generation of human vascular smooth muscle subtypes provides insight into embryological origin–dependent disease susceptibility. Nat Biotechnol. 2012;30(2):165–73.
19. Isselbacher EM, Preventza O, Hamilton Black J, Augoustides JG, Beck AW, Bolen MA, et al. 2022 ACC/AHA guideline for the diagnosis and management of aortic disease: a report of the American Heart Association/American College of Cardiology Joint Committee on Clinical Practice Guidelines. Circulation. 2022;146(24):e334–482.
20. Coady MA, Davies RR, Roberts M, Goldstein LJ, Rogalski MJ, Rizzo JA, et al. Familial patterns of thoracic aortic aneurysms. Arch Surg. 1999;134(4):361–7.
21. Ng CM, Cheng A, Myers LA, Martinez-Murillo F, Jie C, Bedja D, et al. TGF-β–dependent pathogenesis of mitral valve prolapse in a mouse model of Marfan syndrome. J Clin Invest. 2004;114(11):1586–92.
22. Loeys BL, Chen J, Neptune ER, Judge DP, Podowski M, Holm T, et al. A syndrome of altered cardiovascular, craniofacial, neurocognitive and skeletal development caused by mutations in TGFBR1 or TGFBR2. Nat Genet. 2005;37(3):275–81.
23. Germain DP. Clinical and genetic features of vascular Ehlers-Danlos syndrome. Ann Vasc Surg. 2002;16(3):391–7.
24. Ouzounian M, LeMaire SA, Milewicz DM. Heritable aortic root aneurysms. Ann Cardiothorac Surg. 2023;12(3):265–7.
25. Michelena HI, Della Corte A, Evangelista A, Maleszewski JJ, Edwards WD, Roman MJ, et al. International consensus statement on nomenclature and classification of the congenital bicuspid aortic valve and its aortopathy, for clinical, surgical, interventional and research purposes. Eur J Cardiothorac Surg. 2021;60(3):448–76.
26. Detaint D, Michelena HI, Nkomo VT, Vahanian A, Jondeau G, Sarano ME. Aortic dilatation patterns and rates in adults with bicuspid aortic valves: a comparative study with Marfan syndrome and degenerative aortopathy. Heart. 2014;100(2):126–34.
27. Saadoun D, Vautier M, Cacoub P. Medium and large vessel vasculitis. Circulation. 2021;143(3):267–82.
28. Phillippi JA. On vasa vasorum: a history of advances in understanding the vessels of vessels. Sci Adv. 2022;8(16):eabl6364.
29. Heggtveit HA. Syphilitic aortitis: a clinicopathologic autopsy study of 100 cases, 1950 to 1960. Circulation. 1964;29(3):346–55.
30. Kuzmik GA, Sang AX, Elefteriades JA. Natural history of thoracic aortic aneurysms. J Vasc Surg. 2012;56(2):565–71.
31. Rodríguez-Palomares JF, Teixidó-Tura G, Galuppo V, Cuéllar H, Laynez A, Gutiérrez L, et al. Multimodality assessment of ascending aortic diameters: comparison of different measurement methods. J Am Soc Echocardiogr. 2016;29(9):819–826.e4.
32. Loeys BL, Dietz HC, Braverman AC, Callewaert BL, De Backer J, Devereux RB, et al. The revised Ghent nosology for the Marfan syndrome. J Med Genet. 2010;47(7):476–85.
33. Germain DP. Ehlers-Danlos syndrome type IV. Orphanet J Rare Dis. 2007;2(1):32.

34. Elefteriades JA, Ziganshin BA. Aortic morphology determines extent of resection. In: Elefteriades JA, Ziganshin BA, editors. Practical tips in aortic surgery: clinical and technical insights. Cham: Springer; 2021. p. 127–8.
35. Czerny M, Grabenwöger M, Berger T, Aboyans V, Della Corte A, Chen EP, et al. EACTS/STS guidelines for diagnosing and treating acute and chronic syndromes of the aortic organ. Ann Thorac Surg. 2024;118(1):5–115.
36. David TE. Chapter 13—aortic valve-sparing operations. In: Sellke FW, Ruel M, editors. Atlas of cardiac surgical techniques. 2nd ed. Elsevier; 2019. p. 199–214.
37. Sarsam MAI, Yacoub M. Remodeling of the aortic valve anulus. J Thorac Cardiovasc Surg. 1993;105(3):435–8.
38. Doty DB, Doty JR. Chapter 38—aortic aneurysm. In: Cardiac surgery: operative technique. 2nd ed. Salt Lake City: Elsevier Inc; 2012. p. 447–515.
39. Erasmi A, Sievers HH, Scharfschwerdt M, Eckel T, Misfeld M. In vitro hydrodynamics, cusp-bending deformation, and root distensibility for different types of aortic valve–sparing operations: remodeling, sinus prosthesis, and reimplantation. J Thorac Cardiovasc Surg. 2005;130(4):1044–9.
40. Hanke T, Charitos EI, Stierle U, Robinson D, Gorski A, Sievers HH, et al. Factors associated with the development of aortic valve regurgitation over time after two different techniques of valve-sparing aortic root surgery. J Thorac Cardiovasc Surg. 2009;137(2):314–9.
41. Stephens EH, Dearani JA, Pochettino A, Vricella LA, Sundt TM, David TE, et al. Valve-sparing aortic root replacement state-of-the-art review, part II: surgical techniques. Ann Thorac Surg. 2024;2024:S0003497524001164.
42. Ikonomidis JS. Valve-sparing aortic root replacement—"T. David V" method. Oper Tech Thorac Cardiovasc Surg. 2009;14(4):281–96.
43. David TE. Aortic valve-sparing operations. Ann Thorac Surg. 2024;117(1):45–53.
44. David TE, David CM, Ouzounian M, Feindel CM, Lafreniere-Roula M. A progress report on reimplantation of the aortic valve. J Thorac Cardiovasc Surg. 2021;161(3):890–899.e1.
45. Hess PJ, Klodell CT, Beaver TM, Martin TD. The Florida Sleeve: a new technique for aortic root remodeling with preservation of the aortic valve and sinuses. Ann Thorac Surg. 2005;80(2):748–50.
46. Aalaei-Andabili SH, Martin T, Hess P, Klodell C, Karimi A, Arnaoutakis G, et al. Florida Sleeve procedure is durable and improves aortic valve function in Marfan syndrome patients. Ann Thorac Surg. 2017;104(3):834–9.
47. Tasca G, Selmi M, Votta E, Redaelli P, Sturla F, Redaelli A, et al. Aortic root biomechanics after Sleeve and David sparing techniques: a finite element analysis. Ann Thorac Surg. 2017;103(5):1451–9.
48. Malekan R, Spielvogel D, Saunders PC, Lansman SL, Griepp RB. The completion Bentall procedure. Ann Thorac Surg. 2011;92(1):362–3.
49. Shemin RJ. Chapter 14—Bentall procedure. In: Sellke FW, Ruel M, editors. Atlas of cardiac surgical techniques. 2nd ed. Elsevier; 2019. p. 215–24.
50. Bentall H, De Bono A. A technique for complete replacement of the ascending aorta. Thorax. 1968;23(4):338–9.
51. Stamou SC, Williams ML, Gunn TM, Hagberg RC, Lobdell KW, Kouchoukos NT. Aortic root surgery in the United States: a report from the Society of Thoracic Surgeons database. J Thorac Cardiovasc Surg. 2015;149(1):116–122.e4.
52. Arnaoutakis GJ, Sultan I, Siki M, Bavaria JE. Bicuspid aortic valve repair: systematic review on long-term outcomes. Ann Cardiothorac Surg. 2019;8(3):302–12.
53. Mastrobuoni S, Govers PJ, Veen KM, Jahanyar J, Saane SV, Segreto A, et al. Valve-sparing aortic root replacement using the reimplantation (David) technique: a systematic review and meta-analysis on survival and clinical outcome. Ann Cardiothorac Surg. 2023;12(3):149–58.
54. Sá MP, Jacquemyn X, Awad AK, Brown JA, Chu D, Serna-Gallegos D, et al. Valve-sparing aortic root replacement with reimplantation vs remodeling: a meta-analysis. Ann Thorac Surg. 2024;117(3):501–7.

55. Chauvette V, Kluin J, De Kerchove L, El Khoury G, Schäfers HJ, Lansac E, et al. Outcomes of valve-sparing surgery in heritable aortic disorders: results from the AVIATOR registry. Eur J Cardiothorac Surg. 2022;62(3):ezac366.
56. Aalaei-Andabili SH, Martin TD, Hess PJ, Karimi A, Bavry AA, Arnaoutakis GJ, et al. The Florida sleeve procedure is durable and improves aortic valve function. AORTA. 2019;07(02):049–55.
57. Aalaei-Andabili SH, Beaver TM, Martin TD, Hess PJ, Arnaoutakis GJ. Outcomes of Florida Sleeve procedure in patients with bicuspid versus tricuspid aortic valve. Innov Technol Tech Cardiothorac Vasc Surg. 2020;15(4):361–8.
58. Mookhoek A, Korteland NM, Arabkhani B, Di Centa I, Lansac E, Bekkers JA, et al. Bentall procedure: a systematic review and meta-analysis. Ann Thorac Surg. 2016;101(5):1684–9.
59. Gott VL, Cameron DE, Alejo DE, Greene PS, Shake JG, Caparrelli DJ, et al. Aortic root replacement in 271 Marfan patients: a 24-year experience. Ann Thorac Surg. 2002;73(2): 438–43.
60. Golesworthy T, Lampérth M, Mohiaddin R, Pepper J, Thornton W, Treasure T. The Tailor of Gloucester: a jacket for the Marfan's aorta. Lancet. 2004;364(9445):1582.
61. Kenny LA, Austin C, Golesworthy T, Venugopal P, Alphonso N. Personalized external aortic root support (PEARS) for aortic root aneurysm. Oper Tech Thorac Cardiovasc Surg. 2021;26(2):290–305.
62. Pepper J, Golesworthy T, Utley M, Chan J, Ganeshalingam S, Lamperth M, et al. Manufacturing and placing a bespoke support for the Marfan aortic root: description of the method and technical results and status at one year for the first ten patients. Interact Cardiovasc Thorac Surg. 2010;10(3):360–5.
63. Treasure T, Petrou M, Rosendahl U, Austin C, Rega F, Pirk J, et al. Personalized external aortic root support: a review of the current status. Eur J Cardiothorac Surg. 2016;50(3):400–4.
64. Felipe Gaia D, Bernal O, Castilho E, Baeta Neves Duarte Ferreira C, Dvir D, Simonato M, et al. First-in-human Endo-Bentall procedure for simultaneous treatment of the ascending aorta and aortic valve. JACC Case Rep. 2020;2(3):480–5.
65. Grimm JC, Ibrahim M, Szeto WY. Endo-Bentall: is this feasible? Ann Cardiothorac Surg. 2022;11(1):46–7.
66. Ghoreishi M, Chahal D, Shah A, Kang J, Hirsch J, Tran D, et al. First-in-human endovascular aortic root repair (Endo-Bentall) for acute type a dissection. Circ Cardiovasc Interv. 2023;16(10):e013348.
67. Kubo S, Tanaka A, Omura A, Tsunemi K, Oka T, Okada K, et al. Long-term results of valve-sparing aortic root replacement and aortic cusp repair. Ann Thorac Surg. 2024;117(1):78–85.
68. David TE, Seidman MA, David CM, Lafreniere-Roula M. Outcomes of reimplantation of the aortic valve in patients with aortic cusp fenestration. Ann Thorac Surg. 2023;115(1):106–11.

Chapter 6
Surgery for Ascending Aortic Aneurysm

Sivaveera Kandasamy and Bradley S. Taylor

> Billy was walking up the hall, buckling his belt. His tanned face was now sallow and wet with sweat. 'He says there's a bulge in my aorta. Like a bubble in a car tire. Only car tires don't yell when you poke em'. (Stephen King, from *Doctor Sleep*)

History

One of the earliest descriptions of an arterial aneurysm was in the Ebers papyrus, an ancient Egyptian medical text prepared around 2000 BC, which recognized that this was a vascular lesion that needed to be treated surgically with an instrument [1]. More specifically, it recommended that "when thou meetest a tumor of the vessels in any part of the body of a person and thou findest it round in form, growing under thy finger" to "treat it with a knife and burn it with a fire so that it bleeds not too much" [2]. Around 600 BC, the Sushruta Samhita text from ancient India described various methods of hemostasis and hemorrhage control by utilizing cautery and hemp fibers for ligation of bleeding vessels.

The earliest recorded attempt to cure an aortic aneurysm was by the Greek surgeon Antyllus, considered as the true father of vascular surgery, whose ideas were recorded in the fourth century AD by Oribasius. The "Antyllus method", which was first attempted in 200 AD, consisted of proximal and distal ligation without resecting the aneurysm sac, as amputating the "intervening dilated part…is a dangerous operation. The violent tension of the arterial pneuma often displaces the ligatures" [3, 4]. This same advice was also given in the 1500s by the French barber surgeon Ambroise Paré, who also seemed to agree that opening the sac would result in

S. Kandasamy (✉) · B. S. Taylor
Department of Surgery, University of Maryland School of Medicine, Baltimore, MD, USA
e-mail: skandasamy@som.umaryland.edu; Bradley.Taylor@som.umaryland.edu

G. J. Arnaoutakis et al. (eds.), *Aortic Aneurysms*, Contemporary Cardiology,
https://doi.org/10.1007/978-3-032-13134-8_6

severe and fatal hemorrhage and was also one of the first to describe a ruptured aneurysm of the thoracic aorta.

Several centuries would pass before the earliest description of an operative attempt for an ascending aortic aneurysm would be described by Charles H. Moore in 1864. In his case report titled "On a new method of procuring the consolidation of fibrin in certain incurable aneurisms", he described the introduction of wire threads which induced thrombosis [5]. This concept remained as the standard throughout the nineteenth and early part of the twentieth century. Other attempts included attaching the wires to a battery for electrical-induced coagulation by Alfonso Corradi. Electrothermic coagulation and aneurysm wrapping with cellophane to induce periarterial fibrosis were equally inconsistent to provide a cure and fell out of favor [6].

The next milestone in aortic surgery was a technique entitled endoaneurysmorraphy, introduced by Rudolph Matas. This was first described and performed on a traumatic brachial artery aneurysm in 1888. It borrowed aspects from the "Antyllus method", and included opening of the aneurysm, proximal and distal ligation of the supplying artery to the aneurysm, resection of the sac and thrombus contents, and obliterating the feeding collateral vessels from within the sac by suture ligation [7]. The first successful use of this technique in an abdominal aortic aneurysm was later described by Matas in 1923. It was not until the 1950s that this technique fell out of favor with the introduction of synthetic tube grafts.

Within the next 40–50 years, many advances in endovascular surgery were made, and though these are important discoveries that took place in the realm of thoracic aortic surgery, this chapter will focus on the surgical aspect of ascending aortic aneurysms alone. It is important to recognize, however, that a healthy collaboration between cardiothoracic surgeons, vascular surgeons, and biomedical engineers has played a huge role toward the advancement of thoracic aortic surgery.

Anatomy

It is important to remember the anatomical landmarks prior to discussing surgical management. The thoracic and abdominal portions comprise the two main segments of the aorta, with the thoracic aorta consisting of three parts, which are the ascending, arch, and descending. The annulus, which is a fibrous ring at the aortic orifice, is considered the transition point between the left ventricle and aortic root and the origin of the thoracic aorta. The termination of the thoracic aorta is at the diaphragmatic hiatus.

It is worth noting that the aortic root, which is the most proximal portion, is positioned between the annulus and sinotubular junction and comprises of three Valsalva sinuses: right, left, and noncoronary. The tubular ascending aorta begins at the sinotubular junction and extends to the aortic arch at the level of the innominate artery.

When to Intervene

The complications associated with ascending aortic aneurysms are devastating, with the mortality rate of ruptured thoracic aortic aneurysms approaching 90% [8]. Therefore, a pathologically dilated ascending aorta needs to be diagnosed in a timely fashion. Elective surgery remains the mainstay treatment of all ascending aortic aneurysms and has been demonstrated to reduce mortality. Patients who present to the hospital requiring emergent surgical intervention have a mortality risk of approximately 20%, whereas elective ascending aortic aneurysm replacement has an operative mortality close to 2% [18, 19]. Thus, when the aorta reaches a size with a high risk of complications, prophylactic corrective surgery is highly recommended [9].

Retrospective studies have shown that the median aortic diameter associated with an increased risk of dissection, rupture, or death was 6.0 cm. Coady et al. estimated a statistically significant increase in probability by 32.1 percentage points for ascending aneurysms [10]. Accordingly, a size of 5.5 cm has been used as an acceptable size for elective resection of ascending aortic aneurysms due to the resection being able to be performed with a relatively low mortality (Figs. 6.1 and 6.2). Studies have revealed that the growth rate in patients diagnosed with ascending aortic aneurysms was around 0.6 mm/year [19].

Another method used is the aortic size index (ASI), where the maximal aortic diameter measured by MRI is divided by the body surface area. The three groups that were identified using this method were low risk, moderate risk, and high risk with measurements of 2.75 cm/m^2, 2.75–4.24 cm/m^2, and greater than 4.25 cm/m^2 [11].

Current recommendations for prophylactic ascending aorta repair in patients without predisposing conditions other than hypertension are when the aorta reaches 5.5 cm, or the growth rate exceeds 0.5 cm per year. If the patient is undergoing

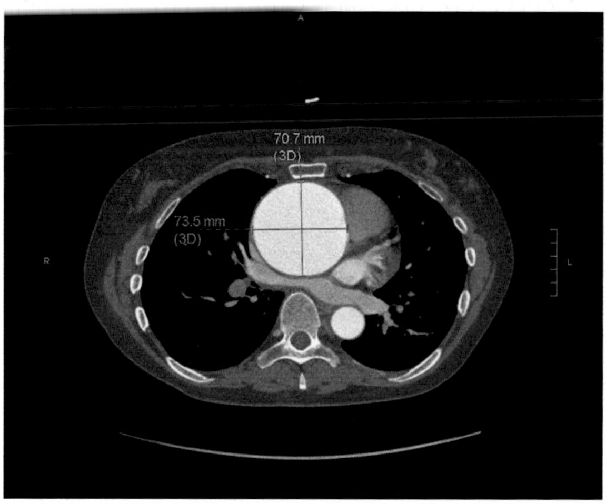

Fig. 6.1 CT angiogram axial view of a high-risk ascending aortic aneurysm

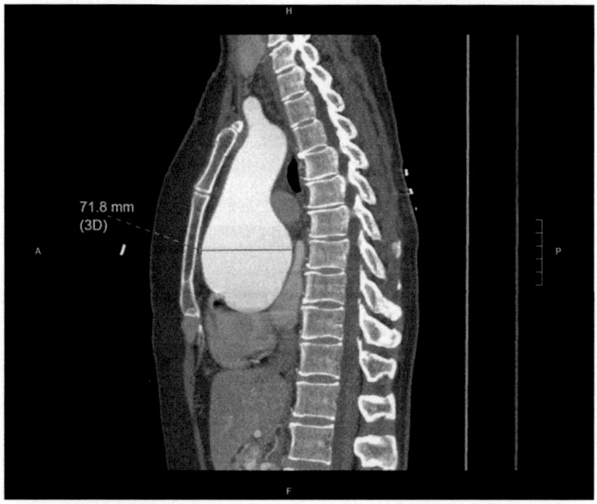

Fig. 6.2 CT angiogram sagittal view of a high-risk ascending aortic aneurysm

another major aortic surgery, ascending aorta repair is recommended at a size over 4.5 cm.

The notable exception to this rule is patients with Marfan syndrome who tend to have complications at a younger age and at smaller aortic diameters. The settings in which patients with Marfan syndrome are recommended for prophylactic surgery are as follows [12]:

1. Aortic diameter of 5.0 cm
2. Aortic diameter of 4.5 cm with a positive family history of complications
3. Aortic diameter exceeding 4.5 cm when undergoing aortic valve replacement
4. Aortic diameter of 4.5 cm with associated significant aortic valve insufficiency
5. Annual aortic diameter growth rate greater than 0.5 cm
6. Women with childbearing potential

For patients with a bicuspid aortic valve, most centers recommend elective aortic replacement when the aortic diameter reaches 5.0 cm [12].

Patients with Loeys-Dietz syndrome require a more aggressive approach to prophylactic surgery. While an aorta size of 4.0 cm was originally recommended, the latest ACCF recommending surgical intervention with an ascending aorta diameter of 4.2 cm when measured by transesophageal ultrasound [13].

Ascending Aortic Replacement

Surgical approach is dependent on two main scenarios: the site of aortic dilation and the functionality of the aortic valve. Although the term ascending aorta replacement may refer to the sinus portion, tubular portion, both, it is important to specify, as the operations involving the aortic root are more complex as they involve repair or replacement of the aortic valve or coronary arteries. Surgical graft replacement of the tubular portion is the most common intervention on the ascending aorta [14]. This, of course, is performed when there is no involvement of the Valsalva sinuses. When the Valsalva sinuses are involved, the Bentall procedure, or a combined valve and graft replacement with reimplant of the coronary arteries, or valve sparing procedure can be performed [15].

Tubular replacement of the ascending aorta is performed with a prosthetic polyethylene terephthalate (Dacron) graft (Fig. 6.1). This operation consists of the usual tenets of cardiothoracic surgery; placing the patient on cardiopulmonary bypass, cross-clamping of the aorta, and cardioplegic arrest (Figs. 6.3, 6.4, 6.5, 6.6, 6.7, 6.8, 6.9 and 6.10). Friable or thin tissue can be reinforced at the aortic suture lines with polytetrafluoroethylene (Teflon) pledgets [14].

In general, ascending aortic replacement is associated with a low morbidity and mortality when performed electively. Concomitant procedures may increase the risk [16, 17].

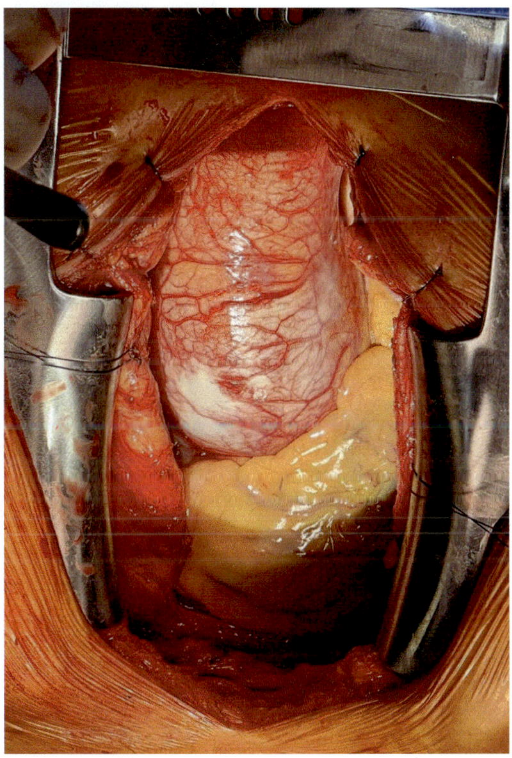

Fig. 6.3 View of an ascending aortic aneurysm after performing a median sternotomy

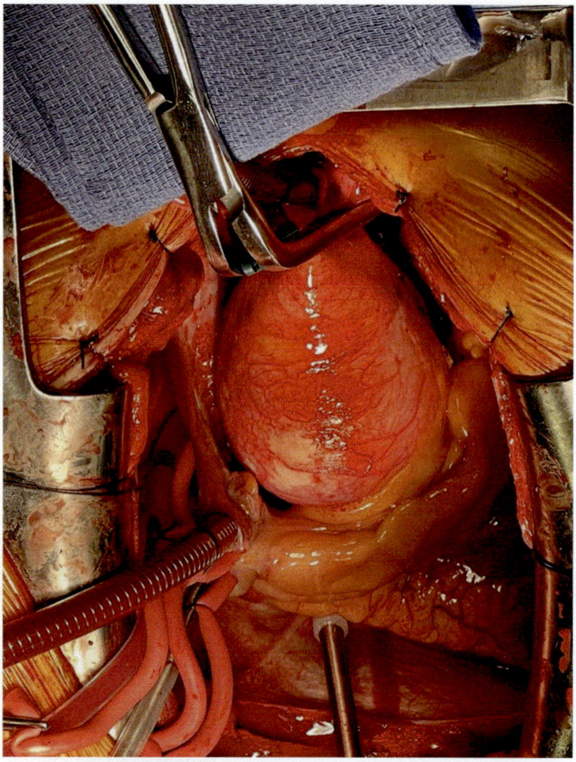

Fig. 6.4 Aortic cross clamp being applied after central aortic, venous, and retrograde cardioplegia cannulation

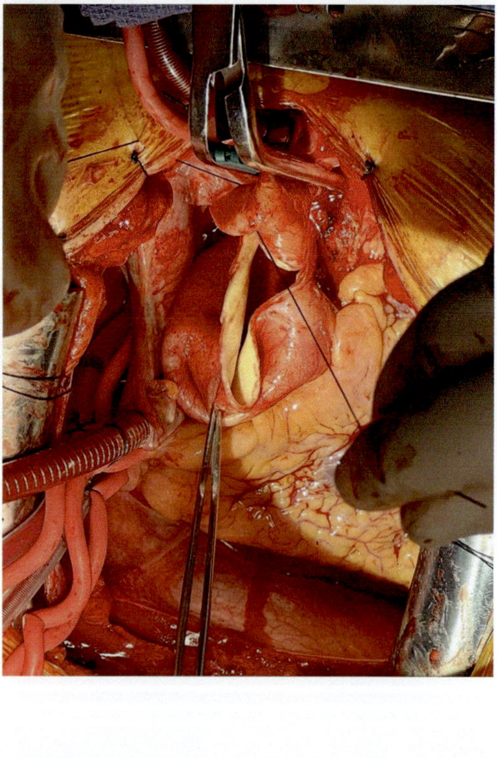

Fig. 6.5 After distal aortic cross clamp and cardiac arrest is achieved, the diseased ascending aorta is being excised

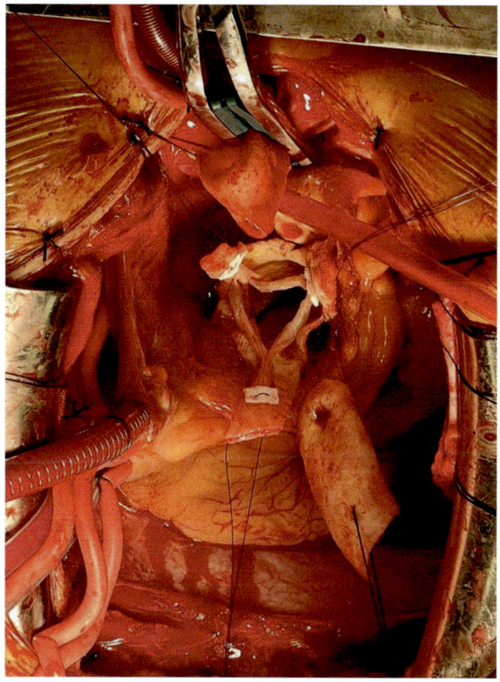

Fig. 6.6 View of aortic valve after excision of diseased ascending aorta. Native aortic valve can be reinforced with polytetrafluoroethylene pledgets when performing a valve-sparing ascending aortic aneurysm replacement

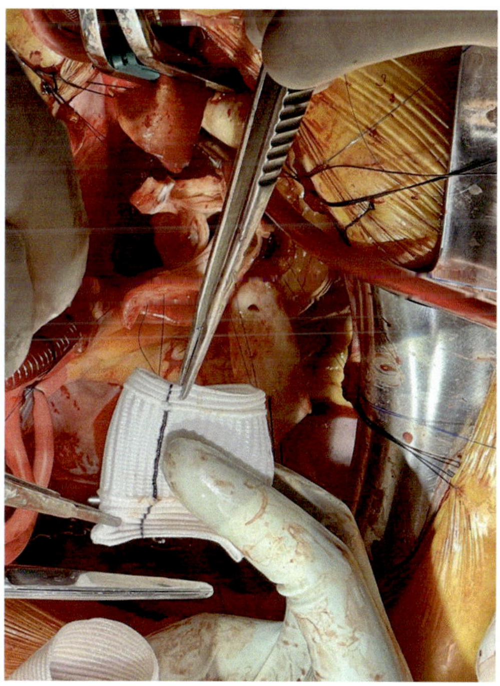

Fig. 6.7 After synthetic tube graft (Dacron) is cut to appropriate size, it is anchored and secured proximally

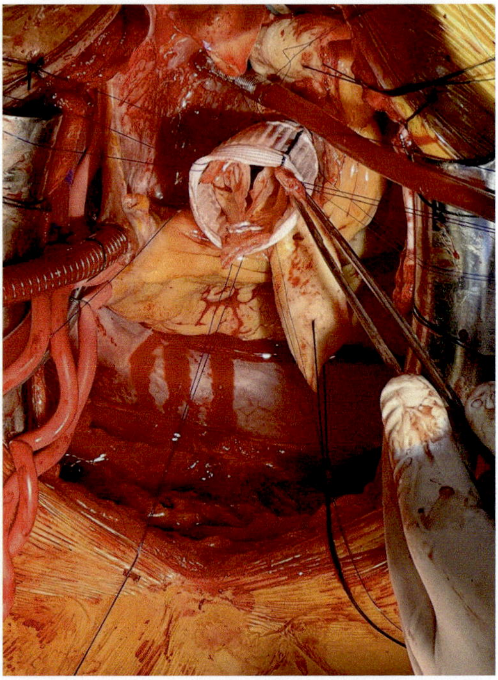

Fig. 6.8 View after proximally securing Dacron graft

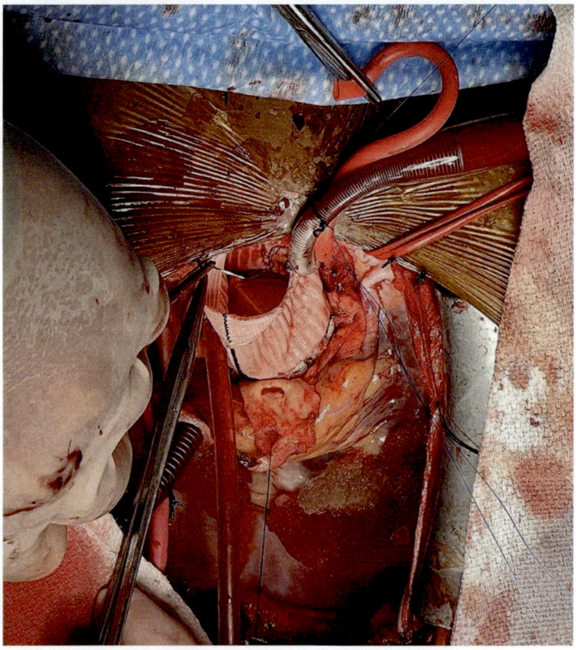

Fig. 6.9 An example of synthetic graft being secured distally

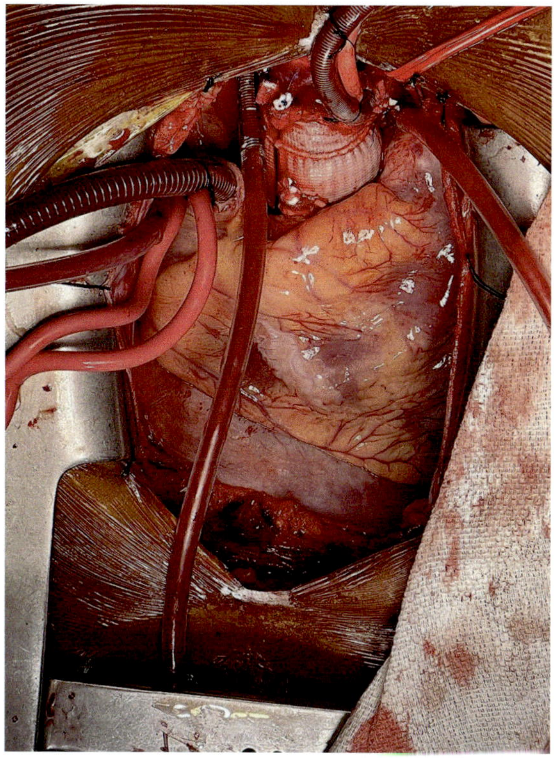

Fig. 6.10 Completion of ascending aortic replacement with synthetic graft

Summary

Though aneurysms of the ascending aorta can be lethal, timely diagnosis and prophylactic corrective surgery have been demonstrated to achieve both low morbidity and mortality. Elective repair remains the mainstay for any symptomatic aneurysm or asymptomatic aneurysm with a diameter greater than 5.5 cm. Notable exceptions to this rule are for patients with congenital abnormalities. Through a combined approach of medical treatment, risk factor control, and screening, timely surgical intervention with graft replacement has been proven to provide excellent results.

References

1. Lippi D. An aneurysm in the Papyrus of Ebers (108, 3-9). Med Secoli. 1990;2(1):1–4.
2. Barker WF. Clio: the arteries. Austin: RG Landers; 1992. p. 2–502.
3. Thompson JE. Early history of aortic surgery. J Vasc Surg. 1998;28(4):746–52.
4. Heidel WA, Raeder I. Oribasii Collectionum medicorum reliquiae. Am J Philol. 1930;51(2):291.

5. Moore CH, Murchison C. On a new method of procuring the consolidation of fibrin in certain incurable aneurisms: with the report of a case in which an aneurism of the ascending aorta was treated by the insertion of wire. Med Chir Trans. 1864;47:129.
6. McFadden PM, Wiggins LM, Boys JA. A history of thoracic aortic surgery. Cardiol Clin. 2017;35(3):307–16.
7. Matas R. Traumatic aneurysm of the left brachial artery. Med News. 1888;53:462–5.
8. Johansson G, Markström U, Swedenborg J. Ruptured thoracic aortic aneurysms: a study of incidence and mortality rates. J Vasc Surg. 1995;21(6):985–8.
9. Saliba E, Sia Y, Dore A, El Hamamsy I. The ascending aortic aneurysm: when to intervene? IJC Heart Vasc. 2015;6:91–100.
10. Coady MA, Rizzo JA, Hammond GL, Mandapati D, Darr U, Kopf GS, Elefteriades JA. What is the appropriate size criterion for resection of thoracic aortic aneurysms? J Thorac Cardiovasc Surg. 1997;113(3):476–91.
11. Davies RR, Gallo A, Coady MA, Tellides G, Botta DM, Burke B, Coe MP, Kopf GS, Elefteriades JA. Novel measurement of relative aortic size predicts rupture of thoracic aortic aneurysms. Ann Thorac Surg. 2006;81(1):169–77.
12. Hiratzka LF, Bakris GL, Beckman JA, Bersin RM, Carr VF, Casey De Jr., et al. ACCF/AHA/AATS/ACR/ASA/SCA/SCAI/SIR/STS/SVM guidelines for the diagnosis and management of patients with thoracic aortic disease: a report; 2010.
13. Loeys BL, Schwarze U, Holm T, Callewaert BL, Thomas GH, Pannu H, De Backer JF, Oswald GL, Symoens S, Manouvrier S, Roberts AE. Aneurysm syndromes caused by mutations in the TGF-β receptor. N Engl J Med. 2006;355(8):788–98.
14. Cameron DE. Surgical techniques: ascending aorta. Cardiol Clin. 1999;17(4):739–50.
15. David TE, Feindel CM, Webb GD, Colman JM, Armstrong S, Maganti M. Long-term results of aortic valve-sparing operations for aortic root aneurysm. J Thorac Cardiovasc Surg. 2006;132(2):347–54.
16. Ergin MA. Early and late results of ascending aorta surgery: risk factors for early and late outcome. World J Surg. 1997;21(6):590–8.
17. Williams JB, Peterson ED, Zhao Y, O'Brien SM, Andersen ND, Miller DC, Chen EP, Hughes GC. Contemporary results for proximal aortic replacement in North America. J Am Coll Cardiol. 2012;60(13):1156–62.
18. Mok SC, Ma WG, Mansour A, Charilaou P, Chou AS, Peterss S, Tranquilli M, Ziganshin BA, Elefteriades JA. Twenty-five year outcomes following composite graft aortic root replacement. J Card Surg. 2017;32(2):99–109.
19. Guo MH, Appoo JJ, Saczkowski R, Smith HN, Ouzounian M, Gregory AJ, Herget EJ, Boodhwani M. Association of mortality and acute aortic events with ascending aortic aneurysm: a systematic review and meta-analysis. JAMA Netw Open. 2018;1(4):e181281.

Chapter 7
Surgical Management of Aortic Arch Aneurysms

R. Wilson King, Michael T. Cain, Yuki Ikeno, and T. Brett Reece

Introduction

Thoracic aortic aneurysms have an incidence of approximately 5–10 per 100,000 patients, and the incidence of aortic arch aneurysms is even lower [1, 2]. The surgical management of these patients is complex, but this chapter will focus on the open surgical management including preoperative assessment, intraoperative monitoring, and surgical techniques.

Preoperative Considerations

Imaging

Diagnosis of aortic arch pathology is generally made with computed tomographic angiography (CTA) of the chest which is highly sensitive and specific [2]. It is prudent to include CTA of the head and neck so that details of the neck vessels and Circle of Willis anatomy can be delineated. Aberrancies or pathology of these vessels will help determine proper cerebral protection and cannulation strategies during preoperative planning. Furthermore, attention to areas of calcium and atheroma should be given in order to characterize the risk of peripheral and visceral embolization from the aorta during manipulation. The degree of atheroma is often referred to

R. W. King (✉)
Department of Surgery, University of Colorado, Boulder, CO, USA
e-mail: ROBERT.3.KING@CUANSCHUTZ.EDU

M. T. Cain · Y. Ikeno · T. B. Reece
Department of Cardiothoracic Surgery, University of Colorado, Boulder, CO, USA
e-mail: michael.cain@cuanschutz.edu; BRETT.REECE@CUANSCHUTZ.EDU

G. J. Arnaoutakis et al. (eds.), *Aortic Aneurysms*, Contemporary Cardiology,
https://doi.org/10.1007/978-3-032-13134-8_7

as a "Shaggy Aorta." The Shaggy Aorta has a higher risk of embolization events, especially during aortic manipulation.

Aberrant anatomy should be noted such as aberrant subclavian artery, right-sided arch, and aberrancy in the vertebral anatomy. This information is important for cannulation planning and cerebral protection planning. If the extent of the pathology is distal enough to where spinal cord ischemia is of concern, then careful evaluation of the intercostals should be done to evaluate the risk of spinal cord ischemia. This may help in making the decision on whether or not to include a lumbar drain preoperatively.

An analysis of the distal extent of the disease should be done so that the surgeon can plan the operation properly. If there is ongoing disease distal to the arch, then a frozen elephant trunk operation should be considered. However, if there is no ongoing disease past the arch then a zone 2 repair or hemiarch is likely feasible.

Swallow

An assessment of the patient's swallow function should be carefully noted in the history and physical exam. In rare instances, the aneurysmal aorta can cause esophageal narrowing leading to dysphagia symptoms, or dysphagia aortica. This can be identified with barium swallow studies. Further, the recurrent laryngeal nerve is at risk in total arch repairs. On the right side, the recurrent laryngeal nerve loops underneath the right subclavian and on the left it loops underneath the arch near the level of the takeoff of the internal carotid and left subclavian (Fig. 7.1). A preoperative assessment of vocal cord function and swallow can help determine how high risk a patient is if damage to one of these nerves occurs.

Diaphragm

The phrenic nerve is also at risk during aortic arch surgery. Specifically, the right phrenic nerve is at risk during dissection of the superior vena cava (SVC) and cannulation of the SVC. The left phrenic nerve passes over the aortic arch distal to the takeoff of the brachiocephalic vessels and courses over the left pulmonary artery and down the pericardium of the heart. Attention is needed to avoid damaging these nerves during the operation.

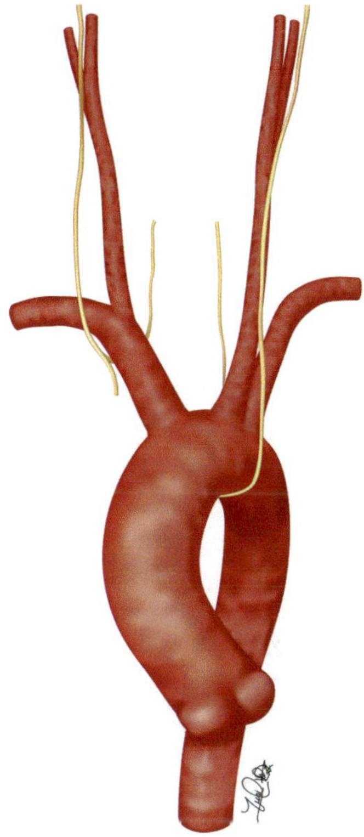

Fig. 7.1 Anatomy of the right and left recurrent laryngeal nerve

Assessing the Risk of Potential Catastrophe

Finally, it is important to assess the risk of potential catastrophe before entering the operating room. In the event of a reoperative case, there can be dense adhesions and an open pericardium that increases the potential for causing catastrophic cardiac or aortic bleeding during sternotomy and dissection. Special care is needed during these cases, including access to peripheral cannulation sites. Fortunately, if the pericardium is intact, then the potential for catastrophe drops tremendously.

Intraoperative Monitoring

Hemodynamics

Hemodynamic monitoring is essential during aortic arch repair. Depending on the location and severity of the aneurysm, the arterial pressures may be different at different sites. Therefore, it is important to have arterial lines in multiple vessels. For example, if there is any malperfusion to the innominate artery, then the right radial arterial pressure may be lower than the left radial arterial pressure. Therefore, an attempt should be made to obtain arterial pressures that are both proximal and distal to the site of the aneurysm. Commonly, arterial lines are inserted in the right radial artery and into the left radial artery and/or left femoral artery. This selection must keep in mind potential sites of malperfusion and overall cannulation strategy. For example, if there is malperfusion in the left iliac, then left femoral artery pressure may not be reliable. Repeated lactate and arterial blood gas measurements should be taken to continuously assess the acid-base status of the patient.

Neuromonitoring

Neurologic injury is one of the most feared complications in aortic arch surgery as there is a high stroke risk and spinal cord injury risk. Because of this, neurophysiologic intraoperative monitoring (NIOM) is essential. Although it is well documented that NIOM is helpful in evaluating spinal cord injury and potentially providing for early intervention, its usefulness in prevention of stroke is still debated [3–5]. However, Ghincea and colleagues found that NIOM modalities can be both highly sensitive and specific in stroke detection during hemiarch repair [6].

One commonly used mechanism is continuous monitoring using electroencephalography (EEG) or bispectral index (BSI) which measure frontal cerebral activity and extrapolates the data to reflect posterior circulation. An important usage of EEG and BSI is to detect the level of hypothermia-mediated cerebral metabolic activity during active cooling. This allows the surgical team to determine when an acceptable amount of cooling has occurred before the initiation of circulatory arrest. Further, alerts from the EEG and BSI can possibly indicate a reversible ischemic insult, such as a malpositioned cannula, that can be quickly intervened on.

Cerebral oximetry by near-infrared spectroscopy (NIRS) is another commonly used method of neuromonitoring. Regional cerebral oxygen saturation levels can be determined by analyzing the absorption of saturated and unsaturated hemoglobin by utilizing near-infrared spectroscopy. NIRS can be used during induction of circulatory arrest to detect cerebral perfusion issues and whether or not perfusion has been restored. One critical use of NIRS has been in detecting contralateral cerebral ischemia during unilateral antegrade cerebral perfusion (ACP). This allows the surgeon to change cannulation strategies and initiate a bilateral perfusion strategy if necessary [7, 8]. Combined with its ease of use and non-invasive technique, NIRS is an attractive NIOM strategy.

Somatosensory evoked potentials (SEPs) and motor evoked potentials (MEPs) are other adjuncts that can be used. One use of these is as an adjunct to EEG during cooling to monitor cerebral metabolic activity. Further, it can be used to help identify reversible spinal cord injuries and allows for surgeons to pre-emptively act to prevent irreversible damage [3, 9].

Procedure

Considerations/Concerns

Reentry

Redo sternotomies are more challenging and come with worse short-term and long-term postoperative outcomes [10]. The potential for catastrophe is greatly increased so peripheral cannulation sites should be prepped into the sterile field in case emergent CPB is needed.

Heart Protection

Although much of the focus during aortic arch repair is on cerebral protection, myocardial protection can be complicated by difficult aortic pathology. In general, surgeons should provide antegrade or retrograde cardioplegia delivery, depending on what the surgeon is most comfortable with. The anatomy and the need for any additional procedures (such as root replacement) drive the decision-making for how to deliver cardioplegia. For short ischemic times, our program prefers antegrade cardioplegia. However, there is a low threshold to use retrograde cardioplegia in cases where antegrade delivery is difficult, especially when there is an inability to clamp the aorta. For longer ischemic times, we often will deliver supplemental cardioplegia down the right coronary os for right ventricular protection. Our bias is also guided by the desire for less frequent delivery of the cardioplegia.

Cerebral Protection

Cerebral protection during aortic surgery, especially during circulatory arrest, remains an evolving science with different modalities. The challenge is most significant during aortic arch surgery as circulation to the brachiocephalic vessels is interrupted during arch reconstruction. Devastating neurological outcomes, including stroke, can occur during any aortic arch surgery. Therefore, the goal of the cerebral perfusion strategy is to limit the metabolic demand to the brain to prevent more global ischemia, limit the total ischemic time, and prevent embolic events through aortic manipulation. Although there is no conclusive strategy that minimizes the risk of adverse neurological outcomes, there are three main methods of cerebral protection during aortic arch surgery.

The first is deep hypothermic circulatory arrest (D-HCA) or moderate hypothermic circulatory arrest (M-HCA). D-HCA is used to lower the metabolic demand from cerebral tissue during circulatory arrest. Cerebral tissue is quite sensitive to hypoxic insult, so lowering the temperature acts to decrease the insult. In fact, it is estimated that for every 10° degree decrease in normal body temperature, there is a

50% reduction in metabolic demand [11]. D-HCA is classified as temperatures between 14.1 and 20 degrees Celsius while M-HCA is defined as temperatures between 20.1 and 28 degrees Celsius. It is estimated that D-HCA provides 20–30 min of HCA, and M-HCA provides only 10–20 min of HCA time. Some surgeons choose to use this strategy in isolation, and has been shown to be safe in circulatory arrest times of up to 30 min [12]; however, others have found that the risk of stroke can be as high as 12% by using D-HCA or M-HCA alone [13]. Other potential issues involved in a D-HCA strategy are prolonged cardiopulmonary bypass (CPB) times related to the time in re-warming and the risk of coagulopathy at lower temperatures, thus increased transfusions and operative time. Because of these issues, surgeons are moving toward M-HCA and away from D-HCA. Surgeons are also using adjunctive antegrade or retrograde perfusion strategies to provide direct oxygen delivery to the tissue.

Selective antegrade cerebral perfusion (SACP) or bilateral antegrade cerebral perfusion (BACP) have been used as adjuncts to hypothermic arrest to try and provide direct oxygen delivery to the cerebral tissue. This strategy was slow to adopt initially as it requires complex arterial cannulation; however, it is becoming more common. Through antegrade cerebral perfusion (ACP), the brain receives physiological arterial blood supply from cannulation of the innominate artery, axillary artery, left common carotid artery, or a combination of these. Because of the complexity, surgeons moved to use SACP, which has been shown to be safe [14]. However, if a patient does not have an intact Circle of Willis, it may be necessary to use BACP, although most patients have adequate collaterals to overcome this. Further, branched grafts can be used for arterial cannulation when there is complex anatomy. Spielvogel and colleagues wrote a review article regarding SACP and found that SACP can be safe and effective, even at moderate hypothermia [15]. A more recent study by Leontyev and colleagues found that the addition of SACP to HCA reduced in-hospital mortality and stroke risk [16].

The previously discussed methods of cerebral protection aim to reduce metabolic demand and increase physiological oxygen delivery; however, they do not do anything to prevent potential embolic events from aortic manipulation. RCP has the potential benefit of washing out embolic debris and is performed by cannulating the superior vena cava (SVC) and perfusing arterial blood from the bypass circuit in a retrograde fashion through the cerebral venous system and back through the arterial system. However, there is the potential for causing cerebral edema at higher perfusion pressures and, thus, poor postoperative neurological outcomes. There is also some concern about metabolic delivery when perfusing in a retrograde fashion. Some studies argue for the use of RCP while others argue against. Ongoing research is needed to find the optimal cerebral protection strategy.

Cannulation

Depending on the cerebral protection strategy during hypothermic circulatory arrest and the patient's anatomy, the surgeon can employ different cannulation strategies. For more proximal disease, the surgeon can employ ACP through central cannulation through the aorta to provide arterial flow. However, this is only feasible if the distal extent of the disease does not reach the innominate artery. If the distal extent of the diseased aorta is into the takeoff of the brachiocephalic vessels, then alternative cannulation strategies should be employed. Firstly, the surgeon can opt to cannulate unilaterally through the innominate artery to deliver ACP. As previously discussed, SACP has been shown to provide adequate arterial blood flow to the brain, even in most patients who have a Circle of Willis that is not intact. However, for the patients who do not seem to tolerate unilateral innominate cannulation, the surgeon can bilaterally cannulate to provide blood flow. Unfortunately, there are many instances in which the innominate artery is diseased and is unable to be cannulated for ACP. In this case, axillary artery cannulation can be employed to provide ACP. In a recent study, the authors found that using axillary artery cannulation versus innominate artery cannulation actually reduces the post-operative risk of embolic stroke [17]. However, there are also studies that suggest that there is no difference in post-operative neurological outcomes when comparing axillary artery cannulation to innominate [18]. Nonetheless, it does seem that axillary artery and innominate cannulation is a safe and effective method of delivering ACP.

With aortic arch pathology that extends into the brachiocephalic vessels, it is often impossible to cannulate the innominate artery for ACP, so more complicated techniques are needed, including the creation of a trifurcated graft. This method was developed by Spielvogel and colleagues in 1999 to avoid the risk of embolization from atherosclerotic brachiocephalic vessels during total arch repair [19].

Our program has instituted what we call the "Shaggy Aorta" protocol that was initially used for cerebral protection with a Shaggy Aorta, but is now used in nearly every open aortic surgery. This protocol begins with central aortic cannulation for the commencement of CPB. Moderate cooling is initiated at 26 degrees C to 28 degrees Celsius. During the construction of the distal anastomosis, HCA is initiated. RCP is administered through the SVC at a rate of 1.5–2 l/min and increased until blood is returned through the carotid artery. If the circulatory arrest time is less than 10 min, then RCP is used without the addition of SACP. However, if the circulatory arrest times extend beyond 10 min, then SACP is delivered, usually through the innominate. Our institution feels that by using RCP initially, much of the atheroembolic debris from aortic manipulation can be washed out before antegrade perfusion. See Fig. 7.2 for the cannulation strategy for the "Shaggy Aorta" protocol.

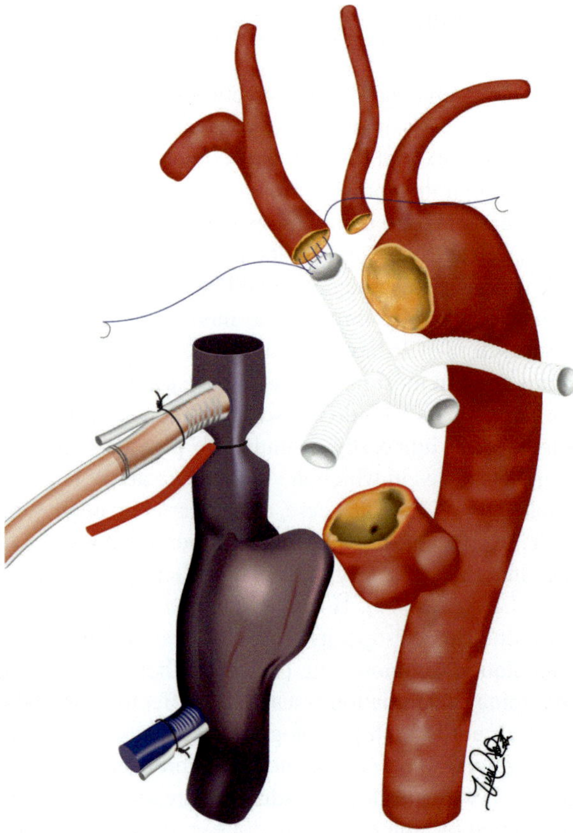

Fig. 7.2 Cannulation strategy for the "Shaggy Aorta" protocol during circulatory arrest with superior vena cava cannulation for retrograde cerebral perfusion and a trifurcated graft for antegrade cerebral perfusion

Complicating Factors

The modern era of aortic surgery and, more specifically, aortic arch surgery is often undertaken for patients in the setting of prior cardiac procedures. Progressive arch degeneration after hemiarch replacement for acute aortic dissection is common, as is prior coronary arterial bypass with subsequent development of intrinsic aortic pathology, among others. These prior procedures induce technical complicating factors which should be carefully considered prior to intervention on the remaining aortic pathology. One such consideration, which is of particular concern in patients with prior ascending aortic intervention (including hemiarch, ascending aortic replacement, and Bentall with associated ascending aortic replacement), is the length of the ascending aortic graft. In those patients whose prior procedure was performed with a short, single segment of synthetic graft (as opposed to separate proximal and distal grafts which are sewn with a graft-to-graft anastomosis), the remaining ascending aortic graft can be prohibitively shortened as it becomes incorporated into the surrounding scar tissue. In these situations, adequate room for aortic cannulation, cross-clamping, and cannulation for antegrade cardioplegic arrest can be challenging without encroaching on the residual diseased aortic arch. Utilization of retrograde cardioplegic arrest can afford some real estate in some individuals, and is useful in those who have root degeneration and aortic insufficiency following prior aortic intervention, however this space increase is not adequate for all. Aortic arch cannulation is tempting in some individuals with residual aneurysmal disease, however caution must be used in this approach given the fragility of the aortic arch tissue, particularly if total arch replacement is not already planned. For individuals with aneurysmal disease or persistent dissection which spares the innominate artery, cannulation of the innominate after end-to-side anastomosis of a 10 mm Dacron graft can be a useful and expedient method for establishing arterial inflow without the need for a separate axillary incision and exposure.

Prior coronary artery bypass grafts provide an additional challenge in reoperative aortic surgery. Preoperative assessment of the patency and lie of these grafts via coronary protocol computed tomography angiography is essential in operative planning, and patent grafts should be preserved if possible. Prior left internal mammary grafts rarely infringe on the operative field, but can be encountered during more distal zone 2 arch dissection and should be mobilized to allow for occlusion during cardiac protection. Patent-free arterial and venous grafts originating from the ascending aorta should be preserved through reimplantation. This is facilitated by excision of a button of native aortic wall, or ascending graft material, which is then reimplanted into the new synthetic aortic graft. Care should be taken to limit mobilize these coronary grafts to a distance required for tension-free reconstruction, as further mobilization only increases the risk of graft injury. All patients should undergo full bilateral lower extremity prep to allow for harvesting of additional vein graft if needed.

Previous felt can prove to be a substantial challenge in the reoperative setting. While useful during the primary procedure, it can severely obscure and hinder reestablishment of dissection planes. For these reasons, we aim to limit felt use during primary aortic procedures for aneurysmal disease, and use it sparingly in the setting of dissection. Preoperative axial imaging can often suggest the presence of significant felt, even when not highlighted in the prior operative records. Careful dissection should be conducted at dense felt locations, and when these areas involve the distal ascending aorta the surgeon should be prepared for inadvertent entry into the aorta and not undertake this mobilization until the patient is in a position where circulatory arrest can be initiated.

Commonly, in reoperative aortic surgery, dense adhesions can develop between the prior ascending aortic graft and both the main pulmonary artery as well as the right pulmonary artery as it passes posterior to the aorta. Early implementation of cardiopulmonary bypass and dissection of these tissue planes facilitates avoidance of injury by decompression of the pulmonary arterial system as well as allows for simple suture repair if injury does occur, as the decompressed pulmonary artery is much less likely to propagate an injury.

Facilitating Factors

When there is ample space for cannulation and cross-clamping, prior ascending aortic grafts can be very helpful both in proximal and distal reoperative aortic surgery. When intervening more distally in the aorta, there is little need for extensive mobilization of the proximal aortic graft; the final graft can be trimmed to an adequate length to join with the previously placed graft. Similarly, in the setting of interval root degeneration or other proximal intervention, a prior distal anastomotic graft should be used and a graft-to-graft anastomosis performed to simplify the overall reconstruction. In the setting of a degenerated prior bioprosthetic Bentall procedure, or replacement of a mechanical Bentall, the prior root graft does not need to be excised completely. Instead, it can be opened distally and the dysfunctional valve can be excised sharply from its attachment to the composite root graft, including all of the valve sewing ring, and a new valve placed directly into this root graft with interrupted mattress sutures similar to a primary aortic valve replacement.

Zone 1 and Zone 2 Arch

Zone 1 and 2 arch replacement for both aneurysmal disease and dissection is approached via a standard median sternotomy with continuous neuro monitoring. In the event of prior cardiac procedures preoperative imaging, specifically the preoperative axial imaging of the chest, is closely studied and the risk for reentry is assessed with planning made for peripheral cardiopulmonary bypass via the femoral arteries if needed emergently. Otherwise, the routine approach is for central cannulation rather than axial cannulation for arterial flow. For root and arch interventions, the heart is mobilized only along the right atrium, superior vena cava, and base of the heart. Mobilization of the left ventricular apex is not necessary for exposure and only poses risk for inadvertent injury.

Cannulation is performed centrally in almost all cases, even in the event of acute or chronic dissection, where epi-aortic ultrasound is utilized for needle and wire-guided cannulation of the true lumen. In the event of a prior hemiarch, the graft is cannulated directly. A standard two-stage venous cannula is placed in the right atrium and the patient is cooled to a temperature of 28 degrees C. During this cooling period, the aortic arch is dissected free for debranching. Judicious use of cautery is performed to avoid inadvertent thermal injury and in the event of deep dissection distally on the arch vessels, avoid injury to recurrent nerve structures. Once dissected free, a 30 mm stapling device is utilized to separate the innominate artery from its aortic origin. This is then suspended using a vascular clamp and trimmed back to reasonable arterial tissue. Prior to division of the artery, attention is directed to the near infrared spectral monitoring on that side to ensure there are no drops in saturation while clamped. A multibranched Spielvogel graft is then anastomosed to the innominate artery and Y'd into the arterial perfusion circuit. This allows antegrade perfusion of the innominate artery once this graft is de-aired that is continuous for the remainder of the procedure. A similar procedure is performed on the left carotid artery at its origin, and an additional limb of the Spielvogel graft is utilized to reperfuse this arch vessel. Importantly, this limb is left somewhat redundant to allow for the predictable retraction of the left carotid artery on release of the vascular clamps to prevent tension at its final resting point.

At this point, the patient has reached a core temperature of 28 degrees C. It is our preference to combine both antegrade cerebral perfusion with retrograde cerebral perfusion during circulatory arrest, and so a purse string is placed in the superior vena cava to allow for a 24 French right-angle cannula at this location. This is connected to the arterial circuit and deaired. Once EEG silence is achieved, circulatory arrest starting with at least 3–10 min of retrograde cerebral protection via the SVC is initiated with free drainage from the Spielvogel graft. A standard parachute distal anastomosis is constructed at zone 2 with a 3-branched Bavaria aortic graft and use of a felt strip reinforcement in the case of dissection. We do not routinely reinforce the anastomosis with felt in the setting of aneurysmal disease. Once 3–10 min of RCP has been achieved, antegrade perfusion is started via the Spielvogel graft for the remainder of circulatory arrest. Upon completion of the distal anastomosis, the aorta is deaired and reperfusion via a side arm is reestablished. A proximal anastomosis is constructed and any other proximal disease is dealt with on rewarming. The Spielvogel graft is then connected to a side branch of the Bavaria graft to reestablish continuity with the neo-aorta. It is important to ensure that you leave a 3–5 cm landing zone in case of future TEVAR. This proximalization of the takeoff of the innominate and left carotid allows for this landing zone for future TEVAR with coverage of the left subclavian. This left subclavian can then be managed with laser fenestration or with carotid subclavian bypass.

Zone 3 Arch

When reconstructing the arch at the zone 3 location, frozen elephant trunk (FET) is often a useful technique. FET can be important in dissection patients as many of these patients will go on to need a distal thoracic aortic repair and abdominal aortic repair. Because of the friability of dissected and aneurysmal tissue, the stent graft from the FET can act as an excellent landing zone for future TEVAR.

When approaching a repair extending through zone 3 of the aortic arch, or involving all branch vessels from the aortic arch, we begin the procedure as previously described for a zone two debranching and proximalization. See Fig. 7.3 for a step-by-step approach. Unlike a zone 2 repair, however, a stiff wire (260 cm Amplatz wire, straight tip) is passed via the common femoral artery into the aortic arch after heparinization for later use for antegrade stent deployment. In the situation of acute or chronic aortic dissection, IVUS is used regularly to confirm true lumen placement of this wire.

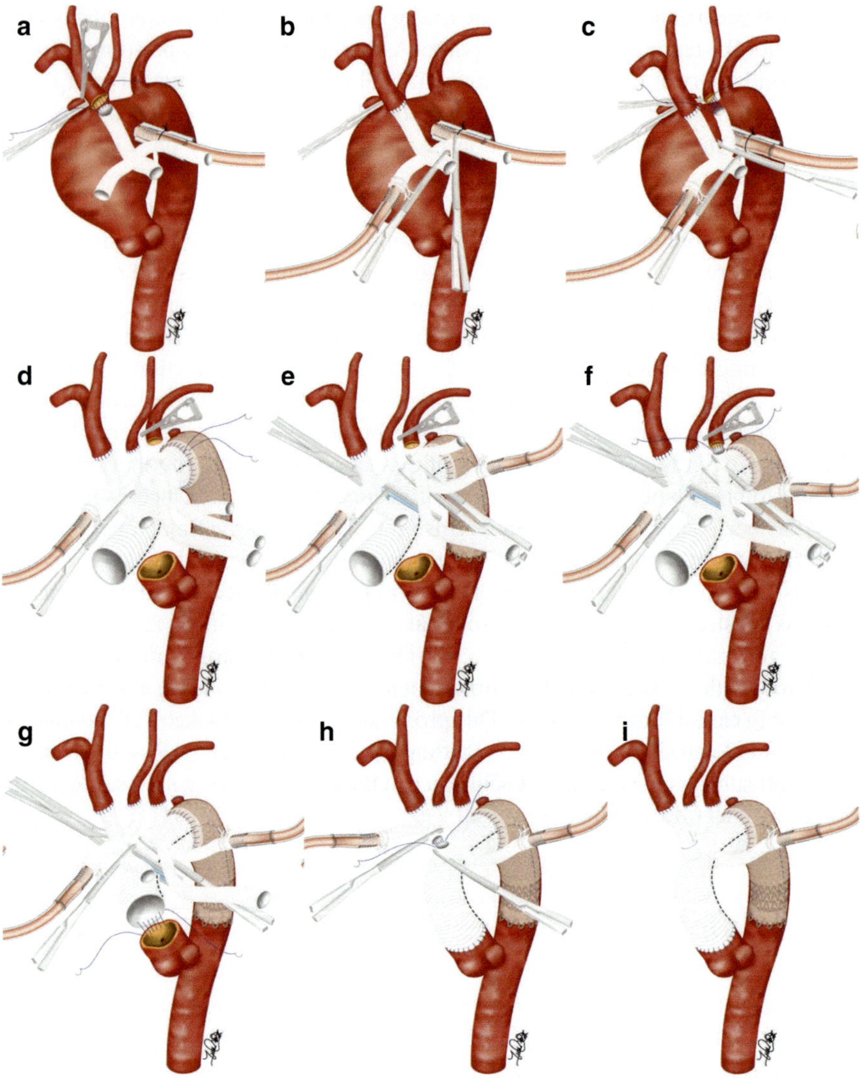

Fig. 7.3 Steps to a Zone 3 arch repair. (**a**) Innominate artery is stapled off and sutured to the branched Spielvogel graft. (**b**) Antegrade perfusion line is attached to the Spielvogel graft. (**c**) An anastomosis to the left carotid is performed to the sidearm of the graft. (**d**) Resection of the diseased aorta and Zone 2 Anastomosis to the elephant trunk graft. (**e**) Reperfusion through sidearm of the aortic graft. (**f**) Anastomosis of the sidearm of the aortic graft to the left subclavian. (**g**) Anastomosis of the proximal graft to the sinotubular junction. (**h**) Anastomosis of the proximal branch of the Spielvogel graft to the aortic graft. (**i**) Staple off the reperfusion limb of the aortic graft

Preoperative planning is critical in this situation, specifically paying close attention to the position and approach to the left subclavian artery as this is often very posterior and difficult to access. Moreover, when you add to the equation the friable nature of this vessel and its diseased character when dissected or aneurysmal, the left subclavian artery can be a point for significant bleeding. Three main options are available for debranching of the left subclavian: (1) direct reimplantation into the previously used Spielvogel graft in an end to end fashion (utilized when this vessel is not displaced posteriorly or leftward), (2) ligation of this vessel at the arch with tunneling of the perfusion limb of the Bavaria graft through the left second intercostal space for left axillary arterial anastomosis after weaning from CPB, or (3) left carotid subclavian bypass. To avoid difficulty with bleeding in the deep posterior mediastinum from this subclavian anastomosis, alternative routes for revascularization should be used somewhat liberally.

Once the arch has been completely debranched and isolated perfusion via the Spielvogel graft has been established, attention is directed to the distal anastomosis. Similar to zone 2 repair, combined antegrade and retrograde cerebral perfusion is utilized during circulatory arrest via the Spielvogel graft and superior vena cava, respectively. A composite graft is fashioned using the Bavaria graft cut approximately 30 mm distal to the 10 mm perfusion side port and a preoperatively selected thoracic endovascular stent graft, most often 10 cm in length. A purse string is placed in the Bavaria graft to facilitate its placement in the transected aorta and adherence to the stent graft during deployment. This device is set aside prepared for circulatory arrest.

During circulatory arrest, the aorta is resected only back to the level of zone 2 to facilitate ease of anastomosis. The previously placed femoral wire is located in the true lumen of the aorta and length is pulled proximally to allow for loading of the antegrade stent over this wire. The Bavaria graft and stent device is then advanced into the aorta over this wire and stent deployed to overlap and sandwich the Bavaria graft between the aorta and stent graft at the level of the transected aorta. The stent is then deployed and a running distal anastomosis reinforced with felt incorporating all layers of the device and aorta is constructed. The aorta is deaired and, similar to a zone 2 repair, the remaining necessary proximal interventions are addressed on rewarming. The debranched head vessels are again anastomosed via the Spielvogel graft to a side limb of the Bavaria graft.

Conclusion

Aortic arch pathology is a challenging clinical situation requiring adequate diagnostic modalities and preoperative planning. CTA of the head, neck, and chest should be utilized in order to fully understand the anatomy before planning the operation. The risk of catastrophe in reoperative cases should be carefully evaluated and planned for if necessary. Swallow evaluation can be done to risk-stratify patients for post-operative recurrent laryngeal nerve injury. Intraoperative monitoring, including multiple locations of arterial lines and NIOM, is important to properly assess hemodynamics and potential ischemic insults. Further, adequate cerebral protection is critical during these cases to limit the intraoperative and postoperative stroke risk. Finally, expert-level understanding of the operative steps of different arch repairs is crucial so that the surgeon is able to decrease operative time and improvise if needed.

References

1. Gouveia EMR, Silva Duarte G, Lopes A, Alves M, Caldeira D, Fernandes EFR, et al. Incidence and prevalence of thoracic aortic aneurysms: a systematic review and meta-analysis of population-based studies. Semin Thorac Cardiovasc Surg. 2022;34(1):1–16.
2. Hiratzka LF, Bakris GL, Beckman JA, Bersin RM, Carr VF, Casey DE Jr, et al. 2010 ACCF/AHA/AATS/ACR/ASA/SCA/SCAI/SIR/STS/SVM guidelines for the diagnosis and management of patients with thoracic aortic disease: executive summary. A report of the American College of Cardiology Foundation/American Heart Association Task Force on Practice Guidelines, American Association for Thoracic Surgery, American College of Radiology, American Stroke Association, Society of Cardiovascular Anesthesiologists, Society for Cardiovascular Angiography and Interventions, Society of Interventional Radiology, Society of Thoracic Surgeons, and Society for Vascular Medicine. Catheter Cardiovasc Interv. 2010;76(2):E43–86.
3. Horiuchi T, Kawaguchi M, Inoue S, Hayashi H, Abe R, Tabayashi N, et al. Assessment of intraoperative motor evoked potentials for predicting postoperative paraplegia in thoracic and thoracoabdominal aortic aneurysm repair. J Anesth. 2011;25(1):18–28.
4. Tanaka Y, Kawaguchi M, Noguchi Y, Yoshitani K, Kawamata M, Masui K, et al. Systematic review of motor evoked potentials monitoring during thoracic and thoracoabdominal aortic aneurysm open repair surgery: a diagnostic meta-analysis. J Anesth. 2016;30(6):1037–50.
5. Weigang E, Hartert M, Siegenthaler MP, Pitzer-Hartert K, Luehr M, Sircar R, et al. Neurophysiological monitoring during thoracoabdominal aortic endovascular stent graft implantation. Eur J Cardiothorac Surg. 2006;29(3):392–6.
6. Ghincea CV, Anderson DA, Ikeno Y, Roda GF, Eldeiry M, Bronsert MR, et al. Utility of neuromonitoring in hypothermic circulatory arrest cases for early detection of stroke: listening through the noise. J Thorac Cardiovasc Surg. 2021;162(4):1035–45.e5.
7. Olsson C, Thelin S. Regional cerebral saturation monitoring with near-infrared spectroscopy during selective antegrade cerebral perfusion: diagnostic performance and relationship to postoperative stroke. J Thorac Cardiovasc Surg. 2006;131(2):371–9.
8. Orihashi K, Sueda T, Okada K, Imai K. Near-infrared spectroscopy for monitoring cerebral ischemia during selective cerebral perfusion. Eur J Cardiothorac Surg. 2004;26(5):907–11.
9. Cheung AT, Pochettino A, McGarvey ML, Appoo JJ, Fairman RM, Carpenter JP, et al. Strategies to manage paraplegia risk after endovascular stent repair of descending thoracic aortic aneurysms. Ann Thorac Surg. 2005;80(4):1280–8; discussion 8–9.
10. Sandhu HK, Tanaka A, Zaidi ST, Perlick A, Miller CC, Safi HJ, et al. Impact of redo sternotomy on proximal aortic repair: does previous aortic repair affect outcomes? J Thorac Cardiov Sur. 2020;159(5):1683–91.
11. Michenfelder JD, Milde JH. The relationship among canine brain temperature, metabolism, and function during hypothermia. Anesthesiology. 1991;75(1):130–6.
12. Ziganshin BA, Rajbanshi BG, Tranquilli M, Fang H, Rizzo JA, Elefteriades JA. Straight deep hypothermic circulatory arrest for cerebral protection during aortic arch surgery: safe and effective. J Thorac Cardiovasc Surg. 2014;148(3):888–98; discussion 98–900.

13. Centofanti P, Barbero C, D'Agata F, Caglio MM, Caroppo P, Cicerale A, et al. Neurologic and cognitive outcomes after aortic arch operation with hypothermic circulatory arrest. Surgery. 2016;160(3):796–804.
14. Milewski RK, Pacini D, Moser GW, Moeller P, Cowie D, Szeto WY, et al. Retrograde and antegrade cerebral perfusion: results in short elective arch reconstructive times. Ann Thorac Surg. 2010;89(5):1448–57.
15. Spielvogel D, Kai M, Tang GH, Malekan R, Lansman SL. Selective cerebral perfusion: a review of the evidence. J Thorac Cardiovasc Surg. 2013;145(3 Suppl):S59–62.
16. Leontyev S, Davierwala PM, Semenov M, von Aspern K, Krog G, Noack T, et al. Antegrade selective cerebral perfusion reduced in-hospital mortality and permanent focal neurological deficit in patients with elective aortic arch surgerydagger. Eur J Cardiothorac Surg. 2019;56(5):1001–8.
17. Kim JH, Lee SH, Lee S, Youn YN, Yoo KJ, Joo HC. Axillary artery cannulation reduces early embolic stroke and mortality after open arch repair with circulatory arrest. J Thorac Cardiovasc Surg. 2020;159(3):772–8.e4.
18. Harky A, Chan JS, Bithas C, Hof A, Sharif M, Froghi S, et al. Innominate vs. axillary artery cannulation in aortic surgery: a systematic review and meta-analysis. Braz J Cardiovasc Surg. 2019;34(2):213–21.
19. Tang GH, Kai M, Malekan R, Lansman SL, Spielvogel D. Trifurcated graft replacement of the aortic arch: state of the art. J Thorac Cardiovasc Surg. 2015;149(2 Suppl):S55–8.

Chapter 8
Hybrid Aortic Arch Reconstruction

Joshua C. Grimm, Karen Kim, and George J. Arnaoutakis

Abbreviations

DTA	descending thoracic aorta
FET	frozen elephant trunk
HCA	hypothermic circulatory arrest
LCCA	left common carotid artery
LSA	left subclavian artery
LZ	landing zone
NIOM	neurophysiologic intraoperative monitoring
TBE	thoracic branch endograft
TEVAR	thoracic endovascular aortic repair

J. C. Grimm (✉) · K. Kim · G. J. Arnaoutakis
Division of Cardiovascular and Thoracic Surgery, Department of Cardiovascular and Thoracic Surgery, University of Texas Dell Medical School at Austin, Austin, TX, USA
e-mail: Joshua.Grimm@austin.utexas.edu; Karen.Kim@austin.utexas.edu; george.arnaoutakis@austin.utexas.edu

G. J. Arnaoutakis et al. (eds.), *Aortic Aneurysms*, Contemporary Cardiology,
https://doi.org/10.1007/978-3-032-13134-8_8

Background

The standard, historical management of arch and descending thoracic aortic (DTA) pathology (acute and chronic dissection and aneurysmal degeneration) had involved a multi-staged procedure, requiring an arch reconstruction utilizing hypothermic circulatory arrest (HCA) followed by a period of convalescence prior to an open thoracoabdominal repair. Even in contemporary series, the intraprocedural mortality remains high and long-term survival low [1].

Accordingly, there has been increased momentum to incorporate endografts into arch and proximal DTA reconstructions. In the late 1990s, Buth described a double transposition of the left subclavian and common carotid arteries, and subsequent retrograde thoracic endovascular aortic repair (TEVAR) [2]. The first report utilizing a stented graft in an antegrade fashion was published by Kato and colleagues [3], while the "frozen elephant trunk" technique gained further popularity following an extensive literature review by Karck [4]. Saleh contributed one of the largest, initial series describing a true hybrid arch repair (HAR) in which patients underwent surgical debranching of all supra-aortic vessels to the native ascending aorta with concomitant external banding of the aorta to ensure secure fixation of the stent graft [5]. While the results were published nearly two decades ago, the excellent short- and intermediate-term outcomes supported the feasibility of marrying open arch techniques with endovascular stenting to tailor operative strategies based on patient-specific factors.

Regardless of the specific strategy employed, the premise of a hybrid technique revolves around proximalizing the supra-aortic branch vessels to create an adequate landing zone for a stent graft. The following will outline the basic anatomic considerations of the various approaches as well as specific technical nuances such as options for management of the left subclavian artery.

Arch Classifications and Zones

When evaluating a patient for a hybrid procedure, the orientation of the supra-aortic branch vessels in relation to the apex of the arch can help dictate the surgical approach. Reference lines (diameter of the left or right common carotid artery) are drawn in a horizontal fashion from the top of the arch downward. In a type 1 arch, all three vessels arise from the same plane at the apex of the arch. This can make debranching without the assistance of cardiopulmonary bypass challenging. In a type 2 arch, the vessels arise within 1 line from the top of the arch. In a type 3, or steepled arch, the vessels arise within 2 lines. The latter is advantageous in regard to branch vessel accessibility, but can prove problematic in ensuring an adequate seal following TEVAR if a portion of the arch is not reconstructed.

The classification system outlined by Ishimaru in 2001 remains the anatomic descriptor of arch zones utilized for open reconstruction and endovascular stenting.

- Zone 0: Ascending aorta and origin of innominate artery
- Zone 1: Origin of the left common carotid artery (LCCA)
- Zone 2: Origin of the left subclavian artery (LSA)
- Zone 3: 2-cm distal to LSA [6]

Hybrid Arch Classification Systems

One of the initial, and perhaps the most straightforward, schemes was proposed by Bavaria et al. [7, 8]. It classified arch interventions into three "types" based on the extent of the open aortic reconstruction performed as well as the adjuncts utilized during the procedure. With ongoing advances in stent-graft design, including branched endoprostheses, Hughes and colleagues introduced the concepts of "zones", in which a landing zone is created and defined by the aforementioned Ishimaru classifications without a median sternotomy [9].

Type 1 HAR

In a Type 1 HAR, the aortopathy is largely limited to the arch and proximal descending thoracic aorta, allowing for debranching of the supra-aortic vessels to "healthy", non-aneurysmal, ascending aorta. This can typically be achieved with a partially occlusive clamp with sequential branch vessel anastomoses. Test clamping with the assistance of neurophysiologic intraoperative monitoring (NIOM, discussed at greater length below) can determine the safety of this approach. An antegrade TEVAR can then be deployed through an additional anteflow limb or in a more conventional, retrograde fashion (concomitant or subsequent procedure).

The success of this strategy is limited by the length and diameter of the proximal landing zone (LZ). The former was elegantly demonstrated by Ganapathi et al., who found that while the proximal endoleak rate (1a) was similar in native aorta and Dacron, results were dependent upon institutional experience and improved when the Dacron LZ was more robust (4–5 cm) [10]. While this study was not limited to complex arch reconstructions, it highlights an important concept which must be considered, especially in the repair of acute, Type A aortic dissections. Failure to create an adequate proximal LZ during any indexed arch procedure could severely limit, or even preclude, endovascular options in the future. In regard to proximal aortic diameter, Williams and colleagues revealed a noticeably high rate of retrograde, Type A aortic dissections in patients with native aortic diameters >40 mm (4.8% v. 0.9%, $p < 0.05$). This devastating complication was more common in the dissection cohort (native aorta >40 mm: 11.8%), especially in Zone 0 cases (25%) [11].

Type II HAR

In patients with ascending or proximal arch pathology, a Type II HAR provides a more reliable proximal LZ for subsequent TEVAR. With this approach, an open distal anastomosis in Zone 0, 1, or 2 is performed with selective debranching, or proximalization, of all, or some portion, of the supra-aortic branch vessels. This is performed under hypothermic circulatory arrest (moderate or deep), typically with some form of adjunctive cerebral perfusion strategy (retrograde or antegrade). The cadence of the operation is highly variable with brain- and body-first approaches both demonstrating excellent outcomes in experienced centers. Multiple studies have illustrated similar outcomes in hemiarch v. extended arch interventions, even in acute, Type A aortic dissection [12, 13]. As in Type I HAR, an appropriate LZ of at least 30 mm should be incorporated into the arch reconstruction.

Type III HAR

This represents the most invasive variant of HAR as it features a conventional, free-floating or frozen elephant trunk (FET) as a component of the total arch repair. Despite it requiring revascularization of all the branch vessels, it does not mandate a Zone 3 anastomosis. The evolution of this strategy to include an endovascular platform during the indexed procedure has simplified access to the trunk during subsequent TEVAR. A meta-analysis published by the Canadian Thoracic Aortic Collaborative suggested lower mortality, but increased spinal cord ischemia, in patients undergoing FET [14]. The frozen technique can be accomplished via antegrade deployment of any of the commercially available TEVAR stents. More recently, the Thoraflex™ Hybrid prosthesis (Terumo Aortic, FL) has obtained US FDA approval for implantation in degenerative aneurysms as well as acute and chronic dissections. It is comprised of a Gelweave™ surgical graft sealed to a nitinol ringed stent graft. In dissection cases, it is critical to ensure the stent is deployed entirely in the true lumen. This can be accomplished with echocardiographic or intravascular ultrasound-guided confirmation of wire position within the correct lumen. It is our strategy to perform these procedures with a "head-first" approach and utilize a debranching limb that serves to both proximalize the head vessels as well as to promptly establish antegrade cerebral perfusion during HCA (Fig. 8.1).

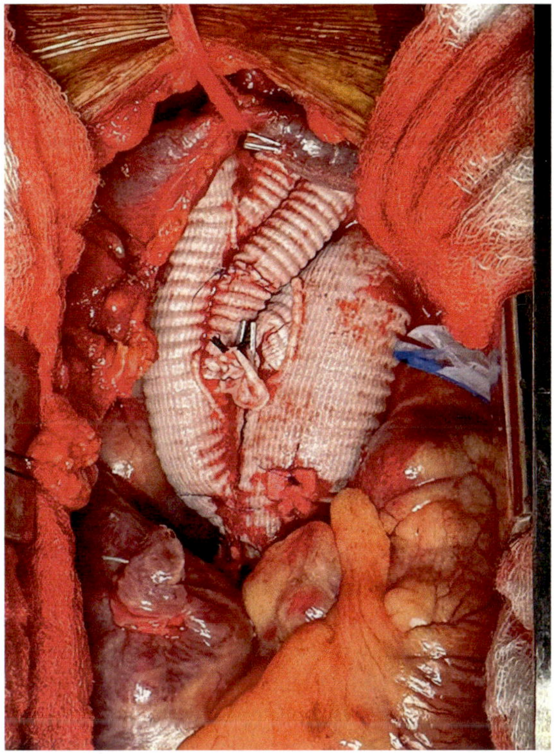

Fig. 8.1 Type III HAR utilizing a debranching limb. Frozen elephant trunk not visualized in image

Considerations for the Left Subclavian Artery

Management of the LSA can complicate HAR, especially in emergent scenarios. There are, however, several options, which can be employed pre-, intra-, and post-operatively to address the LSA in a safe manner. If the procedure is semi-elective, a left carotid-subclavian artery bypass can be performed prior to the planned arch intervention. Additionally, this vessel can be anastomosed during the circulatory arrest if the arch anatomy and the patient's body habitus are favorable. If this is not feasible, an aorto-left axillary bypass can be performed via an infraclavicular incision and a tunneled graft through the left pleural space. Dr. Roselli's group has pioneered a novel technique, termed B-safer, which can be employed in Type III HAR. During hypothermic circulatory arrest, and following deployment of an antegrade TEVAR, a fenestration is fashioned overlying the LSA and a stent is placed into the branch vessel under direct visualization. While the short-term outcomes are promising (operative mortality 5.6%, any stroke 10.7%, disabling stroke 2.9%), this technique is highly nuanced and, therefore, the reproducibility is still unknown [15]. Fenestrations can also be performed with the assistance of laser technology during Zone 2 TEVAR. This is not possible with all stents due to inter-ring distance and stent graft composition. A similar strategy can be achieved with the GORE® TAG®

Thoracic Branch Endograft (TBE, Gore Medical, CA), which has an inner portal that is pre-cannulated for relatively straightforward side-branch stenting. Results from the pivotal study supported FDA approval [16]. Patel et al. published outcomes from the feasibility trial and demonstrated 100% branch vessel patency, 0% 30-day morbidity and mortality, and no persistent 1a endoleaks [17].

Zones 0 and 1 HAR

As previously stated, Hughes et al. proposed a slight modification to the more conventional HAR classification scheme to maintain relevance in an ever-expanding endovascular approach to arch pathology [9]. The "zone" refers to the proximal LZ. In Zone 1 HAR, the LCCA and LSA must be addressed with either carotid-subclavian and carotid-carotid extra-anatomical bypasses or a carotid-subclavian bypass and a branched endograft with a LCCA limb (Fig. 8.2). In Zone 0 HAR, the proximal LZ is within the ascending aorta, so all of the supra-aortic branch vessels require attention. This can be achieved with a double extra-anatomic bypass and an innominate artery snorkel or single-branched endograft. There are several investigational arch devices (i.e., Terumo Aortic Dual Branch and Cook Arch Graft) with multiple channels or branches, but none have achieved FDA approval to date. Haulon and colleagues recently published one of the most exhaustive meta-analyses on the available stent graft options (both single and multi-branch endoprostheses) [18]. Most all of these devices are unavailable in the United States. As briefly mentioned above, the GORE® TBE had excellent outcomes in Zone 2 scenarios and was used off-label in Zones 0 and 1 in a smaller subset of patients [17]. The only

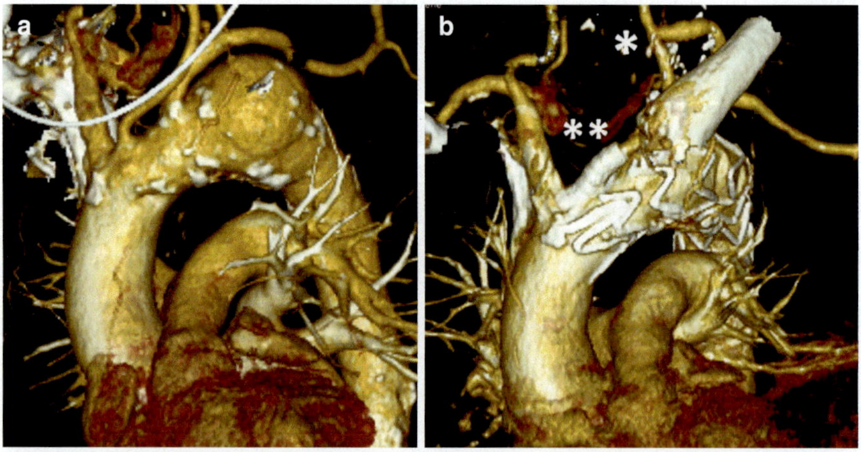

Fig. 8.2 (**a**) Preoperative CTA in high-risk surgical patient demonstrating Type III arch with minimal proximal seal in Zone 2. (**b**) Postoperative CTA following Zone 1 HAR with left carotid-subclavian bypass (*) and Zone 1 TEVAR with left common carotid snorkel (**)

single-branch stent graft currently intended for Zone 0 deployment is the NEXUS (Jotec, GE) arch endograft. The initial, published data on 28 patients revealed a high success rate and acceptable 30-day and 1-year all-cause mortality (7.1% and 10%, respectively) [19].

Complications

In high volume centers, the morbidity and mortality associated with Type II and III HAR remain low and are well documented. Outcomes in endo-forward (Zone 0-1 HAR) approaches are more variable as these techniques are largely institution and operator-dependent. This was illustrated in a large retrospective analysis from Duke, which demonstrated dramatic reductions in mortality (early and late) and stroke in the first and second halves of the study period [20].

Stroke

The etiology of stroke in arch interventions is undoubtedly multifactorial and includes atheromatous disease, branch vessel malperfusion (static or dynamic) and manipulation, and completeness of collateral networks. Several interoperative tools are available to provide NIOM during open and endovascular repairs. While there remains no consensus on the benefit of any of these adjuncts and utilization is highly variable, routine application of NIOM can provide some insight into major intraoperative complications and guide postoperative vigilance. In an extensive, institutional analysis by Ghincea and colleagues, NIOM had a sensitivity of 75%, specificity of 88.5%, PPV of 27.3%, and a NPV 97.9% [21]. Other centers employ BIS and cerebral oximetry to dictate adequate cooling prior to circulatory arrest.

Spinal Cord Ischemia

Spinal cord perfusion relies on a complex array of vessels, including the internal iliacs, intercostals, lumbars, and subclavian. Pathologic involvement in any of these vessels (i.e., dissection) or baseline disease (i.e., atheroma or dense calcium). As such, it is difficult to predict ischemic insults, but extended coverage obviously confers a greater risk for spinal cord injury. This is an especially important consideration during frozen elephant trunk procedures (Type II and III HAR), where stent lengths should be limited to <150 mm to minimize the spinal cord risk [22]. The utilization of elective spinal cord drainage is controversial, especially in circulatory arrest procedures, and the decision should be based on patient-specific factors, such as prior endovascular aortic repair, diseased internal iliac arteries, or complete false lumen thrombosis. Intraoperative hemostasis is critical as postoperative hemorrhage can precipitate hypotension and result in a second-hit to cord perfusion. Moreover, the ability to rescue with hypertension (mean arterial pressure targets 80–100 mmHg) and urgent lumbar drainage is paramount and can salvage patients from this devastating complication.

Summary

HAR has revolutionized the management of aortic arch and proximal descending thoracic aortic pathology. Adverse outcomes can be minimized if the tenets of circulatory arrest and brain and spinal cord protection are followed. As platforms continue to evolve toward a total endovascular solution, it is imperative that appropriate candidates are selected for these procedures as outcomes following conventional, open arch interventions remain favorable.

References

1. Etz CD, Plestis KA, Kari FA, et al. Staged repair of thoracic and thoracoabdominal aortic aneurysms using the elephant trunk technique: a consecutive series of 215 first stage and 120 complete repairs. Eur J Cardiothorac Surg. 2008;34(3):605–14; discussion 614–5. https://doi.org/10.1016/j.ejcts.2008.04.045.
2. Buth J, Penn O, Tielbeek A, Mersman M. Combined approach to stent-graft treatment of an aortic arch aneurysm. J Endovasc Surg. 1998;5(4):329–32. https://doi.org/10.1583/1074-6218(1998)005<0329:CATSGT>2.0.CO;2.
3. Kato M, Ohnishi K, Kaneko M, et al. New graft-implanting method for thoracic aortic aneurysm or dissection with a stented graft. Circulation. 1996;94(9 Suppl):II188–93.
4. Karck M, Kamiya H. Progress of the treatment for extended aortic aneurysms; is the frozen elephant trunk technique the next standard in the treatment of complex aortic disease including the arch? Eur J Cardiothorac Surg. 2008;33(6):1007–13. https://doi.org/10.1016/j.ejcts.2008.02.030.
5. Saleh HM, Inglese L. Combined surgical and endovascular treatment of aortic arch aneurysms. J Vasc Surg. 2006;44(3):460–6. https://doi.org/10.1016/j.jvs.2006.04.057.
6. Mitchell RS, Ishimaru S, Ehrlich MP, et al. First international summit on thoracic aortic endografting: roundtable on thoracic aortic dissection as an indication for endografting. J Endovasc Ther. 2002;9(Suppl 2):II98–105.
7. Bavaria J, Milewski RK, Baker J, Moeller P, Szeto W, Pochettino A. Classic hybrid evolving approach to distal arch aneurysms: toward the zone zero solution. J Thorac Cardiovasc Surg. 2010;140(6 Suppl):S77–80; discussion S86–91. https://doi.org/10.1016/j.jtcvs.2010.07.031.
8. Szeto WY, Bavaria JE. Hybrid repair of aortic arch aneurysms: combined open arch reconstruction and endovascular repair. Semin Thorac Cardiovasc Surg. 2009;21(4):347–54. https://doi.org/10.1053/j.semtcvs.2009.11.007.
9. Hughes GC, Vekstein A. Current state of hybrid solutions for aortic arch aneurysms. Ann Cardiothorac Surg. 2021;10(6):731–43. https://doi.org/10.21037/acs-2021-taes-168.
10. Ganapathi AM, Andersen ND, Hanna JM, Gaca JG, McCann RL, Hughes GC. Comparison of attachment site endoleak rates in Dacron versus native aorta landing zones after tho-

racic endovascular aortic repair. J Vasc Surg. 2014;59(4):921–9. https://doi.org/10.1016/j.jvs.2013.10.086.
11. Williams JB, Andersen ND, Bhattacharya SD, et al. Retrograde ascending aortic dissection as an early complication of thoracic endovascular aortic repair. J Vasc Surg. 2012;55(5):1255–62. https://doi.org/10.1016/j.jvs.2011.11.063.
12. Elbatarny M, Stevens LM, Dagenais F, et al. Hemiarch versus extended arch repair for acute type A dissection: results from a multicenter national registry. J Thorac Cardiovasc Surg. Published online April 20, 2023. https://doi.org/10.1016/j.jtcvs.2023.04.012.
13. Fichadiya A, Gregory AJ, Kotha VK, et al. Extended-arch repair for acute type-A aortic dissection: perioperative and mid-term results. Eur J Cardiothorac Surg. 2019;56(4):714–21. https://doi.org/10.1093/ejcts/ezz071.
14. Hanif H, Dubois L, Ouzounian M, et al. Aortic arch reconstructive surgery with conventional techniques vs frozen elephant trunk: a systematic review and meta-analysis. Can J Cardiol. 2018;34(3):262–73. https://doi.org/10.1016/j.cjca.2017.12.020.
15. Roselli EE, Vargo PR, Bakaeen F, et al. Branched stented anastomosis frozen elephant trunk repair: early results from a physician-sponsored investigational device exemption study. J Thorac Cardiovasc Surg. Published online October 5, 2023. https://doi.org/10.1016/j.jtcvs.2023.09.069.
16. FDA Gore TBE Approval. https://www.accessdata.fda.gov/scripts/cdrh/cfdocs/cfpma/pma.cfm?id=P210032. Accessed 10 Jan 2024.
17. Patel HJ, Dake MD, Bavaria JE, et al. Branched endovascular therapy of the distal aortic arch: preliminary results of the feasibility multicenter trial of the gore thoracic branch endoprosthesis. Ann Thorac Surg. 2016;102(4):1190–8. https://doi.org/10.1016/j.athoracsur.2016.03.091.
18. Nana P, Tyrrell MR, Guihaire J, et al. A review: single and multibranch devices for the treatment of aortic arch pathologies with proximal sealing in Ishimaru Zone 0. Ann Vasc Surg. 2023;94:45–55. https://doi.org/10.1016/j.avsg.2022.09.044.
19. Planer D, Elbaz-Greener G, Mangialardi N, et al. NEXUS arch: a multicenter study evaluating the initial experience with a novel aortic arch stent graft system. Ann Surg. 2023;277(2):e460–6. https://doi.org/10.1097/SLA.0000000000004843.
20. Vekstein AM, Jensen CW, Weissler EH, et al. Long-term outcomes for hybrid aortic arch repair. J Vasc Surg. Published online November 25, 2023. https://doi.org/10.1016/j.jvs.2023.11.032.
21. Ghincea CV, Anderson DA, Ikeno Y, et al. Utility of neuromonitoring in hypothermic circulatory arrest cases for early detection of stroke: listening through the noise. J Thorac Cardiovasc Surg. 2021;162(4):1035–1045.e5. https://doi.org/10.1016/j.jtcvs.2020.01.090.
22. Preventza O, Liao JL, Olive JK, et al. Neurologic complications after the frozen elephant trunk procedure: a meta-analysis of more than 3000 patients. J Thorac Cardiovasc Surg. 2020;160(1):20–33.e4. https://doi.org/10.1016/j.jtcvs.2019.10.031.

Chapter 9
Surgical Management of Type A Aortic Dissection

Derek Serna-Gallegos and Ibrahim Sultan

Past and Present

Acute type A aortic dissection (TAAD) has long been recognized as a deadly ailment. In 1628, Sennertus described an aortic dissection as a rupture of the internal "coat" with elevation and distension of the external "coat", a description that was supported later in 1804 by Scarpa [1]. The death of George II, King of England at Kensington Palace in 1760 may be one of the first documented deaths due to type A aortic dissection, with the diagnosis being made postmortem and reported by Nicholls [2]. Morgagni referenced the George II death as well as several other cases in 1760, yet it was Maunoir in 1802 who initially described the pathogenesis of aortic dissection [3, 4]. Seventeen years after Maunoir's description Laennec echoed the description and gave the condition a name, "aneurysme dissequant" allowing Laennec to take much of the credit for Maunoir's initial work [5]. Shekelton described a healed dissection, which was likely a patient who survived only due to a reentry tear that decompressed the false lumen and Pennock was the first to describe the condition in the American literature [6, 7]. Antemortem diagnosis of an aortic dissection was reported in 1855 by Swain et al. ushering in a new era where treatment as well as diagnosis of aortic dissection became possible [8]. Much of the initial management for aortic dissection was medical [9]. It wasn't until 1954 when Drs Michael DeBakey along with Denton Cooley and Oscar Creech Jr. performed the first successful aortic resection and reconstruction of an aortic dissection, which was a dissection of the descending thoracic aorta [10]. Michael DeBakey was himself affected by the disease late in life requiring colleagues to perform an operation he helped to establish as a treatment for the disease [10, 11].

D. Serna-Gallegos · I. Sultan (✉)
Division of Cardiac Surgery, Heart and Vascular Institute, University of Pittsburgh Medical Center, Pittsburgh, PA, USA
e-mail: Sernagallegosdr@upmc.edu; Sultani@upmc.edu

G. J. Arnaoutakis et al. (eds.), *Aortic Aneurysms*, Contemporary Cardiology,
https://doi.org/10.1007/978-3-032-13134-8_9

Aortic dissection, along with intramural hematoma, penetrating aortic ulcer, and ruptured aneurysm, make up the collection of diagnoses that account for acute aortic syndrome. Figure 9.1 demonstrates the anatomy of the thoracic aorta. The classic teaching regarding acute type A aortic dissection whereby mortality increases 1% per hour initially (with 50% mortality within 3 days and 80% mortality at 2 weeks) demonstrates the importance of prompt and definitive treatment [12]. Improved techniques and institution of neurophysiological monitoring along with cerebral perfusion during lower body circulatory arrest have improved outcomes over time with mortality of 10% or less able to be achieved at high volume centers [13, 14]. Prior reports had demonstrated the in-hospital mortality to be 20–30% [15–17]. Despite these advances persistent mortality rates of 10% in those fit enough to undergo surgery provides many opportunities for improvement in this difficult patient population. The creation of the International Registry of Acute Aortic Dissection (IRAD) in 1996 created a global collaboration that now consists of over 50 centers of excellence, all of whom are contributing to the understanding of aortic dissection and its prevention and treatment.

Several high-volume institutions have begun to explore the option of endovascular therapy for ascending aortic pathology due to the poor outcomes of medical management in patients with prohibitive risk for open surgery. Endovascular options may potentially provide an advantage over medical management for this cohort of patients. A review of 118 ascending endovascular aortic repair cases demonstrated type 1 endoleak in 18.6% of patients with 9.3% requiring reintervention with all-cause mortality of 15.2%, aorta-related mortality of 5% and 3.4% cerebrovascular complications [18]. Other single institution series have demonstrated similar results with the Cleveland Clinic reporting 30-day, 1-year, and 5-year overall survival of

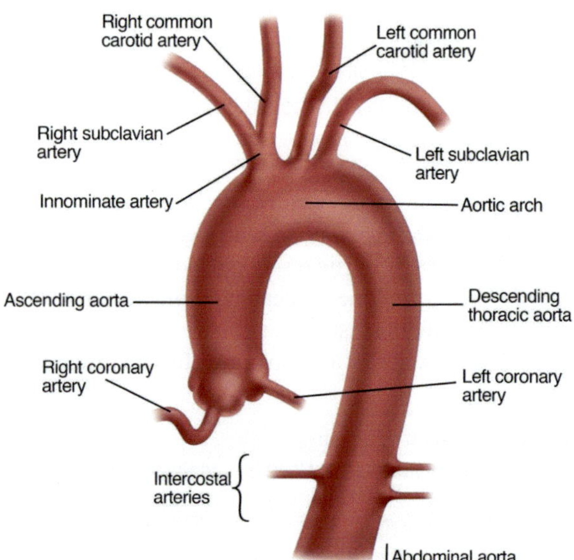

Fig. 9.1 Anatomy of thoracic aorta

81%, 74%, and 64% respectively, with rates of freedom from reintervention at those time periods of 85%, 77%, and 68% respectively [19]. The University of Maryland reported an operative mortality and stroke of 15% and 8% respectively with 70% of patients having no evidence of endoleak [20]. The group at Baylor College of Medicine demonstrated 66% overall survival after a median follow-up of 14.4 months with no aortic-related deaths [21]. Although endovascular treatment has been shown to be feasible, the long-term results are unclear and open surgical management of type A aortic dissection remains the standard of care for patients who can tolerate surgery.

Classification

Classification of ascending aortic dissection relies on two major categorizations: anatomy of the dissection and timing. Acute dissection previously described dissections which had been present for less than 14 days while chronic dissections constituted dissections that had been present for longer than 14 days [22]. Analysis of survival data by the IRAD demonstrated 4 distinct time periods which led to the proposal for a more detailed sub-characterization. The data demonstrated 4 time periods defined as hyperacute (<24 h from symptom onset), acute (2–7 days), subacute (8–30 days), and chronic (>30 days) [23]. Acute on chronic is generally defined as new intimal tears in a patient with a known chronic dissection.

The major anatomic systems for classification of ascending aortic dissection include the Stanford and DeBakey systems [24, 25]. Figure 9.2 demonstrates the Stanford and DeBakey classification systems for aortic dissection. There are advantages and disadvantages to both systems. The Stanford system relies on differentiating the dissection based on involvement of the ascending aorta. The Stanford classification is based on the observation that there are significant differences in mortality and treatment when the ascending aorta is involved in the dissection process. In their initial report of 35 patients with aortic dissection, they reported 25% in hospital mortality for surgically treated ascending aortic dissection versus 67% mortality with medical management. In patients with isolated descending aortic dissection beginning at or distal to the left subclavian artery they reported 28% in hospital mortality with surgical therapy and 20% mortality with medical therapy. These results led to their classification of type A and type B aortic dissection. Ascending aortic replacement for all ascending aortic dissections addresses the two most important complications of acute aortic dissection of the ascending aorta: rupture into the pericardium leading to pericardial tamponade and acute aortic regurgitation. This experience led the group at Stanford to operate emergently on all dissections involving the ascending aorta regardless of involvement of the descending aorta and to treat all isolated descending aortic dissections medically unless malperfusion, rupture, or another complication was present.

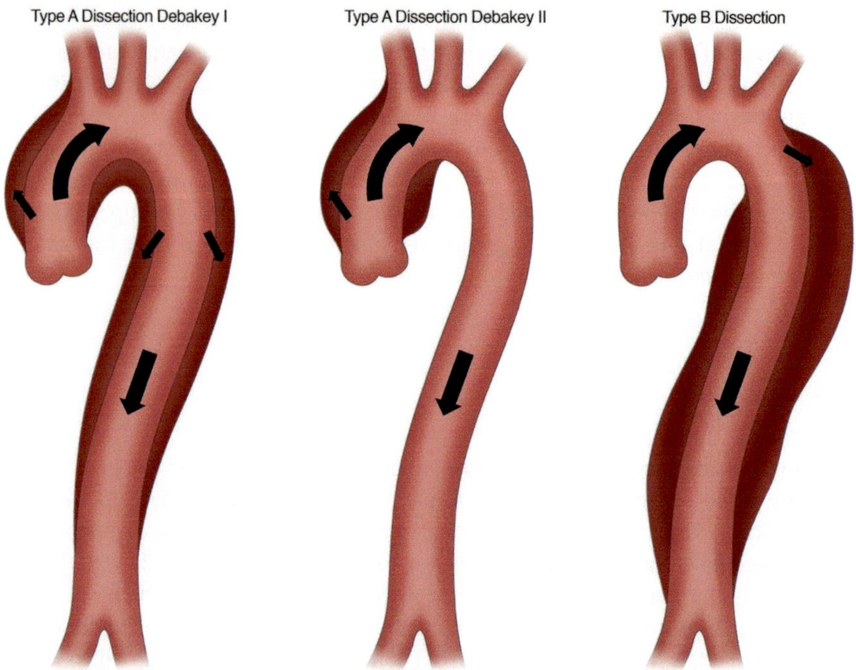

Fig. 9.2 This image demonstrates the Stanford (Type A and B)and DeBakey (I, II, III) classification for aortic dissection

The DeBakey classification includes 3 types of aortic dissection based on the distal extent of the dissection. The Stanford group argued that therapeutic decisions based on prognosis were not made with consideration of the distal extent of the dissection, but instead are made based on the proximal extent of disease. The initial manuscript describing the 3 classifications of aortic dissection described 3 different operations for each classification. For type I the group reported transection of the ascending aorta between clamps, re-approximation of the intima, media, and adventitia with running suture and re-anastomosis of the aorta usually without resection or interposition graft. Interposition graft was used only in cases where there was extensive mural disruption. In type II dissection they describe interposition graft with resection and a clamped distal anastomosis and for type III they describe resection with interposition graft of the descending thoracic aorta [25]. The operation described for type I aortic dissection is largely historical and is not often practiced today as it does not address the most important consideration in aortic dissection surgery which is resection or coverage of the primary intimal tear. While both classifications have value, the Stanford classification is more widely used. When a more accurate anatomical description is necessary the DeBakey classification is useful, however when determining the course of therapy the Stanford classification remains relevant in its simplicity and clinical significance. More recent classifications have also focused on the site of primary intimal tear, yet they have not been utilized to the same extent as the DeBakey and Stanford classification [26, 27].

Presentation and Diagnosis

Aortic dissection has earned its nickname as the "great masquerader" through frequent rates of misdiagnosis. A recent meta-analysis found that 1 in 3 patients with aortic dissection is initially misdiagnosed [28, 29]. The cause for frequent misdiagnosis rests in the variable presentation of the disease, which can include chest pain, back pain, visceral or peripheral malperfusion, syncope, or cerebral infarction. Cardiogenic shock is a particularly dangerous presentation and requires prompt diagnosis and aggressive treatment if the patient is to survive. As many as 1 in 7 patients have been shown to present with shock. In hospital mortality was found to be significantly worse in patients who presented with shock (30.2% vs 23.3% $P = 0.07$) and predictably those treated with surgery had a lower mortality than those medically treated. Outcomes at 5 years demonstrated no differences in post-discharge mortality between patients presenting with shock and those who were stable, suggesting that aggressive and appropriate surgical therapy can rectify pre-presentation deficits caused by shock [30]. In as many as 40% of patients with type A aortic dissection, the presentation to the hospital can be postmortem with cardiac death on presentation [31]. The most common presentation is chest and back pain often described as "tearing" pain and is usually of sudden onset. Patents can usually describe the exact moment when the pain started.

Initial laboratory evaluation usually includes routine labs which can demonstrate anemia, elevated D-dimer, acute kidney injury, elevated lactate, or other labs that demonstrate malperfusion such as elevated creatinine kinase. Physical exam should focus on clinical evidence of malperfusion with evaluation of pulses in all 4 extremities, abdominal exam, neurological exam, and evaluation of the patient's vital signs. Narrowed pulse pressure can signify early pericardial tamponade and conversely a wide pulse pressure may signify severe aortic regurgitation. Altered mental status could be due to low cardiac output or cerebral malperfusion.

Personal and family history are important to ascertain, focused on history of sudden death in family members, connective tissue disease, familial aneurysm history, and personal history of hypertension, aneurysms, or similar symptoms. Family history can be a factor which does affect intraoperative management as the threshold to perform a root replacement is lower in patients with connective tissue disease [32]. Postoperatively, a patient with a significant family or personal history for heritable aortopathy may need to have family members evaluated for aortic disease and followed by appropriate physicians.

Diagnosis was historically made with aortography [33, 34]. Currently, a diagnosis of type A aortic dissection by angiography is typically incidental in the setting of a coronary or aortic valve percutaneous intervention. Chest x-ray can demonstrate a widened mediastinum in the setting of dissected aneurysms, contained rupture with pericardial tamponade, or enlargement of the aortic knob. Computerized tomographic angiography (CTA) is the gold standard for diagnosis and gives the most detailed information on the extent of disease, associated aneurysms, radiologic malperfusion and, in the setting of reoperative surgery, the anatomy of the right ventricle, aorta, and innominate vein in relation to the posterior sternal table as well as patency of any previous coronary grafts. Important considerations that could alter operative planning are listed below.

1. *Site of primary tear:* Will be discussed in more depth later but a tear in the root will likely require some form of root replacement. A tear into the aortic arch will require a more extensive arch replacement whether a zone 2 or 3 depending on extent of tear.
2. *Presence of aneurysms:* A root aneurysm >4.5 cm will require root replacement. Arch aneurysm >4.5 cm will require total arch replacement if the entire aneurysm cannot be resected with hemiarch reconstruction.
3. *Evaluation of branch vessels:* Dynamic or static occlusions of proximal branch vessels may not be clinically evident due to collateral flow but would necessitate interposition graft replacement and would dictate the necessity of total arch replacement. Presence of anomalous subclavian arteries, a bovine arch or a 4-branch arch with the left vertebral as a branch of the aorta are important considerations depending on the extent of arch involvement and planned reconstruction.
4. *Evaluation of the descending thoracic aorta:* Malperfusion with or without pseudocoarctation could require frozen elephant trunk (FET) reconstruction. The CT will help with determining the appropriate size of the thoracic endograft.
5. *Cannulation strategy:* There are numerous options for arterial inflow including central, axillary, or femoral, with recent focus on central cannulation with transesophageal echocardiographic (TEE) guidance. CT is extremely helpful with guiding cannulation strategy in the case of severely dissected axillary or femoral vessels.
6. *Radiologic malperfusion:* Occasionally malperfusion of the viscera can be radiologically evident without being immediately clinically evident depending on how fast the patient was transferred to the referral center, most commonly this situation includes malperfusion of a single kidney in a patient with 2 kidneys.

In patients with severe iodine dye allergy magnetic resonance imaging (MRI) can be a substitute for diagnosis of aortic dissection, however the length of time to get the study can be a serious impediment to referral for appropriate surgical therapy. Magnetic resonance angiography (MRA) has been shown to have similar or improved sensitivity and specify to CTA and MRA may have a role in chronic dissection or in the differentiation of intramural hematoma and dissection in chronically affected patients [35, 36]. The unavailability of MRI in emergent settings as well as issues with the time it takes to perform the procedure in critically ill patients make it an imperfect imaging modality that is not frequently used to make the diagnosis [37].

In cases where CT imaging is not available, either because of allergy or because the images were not sent with the patient from referring center, the diagnosis can be confirmed with TEE. TEE provides much of the needed information including size of the aortic root, valve pathology, descending thoracic aorta morphology and in some circumstances a detailed evaluation of the aortic arch. TEE is plagued by user variability and availability of cardiac anesthesiologists as part of the team taking care of these patients is paramount to obtaining the best outcomes. In the case where TEE is the confirmatory diagnostic test several intraoperative decisions may need to be made during the circulatory arrest portion of the operation when the ascending aorta and arch are opened and evaluated. A large secondary tear in the arch may not be discernable with TEE and may be diagnosed at the time of circulatory arrest necessitating the surgical team to be nimble and able to make rapid changes to perfusion strategies and cerebral protection plans.

Initial Management

The most important consideration in management after the diagnosis has been made is prompt consultation with a cardiothoracic surgeon. Many studies advocate rapid transfer to a high-volume center. A study of all Medicare beneficiaries with acute type A aortic dissection over a 15-year period demonstrated a 7.2% absolute risk reduction for mortality when the patient was transferred to a high-volume center even when the transfer delayed the surgical intervention. The analysis demonstrated that to save an additional life only 14 patients would need to be transferred to a high-volume center [38]. Several other studies have reproduced these findings that experienced centers are able to provide improved outcomes for emergent aortic surgery [39, 40]. These manuscripts emphasize the importance of volume– outcomes relationship in Type A aortic dissection, and the transfer of patients with type A aortic dissection should be viewed as part of the initial management in the same way as blood pressure control and anti-impulse therapy, particularly in centers without cardiac surgery services.

Once interfacility transfer is initiated, the next important consideration is rapid arrival to the operating room by the receiving facility. Several groups have endorsed using the operating room as the first place in the hospital where a transfer is taken upon arrival, without any delay in the intensive care unit [13, 41–43].

Initial medical management often started in the ED on presentation should address the most important goal in medical management of type A aortic dissection; reduction in aortic wall stress. Arterial lines should routinely be placed in the right radial artery for continuous monitoring of arterial blood pressure and to indirectly monitor perfusion of the right carotid artery. Reduction in aortic wall stress is achieved by employing medications which serve to control both the heart rate and blood pressure. In the absence of contraindications such as hypotension or bradycardia, an intravenous beta-adrenergic blocker should be initiated and titrated to a goal heart rate of 60 beats per minute or less. If contraindications to beta-adrenergic blockers are present, the use of a nondihydropyridine calcium channel blocker can be used. Goal systolic blood pressures below 120 mmHg should be obtained [32]. A relatively common mistake that can be made by practitioners who are not familiar with these patients is to initially lower the blood pressure with vasodilator agents which can cause compensatory tachycardia, leading to increased wall stress on the dissected aorta. In patients who require multiple agents to control hypertension, a vasodilator can be added to the regimen once the patient's heart rate is controlled with beta blockade [44].

Patient Selection

Determination of candidacy for surgical repair of a type A aortic dissection requires a definitive decision to be made in many cases with inadequate workup given the emergent circumstances. Careful preoperative cardiopulmonary evaluation is often not possible and often patients are unable to provide important medical details outside from their current symptoms. Family members may not be available to provide medical history. There are no definite contraindications to surgical repair, although debilitating stroke or coma, advanced age, and severe malperfusion are complications of the disease that have informed decision-making as to candidacy for operative therapy. Recent studies suggest that neurological recovery can be obtained with aggressive surgical therapy of type A aortic dissection patients who present with a neurological deficit, and cerebral malperfusion should not be an absolute contraindication to operative therapy [45–47]. Certain prognostic factors such as internal carotid artery occlusion versus common carotid artery occlusion have demonstrated worse prognosis and could be useful in informing a thoughtful decision about offering surgery [48]. Age alone has previously been viewed by some centers as a relative contraindication to surgical repair of TAAD. Studies investigating outcomes of octogenarians and nonagenarians have been mixed, with some suggesting significantly increased mortality and morbidity in patients over 80 years of age while other studies have suggested that with proper selection acceptable outcomes of octogenarians can be achieved [49–52]. Similarly, acceptable outcomes have been achieved in patients with previous cardiac surgery undergoing repair of TAAD [53, 54]. No set of definitive rules exist and there is no replacement for a thoughtful and thorough evaluation on an individualized basis.

Cannulation Strategies

The ability to achieve a safe short-term and durable long-term outcome begins as soon as the diagnosis of TAAD is made. Planning for the cadence of the operation is often standardized institutionally but often individualized adjustments to the technical aspects of the operation are required. Any successful cannulation strategy in type A aortic dissection must address several considerations that are listed below:

1. Time to initiation of cardiopulmonary bypass
2. Reliable true lumen perfusion during cooling to minimize malperfusion
3. Minimization of cerebral embolism and prevention of progression of the dissection flap
4. Cerebral perfusion during lower body circulatory arrest
5. Reliable perfusion after circulatory arrest when rewarming

Arterial cannulation is usually performed through one of three routes: right axillary artery, femoral artery, or central cannulation. Right axillary artery cannulation, either directly or through a graft anastomosed to the artery, has several benefits. When performing right axillary arterial cannulation, the patient is already prepared for selective right carotid artery antegrade cerebral perfusion at the time of lower body circulatory arrest by simply clamping the innominate artery and continuing to perfuse the right cerebral circulation. Right axillary cannulation has been demonstrated to be a safe strategy even in cases of dissection involvement of the right axillary artery [55, 56]. The main drawbacks of right axillary arterial cannulation are the time it takes to expose the right axillary artery, additional time to perform an end to side graft for perfusion or if a graft is not used the possibility of right upper extremity ischemia from the cannula impeding distal flow down the right upper extremity. Patients suffering from cardiac tamponade or those undergoing active CPR resuscitation may not tolerate the extra time it takes for axillary arterial cannulation. For those who perform an "arch first" technique for either zone 2 or zone 3 arch reconstruction, the sequence of arch vessel reconstruction must be altered since flow to the entire body will be coming from the innominate artery requiring that reconstruction of the left common carotid and left subclavian arteries be performed prior to clamping of the innominate artery for reinstruction. In the setting of right axillary arterial cannulation bilateral radial artery pressure monitoring lines are helpful.

First described in 1998 central aortic cannulation has become a reliable and expeditious strategy for arterial cannulation in TAAD [57]. Central aortic cannulation requires both a surgeon who is familiar with the technique as well as anesthesia colleagues who are comfortable with aiding the surgeon using transesophageal echocardiography (TEE). The technique involves using Seldinger technique to advance an arterial canula through the ascending aorta into the distal arch or proximal descending aorta after confirming that the wire is within the true lumen of the descending thoracic aorta using TEE guidance. Early concerns regarding aortic rupture with central cannulation have proven to be unfounded with safety demonstrated in multiple studies [58–60]. Kreibich et al. found that central cannulation was safe and had similar outcomes of stroke and mortality compared to right axillary and femoral cannulation in a study of 584 patients [55]. Many centers employ central aortic cannulation almost exclusively due to its expeditious implementation and the ability to quickly relieve tamponade and improve malperfusion through a single incision. Cannulation centrally can be tailored to retrograde or antegrade cerebral perfusion easily with an "arch first" technique for debranching the arch with a second arterial perfusion line perfusing a trifurcated graft that is sequentially anastomosed to each arch branch prior to lower body circulatory arrest or with balloon tipped cannulas at the time of lower body circulatory arrest if not performing aortic arch debranching or when performing hemiarch reconstruction. Retrograde cerebral perfusion can simply be performed through a snared superior vena cava cannula. The merits of central cannulation have led to an increasing experience with the technique over the years.

Femoral arterial cannulation is routinely performed in many centers, demonstrates time efficiency similar to central cannulation, and is especially useful in the situation where a patient is undergoing CPR at the time of arrival. The theoretical concern of embolic stroke due to retrograde flow of blood in the aorta has been investigated and several studies have validated the concern [60–62]. A meta-analysis comparing right axillary arterial cannulation to femoral cannulation demonstrated statistically significantly reduced permanent neurologic deficit in patients undergoing right axillary arterial cannulation [61]. A recent study of over 1500 patients demonstrated increased incidence of stroke and acute brain infarction (stroke, 11.7% vs 7.0%, $P = .03$; acute brain infarction, 6.0% vs 2.7%, $P < .01$) when femoral cannulation was used in type A aortic dissection [63]. Evaluations using the STS database and a separate study of over 25,000 patients by Helder et al. reported increased risk of stroke when compared to axillary or central aortic cannulation [64, 65]. It is important to note that there is very little prospective data, and some of these findings may reflect selection bias. Femoral arterial cannulation is most appropriate in situations where there is not adequate time for axillary dissection and cannulation, for surgeons, anesthesiologists, and institutions unfamiliar with central cannulation, or as previously mentioned in which the patient is actively undergoing cardiopulmonary resuscitation on arrival to the operating room.

Preoperative Planning of the Extent of Resection

Comprehensive preoperative planning in TAAD includes the expected extent of reconstruction that will be necessary. Preoperative CTA can almost always provide enough information for planning the extent of resection. The combination of CTA, which should include the abdomen and pelvis, and TEE can reliably localize the primary intimal tear and diagnose the presence of any root, ascending, or arch aneurysms as well as any radiological evidence of either visceral or cerebral malperfusion.

Management of the Aortic Arch

Although hemiarch reconstruction with aortic valve preservation and resuspension of the commissures is commonly all that is required to achieve the goals of dissection management, there are circumstances when a more extensive arch intervention is warranted [66]. A hemiarch reconstruction is demonstrated in Fig. 9.3. The principals of any dissection operation include resection of the primary or any major secondary tears and reconstitution of true lumen flow. In TAAD, the mortality has historically been high compared to other elective cardiac operations such that theoretical concerns for later reoperation and long-term disease-related mortality have been secondary to achieving in-hospital and short-term survival. As mortality has improved in some series to below 10%, concerns over long-term need for reoperation have increased leading many surgeons to undertake more extensive arch reconstruction to minimize need for reoperation and promote favorable aortic remodeling [13].

The use of lower body circulatory arrest to achieve complete resection of the entire ascending aorta and primary entry tear is of utmost importance. Performing an open distal anastomosis allows for proper preparation of the distal aorta with either felt neomedia technique, felt "sandwich" strips for enforcement or adventitial flap reinforcement. The specific technique for reinforcement is not as important as the meticulous technique used to minimize or exclude intimal tears from torque placed when passing the suture through friable aortic tissue. In addition to resection of the primary tear and reconstitution of true lumen flow, open distal anastomosis should also be considered one of the important principles of TAAD therapy in order to achieve a durable distal reconstruction. Distal reentry tears and persistent perfusion of the false lumen have both been shown to portend worse prognosis specifically related to late events of the distal aorta [67]. Moon et al. reported 97% freedom

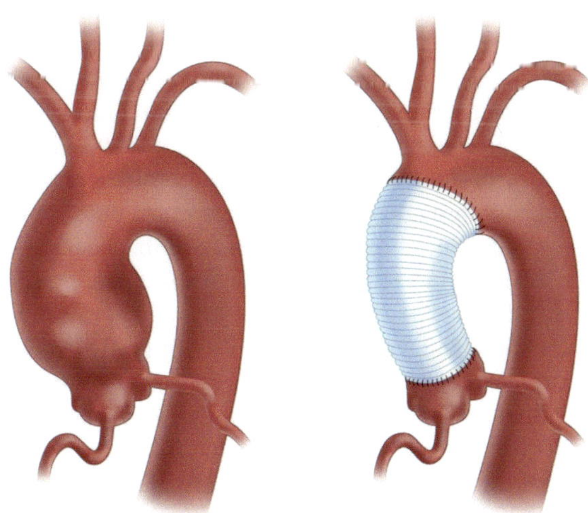

Fig. 9.3 Hemiarch reconstruction of the ascending aorta and proximal aortic arch

from reoperation when open hemiarch distal reconstruction was used compared to 76% freedom from reoperation when a clamped ascending only reconstruction was performed [68]. Rylski and colleagues reported similar results with 90% and 85% freedom from distal aortic reintervention after hemiarch reconstruction at 10 years for DeBakey II and DeBakey I TAAD respectively [69].

The extent of resection of the arch is determined by several factors including arch tear locations, presence of aneurysm, malperfusion, and distal arch anatomy. The prolonged operative and circulatory arrest times should be balanced against the benefits of more extensive arch resection. Several centers have reported that the risks of more extensive arch reconstruction are similar to standard hemiarch reconstruction [70, 71]. Recommended indications for extended (zone 2 or zone 3) aortic arch resection and reconstruction include primary or large secondary tear that cannot be resected by hemiarch, arch aneurysm or rupture, malperfusion from arch vessel dissection or circumferential arch dissection [44, 72]. Other accepted indications include the need for FET to promote aortic remodeling if pseudo coarctation of the descending thoracic aorta is present, young patients with hereditary disorders, retrograde dissections whose primary tear is in the descending thoracic aorta or in patients with circumferential arch dissection [44]. Particularly in patients with hereditary disorders, who will likely require multiple operations to manage ongoing thoracic aortic disease, performing an extensive operation at the time of dissection (such as a total arch with frozen or classical elephant trunk) could decrease future interventions. When FET is utilized the risk of spinal ischemia must be considered. Several investigations have suggested that using a stent graft that does not extend below the sixth thoracic vertebrae or stent grafts that are less than 15 cm in length can avoid spinal cord ischemia [73–75]. One of the most important principles of FET technique involves reliably gaining true lumen access for the entirety of the stent graft deployment. True lumen access can be approached 2 distinct ways; with access of the femoral artery true lumen where a wire passed retrograde into the open arch at the time of lower body circulatory arrest or in an antegrade fashion by passing a pigtail catheter into the true lumen during lower body circulatory arrest and then exchanging the pigtail for a wire over which the stent graft is deployed. With antegrade deployment often the tip of the wire cannot be reliably visualized and if secondary tears exist in the descending thoracic aorta the antegrade wire passing into the false lumen through a secondary tear could lead to false lumen deployment of the stent graft. Likewise, a wire used to access the femoral arterial true lumen could pass through a secondary tear in the descending thoracic aorta and then into the open arch leading to deployment of the stent graft into the false lumen. In general when a short (100 or less mm graft) is deployed with an antegrade pigtail and wire technique the distal extent of the stent graft can be visualized directly to ensure true lumen deployment. The EFT stent graft is incorporated into the distal aortic anastomosis effectively eliminating the risk of stent migration or type 1a endoleak.

Although not uncommon intimal tears in the arch can comprise between 9% and 31% of TAAD and present particular dilemmas in how to safely excise or cover the intimal tear [76]. Arch aneurysms are present in 6% of patients who present with TAAD [77]. Retrograde TAAD emanating from a type B intimal tear presents a situation where a total arch and FET are strongly encouraged to cover and exclude the primary tear.

Replacement of arch branch vessels beyond the thoracic inlet can also be performed. In selected circumstances, such as cerebral malperfusion with extrathoracic carotid dissection and neurologic dysfunction, common carotid replacement in the neck is a safe procedure and can improve neurologic outcomes [72, 78].

Management of the Aortic Root

The aortic root must be managed carefully and thoughtfully in patients suffering from TAAD. The guiding principles remain the same as with the ascending aorta and arch, which are to restore true lumen flow, minimize malperfusion, and resect any intimal tears. Similar to the aortic arch, more aggressive management at the time of the initial operation may increase operative, cardiopulmonary bypass, and myocardial ischemia times with a decreased need for future interventions. There are 3 distinct options for management of the aortic root in TAAD: aortic root preservation (ARP) with reconstruction of the dissected sinuses and resuspension of the valve commissures, aortic root replacement (ARR) with a composite valve conduit, and valve sparing root replacement (VSRR). Key considerations include patient age, dissection anatomy, hemodynamic stability, presence of malperfusion, and surgeon familiarity with root operations. The crux of the issue pertains to the durability of the patient's native aortic root and likelihood for need for future intervention. Cross-sectional imaging with CTA in addition to TEE can provide much of the information necessary to determine the extent of reconstruction that is required even before an incision is made.

A majority of patients can be managed with root preservation consisting of evacuation of thrombus between the intima and adventitia in any of the dissected sinuses and repair of the affected sinuses with either felt neomedia or felt "sandwich" technique and resuspension of each valve commissure [79]. Long-term results of root preservation in patients who did not have an indication for root replacement demonstrate durability with a study of 489 patients demonstrating 96%, 92% and 89% freedom from proximal aortic reoperation at 5, 10, and 15 years respectively [80]. Twenty-three-year follow-up from the University of Genova echoed the same results with freedom from proximal aortic reoperation in 319 patients of 97%, 92% and 82% at 5, 10, and 23 years [81]. These results reinforce the principle of appropriate root preservation in TAAD given the complication rates of patients with mechanical aortic valves requiring anticoagulation and structural degeneration of bioprosthetic valves.

Clearly defined indications for root replacement include aortic root aneurysm >4.5 cm, intimal tear extending into the aortic sinuses, extensive destruction of the aortic sinuses, coronary malperfusion, and heritable aortic disease [32, 44]. A root replacement with either a composite valved conduit or with a VSRR reimplantation technique involves significantly more complexity than root preservation. More extensive dissection around an aortic root where tissue planes are often abolished due to edema and hematoma makes mobilization of the coronary buttons difficult. Despite the increased complexity of aortic root replacement, several series have demonstrated safety comparable to root preservation. The largest series of patients comparing aortic root replacement and root preservation comes from the International Registry of Acute Dissection (IRAD). This group evaluated 699 root replacement patients and 1296 root preservation patients with no difference in operative mortality (ARP 18% vs ARR 21.3%; $P = 0.07$) or 3-year survival (ARP 91.6% vs ARR 92.5% $P = 0.62$). There was also 99% freedom from root reintervention in both groups demonstrating that both root replacement and root preservation can have favorable short- and mid-term outcomes in properly selected patients [82]. Patients with Marfan syndrome and other heritable thoracic aortic diseases (HTAD) benefit from root replacement instead of root preservation given the high need for reintervention when valve preservation is performed. A series of 74 patients with Marfan syndrome who underwent TAAD repair demonstrated freedom from aortic root reoperation rates of 95%, 88%, and 79% for patients undergoing root replacement and 83%, 60%, and 20% in patients undergoing root preservation at 5-, 10-, and 20-year follow-up respectively [83].

Valve sparing root replacement techniques involve even more technical complexity than a valved conduit due to the more extensive dissection of the aortic root to below the level of the aortic valve annulus and the proper sizing and reimplantation of the valve inside a conduit. The group at Emory University demonstrated promising findings with their series of VSRR in TAAD between the years of 2005 and 2013 with 43 patients undergoing VSRR. Of the 43 patients who underwent VSRR there was a 4.7% rate of operative mortality. After 9-year follow-up freedom from > mild aortic regurgitation was 94% and freedom from root reintervention including aortic valve replacement was 100% [84]. Current guidelines recommend VSSR as a reasonable option in well-selected patients, usually young patients with normal ventricular function and normal valve cusps [44].

Circulatory Arrest and Cerebral Perfusion Strategies

The ability to perform an open distal aortic anastomosis requires temporarily halting the perfusion of the aorta to create a bloodless field where the surgeon can perform an adequate aortic resection and reconstruction. To safely achieve circulatory arrest required adjuncts for lower body and cerebral perfusion, which have evolved over the last four decades. In the 1970s Griepp and colleagues provided evidence that deep hypothermic circulatory arrest (DHCA) provided cerebral and visceral protection for thoracic aortic reconstruction [85]. Several considerations have arisen over time and are listed below:

1. What is the appropriate temperature for circulatory arrest?
2. Is cerebral perfusion necessary?
3. Is antegrade or retrograde cerebral perfusion superior?

In the original report of 4 patients by Griepp, the average lowest esophageal and rectal temperatures were 14 and 18 °C, respectively [85]. In subsequent studies, the definition of deep hypothermia is generally accepted as <20 °C. As the nadir temperature decreases, the metabolic demands of end organs also decrease, yet deeper hypothermia has been associated with complications related to coagulopathy, organ dysfunction, respiratory failure, neuronal cell loss, and systemic inflammatory responses [86–88]. A study comparing moderate hypothermic circulatory arrest (MHCA) (nadir temperature > 20 °C) and DHCA has demonstrated less blood loss when MHCA is employed compared to DHCA [86, 89]. Data from the Society of Thoracic Surgeons database evaluated the optimal temperature for hypothermic circulatory arrest in elective hemiarch replacement and demonstrated that a nadir temperature of 27 °C when combined with selective antegrade cerebral perfusion led to the greatest early survival benefit with the lowest perioperative risk. Patients cooled to between 21 and 23 °C had higher risks of mortality and major morbidity when compared to those cooled to 24 °C [90]. A study of the IRAD database found the combination of MHCA and antegrade cerebral perfusion to be as safe as DHCA in TAAD with regard to in-hospital mortality and perioperative stroke even in the setting of longer circulatory arrest times with MHCA after propensity matching [91]. The safety of MHCA when combined with cerebral perfusion allows patients to avoid the risks of DHCA while mitigating the metabolic risks of warmer ischemia. This trend toward MHCA with cerebral perfusion has been echoed in consensus documents of respected thoracic surgical societies [44].

Cerebral perfusion during the period of lower body circulatory arrest has largely replaced isolated total body circulatory arrest. Antegrade cerebral perfusion (ACP) can be achieved through an open arch during the time of lower body circulatory arrest with the use of balloon tipped cannulas or can be performed through a trifurcated arch graft and an additional arterial line from the cardiopulmonary bypass pump if an "arch first" technique is employed. In an "arch first" technique, with cerebrovascular reconstruction during the period of cooling, the only anastomosis that needs to be completed under lower body circulatory arrest is the distal aortic anastomosis. When the lower body is ischemic, the arterial pressure to the arch vessels is maintained with a mean arterial pressure goal of 60 70 mm Hg.

Retrograde cerebral perfusion (RCP) can be achieved by placing an angled superior vena cava (SVC) cannula in addition to a dual-stage right atrial cannula. At the time of lower body circulatory arrest, the superior vena cava is snared around the cannula. The inflow to the cannula for RCP is from the microplegia system which is connected to a three-way stopcock that is integrated into the tubing of the SVC cannula between the cannula and the Y connection to the right atrial cannula. The SVC cannula is isolated from the venous drainage reservoir with a tubing clamp and RCP is begun with cold, 4 °C blood to achieve a central venous pressure of 30 mm Hg as measured by the right internal jugular central venous catheter. It is important to thoroughly flush cardioplegia from the circuit prior to initiating RCP. When the arch is open, the surgeon should be able to see dark deoxygenated blood emanating from the arch vessels. Any lack of blood draining from the arch vessels requires immediate troubleshooting, and is most frequently because the SVC cannula is not snared or the tubing between the SVC cannula and the Y connector is not clamped. Another possibility for a lack of blood draining from the arch vessels is that the SVC cannula has been misdirected into the azygous vein rather than the SVC and this possibility must also be ruled out.

Both ACP and RCP have their theoretical benefits, with RCP promoting the ability to flush air, debris, or thrombus that has entered the arch vessels prior to or during the operation and advocates of ACP promoting the normal physiology of antegrade cerebral perfusion. One evaluation of the STS database suggested that cerebral perfusion compared with no cerebral perfusion, in both deep and moderate hypothermia, had better outcomes with regard to mortality and neurologic compromise, but the number of deep hypothermia without cerebral perfusion was small. Further, this study did not demonstrate any difference in outcomes between ACP and RCP [92]. Comparisons of both ACP and RCP have not been definitive and only 1 randomized trial has examined the outcomes of each approach in elective arch surgery which demonstrated no difference in clinical stroke, MRI, or neurocognitive studies after total arch replacement [93, 94].

Our strategy employs both ACP and RCP with the degree of cooling determined by intraoperative neurological monitoring (IONM). We perform an "arch first" approach to total arches which lends itself to selective ACP as the arch branches are grafted using a trifurcated arch graft that is later proximalized and anastomosed to the neoascending aortic graft. We use the same strategy for both zone 2 and zone 3 total arches. The proximalized arch graft sets up any later endovascular work if a thoracic endograft needs to be deployed with a long and stable proximal landing zone in the aortic graft. In the setting of a zone 2 total arch where a descending thoracic endograft is needed, a left subclavian transposition to the left common carotid artery is all that is needed to be able to utilize the aortic graft for a landing zone. We routinely utilize RCP for all hemiarch reconstructions. Both ACP and RCP are utilized when a hemiarch is initially planned but findings during evaluation of the arch, such as a tear in the arch, necessitate total arch repair. In the setting of planned hemiarch reconstruction which changes to total arch reconstruction, RCP is initially utilized during the anastomosis of the trifurcated arch graft to the innominate artery after which selective ACP is begun.

In all aortic dissections, we employ IONM, specifically 4-limb somatosensory evoked potentials (SSEPs) and electroencephalography (EEG) to dictate when we can safely commence lower body circulatory arrest. Once there is absence of SSEPs and electrocerebral silence has been achieved we cool for an additional 4 min then begin a period of lower body circulatory arrest [78]. These parameters are usually achieved between 45 and 60 min of cooling and the bladder temperature is usually between 18 and 21 °C. Data from the University of Pennsylvania demonstrate that at 45 min of cooling 90% of patients have lost all EEG activity and that by 60 min of cooling nearly 100% of patients have lost all EEG activity [13]. This approach requires real-time collaboration with a neurophysiology team who is on call 24 h a day for TAAD.

Postoperative Complications

Bleeding

The risk of coagulopathy has long been recognized in patients with aortic dissection [95]. Several publications over the last few decades have demonstrated worse outcomes in elective cardiac surgery patients who receive blood transfusions and many institutions have embarked on campaigns to limit blood product utilization after cardiac surgery [96–99]. Specifically in elective aortic surgery requiring deep hypothermic lower body circulatory arrest (DHLBCA) worse short- and long-term outcomes were demonstrated in patients that required blood transfusion with regard to operative and long-term mortality as well as stroke and renal complications [100]. There are limited data on the effects of blood transfusion in the setting of TAAD but two studies have examined these outcomes. A study of 3209 patients in Taiwan who presented with TAAD demonstrated worse late outcomes with increases in all-cause mortality, renal disease, and respiratory failure which increased in a dose-dependent manner with the administration of packed red blood cells (PRBCs) [101]. Schafigh and colleagues identified several preoperative and intraoperative risk factors for high blood transfusion requirement. Preoperative risk factors include age, INR at admission, dual antiplatelet therapy, presence of hemopericardium, and hyperlipidemia. Intraoperative risk factors included lower temperatures for circulatory arrest, contained rupture of the ascending aorta and open chest requirement after surgery [102].

Stroke

Stroke continues to be the most dreaded and debilitating postoperative complication of surgery for TAAD. Rates for postoperative stroke in the setting of TAAD range from 13% to 19%. An STS database evaluation found the incidence of postop stroke was 13% overall with axillary cannulation being associated with a lower incidence than femoral cannulation (OR 0.6 $P < 0.001$) [64]. Data such as this helps to inform the guidelines from the American Association of Thoracic Surgery which have class IIa recommendations for axillary and direct aortic cannulation vs a IIb recommendation for femoral artery cannulation for TAAD [44]. A study from the Nordic Consortium Registry found a postoperative stroke incidence of 18.6% [103]. The German Registry for Acute Aortic Dissection identified 9.6% of patients who developed new neurological dysfunction (ND) after surgery but also demonstrated resolution of ND in 12.6% of the 20.3% of patients who presented with preoperative ND, adding to the evidence that preoperative cerebral malperfusion can be reversible. Ischemic stroke is the predominant etiology of postoperative stroke accounting for 18.6% of the strokes in a single institution series but hemorrhagic stroke accounted for worse neurological outcomes and lower survival than ischemic stroke

[104]. In the single institution series risk factors for hemorrhagic stroke included patients who underwent complex arch replacement, longer cardiopulmonary bypass times, and longer aortic cross clamp times.

Postoperative Management

Postoperative blood pressure management can have direct effects on the long-term outcomes of patients who survive and recover from TAAD. A strategy to minimize aneurysmal degeneration of the ongoing dissection flap of the descending thoracic aorta is of the utmost importance as well as to preserve the aortic root when root preservation techniques are employed. Β-adrenergic blockade helps to control blood pressure and heart rate, in turn leading to improved impulse control and decreased wall stress on the aorta. Improved outcomes with use of beta blockers in this cohort have been demonstrated, including reduced all-cause mortality at 8 years with strict adherence to beta-blocker therapy (22/7% vs 14.4% $P = 0.008$) [105]. Other studies have also demonstrated a decreased rate of dissection-related surgery, and decreased incidence of increasing aortic diameter in chronic type B dissection [106]. The importance of beta blockade and strict blood pressure control has been reinforced by findings in other studies [107, 108].

Use of angiotensin receptor blockers (ARB) and angiotensin-converting enzyme inhibitors (ACEI) has previously been suggested to be important in slowing progression of ascending aortic and aortic root aneurysms particularly in patients with Marfan Syndrome. Of note 2 studies that had previously been used to demonstrate the effect of ARB and ACEI to decrease growth in ascending aorta in systole and reduction in aortic diameter in diastole in MF patients and to reduce aortic dissection risk in patients with risk factors have been retracted since their publication due to data inadequacies [109, 110]. An IRAD registry analysis did not find an association between ACEI use and mortality [111, 112].

Imaging Surveillance

Lifelong surveillance is an important facet in the care of TAAD patients. Depending on the initial extent of reconstruction patients can be at risk for aneurysmal degeneration of an ongoing descending thoracic aortic dissection or a need for proximal root or aortic valve intervention. Pseudoaneurysms can also occur at sites of anastomoses. At our institution in the initial postoperative period cross-sectional imaging usually with CTA is completed prior to index hospitalization discharge and at postoperative periods of 1, 3, 6, and 12 months postop. If the imaging findings remain stable annual CTA evaluation is continued for the entirety of the patient's life. Transthoracic echocardiography is performed at 1 month follow-up and then annually.

Development of descending thoracic aortic aneurysmal disease can often be managed with endovascular stenting particularly in the setting of a frozen elephant trunk or total arch with proximalization of the arch vessels. If a zone 2 total arch had been performed then a left subclavian to left carotid transposition can allow for a stable landing zone in the aortic graft without compromising any arch vessels.

Special Situations

Management of Malperfusion

Pulse deficit has been reported as frequently as 30% in patients with TAAD, with overt limb-threatening ischemia being substantially more rare and mesenteric ischemia occurring with a frequency of <5% in patients with TAAD [113]. Malperfusion defects are often categorized as static obstructions or dynamic obstructions. Static obstructions are usually not improved with reconstitution of true lumen blood flow whereas dynamic obstructions occur from pressurization of the false lumen and occlusion of true lumen blood flow which often resolves after reconstruction of the aorta and reconstitution of true lumen flow. Extremity malperfusion can often be resolved with repair of the dissection and reconstitution of true lumen blood flow and placement of arterial lines in the affected limbs can help to determine if true lumen flow will resolve the issue. Once on cardiopulmonary bypass with true lumen flow reconstituted, the arterial lines in the affected limb will often equilibrate to the blood pressure of the nonaffected limbs. If, after the proximal aortic reconstruction, the malperfusion of a limb is not resolved a static obstruction should be suspected and a femoral bypass is indicated or another reconstruction for the upper extremities such as a subclavian carotid transposition.

Visceral Malperfusion

Malperfusion of the abdominal viscera is a much more ominous preoperative finding in patients with TAAD and occurs in 3.7–7% of patients with TAAD [113, 114]. Often these patients are not surgical candidates if their lactate is extremely elevated with evidence of sepsis and if there is concern for overt abdominal catastrophe given poor postoperative outcomes with operative mortality as high as 43% [115]. Several groups have championed a new paradigm to deal with visceral malperfusion, which is to treat the specific visceral vessels, usually the celiac and superior mesenteric arteries with fenestrations and stents to reconstitute perfusion and resolve the malperfusion of the vascular bed [116–119]. After a delay and once the malperfusion is improved, if the patient survives the initial malperfusion and does not suffer rupture or another aortic complication of the TAAD, central aortic repair is performed. This strategy demonstrated a 15% mortality in patients waiting for central aortic repair after intervention for malperfusion in a small series [118]. It is impossible to reliably predict malperfusion that will improve with central aortic repair alone or which patients will not survive the delay to central aortic repair when a malperfusion first approach is employed. The malperfusion first approach also requires a dedicated team of interventionalists with experience in dissection flap fenestration and stenting.

Type A Aortic Dissection in Patients with Previous Cardiac Surgery

Type A aortic dissection in patients with previous cardiac surgery occurs in as many as 9–15% of patients presenting with TAAD [53, 54, 120]. Etiology of dissection in these patients can be the same as in patients without a history of cardiac surgery but can also include sites of aortotomy with previous aortic valve replacement, sites of anastomoses with root replacement or the sites of proximal anastomoses in the case of previous coronary bypass grafting. Reports of outcomes have demonstrated comparable outcomes to patients who have not had previous cardiac surgery when performed at centers with experience and the history of previous cardiac surgery should not contraindicate offering surgery to a patient who is otherwise a candidate [53]. In a multicenter study history of previous coronary bypass with patent grafts carried the highest mortality risk [120]. The adhesions from previous cardiac surgery are not protective from rupture and tamponade as these complications were similar to patients without a history of previous cardiac surgery in a single-center study of 330 patients [54].

References

1. Levinson DC, Edmeades DT, Griffith GC. Dissecting aneurysms of the aorta: its clinical, electrocardiographic and laboratory features a report of fifty-eight autopsied cases. Circulation. 1950;1:360–87.
2. Nicholls F. Observations concerning the body of his late Majesty: October 26, 1760. London; 1762.
3. Maunoir JP. Memoires Physiologiques et Pratiques sur l'Anevrisms et la Ligature ses Arteres. A Geneve: chez J.J. Paschoud; 1802.
4. Morgagni G. The seats and causes of diseases: investigated by anatomy, containing a great variety of dissections and accompanied with remarks, vol. 1. Boston: Wells and Lilly; 1769. p. 808.
5. Laennec RTH. Traite de l'Auscultation Mediate et des maladies des poumons et du coeur, vol. 2. New York: Samuel S. and William Wood; 1819. p. 411.
6. Shekelton J. Healed dissecting aneurysm, vol. 3. Dublin Hospital Report; 1822. p. 231.
7. Pennock CW. Case of anomalous aneurysm of the aorta resulting form effususion of blood composing the middle coat of that vessel. Am J Med Sci. 1838;23:13.

8. Swaine L. A case of dissecting aneurysm of the aorta. Trans Path Soc Lond. 1855;7(106):186.
9. Wheat MW Jr, et al. Treatment of dissecting aneurysms of the aorta without surgery. J Thorac Cardiovasc Surg. 1965;50:364–73.
10. De Bakey ME, Cooley DA, Creech O Jr. Surgical considerations of dissecting aneurysm of the aorta. Ann Surg. 1955;142(4):586–610; discussion, 611–2.
11. Altman LK. The man on the table devised the surgery. New York Times; 2006. New York.
12. Coady MA, et al. Natural history, pathogenesis, and etiology of thoracic aortic aneurysms and dissections. Cardiol Clin. 1999;17(4):615–35; vii.
13. Bavaria JE, et al. New paradigms and improved results for the surgical treatment of acute type A dissection. Ann Surg. 2001;234(3):336–42; discussion 342–3.
14. Sultan I, et al. Intraoperative neurophysiologic monitoring during aortic arch surgery. J Thorac Cardiovasc Surg. 2021;165(6):1971–1981.e2.
15. Bavaria JE, et al. Circulatory management with retrograde cerebral perfusion for acute type A aortic dissection. Circulation. 1996;94(9 Suppl):II173–6.
16. David TE, et al. Surgery for acute type A aortic dissection. Ann Thorac Surg. 1999;67(6):1999–2001; discussion 2014–9.
17. Fann JI, et al. Surgical management of aortic dissection during a 30-year period. Circulation. 1995;92(9 Suppl):II113–21.
18. Muetterties CE, Menon R, Wheatley GH 3rd. A systematic review of primary endovascular repair of the ascending aorta. J Vasc Surg. 2018;67(1):332–42.
19. Roselli EE, et al. Zone zero thoracic endovascular aortic repair: a proposed modification to the classification of landing zones. J Thorac Cardiovasc Surg. 2018;155(4):1381–9.
20. Ghoreishi M, et al. Endovascular repair of ascending aortic disease in high-risk patients yields favorable outcome. Ann Thorac Surg. 2020;109(3):678–85.
21. Preventza O, et al. Endovascular repair of the ascending aorta: when and how to implement the current technology. Ann Thorac Surg. 2014;97(5):1555–60.
22. Criado FJ. Aortic dissection: a 250-year perspective. Tex Heart Inst J. 2011;38(6):694–700.
23. Booher AM, et al. The IRAD classification system for characterizing survival after aortic dissection. Am J Med. 2013;126(8):730.e19–24.
24. Daily PO, et al. Management of acute aortic dissections. Ann Thorac Surg. 1970;10(3):237–47.
25. Debakey ME, et al. Surgical management of dissecting aneurysms of the aorta. J Thorac Cardiovasc Surg. 1965;49:130–49.
26. Sievers HH, et al. Aortic dissection reconsidered: type, entry site, malperfusion classification adding clarity and enabling outcome prediction. Interact Cardiovasc Thorac Surg. 2020;30(3):451–7.
27. Lombardi JV, et al. Society for Vascular Surgery (SVS) and Society of Thoracic Surgeons (STS) reporting standards for type B aortic dissections. J Vasc Surg. 2020;71(3):723–47.
28. Lovatt S, et al. Misdiagnosis of aortic dissection: a systematic review of the literature. Am J Emerg Med. 2022;53:16–22.
29. Arnaoutakis GJ, et al. Misdiagnosis of thoracic aortic emergencies occurs frequently among transfers to aortic referral centers: an analysis of over 3700 patients. J Am Heart Assoc. 2022;11(13):e025026.
30. Bossone E, et al. Shock complicating type A acute aortic dissection: clinical correlates, management, and outcomes. Am Heart J. 2016;176:93–9.
31. Cohn LH, Adams DH. Cardiac surgery in the adult, vol. 5e. McGraw Hill; 2017.
32. Hiratzka LF, et al. 2010 ACCF/AHA/AATS/ACR/ASA/SCA/SCAI/SIR/STS/SVM guidelines for the diagnosis and management of patients with thoracic aortic disease: executive summary. A report of the American College of Cardiology Foundation/American Heart Association Task Force on Practice Guidelines, American Association for Thoracic Surgery, American College of Radiology, American Stroke Association, Society of Cardiovascular Anesthesiologists, Society for Cardiovascular Angiography and Interventions, Society of Interventional Radiology, Society of Thoracic Surgeons, and Society for Vascular Medicine. Catheter Cardiovasc Interv. 2010;76(2):E43–86.

33. Shuford WH, Sybers RG, Weens HS. Problems in the aortographic diagnosis of dissecting aneurysm of the aorta. N Engl J Med. 1969;280(5):225–31.
34. Dinsmore RE, et al. Angiographic findings in dissecting aortic aneurysm. N Engl J Med. 1966;275(21):1152–7.
35. Murray JG, et al. Intramural hematoma of the thoracic aorta: MR image findings and their prognostic implications. Radiology. 1997;204(2):349–55.
36. Baliga RR, et al. The role of imaging in aortic dissection and related syndromes. JACC Cardiovasc Imaging. 2014;7(4):406–24.
37. Moore AG, et al. Choice of computed tomography, transesophageal echocardiography, magnetic resonance imaging, and aortography in acute aortic dissection: International Registry of Acute Aortic Dissection (IRAD). Am J Cardiol. 2002;89(10):1235–8.
38. Goldstone AB, et al. Interfacility transfer of medicare beneficiaries with acute type A aortic dissection and regionalization of care in the United States. Circulation. 2019;140(15):1239–50.
39. Knipp BS, et al. A contemporary analysis of outcomes for operative repair of type A aortic dissection in the United States. Surgery. 2007;142(4):524–8; discussion 528.e1.
40. Chikwe J, et al. National outcomes in acute aortic dissection: influence of surgeon and institutional volume on operative mortality. Ann Thorac Surg. 2013;95(5):1563–9.
41. Bavaria JE, et al. Advances in the treatment of acute type A dissection: an integrated approach. Ann Thorac Surg. 2002;74(5):S1848–52; discussion S1857-63.
42. Mehta CK. Impact of a direct-to-operating room aortic emergency transfer program for type A aortic dissection. Socitey of Thoracic Surgeons Annual Meeting 2022; 2022.
43. Chavanon O, et al. Direct admission to the operating room: an efficient strategy for patients with diagnosed or highly suspected acute type A aortic dissection. Can J Cardiol. 2011;27(6):685–91.
44. Malaisrie SC, et al. 2021 The American Association for Thoracic Surgery expert consensus document: surgical treatment of acute type A aortic dissection. J Thorac Cardiovasc Surg. 2021;162(3):735–758 e2.
45. Most H, et al. Is surgery in acute aortic dissection type A still contraindicated in the presence of preoperative neurological symptoms? Eur J Cardiothorac Surg. 2015;48(6):945–50; discussion 950.
46. Sultan I, et al. Surgery for type A aortic dissection in patients with cerebral malperfusion: results from the International Registry of Acute Aortic Dissection. J Thorac Cardiovasc Surg. 2021;161(5):1713–1720.e1.
47. Di Eusanio M, et al. Patients with type A acute aortic dissection presenting with major brain injury: should we operate on them? J Thorac Cardiovasc Surg. 2013;145(3 Suppl):S213–21.e1.
48. Fukuhara S, et al. Type A aortic dissection with cerebral malperfusion: new insights. Ann Thorac Surg. 2021;112(2):501–9.
49. Kageyama S, et al. Early mortality of emergency surgery for acute type A aortic dissection in octogenarians and nonagenarians: a multi-center retrospective study. J Thorac Cardiovasc Surg. 2022;167(1):65–75.e8.
50. Nakai Y, et al. Surgical outcomes of acute type A aortic dissection in septuagenarians and octogenarians. Asian Cardiovasc Thorac Ann. 2022;30(7):2184923221083369.
51. Hemli JM, et al. Management of acute type A aortic dissection in the elderly: an analysis from IRAD. Eur J Cardiothorac Surg. 2022;61(4):838–46.
52. Chen JW, Sainbayar N, Hsu RB. Outcome of emergency surgery for acute type A aortic dissection in octogenarians. J Card Surg. 2022;37(3):610–5.
53. Rylski B, et al. Type A aortic dissection after previous cardiac surgery: results of an integrated surgical approach. Ann Thorac Surg. 2014;97(5):1582–8; discussion 1588–9.
54. Estrera AL, et al. Outcomes of acute type A aortic dissection after previous cardiac surgery. Ann Thorac Surg. 2010;89(5):1467–74.
55. Kreibich M, et al. Outcome after aortic, axillary, or femoral cannulation for acute type A aortic dissection. J Thorac Cardiovasc Surg. 2019;158(1):27–34.e9.

56. Rylski B, et al. Is right axillary artery cannulation safe in type A aortic dissection with involvement of the innominate artery? J Thorac Cardiovasc Surg. 2016;152(3):801–807.e1.
57. Lijoi A, et al. Stanford type A aortic dissection. A new surgical approach. Tex Heart Inst J. 1998;25(1):65–7.
58. Suzuki T, et al. Safety and efficacy of central cannulation through ascending aorta for type A aortic dissection. Interact Cardiovasc Thorac Surg. 2010;11(1):34–7.
59. Reece TB, et al. Central cannulation is safe in acute aortic dissection repair. J Thorac Cardiovasc Surg. 2007;133(2):428–34.
60. Kamiya H, et al. Comparison of ascending aorta versus femoral artery cannulation for acute aortic dissection type A. Circulation. 2009;120(11 Suppl):S282–6.
61. Benedetto U, et al. Axillary versus femoral arterial cannulation in type A acute aortic dissection: evidence from a meta-analysis of comparative studies and adjusted risk estimates. Eur J Cardiothorac Surg. 2015;48(6):953–9.
62. Klotz S, et al. Is the outcome in acute aortic dissection type A influenced by of femoral versus central cannulation? Ann Cardiothorac Surg. 2016;5(4):310–6.
63. Wang X, et al. Femoral artery cannulation increases the risk of postoperative stroke in patients with acute DeBakey I aortic dissection. J Thorac Cardiovasc Surg. 2022;166(4):1023–1031.e15.
64. Ghoreishi M, et al. Factors associated with acute stroke after type A aortic dissection repair: an analysis of the Society of Thoracic Surgeons National Adult Cardiac Surgery Database. J Thorac Cardiovasc Surg. 2020;159(6):2143–2154.e3.
65. Helder MRK, et al. Regional and temporal trends in the outcomes of repairs for acute type A aortic dissections. Ann Thorac Surg. 2020;109(1):26–33.
66. Sultan I, et al. Routine use of hemiarch during acute type A aortic dissection repair. Ann Cardiothorac Surg. 2016;5(3):245–7.
67. Tamura K, et al. The prognostic impact of distal anastomotic new entry after acute type I aortic dissection repair. Eur J Cardiothorac Surg. 2017;52(5):867–73.
68. Moon MR, et al. Does the extent of proximal or distal resection influence outcome for type A dissections? Ann Thorac Surg. 2001;71(4):1244–9; discussion 1249–50.
69. Rylski B, et al. Long-term results of aggressive hemiarch replacement in 534 patients with type A aortic dissection. J Thorac Cardiovasc Surg. 2014;148(6):2981–5.
70. Salem M, et al. Is total arch replacement associated with an increased risk after acute type A dissection? J Thorac Dis. 2020;12(10):5517–31.
71. Yang B, et al. Late outcomes of strategic arch resection in acute type A aortic dissection. J Thorac Cardiovasc Surg. 2019;157(4):1313–1321.e2.
72. Sultan I, et al. Outcomes of carotid artery replacement with total arch reconstruction for type A aortic dissection. Ann Thorac Surg. 2021;112(4):1235–42.
73. Flores J, et al. Extensive deployment of the stented elephant trunk is associated with an increased risk of spinal cord injury. J Thorac Cardiovasc Surg. 2006;131(2):336–42.
74. Katayama K, et al. Multiple factors predict the risk of spinal cord injury after the frozen elephant trunk technique for extended thoracic aortic disease. Eur J Cardiothorac Surg. 2015;47(4):616–20.
75. Preventza O, et al. Neurologic complications after the frozen elephant trunk procedure: a meta-analysis of more than 3000 patients. J Thorac Cardiovasc Surg. 2020;160(1):20–33.e4.
76. Ma WG, et al. Type A aortic dissection with arch entry tear: surgical experience in 104 patients over a 12-year period. J Thorac Cardiovasc Surg. 2016;151(6):1581–92.
77. Evangelista A, et al. Insights from the international registry of acute aortic dissection: a 20-year experience of collaborative clinical research. Circulation. 2018;137(17):1846–60.
78. Trivedi D, et al. Aggressive aortic arch and carotid replacement strategy for type A aortic dissection improves neurologic outcomes. Ann Thorac Surg. 2016;101(3):896–903; Discussion 903–5.

79. Klaus K, Büsch C, Bartosz R, Daniel-Sebastian D, Tobias K, Thomas H, Jens B, Jochen P, Thilo N, Christian H, Phillip J, Andreas B, Khaled C, Matthias K, Rawa A. Treatment of the aortic root in acute aortic dissection type A: insights from the German Registry for Actue Dissection Type A (GERAADA) Registry. Eur J Cardiothorac Surg. 2022;20:ezac261. Ahead of Print.
80. Rylski B, et al. Long-term results of neomedia sinus valsalva repair in 489 patients with type A aortic dissection. Ann Thorac Surg. 2014;98(2):582–8; discussion 588–9.
81. Dell'Aquila AM, et al. Fate of the preserved aortic root after treatment of acute type A aortic dissection: 23-year follow-up. J Thorac Cardiovasc Surg. 2013;146(6):1456–60.
82. Di Eusanio M, et al. Root replacement surgery versus more conservative management during type A acute aortic dissection repair. Ann Thorac Surg. 2014;98(6):2078–84.
83. Rylski B, et al. Type A aortic dissection in Marfan syndrome: extent of initial surgery determines long-term outcome. Circulation. 2014;129(13):1381–6.
84. Leshnower BG, Chen EP. When and how to replace the aortic root in type A aortic dissection. Ann Cardiothorac Surg. 2016;5(4):377–82.
85. Griepp RB, et al. Prosthetic replacement of the aortic arch. J Thorac Cardiovasc Surg. 1975;70(6):1051–63.
86. Kamiya H, et al. The safety of moderate hypothermic lower body circulatory arrest with selective cerebral perfusion: a propensity score analysis. J Thorac Cardiovasc Surg. 2007;133(2):501–9.
87. Jabagi H, Wells G, Boodhwani M. COMMENCE trial (Comparing hypOtherMic teMperaturEs duriNg hemiarCh surgEry): a randomized controlled trial of mild vs moderate hypothermia on patient outcomes in aortic hemiarch surgery with anterograde cerebral perfusion. Trials. 2019;20(1):691.
88. Rohrer MJ, Natale AM. Effect of hypothermia on the coagulation cascade. Crit Care Med. 1992;20(10):1402–5.
89. Keenan JE, et al. Does moderate hypothermia really carry less bleeding risk than deep hypothermia for circulatory arrest? A propensity-matched comparison in hemiarch replacement. J Thorac Cardiovasc Surg. 2016;152(6):1559–1569.e2.
90. Seese L, et al. Optimal circulatory arrest temperature for aortic hemiarch replacement with antegrade brain perfusion. J Thorac Cardiovasc Surg. 2021;165(5):1759–1770.e3.
91. Pupovac SS, et al. Moderate versus deep hypothermia in type A acute aortic dissection repair: insights from the international registry of acute aortic dissection. Ann Thorac Surg. 2021;112(6):1893–9.
92. Englum BR, et al. Hypothermia and cerebral protection strategies in aortic arch surgery: a comparative effectiveness analysis from the STS Adult Cardiac Surgery Database. Eur J Cardiothorac Surg. 2017;52(3):492–8.
93. Hu Z, et al. Similar cerebral protective effectiveness of antegrade and retrograde cerebral perfusion combined with deep hypothermia circulatory arrest in aortic arch surgery: a meta-analysis and systematic review of 5060 patients. J Thorac Cardiovasc Surg. 2014;148(2):544–60.
94. Svensson LG, et al. Implications from neurologic assessment of brain protection for total arch replacement from a randomized trial. J Thorac Cardiovasc Surg. 2015;150(5):1140–7 e11.
95. Fine NL, et al. Multiple coagulation defects in association with dissecting aneurysm. Arch Intern Med. 1967;119(5):522–6.
96. Whitson BA, et al. Risk of adverse outcomes associated with blood transfusion after cardiac surgery depends on the amount of transfusion. J Surg Res. 2010;158(1):20–7.
97. Surgenor SD, et al. The association of perioperative red blood cell transfusions and decreased long-term survival after cardiac surgery. Anesth Analg. 2009;108(6):1741–6.
98. Engoren MC, et al. Effect of blood transfusion on long-term survival after cardiac operation. Ann Thorac Surg. 2002;74(4):1180–6.
99. Moskowitz DM, et al. The impact of blood conservation on outcomes in cardiac surgery: is it safe and effective? Ann Thorac Surg. 2010;90(2):451–8.

100. Sultan I, et al. The use of blood and blood products in aortic surgery is associated with adverse outcomes. J Thorac Cardiovasc Surg. 2021;165(2):544–551.e3.
101. Chen FT, et al. Effect of massive blood transfusion on late outcomes after surgical repair of acute type A aortic dissection. Medicine (Baltimore). 2019;98(45):e17816.
102. Schafigh M, et al. Risk factors for high blood product use in patients with stanford type A dissection. Thorac Cardiovasc Surg. 2022;70(4):306–13.
103. Pan E, et al. Low rate of reoperations after acute type A aortic dissection repair from the Nordic Consortium Registry. J Thorac Cardiovasc Surg. 2018;156(3):939–48.
104. Lin CY, et al. Postoperative stroke after type A aortic dissection repair: hemorrhage versus ischemia. World J Surg. 2022;46(3):690–700.
105. Chen SW, et al. Effect of beta-blocker therapy on late outcomes after surgical repair of type A aortic dissection. J Thorac Cardiovasc Surg. 2020;159(5):1694–1703 e3.
106. Genoni M, et al. Chronic beta-blocker therapy improves outcome and reduces treatment costs in chronic type B aortic dissection. Eur J Cardiothorac Surg. 2001;19(5):606–10.
107. Melby SJ, et al. Importance of blood pressure control after repair of acute type A aortic dissection: 25-year follow-up in 252 patients. J Clin Hypertens (Greenwich). 2013;15(1):63–8.
108. Zierer A, et al. Aortic enlargement and late reoperation after repair of acute type A aortic dissection. Ann Thorac Surg. 2007;84(2):479–86; discussion 486–7.
109. Lancet E. Retraction—valsartan in a Japanese population with hypertension and other cardiovascular disease (Jikei Heart Study): a randomised, open-label, blinded endpoint morbidity-mortality study. Lancet. 2013;382(9895):843.
110. Notice of Retraction: Ahimastos AA, et al. Effect of perindopril on large artery stiffness and aortic root diameter in patients with Marfan syndrome: a randomized controlled trial. JAMA. 2007;298(13):1539–47. JAMA. 2015;314(24):2692–3.
111. Suzuki T, et al. Type-selective benefits of medications in treatment of acute aortic dissection (from the International Registry of Acute Aortic Dissection [IRAD]). Am J Cardiol. 2012;109(1):122–7.
112. Zeng D, et al. Du1, encoding a novel Prp1 protein, regulates starch biosynthesis through affecting the splicing of Wxb pre-mRNAs in rice (*Oryza sativa* L.). Plant Mol Biol. 2007;65(4):501–9.
113. Erbel R, et al. 2014 ESC Guidelines on the diagnosis and treatment of aortic diseases: document covering acute and chronic aortic diseases of the thoracic and abdominal aorta of the adult. The Task Force for the Diagnosis and Treatment of Aortic Diseases of the European Society of Cardiology (ESC). Eur Heart J. 2014;35(41):2873–926.
114. Di Eusanio M, et al. Clinical presentation, management, and short-term outcome of patients with type A acute dissection complicated by mesenteric malperfusion: observations from the International Registry of Acute Aortic Dissection. J Thorac Cardiovasc Surg. 2013;145(2):385–390.e1.
115. Fann JI, et al. Treatment of patients with aortic dissection presenting with peripheral vascular complications. Ann Surg. 1990;212(6):705–13.
116. Kamman AV, et al. Visceral malperfusion in aortic dissection: the Michigan experience. Semin Thorac Cardiovasc Surg. 2017;29(2):173–8.
117. Lauterbach SR, et al. Contemporary management of aortic branch compromise resulting from acute aortic dissection. J Vasc Surg. 2001;33(6):1185–92.
118. Deeb GM, et al. Surgical delay for acute type A dissection with malperfusion. Ann Thorac Surg. 1997;64(6):1669–75; discussion 1675–7.
119. Slonim SM, et al. Percutaneous balloon fenestration and stenting for life-threatening ischemic complications in patients with acute aortic dissection. J Thorac Cardiovasc Surg. 1999;117(6):1118–26.
120. Stanger O, et al. Type A aortic dissection after nonaortic cardiac surgery. Circulation. 2013;128(15):1602–11.

Chapter 10
Endovascular Management of Acute Type A Aortic Dissections

Adam Daly and Eric E. Roselli

Introduction

Acute type A dissection is a life-threatening emergency, with International Registry Aortic Dissection (IRAD) data highlighting a 1–2% per hour mortality risk in surgically untreated patients [1, 3]. Operative mortality rates of 18–25% are commonly described although this may be reduced to 5–8% in expert aortic centers [7]. Up to one-third of patients may be deemed inoperable due to co-morbidities, critical status, or due to complications of dissection [2, 8]. As such, these patients who are denied a mechanical treatment option for acute dissection suffer a medically treated mortality rate of 57–67%, which has not improved overtime [3, 4, 8]. In a detailed analysis of these patients turned down at our center, we found that two-thirds were related to very high, but not necessarily prohibitive, risk considerations (e.g., elderly and frail versus end-stage disease) [8]. The role of endovascular management in treating descending aortic dissection has now superseded open surgery and forms the basis upon which off-label use of endovascular treatment in the proximal aorta should be considered. Over the last two decades, our group and many others have described their anecdotal experiences with the off-label use of endovascular devices for treating ascending aortic pathology including acute dissection [6, 8–14]. As Michael Dake pointedly describes in a recent editorial on the subject, "…moving the discussion beyond the novelty level of "look, it can be done" to the next stage … of a clinical trial … I wonder … if the current TEVAR technology is ready" [15].

A. Daly · E. E. Roselli (✉)
Aortic Center, Department of Thoracic and Cardiovascular Surgery, Heart, Vascular, and Thoracic Institute, Cleveland Clinic, Cleveland, OH, USA
e-mail: RosellE@ccf.org

G. J. Arnaoutakis et al. (eds.), *Aortic Aneurysms*, Contemporary Cardiology, https://doi.org/10.1007/978-3-032-13134-8_10

Endovascular Management of Dissection

The accepted benefit of TEVAR in distal aortic dissection has led to subspecialization, increased operator skillset, and expanded ability to treat increasingly complex aortic disease. The potential benefit of endovascular surgery in the arch and more proximal aorta is being explored, especially in the face of dismal outcomes in medically treated patients with aortic dissection who are deemed unsuitable for open surgery. Figure 10.1 demonstrates our treatment algorithm for patients with acute Type A dissection. Endovascular surgery avoids sternotomy, cardiopulmonary bypass, and circulatory arrest and avoids or reduces the associated sequelae of open surgery such as coagulopathy, myocardial, cerebral, and renal ischemia. Certainly, in the acute complicated type B aortic dissection cohort, TEVAR has shown favorable mortality and morbidity outcomes relative to open surgery or medical management [5]. Can adherence to the important principles of care in this subset of patients translate to successful TEVAR in patients with acute ascending aortic dissection?

The principal objective of endovascular surgery in acute aortic dissection is sealing the entry-tear and redirecting flow through the true lumen using covered stent-grafts to optimize end-organ perfusion and reduce the risk of aortic rupture. Other important technical considerations learned from the experience with TEVAR for distal aortic dissection include achieving this seal within an adequate proximal landing zone measuring at least 15–20 mm in length of coverage with a parallel lie to the proximal sealing stent portion and minimal oversizing (i.e., <10%) so as to reduce the risk of focal aortic injury and retrograde dissection. Bare metal stents have been implicated in the risk of intimal injury and coverage of the left subclavian artery has been readily tolerated to achieve these other more pressing goals.

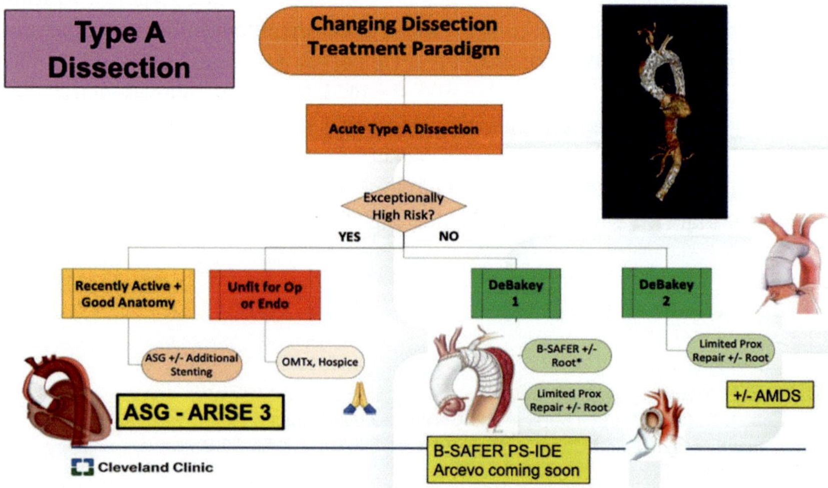

Fig. 10.1 Current treatment algorithm for acute type A aortic dissection at the Cleveland Clinic

Although the principal objective of covering the entry tear is maintained when performing TEVAR for ascending aortic dissection, the biologic and physiologic behavior of the ascending aorta is very different from the descending aorta. TEVAR in this space requires a unique understanding of the pathology, hemodynamic boundary conditions, and additional considerations posed by the patient prosthesis interface in this location. In fact, we have demonstrated that even along the length of the ascending aorta that there exist important regional differences in both clinical behavior and in-vitro tissue biomechanics [16, 17].

With this in mind, there are several morphological and technical aspects that must be considered when determining suitability for endovascular surgery in the ascending aorta that differ from descending TEVAR. The use of endovascular stenting in acute type A aortic dissection as an off-label procedure has provided important insights into the development of a sight-specific device and delivery system designed for treating the ascending aorta that has gone through an initial first-in-human trial for treating ascending aortic dissection and is currently being investigated as part of two additional pivotal studies focused on elective and emergency indications, respectively (ASG devices, ARISE, ARISE2, and ARISE3 trials; W.L. Gore, Flagstaff, AZ, USA) [6, 17].

Aorta and Patient-Related Challenges

The morphologic characteristics and the hemodynamic environment of the proximal aorta differ greatly from those of the descending thoracic aorta. The proximal aorta is more curved than the distal aorta. On average, the greater curvature of the ascending aorta is about 30% longer than the lesser curvature of the ascending aorta [17]. This complex shape and variability among patients can lead to variability in device conformations and angulation. Furthermore, the ascending aorta is relatively short, averaging 7 cm in the center line of flow length which is 3 cm shorter than most commercially available descending stentgrafts [18]. However, the devices tend to foreshorten and the length along the greater curve may be more accurate to use during planning.

In endovascular surgery, the aorta is subdivided into sequential zones to allow for a standardized method of designating the device landing zone and extent of treatment. Using this convention, zone zero vaguely refers to the aorta proximal to the innominate artery. Previously, we further subcategorized zone zero into three segments (0A, 0B, 0C) as demonstrated in Fig. 10.2 which we found to be useful in assessing the complexity of the lesion and prognosis [17]. In our early experience with off-label use of devices, 71% of acute aortic syndromes undergoing ascending endovascular intervention involved zone 0A, which conferred a worse survival advantage compared to the 29% that only extended to zone 0B. The patients with the distribution of disease beyond zone 0A were more likely to have an aortic entry tear that was amenable to coverage with the

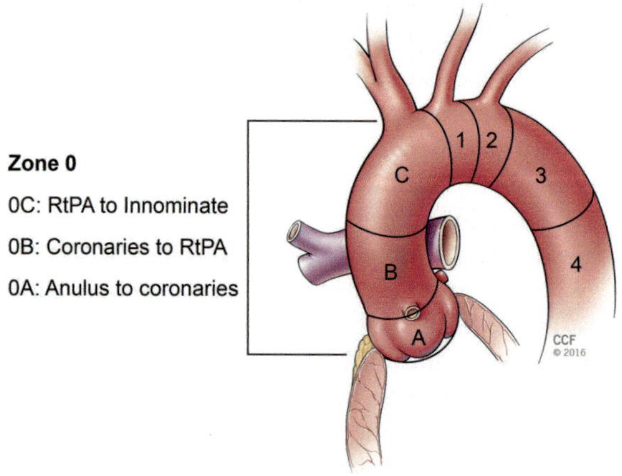

Fig. 10.2 Subcategorization of Zone 0. (Adapted from Ref. [17], used with permission)

stentgraft device, a factor that is critical to success. Although it has not been well described, it is generally accepted that a large proportion of entry tears in acute ascending aortic dissections occur in the proximal half of the ascending aorta on the greater curve.

In addition to anatomic and morphologic details of disease involving the ascending aorta, one must consider the volatility of the hemodynamic environment in the ascending aorta and how this may affect TEVAR devices placed in this location. The boundary conditions of the aorta in this location and how they may affect the patient prosthesis interface are still incompletely understood, but the elasticity and compliance of the ascending aorta is clearly greater than that which is encountered in the more distal thoracic aorta. This may be accentuated in patients with aortic valve insufficiency and younger patients with greater elastic energy [16]. Additionally, patients with acute dissection are often severely hypertensive placing additional stress and displacement forces upon TEVAR devices in this location. After ascending stentgrafting, it will also be important to understand how the patient prosthesis interface affects flow dynamics and aortic wall biomechanics.

Device and Procedure-Related Challenges

A fundamental principle for achieving satisfactory technical outcome with endovascular surgery is ensuring adequate seal and fixation. To facilitate this, adequate proximal and distal landing zone locations are required. Typically, this is defined as a length of aorta of at least 15–20 mm with a shape and contour that allows for a parallel lie of the device's sealing stent to optimize circumferential apposition. In other aortic locations, securing the stentgrafts within proper landing zone may require coverage of a branch vessel (e.g., left subclavian artery or celiac artery), but in the ascending aorta it is critical not to compromise flow into the left and right

Table 10.1 Characteristics favoring endovascular surgery

Favors endosurgery	Against endosurgery
High/prohibitive open surgical risk	Suitable for open surgery
Entry tear in mid-ascending aorta, >2 cm from sinotubular junction	Moderate-severe aortic incompetence
Ascending aorta diameter <38 mm (may be <48 mm with investigational devices)	Aorto-coronary bypass grafts
Adequate peripheral access (femoral or axillary artery >8 mm, limited calcification, limited tortuosity)	

main coronary arteries proximally. Distally, partial coverage of the innominate artery may be tolerated without compromising perfusion, but it cannot be totally covered. A suitably sized stent to provide the necessary radial force relative to aortic size is required. Due to the greater displacement forces and compliance of the ascending aorta as compared to the more distal aorta, a greater percentage of oversizing has been recommended in the ascending aorta as compared to the descending thoracic aorta (10–30% versus <10% for acute dissections). Table 10.1 demonstrates important patient characteristics favorable for endovascular surgery.

Relative to stentgrafting in the descending aorta, stenting in the ascending aorta or arch is more complicated. The relatively short and asymmetrical ascending aorta can pose difficulties for commercially available stents designed for the descending aorta which are at minimum 10 cm in length, and which generally have equidistant sides. Obtaining an adequate landing zone can be difficult given the oftentimes relatively short ascending aorta, proximal location of the entry tear, and relative proximity of the aortic root (i.e., coronary arteries and aortic valve). Furthermore, due to the 270° angulation that must be achieved to access the ascending aorta from the descending thoracic aorta and the increased hemodynamic force due to relative proximity to the contractile forces from the left ventricle, accurate placement and deployment of the stent can be challenging [2]. These challenges are not insurmountable however and specific technical considerations are addressed below.

Imaging A gated CT scan of the aorta is recommended for preoperative assessment and planning, to reduce motion artefact, to accurately identify the site of entry tear, and to accurately assess center-line cross-sectional area measurements and greater curvature length.

Entry Tear Site Accurate identification of the entry tear is critical to the success of the procedure as the goal is to occlude flow into the entry site. Approximately 75% of tears in acute type A dissection are in the ascending aorta; 66% of these are along the greater curvature, 14% along the lesser curvature, 10% anteriorly located, and 10% posteriorly located [18]. Because of the proximity of many entry tears to the sinotubular junction (STJ) of the aorta, an ideal deployment would allow for precise and circumferential alignment of the stentgrafts device at the STJ. For patients with persistent true lumen compression after coverage of the proximal entry tear, additional stentgrafting to cover additional entry tears and/or the use of bare metal stents (Zenith-D, Cook, Indiana, USA) may be considered to promote flow through the true lumen and aortic remodeling in certain cases, particularly if there is persistent distal malperfusion [19].

Aortic Diameter The aortic diameter should be measured perpendicular to the center line. Current commonly used stentgrafts enable stenting in aortas ranging from 18 to 42 mm. Aortic diameters in the ascending aorta are larger than other more distal segments of the aorta and in the diseased state commonly exceed 4 cm. To achieve seal and fixation in these larger caliber aortic segments with greater oversizing requirements dedicated ascending stentgraft devices may need to come in larger sizes than what is currently available. Currently, work is underway to design a version of the ASG device (WL Gore, Flagstaff, AZ, USA) that comes in a diameter up to 53 mm. If the proximal landing zone is adequately sized to achieve seal, but the distal ascending aorta is too large, more complex endovascular surgery can be performed to circumnavigate the issue by extending the stentgraft across the arch with branched stentgrafting into the supra-aortic vessels. These branched arch grafts are currently investigational for some devices in zones zero and one, but the Gore TBE device has recently been FDA-approved for commercial use in zone 2 and zone 0 but without the proximal ascending component.

Stentgraft Considerations No dedicated ascending aorta stentgraft is currently commercially available, and the ASG device is still in early-phase studies. A review of published ascending stentgrafting experiences demonstrated 13 different devices were used for 118 patients, 71% of which were thoracic endovascular stentgrafts, highlighting the variability of equipment used to accommodate anatomical variation [20]. In the acute aortic syndrome setting delay is often not safe, so customized devices do not offer a reasonable option. The complex and varying morphology of the ascending aorta requires a device that can be modified to fit the patient as is available to some extent in the novel ASG device. To accommodate the short ascending aorta, the device lengths should be limited to 5–10 cm.

In our earlier series with mostly off-label use of devices, most patients had a proximal landing zone in 0B providing adequate territory for landing with less than ideal device accuracy. In the subset of patients requiring proximal landing in zone 0A, more intraoperative complications and poorer outcomes occurred. Coronary occlusion required conversion to open procedure and early mortality in one, and in others the device was repositioned distally using a technique of rapid pacing for balloon capture of the device followed by cardiac ejection to shift the position of the device internally [17]. We have also used this balloon repositioning technique to address significant aortic valve incompetence caused by leaflet capture from the edge of stentgrafts extending too far into the aortic root.

Access Retrograde delivery of the stentgrafts is preferred. As with any endovascular procedure, adequate peripheral access is required and vessel requirements are similar to what has been described for other TEVAR procedures (>7 mm). Alternative access site options have been described including the left axillary artery and the left ventricular apex [9, 21].

Technique

Endovascular treatment of acute type A dissections should be managed in a hybrid operating room with high-resolution fluoroscopy and mechanical circulatory support and open conversion equipment readily available. Preoperative anesthesiology preparation includes placement of two arterial lines, pre- and post-arch, central venous access, general anesthesia, and intubation with single lumen tube. Both transesophageal echocardiography (TEE) and intravascular ultrasound (IVUS) are crucial both for pre- and postoperative assessment of ventricular and valvular function and to guide aortic navigation and stent deployment.

Access is determined based on preoperative imaging, but typically large-bore femoral access is obtained for device delivery and a 5Fr sheath is placed in the right arm for delivery of the angiography catheter into the aortic root across the innominate artery. Additionally, a 5 or 6Fr sheath is placed into a femoral vein for placement of the temporary transvenous pacing wire. Heparin is given to achieve an activated clotting time of approximately 250–300 s once access is secured. In our early experience, transfemoral access was most commonly used (56%), followed by axillary artery (23%) and left ventricle apex (22%) [6, 17]. Transfemoral delivery is performed over a stiff wire (Lunderquist, Cook, Indiana, USA) with access across the aortic valve [17]. Fluoroscopy and TEE guidance are critical to accurate wire placement and to assess aortic valve function in the setting of a transvalvular wire. During stentgraft deployment, rapid ventricular pacing is performed to reduce the ejection force of the ventricle and therefore reduce the potential for malpositioning. With the ASG device, deployment is staged into four components, as demonstrated in Fig. 10.3. During the first stage, the device is partially deployed allowing for longitudinal repositioning and creating a curvature of the device by foreshortening the lesser curve, and during the second stage the device is fully expanded and then may be further foreshortened along the lesser curve to optimize the lie in relation to the STJ before final release from the delivery system. Completion angiogram is performed to ensure adequate placement, seal of the tear, coronary and arch branch patency, and to rule out endoleak [6, 17]. Completion TEE confirms maintenance (or improvement) of aortic valve function.

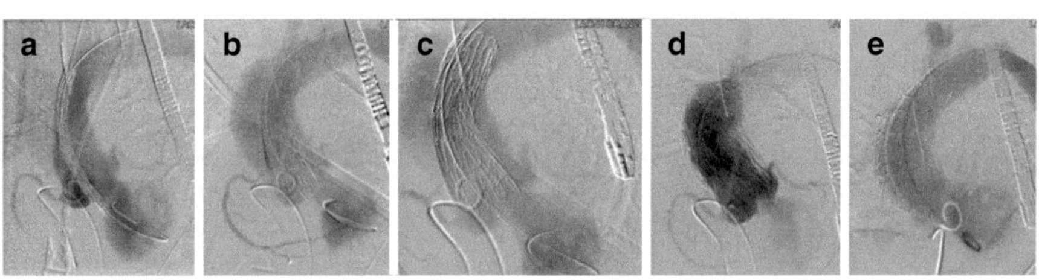

Fig. 10.3 Intraoperative fluoroscopy demonstrating the staged delivery of the ASG device. (Adapted from Ref. [6], used with permission). (**a**) delivery into the ascending aorta, (**b**) first-stage deployment with partial expansion, (**c**) device curvature aligned with coronary origins, (**d**) second-stage deployment with full expansion, (**e**) and completion aortogram after delivery and full deployment of the second distal device

The extent of endovascular repair can range from a limited repair sealing the entry tear in the ascending aorta to a total endovascular aortic repair of the entire thoracic aorta. More extensive distal endovascular surgery may include the use of a hybrid strategy with the use of covered proximal stentgrafts to seal the ascending aortic entry tear, combined with investigational branched devices to span across the aortic arch, and potentially, additional bare metal stenting across the thoracoabdominal segments of the aorta to counteract true lumen compression and promote aortic wall remodeling [19]. More extensive proximal repair including "Endo-Bentall" repairs has also been described [22]. In our experience, the use of endovascular surgery may be extended to other high-risk cases including intramural hematoma, pseudoaneurysm and chronic dissection, either as definitive surgery or as a bridge to completion surgery, with satisfactory results including an 81% operative survival and 64% five-year survival [17, 21].

Outcomes and Specific Risks

Endovascular treatment in acute type A aortic dissection is novel and outcome data is limited. Limited case series describing endovascular surgery for the management of type A dissection and other high-risk conditions demonstrate satisfactory operative survival of up to 85% and therefore this remains a viable option for high-risk operative candidates [21]. We previously demonstrated that survival in patients with pathology in Zone 0A was significantly worse compared to Zone 0B or Zone 0C [17].

While the proposed benefits of endovascular surgery include avoidance of sternotomy, avoidance of cardiopulmonary bypass and circulatory arrest which enable high-risk candidates to be offered a treatment other than medical management, there are indeed risks particular to endovascular surgery that must be considered. Overall, one meta-analysis reported the most common complication was that of Type 1 endoleak which occurred in 18.2% of cases [8]. Complications such as stent migration, retrograde extension of the dissection into the aortic root, and aortic rupture can occur [20]. The risk of embolic cerebrovascular events, akin to the TAVR population, still exists and can be expected in proximal aortic pathology. Cases of severe aortic incompetence due to interference of the stent-graft with the aortic valve have been described but will hopefully become less of an issue with the development of more accurate dedicated site-specific devices [23]. Rarely, conversion to open procedure due to retained delivery system can also occur and highlights the importance of creating a multi-disciplinary team to perform these operations safely [21, 24].

The Future

Endovascular surgery remains in its infancy and limited to high- or prohibitive-risk patients with acute type A aortic dissection. The promising role of endovascular surgery in complicated type B dissection and evolving role of transcatheter aortic valve replacement provides an exciting insight into the potential role of endosurgery in the acute type A population. Concomitant TAVR has been described and discussed as a potential adjunct for some patients; however, we know outcomes of TAVR for aortic incompetence are not as promising as in those who present with stenosis and there may be a risk of device migration or embolization [25, 26]. In 2020, there was a single case of a customized device created for the performance of a so-called endo-Bentall procedure, but this was a very unique case of chronic aneurysm and the everyday use of such technology is still far from reality as an emergency off-the-shelf option. It is important to remember that with the current state of TAVR technology that even the latest iterations of these devices have a significant occurrence of minimal to mild paravalvular leak that would manifest as a serious endoleak in a patient with ascending aortic disease [27, 28].

Limitations in acute type A dissection endovascular repair remain individual patient anatomical variability and precise imaging of such, a lack of commercially available stentgrafts, and endovascular technical expertise. Open surgical repair will remain the gold standard for the general population with acute type A dissection repair until endovascular repair is proven to provide similar long-term outcomes, but it is likely that it will eventually play a complementary role to open repair.

"The next-generation ascending stent-graft device needs to be highly conformable and elastic with adequate strength of fixation in what is a hostile environment. The device likely needs to be curved like the ascending aorta. It should have a relatively flush edge proximally so that it does not impose on the origins of the coronaries or the commissures of the aortic valve despite the need to abut them. As we learn more about the endovascular treatment of ascending disease, we will better understand the need for branched devices to accommodate the brachiocephalic and other arch branch vessels so that distal seal and fixation are achieved. The novel delivery systems will need to be exceedingly precise to allow for controlled deployment at the sinotubular junction in a coaxial plane. This may require a repositionable system that is steerable. The tip of the delivery system needs to be short because of the proximity to the aortic valve. The least-invasive delivery options are retrograde." [17]. As industry continues to develop site specific devices and study their use in the ascending aorta, we will continue to improve our understanding of the role for this novel technology.

Author Disclosures Dr. Roselli speaks and serves as a consultant and investigator for Artivion, Cook, Edwards Lifesciences, W.L. Gore, Medtronic, and Terumo Aortic.

Funding None to disclose.

References

1. Malaisrie SC, Szeto WY, Halas M, Girardi LN, Coselli JS, Sundt TM, et al. 2021 The American Association for Thoracic Surgery expert consensus document: surgical treatment of acute type A aortic dissection. J Thorac Cardiovasc Surg [Internet]. 2021 [cited 2022 Aug 24];162(3):735–758.e2. Available from: http://www.jtcvs.org/article/S0022522321007376/fulltext
2. Nordon IM, Hinchliffe RJ, Morgan R, Loftus IM, Jahangiri M, Thompson MM. Progress in endovascular management of type A dissection. Eur J Vasc Endovasc Surg [Internet]. 2012 [cited 2022 Mar 13];44(4):406–10. Available from: https://pubmed.ncbi.nlm.nih.gov/22921418/
3. Evangelista A, Isselbacher EM, Bossone E, Gleason TG, di Eusanio M, Sechtem U, et al. Insights from the international registry of acute aortic dissection: A 20-year experience of collaborative clinical research. Circulation [Internet]. 2018 [cited 2022 Mar 13];137(17):1846–60. Available from: https://www.ahajournals.org/doi/abs/10.1161/CIRCULATIONAHA.117.031264
4. Inoue Y, Matsuda H, Uchida K, Komiya T, Koyama T, Yoshino H, et al. Analysis of acute type A aortic dissection in Japan Registry of Aortic Dissection (JRAD). Ann Thorac Surg. 2020;110(3):790–8.
5. MacGillivray TE, Gleason TG, Patel HJ, Aldea GS, Bavaria JE, Beaver TM, et al. The Society of Thoracic Surgeons/American Association for Thoracic Surgery Clinical Practice Guidelines on the management of type B aortic dissection. Ann Thorac Surg [Internet]. 2022 [cited 2022 Mar 13];0(0). Available from: http://www.annalsthoracicsurgery.org/article/S0003497521019743/fulltext
6. Roselli EE, Atkins MD, Brinkman W, Coselli J, Desai N, Estrera A, et al. ARISE: first-in-human evaluation of a novel stent graft to treat ascending aortic dissection. J Endovasc Ther [Internet]. 2022 [cited 2022 Aug 24]. Available from: https://journals.sagepub.com/doi/abs/10.1177/15266028221095018?journalCode=jeta
7. Aggarwal B, Raymond CE, Randhawa MS, Roselli E, Jacob J, Eagleton M, et al. Transfer metrics in patients with suspected acute aortic syndrome. Circ Cardiovasc Qual Outcomes [Internet]. 2014 [cited 2022 Aug 24];7(5):780–2. Available from: https://pubmed.ncbi.nlm.nih.gov/25205785/
8. Roselli EE, Hasan SM, Idrees JJ, Aftab M, Eagleton MJ, Menon V, et al. Inoperable patients with acute type A dissection: are they candidates for endovascular repair? Interact Cardiovasc Thorac Surg [Internet]. 2017 [cited 2022 Aug 24];25(4):582–8. Available from: https://pubmed.ncbi.nlm.nih.gov/28962505/
9. Roselli EE, Brozzi N, Albacker T, Lytle BW. Transapical endovascular ascending repair for inoperable acute type A dissection. JACC Cardiovasc Interv [Internet]. 2013 [cited 2022 Aug 24];6(4):425–6. Available from: https://www.jacc.org/doi/10.1016/j.jcin.2012.10.021
10. Ghoreishi M, Shah A, Jeudy J, Pasrija C, Lebowitz J, Kaczorowski D, et al. Endovascular repair of ascending aortic disease in high-risk patients yields favorable outcome. Ann Thorac Surg [Internet]. 2020 [cited 2022 Aug 24];109(3):678–85. Available from: https://pubmed.ncbi.nlm.nih.gov/31472140/
11. Kölbel T, Reiter B, Schirmer J, Wipper S, Detter C, Debus ES, et al. Customized transapical thoracic endovascular repair for acute type A dissection. Ann Thorac Surg. 2013;95(2):694–6.
12. Metcalfe MJ, Karthikesalingam A, Black SA, Loftus IM, Morgan R, Thompson MM. The first endovascular repair of an acute type A dissection using an endograft designed for the ascending aorta. J Vasc Surg. 2012;55(1):220–2.
13. Lu Q, Feng J, Zhou J, Zhao Z, Bao J, Feng R, et al. Endovascular repair of ascending aortic dissection: a novel treatment option for patients judged unfit for direct surgical repair. J Am Coll Cardiol [Internet]. 2013 [cited 2022 Aug 24];61(18):1917–24. Available from: https://pubmed.ncbi.nlm.nih.gov/23122798/

14. Vallabhajosyula P, Gottret JP, Bavaria JE, Desai ND, Szeto WY. Endovascular repair of the ascending aorta in patients at high risk for open repair. J Thorac Cardiovasc Surg. 2015;149(2):S144–50.
15. Dake MD. On the endovascular climb to the type A dissection summit, reaching a new base camp*. J Am Coll Cardiol [Internet]. 2016 [cited 2022 Aug 24];68(18):1955–7. Available from: https://www.jacc.org/doi/10.1016/j.jacc.2016.07.772
16. Durbak E, Tarraf S, Gillespie C, Germano E, Cikach F, Blackstone E, et al. Ex vivo biaxial load testing analysis of aortic biomechanics demonstrates variation in elastic energy distribution across the aortic zone zero. J Thorac Cardiovasc Surg. 2021;166(3):701–712.e7.
17. Roselli EE, Idrees JJ, Johnston DR, Eagleton MJ, Desai MY, Svensson LG. Zone zero thoracic endovascular aortic repair: a proposed modification to the classification of landing zones. J Thorac Cardiovasc Surg [Internet]. 2018 [cited 2022 Mar 20];155(4):1381–9. Available from: http://www.jtcvs.org/article/S0022522317327411/fulltext
18. Moon MC, Greenberg RK, Morales JP, Martin Z, Lu Q, Dowdall JF, et al. Computed tomography-based anatomic characterization of proximal aortic dissection with consideration for endovascular candidacy. J Vasc Surg [Internet]. 2011 [cited 2022 Mar 18];53(4):942–9. Available from: https://pubmed.ncbi.nlm.nih.gov/21345636/
19. Vargo PR, Tarola CL, Durbak E, Doh CY, Caputo FJ, Smolock CJ, et al. Early results of bare metal extension stent for thoracoabdominal aortic dissection. JTCVS Tech [Internet]. 2022 [cited 2022 Aug 24];14:1–8. Available from: http://www.jtcvstechniques.org/article/S2666250722002371/fulltext
20. Muetterties CE, Menon R, Wheatley GH. A systematic review of primary endovascular repair of the ascending aorta. J Vasc Surg [Internet]. 2018 [cited 2022 Mar 18];67(1):332–42. Available from: https://pubmed.ncbi.nlm.nih.gov/28844469/
21. Roselli EE, Idrees J, Greenberg RK, Johnston DR, Lytle BW. Endovascular stent grafting for ascending aorta repair in high-risk patients. J Thorac Cardiovasc Surg [Internet]. 2015 [cited 2022 Mar 18];149(1):144–54. Available from: https://pubmed.ncbi.nlm.nih.gov/25312226/
22. Felipe Gaia D, Bernal O, Castilho E, Baeta Neves Duarte Ferreira C, Dvir D, Simonato M, et al. First-in-human Endo-Bentall procedure for simultaneous treatment of the ascending aorta and aortic valve. JACC Case Rep. 2020;2(3):480–5.
23. Palma JH, Gaia DF, Guilhen JS, Buffolo E. Endovascular treatment of chronic type A dissection. Interact Cardiovasc Thorac Surg [Internet]. 2008 [cited 2022 Mar 18];7(1):164–6. Available from: https://pubmed.ncbi.nlm.nih.gov/17933835/
24. Roselli EE, Idrees J, Mick S, Kapadia S, Tuzcu M, Svensson LG, et al. Emergency use of cardiopulmonary bypass in complicated transcatheter aortic valve replacement: importance of a heart team approach. J Thorac Cardiovasc Surg. 2014;148(4):1413–6.
25. Arias EA, Bhan A, Lim ZY, Mullen M. TAVI for pure native aortic regurgitation: are we there yet? Interv Cardiol. 2019;14(1):26–30. https://doi.org/10.15420/icr.2018.37.1 Available from: /pmc/articles/PMC6406131/
26. TAVR for Aortic Regurgitation—American College of Cardiology [Internet]. [cited 2022 Aug 24]. Available from: https://www.acc.org/latest-in-cardiology/articles/2017/12/21/08/16/tavr-for-aortic-regurgitation
27. Franzone A, Piccolo R, Siontis GCM, Lanz J, Stortecky S, Praz F, et al. Transcatheter aortic valve replacement for the treatment of pure native aortic valve regurgitation: a systematic review. JACC Cardiovasc Interv [Internet]. 2016 [cited 2022 Aug 24];9(22):2308–17. Available from: https://pubmed.ncbi.nlm.nih.gov/28026742/
28. Montalto C, Sticchi A, Crimi G, Laricchia A, Khokhar AA, Giannini F, et al. Outcomes after transcatheter aortic valve replacement in bicuspid versus tricuspid anatomy: a systematic review and meta-analysis. Cardiovasc Interv [Internet]. 2021 [cited 2022 Aug 24];14(19):2144–55. Available from: https://www.jacc.org/doi/10.1016/j.jcin.2021.07.052

Chapter 11
Nonoperative Management of Type B Aortic Dissection

John R. Spratt and George J. Arnaoutakis

Introduction

Historically, uncomplicated type B aortic dissection has been managed through vigilant imaging monitoring and the administration of anti-impulse medications, aimed at averting both immediate and delayed aortic complications.

Definitions

Classification of Aortic Dissection

Aortic dissection (AD) results from a weakness of the aortic media that is aggravated by an intimal tear that results in the progressive mechanical destruction of the medial layer by pulsatile blood flow [1]. The destruction of the medial layer creates a second (false) lumen (FL) which flows in parallel to the native (true) lumen (TL) separated by an intimomedial septum referred to most commonly as an "intimal flap" or "dissection flap," creating a characteristic double-barrel appearance of the aorta on cross-sectional imaging [2]. The dissection flap can develop fenestrations

J. R. Spratt (✉)
Division of Cardiovascular Surgery, Department of Surgery, University of Florida, Gainesville, FL, USA
e-mail: john.spratt@surgery.ufl.edu

G. J. Arnaoutakis
Division of Cardiovascular and Thoracic Surgery, Department of Cardiovascular and Thoracic Surgery, University of Texas at Austin Dell Medical School, Austin, TX, USA
e-mail: george.arnaoutakis@austin.utexas.edu

G. J. Arnaoutakis et al. (eds.), *Aortic Aneurysms*, Contemporary Cardiology,
https://doi.org/10.1007/978-3-032-13134-8_11

as the false lumen propagates distally by shearing off the intimal component of branch vessel ostia, allowing re-entry of flow into the true lumen and maintaining false lumen patency.

Historically, aortic dissection has been classified based on the location of the entry tear and the anatomic extent of the dissection under one of two classification systems. Under the Stanford classification system, dissections involving the ascending aorta are considered "type A." Dissections limited to the descending aorta at or distal to the level of the left subclavian artery (LSA) are considered "type B." The simplicity of this classification has contributed to its wide adoption but also creates a set of specific exceptions for presentations not captured by this binary system. Dissections confined purely to the aortic arch without extension into the ascending aorta or beyond the LSA are considered "non-A, non-B" dissections and those with the primary entry tear beyond the ascending aorta but with ascending involvement by retrograde extension are considered "retrograde type A" dissections [3].

Alternatively, the DeBakey classification system provides more anatomic detail. Dissections originating in and extending beyond the ascending aorta are considered type I, whereas those confined to the ascending aorta are considered type II. Dissections originating in the descending aorta beyond the LSA are considered type III, with subtypes for those confined to (IIIa) and extending beyond (IIIb) the thoracic aorta [3].

A 2020 joint guideline issued by the Society of Vascular Surgery (SVS) and Society of Thoracic Surgeons (STS) offers a detailed classification system that avoids much of the ambiguity of the Stanford and DeBakey classifications (Fig. 11.1) [4]. Based on the location of the entry tear, dissections are grouped into three distinct categories, "A" (entry tear in zone 0), "B" (entry tear in zone ≥1), and "I" (unidentified entry tear in dissection involving zone 0). Beyond these three main

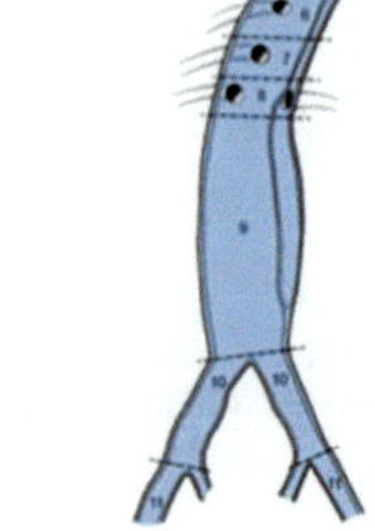

Type	Proximal Extent	Distal Extent
A_D Entry tear: Zone 0	0	0
	1	1
	2	2
	3	3
B_{PD} Entry tear: ≥Zone 1	4	4
	5	5
	6	6
	7	7
	8	8
I_D Unidentified entry tear involving Zone 0	9	9
	10	10
	11	11
	12	12

Fig. 11.1 STS/SVS aortic dissection classification system. (Adapted from Fig. 3 of Ann Thorac Surg 113, P1073)

groups, subscript descriptors are added to specify the extent of dissection. For example, dissections originating in the ascending aorta and terminating in the infrarenal aorta are considered "A_9", whereas a dissection with an entry tear in the mid-descending aorta extending distally into the common iliac arteries and proximally to the level of the innominate artery would be considered "$B_{10,1}$". Non-A, non-B dissections may be more precisely described as "$B_{1,2}$" and retrograde type A dissections can be described based on the ability to identify the entry tear on imaging (e.g., $B_{0,4}$ vs. I_4).

Malperfusion

The phenomenon of malperfusion is defined by the impairment of blood flow to an end organ as the result of a dissection. Depending on the extent of the dissection, the propagation of the false lumen within the aortic wall may narrow or completely obstruct the inflow to any aortic branch. "Malperfusion syndrome" refers to clinical manifestation(s) of end-organ ischemia (e.g., acute kidney injury from diminished renal blood flow, lower extremity neurovascular impairment from iliac involvement, or lactic acidosis from compromised mesenteric inflow) associated with malperfusion [1].

Complicated vs. Uncomplicated Type B Aortic Dissection

Type B dissections may be considered "complicated" or "uncomplicated" based on the presence of certain radiographic and clinical features (Table 11.1). Complicated dissections are those with clear evidence of rupture or a clinically evident malperfusion syndrome. TBAD may also be included in a third category, "high-risk", based on several specific features, which include refractory pain/hypertension, large aortic (>40 mm) or false lumen (>22 mm) diameters, and readmission. The presence of a bloody-appearing pleural effusion on imaging is also considered high-risk. TBAD without rupture, malperfusion, or high-risk features is considered uncomplicated [1].

Table 11.1 Type B aortic dissection characteristics

Uncomplicated
No rupture
No malperfusion
No high-risk features
High-risk
Refractory pain
Refractory hypertension
Bloody pleural effusion
Aortic diameter > 40 mm
Radiographic-only malperfusion
Readmission
Entry tear on lesser curve of arch
False lumen diameter > 22 mm
Complicated
Rupture
Malperfusion

Other Acute Aortic Syndromes

Intramural Hematoma

Intramural hematoma (IMH) is defined as a crescentic or circumferential thickening of the aortic wall without evidence of intimal defect and is thought to result from spontaneous hemorrhage of vaso vasora into the aortic media. A disease seen primarily in older patients, risk factors include longstanding hypertension, atherosclerosis, and tobacco use, which may contribute to degeneration and structural instability of aortic media and vaso vasorum [5]. IMH preferentially affects the descending aorta and is anatomically classified by the same systems used for true aortic dissections. However, in a subtle shift from the Stanford classification, "type B" is used to describe IMH in both the arch and the descending aorta. Malperfusion and its sequelae are uncommon in IMH because of its more focal nature and lower tendency to propagate within the aortic wall than dissection, although spinal cord ischemia can affect as many as 9.8% of patients with type B IMH because of local effects on intercostal vessels. IMH can progress to a more typical dissection and may also lead to aneurysmal dilation and/or aortic rupture. There are certain "high-risk" radiographic and clinical features of type B IMH are associated with worse outcomes without intervention, including maximum aortic diameter greater that 47–55 mm, wall thickness >11–13 mm, increasing or recurrent pleural effusion, progressive aortic or hematoma enlargement, poor blood pressure control, focal intimal disruption, ulcer-like projections, progression to dissection and persistent pain [5, 6].

Penetrating Atherosclerotic Ulcer

Penetrating atherosclerotic ulcer (PAU) is an atherosclerotic lesion of the aorta with ulceration penetrating the elastic lamina, allowing hematoma formation within the aortic media and possible progression to dissection, IMH, or rupture [6]. Anatomic classification and risk factors for PAU are similar to those for IMH. High-risk radiographic and clinical features of PAU include maximum PAU diameter >13–20 mm, maximum PAU depth >10 mm, significant increase in PAU depth and/ or diameter, association with saccular aneurysm, and presence of an increasing pleural effusion. PAU with adjacent IMH is also associated with high (15–20%) risk of early rupture [6].

Incidence

Overall

The global incidence of acute aortic dissection is approximately 3–14 cases per 100,000 persons per year, of which about 30% are type B dissections. Of these, approximately one-third of type B dissections (10% of total dissection cohort) are considered complicated at presentation based on the presence of clinical evidence of rupture and/ or malperfusion [7]. These population-level statistics may underestimate the true incidence, however, due to the fact that many of these patients die before reaching a hospital with the cause of death either never determined or erroneously attributed to myocardial infarction or other non-aortic pathology [1, 8]. IMH is less common than true dissection but still represents a significant minority of patients presenting with acute aortic syndromes (AAS). Among patients presenting with AAS, IMH is present in 6–23% in North America and Europe and 26–44% in Asia [6]. PAU is a relatively rare cause of AAS (2.3–11%) [9].

Risk Factors for Dissection

The dominant risk factor for aortic dissection is hypertension. Other risk factors include increased age and structural abnormalities of the aortic wall (e.g., Marfan syndrome and other connective tissue disorders). Men are more affected than women; one series from the International Registry of Acute Aortic Dissection (IRAD) reported a male-female ratio of 4:1. While the incidence of Type A dissection appears highest in patients 50–60 years of age, type B dissections most frequently affect patients 60–70 years of age [2, 8].

Clinical Presentation

The most common presenting feature of acute aortic syndromes, regardless of location, is severe sharp and/or stabbing pain in the chest, back, or abdomen. While pain is often the sole complaint, other accompanying symptoms may be present based on the location and extent of the dissection. These include differential extremity blood pressures (unilateral subclavian or iliofemoral inflow compromise), abdominal pain/gastrointestinal bleeding (celiac and/or superior mesenteric malperfusion), dyspnea (airway compression, aortic regurgitation, cardiac tamponade), myocardial ischemia (coronary malperfusion), paraplegia (spinal cord malperfusion from intercostal and/or left subclavian malperfusion), and shock, which may be multifactorial (cardiac tamponade, hemothorax, aortic rupture, acute severe aortic insufficiency, severe myocardial ischemia) [6].

Diagnosis

All acute aortic syndromes, including TBAD, are best visualized by contrasted computed tomographic angiography (CTA) because it is widely available, rapidly performed, and provides high-fidelity images of the entire aorta. A high-quality arterial-phase CTA of the chest, abdomen, and pelvis will demonstrate the extent of dissection, branch vessel involvement, associated pleural and pericardial effusion, and periaortic hematoma, along with secondary evidence of malperfusion (e.g., pneumatosis intestinalis in the setting of superior mesenteric inflow compromise). Anatomic features of other AAS, including IMH and PAU, are readily visualized [3, 6].

Other imaging modalities are also useful in visualizing acute aortic pathology. Transthoracic echocardiography (TTE) is portable, non-invasive, and does not require the administration of IV contrast. TTE does not effectively visualize the arch and thoracoabdominal aorta but can demonstrate proximal ascending/root pathology, including aortic insufficiency, and pericardial effusion. Transesophageal echocardiography (TEE) provides greater sensitivity and anatomic resolution and, although the mid arch is obscured by the trachea, allows visualization of nearly the entire thoracic aorta. Magnetic resonance imaging (MRI) provides diagnostic aortic imaging without the use of iodinated contrast but can be time-consuming to perform, may have limited availability in some settings, and magnetic safety precautions may interfere with the ongoing care of a critically ill patient [6].

Laboratory evaluation does not play a primary role in the diagnosis of AAS. However, certain clusters of findings may be suggestive of patterns of malperfusion or overall acuity of presentation. Lactic acidosis may be seen in the setting of visceral or extremity malperfusion (especially in combination with elevate creatine kinase) or shock caused by cardiac tamponade or aortic rupture. Elevated blood urea nitrogen and creatinine suggestive of acute kidney injury may indicate renal malperfusion. Troponin elevation may be caused by a dissection with coronary involvement.

Medical Management

Initial Management

Following the diagnosis of acute TBAD, the initial therapeutic priority for patients not in extremis is initiation of anti-impulse therapy and pain control, discussed below. Generally, patients presenting in extremis with TBAD are suffering from complicated disease and are likely to require early operative intervention. Patients should be admitted to an ICU setting and reliable large-bore intravenous access and an arterial line for blood pressure monitoring should be established. Once this initial clinical stabilization is underway, it must be determined whether the TBAD is complicated or uncomplicated, described previously, to determine the appropriate therapeutic strategy.

Goals of Therapy

The initial therapeutic objective in patients with uncomplicated TBAD is the prevention of progression of the dissection through the use of anti-impulse therapy [1]. Diligent examination at presentation for any clinical or radiographic signs suggestive of the presence of complicated dissection at initial presentation is essential to prevent patients from being inappropriately assigned to nonoperative treatment. Finally, patients must be continually re-assessed for signs of complicated disease, which may indicate a failure of medical management and the need for procedural intervention.

Anti-impulse Therapy

Medical management of aortic dissection is intended to reduce the hemodynamic forces responsible for creating and propagating the dissection. This is achieved by reducing the systolic blood pressure and the dP/dt, which has the combined effect of reducing the force and duration of the antegrade pressure head within the false lumen responsible for dissection propagation [2]. This is most commonly achieved with the use of infusions of a beta blocker and a vasodilator. Beta blockade is initiated first and titrated to effect, usually a goal heart rate of 60–80 beats per minute, which will likely carry a secondary antihypertensive effect. Following achievement of satisfactory beta blockade, intravenous arterial vasodilator therapy should be used to obtain a systolic blood pressure of 100–120 mmHg. Pain management, usually with opioids, is also essential for patients with acute dissection and may also help with blood pressure control.

Choice of specific agents for anti-impulse therapy may be driven by patient and institutional factors. Labetalol is useful in this setting due to its combined alpha- and beta-antagonism, which can reduce both heart rate and blood pressure. Esmolol is shorter-acting and may be useful as a trial of beta blockade in patients with history of bronchospasm or COPD exacerbation [2]. Sodium nitroprusside and clevidipine are both effective arterial vasodilators and are appropriate for use in this setting.

Once appropriate hemodynamic parameters are achieved and no procedural intervention is planned, patients can be transitioned to oral beta blockade and antihypertensive therapy. Oral labetalol, metoprolol, or atenolol are suitable for beta blockade. Angiotensin-converting enzyme inhibitors, angiotensin receptor blockers, and dihydropyridine calcium channel blockers can be useful for adjunct long-term blood pressure control [1].

Repeat Imaging

During the index hospitalization, patients should undergo emergent repeat CTA if there are new clinical signs concerning for development of complicated disease. These may include pain that is new in location/character that had previously been well controlled, hemodynamic compromise, or evidence of malperfusion. In the absence of these, patients should undergo repeat CTA prior to discharge to document stability of the dissection. Repeat CTA should then be performed at 1 month after discharge and then every 6 months, converting to annual surveillance once stability of the dissection and any associated aneurysm is observed on two or more consecutive studies [2].

Surgical Intervention

Traditionally, surgical intervention for acute type B aortic dissection has been reserved for patients with complicating features such as rupture or malperfusion. Recently, there has been increased focus on high-risk radiographic features, such as large entry tear or large false lumen to true lumen ratio, that have prompted some surgeons to perform early endovascular repair. The benefit of this approach is under active investigation.

Expected Outcomes

Following the acute phase of dissection, the flap will thicken and fibrose and the dissection enters a chronic phase. The new comparative stiffness of the flap will usually prevent propagation of the dissection and cause the flap to become relatively static compared to the dynamic motion of the flap seen in acute dissections. The false lumen, contained primarily by the aortic adventitia and remnant media, is prone to aneurysmal dilation caused by the exposure of its noncompliant wall to continued antegrade blood flow, making diligent surveillance essential [1].

Although long-term outcomes of medical therapy for TBAD are good, a significant number of patients suffer late events attributable to the dissection. Fattori et al. reported a pooled analysis of 1480 patients with TBAD treated medically. Among this group, the pooled early mortality rate was 6.4% with early rates of stroke and spinal cord ischemia of 4.2% and 5.3%. Survival at 5 years was 70.2–89%. Freedom from adverse aortic events (aortic death, rupture, new dissection, aneurysm enlargement, and reintervention) was 75–88.5% at 5 years [10].

Conclusion

Uncomplicated type B aortic dissection has historically been treated with careful imaging surveillance and anti-impulse medical therapy, to prevent both acute and late aortic complications.

References

1. Macgillivray TE, Gleason TG, Patel HJ, et al. The Society of Thoracic Surgeons/American Association for Thoracic Surgery Clinical Practice Guidelines on the management of type B aortic dissection. Ann Thorac Surg. 2022;113(4):P1073–92. https://doi.org/10.1016/j.athoracsur.2021.11.002.
2. Conrad MF, Cambria RP. Chapter 138: aortic dissection. In: Cronenwett JL, Johnston KW, editors. Rutherford's vascular surgery. 8th ed. Saunders; 2014.
3. Hiratzka LF, Bakris GL, Beckman JA, et al. 2010 ACCF/AHA/AATS/ACR/ASA/SCA/SCAI/SIR/STS/SVM guidelines for the diagnosis and management of patients with thoracic aortic disease. J Am Coll Cardiol. 2010;55(14):e27–e129. https://doi.org/10.1016/j.jacc.2010.02.015.
4. Lombardi JV, Hughes GC, Appoo JJ, et al. Society for Vascular Surgery (SVS) and Society of Thoracic Surgeons (STS) reporting standards for type B aortic dissections. J Vasc Surg. 2020;71(3):723–47. https://doi.org/10.1016/J.JVS.2019.11.013.
5. Brown JA, Arnaoutakis GJ, Kilic A, Gleason TG, Aranda-Michel E, Sultan I. Medical and surgical management of acute type B aortic intramural hematoma. J Card Surg. 2020;35(9):2324–30. https://doi.org/10.1111/jocs.14823.
6. Isselbacher EM, Preventza O, Hamilton Black J 3rd, et al. 2022 ACC/AHA guideline for the diagnosis and management of aortic disease: a report of the American Heart Association/

American College of Cardiology Joint Committee on Clinical Practice Guidelines. Circulation. 2022;146(24):e334–482. https://doi.org/10.1161/cir.0000000000001106.
7. Fattori R, Tsai TT, Myrmel T, et al. Complicated acute type B dissection: is surgery still the best option? J Am Coll Cardiol Intv. 2008;1(4):395–402. https://doi.org/10.1016/j.jcin.2008.04.009.
8. Patel AY, Eagle KA, Vaishnava P. Acute type B aortic dissection: insights from the International Registry of Acute Aortic Dissection. Ann Cardiothorac Surg. 2014;3(4):368–74. https://doi.org/10.3978/j.issn.2225-319X.2014.07.06.
9. Meharban N, Munir W, Idhrees M, Bashir A, Bashir M. Management of the penetrating atherosclerotic ulcer in the descending thoracic aorta. Asian Card Thorac Ann. 2021;29(7):661–8. https://doi.org/10.1177/02184923211033166.
10. Fattori R, Cao P, Rango PD, et al. Interdisciplinary Expert Consensus Document on management of type B aortic dissection. J Am Coll Cardiol. 2013;61(16):1661–78. https://doi.org/10.1016/j.jacc.2012.11.072.

Chapter 12
Operative Management of Type B Dissection

Alexander P. Nissen and Bradley G. Leshnower

Introduction

Pathophysiology and Epidemiology

Acute aortic dissection (AAD) is a failure of the biomechanical properties of the aortic wall. A disruption of the aortic intimal layer results in division of the medial layer and the creation of "true" and "false" lumens. Propagation of the dissection may result in diminished or absent blood flow to aortic branch vessels with resultant end-organ ischemia. Furthermore, the pressurized false lumen is at risk for rupture at sites of weakness, with subsequent hemorrhage. AAD is a life-threatening medical catastrophe associated with significant morbidity, and an in-hospital mortality of 25–30% [1]. The incidence of AAD is approximately 15 per 100,000 person-years [2]. Acute Type B aortic dissection (aTBAD) accounts for approximately 25–40% of aortic dissections, 10–30% of which are complicated by malperfusion or rupture (see below) [3–5]. Recent trends have demonstrated that patients with aTBAD are often transferred to a tertiary referral center, and increasingly treated with thoracic endovascular aortic repair (TEVAR) as opposed to medical therapy alone [6].

A. P. Nissen · B. G. Leshnower (✉)
Department of Surgery, Division of Cardiothoracic Surgery, Emory University School of Medicine, Atlanta, GA, USA
e-mail: alexander.paul.nissen@emory.edu; bleshno@emory.edu

G. J. Arnaoutakis et al. (eds.), *Aortic Aneurysms*, Contemporary Cardiology,
https://doi.org/10.1007/978-3-032-13134-8_12

Clinical Features and Diagnosis

The most common chief complaint in a patient presenting with aTBAD is chest or back pain, which may be described as tearing in character, and of sudden onset. Patients frequently have uncontrolled hypertension; however, important components of the patient history include: (1) family history of aortic disease/dissection, (2) connective tissue disease history, and (3) recent drug use such as cocaine or methamphetamines which may cause acute severe hypertension [7, 8]. Additional comorbidities such as kidney disease, diabetes, smoking, chronic obstructive pulmonary disease (COPD), peripheral and cerebrovascular disease should be assessed for and noted. The test of choice for diagnosing any acute aortic syndrome is a contrasted computed tomography (CT) scan of the entire aorta, given its widespread availability, speed, and accuracy [7]. Additional CT scans of the head/neck, and lower extremities may be added for clinical concerns. Transesophageal echocardiography (TEE) and magnetic resonance imaging (MRI) are alternative imaging modalities in certain clinical scenarios, but should not supplant CT for rapid diagnosis and characterization.

Important clinical findings when assessing patients need for operative intervention with aTBAD include: (1) acute limb pain, weakness, blood pressure or pulse exam asymmetry indicating extremity malperfusion; (2) acute abdominal pain or tenderness out of proportion to exam concerning for mesenteric ischemia; (3) oliguria and/or an elevation of the serum creatinine indicating renal malperfusion; (4) paraplegia or paraparesis indicating spinal cord malperfusion; (5) syncope or shortness of breath which may be the result of a pericardial effusion and cardiac tamponade. The presence of a pericardial effusion mandates a careful inspection of the imaging to exclude ascending aortic dissection.

Classification

Based on the location of the proximal-most intimal tear and extent of aortic involvement, AAD can be further classified according to either the DeBakey [9] or Stanford [10] classifications. The Stanford classification is commonly used and stratifies patients with dissection involving any portion of the aorta proximal to the left subclavian artery (LSCA) as type A, and patients with dissection exclusively involving the aorta distal to the LSCA as Type B. The DeBakey classification similarly describes patients with dissection beginning distal to the LSCA as DeBakey III (DeBakey I and II involving the ascending aorta), further divided into DeBakey IIIa dissections which terminate at or above the level of the diaphragm, vs. DeBakey IIIb dissections which extend below the diaphragm. This chapter will primarily refer to dissections using the Stanford classification, with occasional description of differences between DeBakey IIIa vs. IIIb dissections as needed.

In 2020, the Society for Vascular Surgery (SVS) and Society of Thoracic Surgeons (STS) established a novel reporting system for aortic dissection. In this new nomenclature, any dissection which begins after the origin of the innominate artery (Ishimaru Zone 1 or beyond) is classified as Type B, with additional detail provided by listing the proximal and distal aortic zones of involvement [11].

Timing of presentation is also critical in treatment decisions. Acuity of dissection is currently defined as the following: Hyperacute, <24 h from symptom onset; Acute, 1–14 days; Subacute, 15–90 days; and Chronic, >90 days [11]. For the purposes of the chapter, the term "acute" will include both hyperacute and acute dissections.

Malperfusion may be diagnosed either radiographically and/or clinically. Radiographic malperfusion is defined by a diminished or absence of contrast enhancement in an aortic branch vessel or end-organ (e.g., kidney), which may indicate end-organ ischemia. Clinical malperfusion occurs when there is a physical exam (e.g., diminished femoral pulse) or laboratory indicator (e.g., elevated serum creatinine or lactate level) of a lack of blood flow to an end-organ. Malperfusion is also characterized as either "dynamic" or "static." Dynamic malperfusion occurs when an aortic branch vessel is obstructed by the dissection flap at its origin from the aorta secondary to changes in blood flow and pressure between the true and false lumen during the cardiac cycle. Static malperfusion results from the dissection propagating into the branch vessel with subsequent complete obstruction of the true lumen due to pressurization or thrombosis of the false lumen. Distinguishing dynamic from static malperfusion is important in guiding the endovascular treatment of TBAD.

A final critical aspect in the diagnosis and subsequent treatment of aTBAD is evaluating whether the dissection is "complicated" or "uncomplicated." The term "complicated" refers to TBAD with aortic rupture or malperfusion. All other TBADs are considered "uncomplicated" [11].

Acute Complicated Type B Dissection

Endovascular Management

Nonoperative management of aTBAD is covered in Chap. 11. In patients with complicated aTBAD, and anatomy suitable for endovascular intervention, TEVAR is the standard of care (Class 1 recommendation) [7]. TEVAR has revolutionized the management of aTBAD as well as treatment of descending thoracic aortic aneurysms. In the setting of complicated aTBAD, coverage of the primary intimal tear and all large secondary tears within the descending thoracic aorta remains the primary goal, in order to eliminate antegrade false lumen perfusion and restore perfusion to all end-organs. While there are various technical options to the procedure, the following description will focus upon the salient points of our technique at Emory for performing TEVAR for complicated aTBAD [13].

After careful review of all preoperative imaging, including confirming adequate iliofemoral vascular size to accommodate the delivery system, bilateral common femoral artery access is obtained. After ultrasound-guided bilateral femoral access is obtained, the side designated for device delivery is typically prepared with two percutaneous closure devices and then an 8 French (Fr) sheath is initially placed. A 5 Fr sheath (Fig. 12.1) is placed in the contralateral side. It should be noted that in cases of iliofemoral malperfusion, the device side should always be placed in the malperfused side as this artery always originates from the true lumen. Next, a 0.035″ Benson or Glide wire is advanced into the true lumen of the dissected aorta guided by the use of intravascular ultrasound (IVUS). IVUS is mandatory in TEVAR for TBAD as it enables accurate wire placement into the true lumen. It is also used to evaluate aortic diameter measurements for final endograft sizing. After IVUS-guided advancement of both wires into the ascending aorta, the device delivery side is exchanged for a stiff 0.035″ Lunderquist wire and the contralateral side exchanged for a marker pigtail catheter, to be connected to a contrast injector. An initial aortogram is obtained, further delineating branch vessel anatomy, true lumen compression, and may also show areas of rapid false lumen filling or rupture (Fig. 12.2). Based on preoperative CT measurements and IVUS, an endograft is selected that is ≤10% oversized for the total aortic diameter of the proximal landing zone. If the

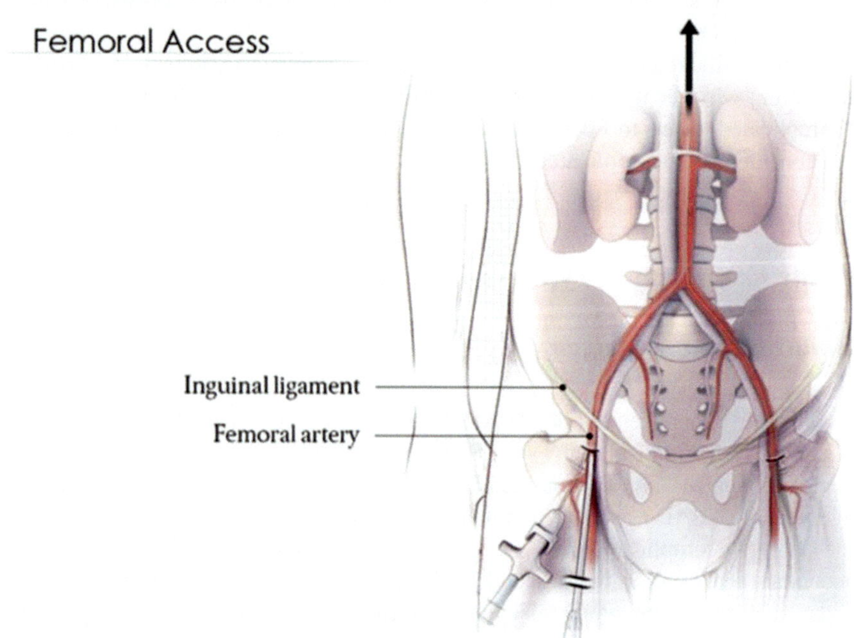

Fig. 12.1 Initial femoral access for TEVAR

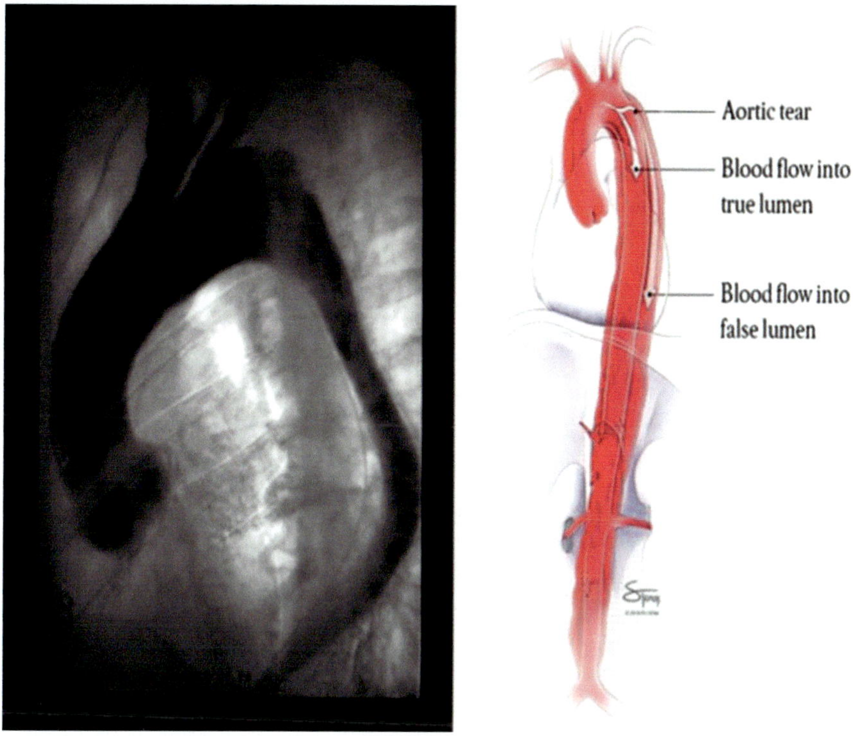

Fig. 12.2 Wire positioning in the ascending aorta and initial aortography

primary intimal tear is at the origin of the LSCA, then Zone 2 is chosen for the non-dissected proximal landing zone with left subclavian coverage. Otherwise, the graft is placed at the distal edge of the LSCA origin in Zone 3.

In the emergent setting, revascularization of the LSCA prior to TEVAR is not required except in cases of (1) a patent left internal mammary artery to left anterior descending artery (LIMA-LAD) bypass graft, (2) a dominant left vertebral artery with incomplete circle of Willis or atretic right vertebral artery, or (3) a patent left axillary-femoral bypass. A full list of additional relative indications in the non-emergent setting have been delineated by the Society for Vascular Surgery [12]. Ultimately, a plan for LSCA management should be determined based upon preoperative imaging analysis, with options for partial or full coverage, and open or endovascular revascularization [13].

The delivery system is advanced into the aortic arch. The image intensifier is positioned in a steep left anterior oblique (LAO) position to optimize visualization of the arch vessel origins. The degree of obliquity is dictated by the anatomy of the arch angulation. A magnified aortogram is performed for precise proximal endograft deployment. At this point, the systolic blood pressure is lowered to <100 mmHg with short-acting anti-hypertensives to facilitate accurate endograft deployment, and the graft is deployed landing just distal to the LSCA (Fig. 12.3). After

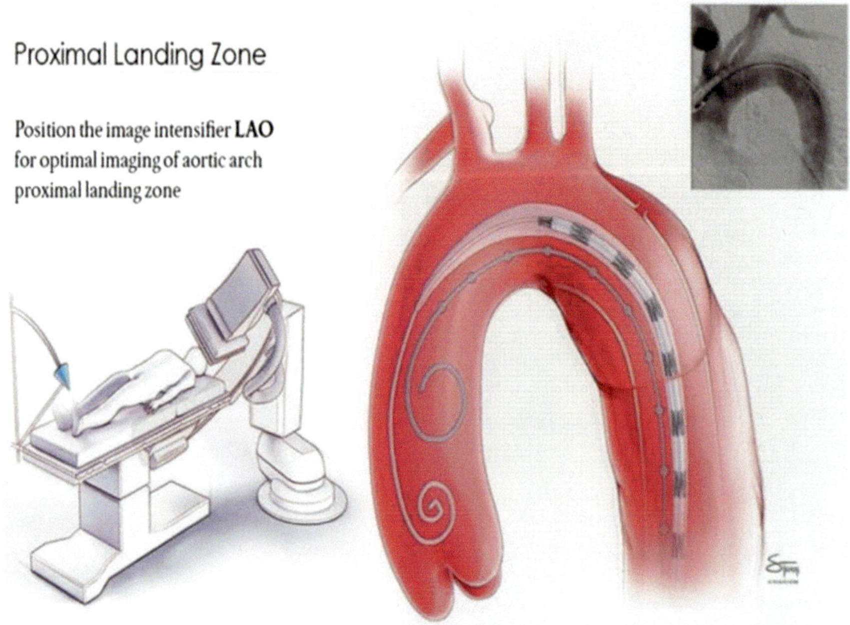

Fig. 12.3 Proxima landing zone endograft positioning

deployment of the first endograft, systolic blood pressure is intentionally augmented to a range of 160–200 mmHg. The purpose of this maneuver is to optimize spinal cord perfusion to mitigate the risk of spinal cord ischemia. A second stent graft is typically added to extend coverage to the celiac axis, thereby covering all secondary intimal tears within the descending thoracic aorta. Sizing of the second endoprosthesis is based on both the aortic size at the level of the celiac, and the size of the first endograft. The second endograft is telescoped within the first, the key landmark for deployment being the origin of the celiac artery distally, which is best visualized with the image intensifier in the steep lateral view on aortography (Fig. 12.4). Once appropriately positioned, the endograft is deployed with the distal end terminating just proximal to the celiac origin. At the completion of the procedure, all sheaths are removed with the stiff wire on the delivery side remaining in place. The pigtail catheter in the contralateral side is used to obtain a distal aortogram with iliofemoral runoff to evaluate for access vessel dissection or rupture. Once vessel integrity is confirmed, the stiff wire is removed and the previously placed closure devices are tightened. The contralateral pigtail catheter is rewired for removal, and all devices removed from this side as well with application of a closure device. After procedural completion, patients are extubated in the operating room for immediate neurologic assessment. If there are any signs of spinal cord ischemia a lumbar drain is emergently placed. We also routinely institute a period of blood pressure augmentation to a systolic blood pressure (SBP) of at least 160 mmHg for the first 48 h after

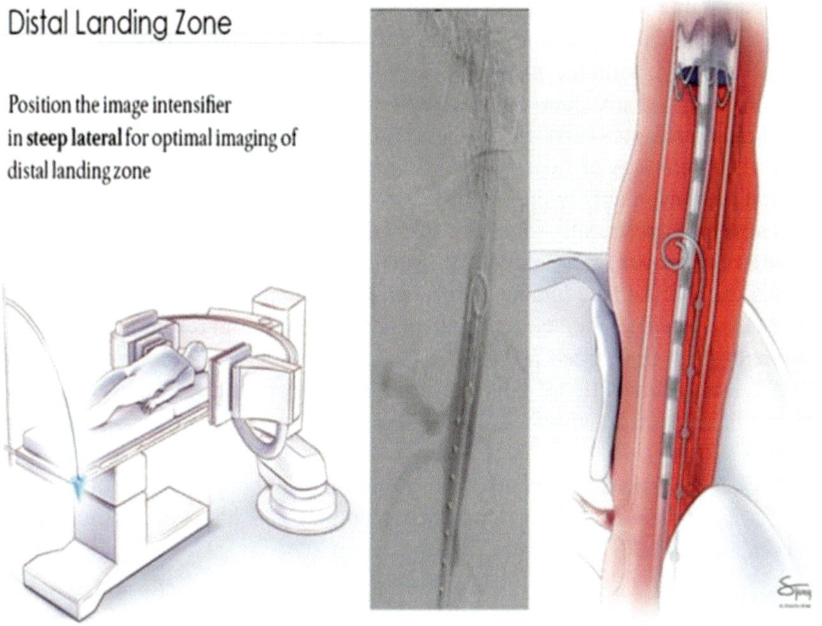

Fig. 12.4 Distal landing zone measurement and endograft positioning

TEVAR to maximize spinal cord perfusion. Patients may then be medically titrated to a SBP of 130–150 mmHg on oral medications by the time of discharge.

In addition to the above description, one should consider specific planning/technical modifications in cases of rupture and/or static malperfusion. In cases of aTBAD complicated by rupture, it may be difficult to determine the precise location of false lumen rupture. Therefore, our strategy in rupture cases is to perform emergent coverage beginning at the distal edge of the left common carotid artery (Zone 2) and extending to the origin of the celiac, in order to cover all possible thoracic intimal tears as sites of possible false lumen communication and pressurization. Although retrograde filling from the abdominal aorta may persist, typically the thoracic false lumen will completely thrombose with this approach and control hemorrhage. Additionally, in cases of rupture or hemodynamic instability, awake TEVAR can be safely accomplished to minimize the rupture risk associated with induction and emergence from anesthesia [14].

In cases of aTBAD with dynamic malperfusion, TEVAR alone will typically resolve the malperfusion by eliminating antegrade false lumen perfusion, thus restoring blood flow and pressurization of the true lumen. In contrast, static malperfusion with dissection extension into a branch vessel that is causing static true lumen occlusion or thrombus formation will require branch vessel stenting [15, 16].

TEVAR can be a life-saving therapy, but it is also associated with specific risks. Spinal cord ischemia with paraparesis/paraplegia is reported in 1–6%, with conflicting data regarding the use of prophylactic vs. selective lumbar drain placement [17, 18]. Our group has also demonstrated excellent safety with extended TEVAR coverage without an increased risk of spinal cord ischemia when using protocolized blood pressure augmentation and selective lumbar drainage [19, 20]. TEVAR also promotes early and sustained aortic remodeling across the stented segment, with high rates of false lumen obliteration during late follow-up (Fig. 12.5) [21, 22]. Advancements in endograft technology have produced a bare metal stent that is designed specifically for use in aortic dissection. This device is intended to be used after the primary intimal tear has been covered with a traditional stent graft, in order to expand the true lumen distally while maintaining perfusion to intercostal arteries that provide spinal cord perfusion [23]. While initial results with bare metal stent extensions have been promising, the late remodeling outcomes of extended TEVAR using conventional covered stent grafts from the left subclavian to the celiac appear superior, with the caveat of inherent limitations of cross-trial comparisons [20, 23].

Over the past two decades, outcomes reported from both single institution experiences, and multi-center trials have confirmed that TEVAR is the optimal therapy for complicated aTBAD. Survival ranges from 95% to 99%, with high rates of

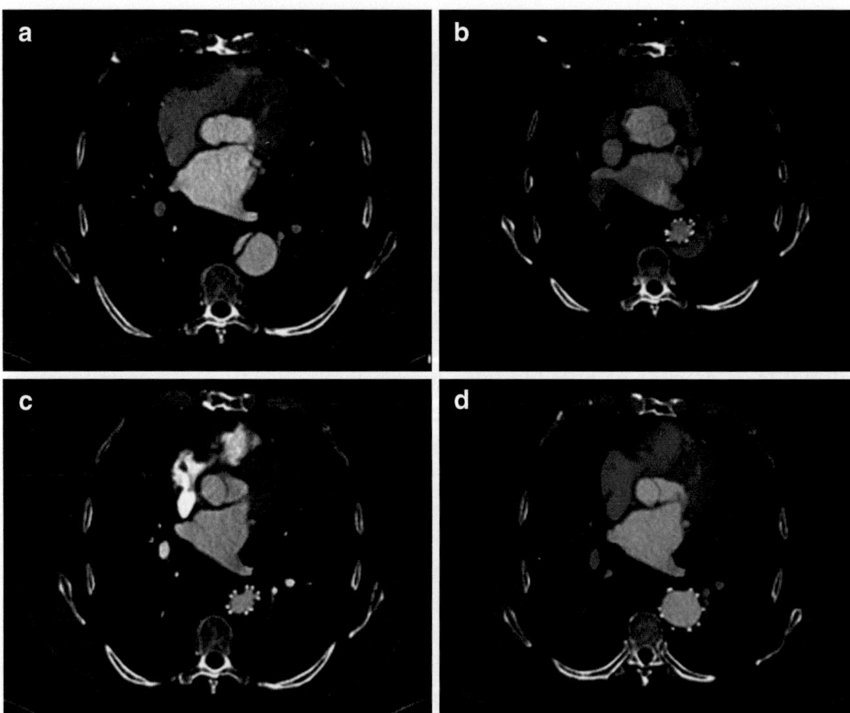

Fig. 12.5 False lumen thrombosis and obliteration before and after TEVAR. (**a**) Preoperative, (**b**) Partial thrombosis, (**c**) Complete thrombosis, (**d**) Obliteration

technical success (95–100%), and low rates of stroke (2–5%), and retrograde type A aortic dissection (rTAAD) (1–4%) [19, 20, 24–27].

Open Surgical Management

Open repair of complicated aTBAD with either descending aortic replacement or total arch replacement with frozen elephant trunk, has become increasingly uncommon since the advent of TEVAR, but remains an option for patients without a feasible proximal landing zone for a stent graft. In these instances, open replacement using either left heart bypass or full cardiopulmonary bypass with deep hypothermic circulatory arrest can be completed in an emergent setting with good results reported by experienced centers and surgeons [28, 29]. Early mortality for open replacement of complicated aTBAD ranges from 5% to 10%, with risk of spinal cord ischemia in 4–8%, stroke in 5–10%, postoperative renal failure in 2–13%, and bleeding. Independent predictors of mortality after open replacement include preoperative rupture, visceral malperfusion, COPD, and renal dysfunction (measured by admission glomerular filtration rate). Despite the increased short-term morbidity of open aortic replacement, compared to TEVAR, 5-year survival remains approximately 70% with low rates of late reintervention (10–12% at 10 years), highlighting the durability of open aortic replacement [28, 29]. Open operative therapy for the descending and thoracoabdominal aorta is further discussed in Chap. 14.

Acute Uncomplicated Type B Dissection

Natural History and Predicting Failure of Medical Management

Medical management with anti-hypertensives and anti-impulse control remains the cornerstone of optimal medical therapy (OMT), used for initial management of uncomplicated aTBAD [7, 8]. This is discussed in detail in Chap. 11. Despite low in-hospital mortality for uncomplicated aTBAD, natural history studies have demonstrated continued attrition of patients and accumulation of late reinterventions, with intervention-free survival of only 41% at 6 years [30]. In fact, late intervention-free survival for uncomplicated aTBAD has been shown to be inferior to complicated aTBAD treated with TEVAR at the index hospitalization [27]. Given these poor long-term results, efforts have been focused upon the identification of predictors of failure of OMT for uncomplicated aTBAD. Thus far, aortic size greater than 44 mm in one series, and greater than 45 mm in another large series have each predicted late reintervention [31, 32]. Proximal descending aortic false lumen diameter of >22 mm, and proximity of the intimal tear to the LSCA on initial imaging appear to be additional risk factors for late complications or need for intervention [31, 33].

TEVAR vs. Optimal Medical Therapy (OMT) in Uncomplicated Type B Dissection

Given the above-described limitations of OMT in the long-term management of uncomplicated aTBAD, compared against the favorable short-term safety profile of TEVAR and long-term benefits of aortic remodeling and survival, there has been growing interest in early prophylactic TEVAR in the uncomplicated aTBAD population. The first trial to demonstrate a survival benefit of TEVAR compared to OMT was the INSTEAD-XL trial. At 5 years, the TEVAR group had an aortic-related mortality of 6.9% compared to 19.3% for OMT ($p = 0.04$) [34]. The ADSROB trial also reported favorable outcomes with TEVAR compared to OMT at 1 year, though the primary composite endpoint under evaluation was a combination of aortic remodeling, dilatation, or rupture, and statistical significance was driven almost entirely by rates of false lumen thrombosis without differences in dilatation, rupture, or survival between groups [35, 36]. Nonrandomized studies have also demonstrated a survival benefit for TEVAR in uncomplicated aTBAD patients. A California state-wide database analysis reported a 5-year survival of 76% with TEVAR compared to 60% with OMT ($p < 0.01$) for uncomplicated aTBAD [37]. Our center has also confirmed both the high rate of failure of medical management and improved long-term survival comparing complicated aTBAD treated with early TEVAR vs. uncomplicated aTBAD treated with late TEVAR in the chronic phase [27]. A follow-up analysis of uncomplicated aTBAD patients treated at Emory comparing TEVAR vs. OMT again demonstrated improved aortic remodeling with a trend toward improved 5-year survival (91% after TEVAR vs. 82% for OMT) [38]. A new NIH-funded trial, IMPROVE-AD, will randomize patients with uncomplicated aTBAD to either OMT or TEVAR, and should provide novel information regarding the optimal therapy for uncomplicated aTBAD [39].

Chronic Type B Dissection

Endovascular Management

TEVAR

Open descending/thoracoabdominal aortic replacement remains the definitive therapy for the treatment of aneurysms secondary to chronic type B aortic dissection (cTBAD). However, many patients are poor candidates for open repair due to age and medical comorbidities. TEVAR for cTBAD has been shown to be safe with a low risk of mortality (0–5%) and attendant complications including stroke (1–5%), and paraplegia (1–4%) [40–42]. Positive aortic remodeling with true lumen expansion and false lumen thrombosis or obliteration has been reported in approximately 80% of cases.

In cTBAD, the presence of a rigid aortic septum presents a significant challenge for complete relamination of the aortic wall with TEVAR, resulting in persistent retrograde false lumen perfusion and pressurization from distal aortic fenestrations. Retrograde false lumen perfusion remains the "Achilles' heel" of endovascular therapy for cTBAD and represents the most common mechanism of failure which leads to persistent false lumen pressurization, expansion, and rupture. Recognizing this key limitation has led to increased interest in more extensive aortic coverage with fenestrated and branched endografts, as well as a host of management techniques for distal landing zone optimization for the purpose of inducing false lumen thrombosis [43–45].

Distal Landing Zone Optimization and False Lumen Management

Two general concepts have been developed for distal landing zone optimization and false lumen management: (1) false lumen embolization, and (2) the creation of a single lumen at the distal landing zone. False lumen embolization represents a relatively non-specific strategy that involves deployment of coils, plugs, modified stent grafts and/or glue into the false lumen to induce thrombosis [46, 47]. Limitations of this technique are well-reported, and subsequent difficulties with endovascular reintervention and aortic surveillance (due to metallic artifact on imaging) should be considered [48, 49].

Creation of a single lumen at or near the distal landing zone, in order to achieve apposition between the endograft and outer aortic wall circumferentially, thereby eliminating retrograde false lumen flow has shown promise. The first iteration of this concept was described by Kobel and colleagues with the "Knickerbocker" technique in which an aortic balloon is inflated to intentionally rupture the dissection flap and expand the stent graft to the outer aortic wall following TEVAR [50]. Efficacy of this technique is variable, as the rigid dissection flap frequently prevents complete TEVAR expansion and relamination of the aortic wall, even with aggressive balloon dilation of the septum. Furthermore, there is a lack of control with respect to the extent of septal rupture both proximal and distal to the segment of aorta that is undergoing aortoplasty. This can result in a stent graft-induced new entry tear (SINE) at the distal aspect of the endograft which can lead to increased false lumen perfusion and rapid expansion. Modifications of the Knickerbocker technique have involved more extensive endograft coverage and balloon fracture fenestration, with some improvements [51, 52]. In order to improve precision with regard to the level and extent of fenestration, wire fenestration has been reported, but was first limited by only utilizing existing entry tears for access between the true and false lumen [53]. More complex techniques utilizing laser fenestration and electrosurgical techniques for precise aortic septostomy have since been reported, with excellent early safety and efficacy, as well as promising aortic remodeling outcomes [54, 55]. In our initial series, utilizing electrosurgical aortic septostomy for balloon fenestration and TEVAR in cTBAD, elimination of retrograde false lumen perfusion was accomplished in 100% of patients, and 91% demonstrated complete false lumen thrombosis or obliteration [55]. While early outcomes remain promising, long-term follow-up, continued experience, and research in this area remain critical to improving endovascular therapy for cTBAD.

Open Surgical Management

For patients with cTBAD and aneurysmal degeneration, who are able to tolerate open aortic replacement, open repair of the descending thoracic aorta (DTA) or thoracoabdominal aorta (TAA) remains the gold standard in terms of definitive management and durability, against which all other treatment options are traditionally compared [56]. Open DTA and TAA replacement has become increasingly centralized at centers with accumulated experience and continues to be performed with excellent outcomes. The utilization of distal aortic perfusion combined with cerebrospinal fluid drainage has significantly improved the safety of these repairs [57]. When performed at high volume aortic centers, open DTA/TAA replacement can be accomplished with mortality of 7–15% overall, though extent of aortic replacement, preoperative renal function, age, emergency operation, and postoperative spinal cord ischemia remain independent risk factors for mortality [57, 58]. The durability of open DTA/TAA is excellent, with freedom from reoperation as high as 95% at 10 year follow-up [58]. Please also see Chap. 14 for a dedicated discussion of open operative therapy for the descending and thoracoabdominal aorta.

Conclusions

Type B aortic dissection remains a complex and potentially lethal pathology. Great strides have been made in all areas of diagnosis and treatment. In the acute phase, successful management still hinges on rapid assessment and diagnosis of all attendant complications, elimination of malperfusion or risk of rupture, and restoration of true lumen flow while minimizing morbidity. Treatment strategies in complicated aTBAD are also being increasingly applied to patients with uncomplicated aTBAD. In the chronic phase, open replacement remains an excellent and durable option in patients fit for surgery, while application of TEVAR is growing but continues to face unique challenges for false lumen management to achieve successful aortic remodeling. Areas of continued active investigation in both the acute and chronic setting include TEVAR best practices, management for uncomplicated aTBAD patients, TEVAR modifications and additional endovascular therapies for chronic dissection, and end-organ protection during open aortic replacement. Practicing and aspiring cardiac and vascular surgeons remain poised to tackle these challenges moving forward.

Acknowledgements The authors would like to thank Satyen Tripathi for providing illustrations for this chapter.

References

1. Hagan PG, Nienaber CA, Isselbacher EM, Bruckman D, Karavite DJ, Russman PL, et al. The International Registry of Acute Aortic Dissection (IRAD): new insights into an old disease. JAMA. 2000;283(7):897–903.
2. Landenhed M, Engstrom G, Gottsater A, Caulfield MP, Hedblad B, Newton-Cheh C, et al. Risk profiles for aortic dissection and ruptured or surgically treated aneurysms: a prospective cohort study. J Am Heart Assoc. 2015;4(1):e001513.
3. Fattori R, Cao P, De Rango P, Czerny M, Evangelista A, Nienaber C, et al. Interdisciplinary expert consensus document on management of type B aortic dissection. J Am Coll Cardiol. 2013;61(16):1661–78.
4. Jonker FH, Patel HJ, Upchurch GR, Williams DM, Montgomery DG, Gleason TG, et al. Acute type B aortic dissection complicated by visceral ischemia. J Thorac Cardiovasc Surg. 2015;149(4):1081–6.e1.
5. Suzuki T, Mehta RH, Ince H, Nagai R, Sakomura Y, Weber F, et al. Clinical profiles and outcomes of acute type B aortic dissection in the current era: lessons from the International Registry of Aortic Dissection (IRAD). Circulation. 2003;108(Suppl 1):II312–7.
6. Pape LA, Awais M, Woznicki EM, Suzuki T, Trimarchi S, Evangelista A, et al. Presentation, diagnosis, and outcomes of acute aortic dissection: 17-year trends from the International Registry of Acute Aortic Dissection. J Am Coll Cardiol. 2015;66(4):350–8.
7. Isselbacher EM, Preventza O, Hamilton Black J 3rd, Augoustides JG, Beck AW, Bolen MA, et al. 2022 ACC/AHA guideline for the diagnosis and management of aortic disease: a report of the American Heart Association/American College of Cardiology Joint Committee on Clinical Practice Guidelines. Circulation. 2022;146(24):e334–482.
8. MacGillivray TE, Gleason TG, Patel HJ, Aldea GS, Bavaria JE, Beaver TM, et al. The Society of Thoracic Surgeons/American Association for Thoracic Surgery clinical practice guidelines on the management of type B aortic dissection. J Thorac Cardiovasc Surg. 2022;163(4):1231–49.
9. De Bakey ME, Cooley DA, Creech O Jr. Surgical considerations of dissecting aneurysm of the aorta. Ann Surg. 1955;142(4):586–610; discussion, 1–2.
10. Daily PO, Trueblood HW, Stinson EB, Wuerflein RD, Shumway NE. Management of acute aortic dissections. Ann Thorac Surg. 1970;10(3):237–47.
11. Lombardi JV, Hughes GC, Appoo JJ, Bavaria JE, Beck AW, Cambria RP, et al. Society for Vascular Surgery (SVS) and Society of Thoracic Surgeons (STS) reporting standards for type B aortic dissections. Ann Thorac Surg. 2020;109(3):959–81.
12. Matsumura JS, Lee WA, Mitchell RS, Farber MA, Murad MH, Lumsden AB, et al. The Society for Vascular Surgery Practice Guidelines: management of the left subclavian artery with thoracic endovascular aortic repair. J Vasc Surg. 2009;50(5):1155–8.
13. Charlton-Ouw KM, Estrera AL. Thoracic endovascular aortic repair for aneurysm: how I teach it. Ann Thorac Surg. 2018;106(3):646–50.
14. Forcillo J, Duwayri YM, Jordan WD Jr, Leshnower BG. Awake thoracic endovascular aneurysm repair for aortic rupture: a case series. Semin Thorac Cardiovasc Surg. 2018;30(1):36–9.
15. Leshnower BG, Chen EP. TEVAR for acute complicated type B aortic dissection. Oper Tech Thorac Cardiovasc Surg. 2018;23(1):21–33.
16. Norton EL, Williams DM, Kim KM, Khaja MS, Wu X, Patel HJ, et al. Management of acute type B aortic dissection with malperfusion via endovascular fenestration/stenting. J Thorac Cardiovasc Surg. 2020;160(5):1151–61.e1.

17. Feezor RJ, Martin TD, Hess PJ Jr, Daniels MJ, Beaver TM, Klodell CT, et al. Extent of aortic coverage and incidence of spinal cord ischemia after thoracic endovascular aneurysm repair. Ann Thorac Surg. 2008;86(6):1809–14; discussion 14.
18. Hanna JM, Andersen ND, Aziz H, Shah AA, McCann RL, Hughes GC. Results with selective preoperative lumbar drain placement for thoracic endovascular aortic repair. Ann Thorac Surg. 2013;95(6):1968–74; discussion 74–5.
19. Lou X, Duwayri YM, Jordan WD Jr, Chen EP, Veeraswamy RK, Leshnower BG. The safety and efficacy of extended TEVAR in acute type B aortic dissection. Ann Thorac Surg. 2020;110(3):799–806.
20. Nissen AP, Huckaby LV, Duwayri YM, Jordan WD Jr, Farrington WJ, Keeling WB, et al. Extended thoracic endovascular aortic repair is optimal therapy in acute complicated type B dissection. J Vasc Surg. 2024;80(4):1055–63.
21. Conrad MF, Carvalho S, Ergul E, Kwolek CJ, Lancaster RT, Patel VI, et al. Late aortic remodeling persists in the stented segment after endovascular repair of acute complicated type B aortic dissection. J Vasc Surg. 2015;62(3):600–5.
22. Leshnower BG, Duwayri YM, Chen EP, Li C, Zehner CA, Binongo JN, et al. Aortic remodeling after endovascular repair of complicated acute type B aortic dissection. Ann Thorac Surg. 2017;103(6):1878–85.
23. Lombardi JV, Gleason TG, Panneton JM, Starnes BW, Dake MD, Haulon S, et al. Five-year results of the STABLE II study for the endovascular treatment of complicated, acute type B aortic dissection with a composite device design. J Vasc Surg. 2022;76(5):1189–97.e3.
24. Azizzadeh A, Valdes JA, Estrera AL, Charlton-Ouw KM, Safi HJ. Thoracic endovascular repair (TEVAR): a focus on complications. Cir Cardiovasc. 2010;17:11–23.
25. Bavaria JE, Brinkman WT, Hughes GC, Shah AS, Charlton-Ouw KM, Azizzadeh A, et al. Five-year outcomes of endovascular repair of complicated acute type B aortic dissections. J Thorac Cardiovasc Surg. 2022;163(2):539–48.e2.
26. Hanna JM, Andersen ND, Ganapathi AM, McCann RL, Hughes GC. Five-year results for endovascular repair of acute complicated type B aortic dissection. J Vasc Surg. 2014;59(1):96–106.
27. Lou X, Chen EP, Duwayri YM, Veeraswamy RK, Jordan WD Jr, Zehner CA, et al. The impact of thoracic endovascular aortic repair on long-term survival in type B aortic dissection. Ann Thorac Surg. 2018;105(1):31–8.
28. Estrera AL, Miller CC, Goodrick J, Porat EE, Achouh PE, Dhareshwar J, et al. Update on outcomes of acute type B aortic dissection. Ann Thorac Surg. 2007;83(2):S842–5; discussion S6–50.
29. Lau C, Soletti GJ, Lawrence KM, Rahouma M, Iannacone E, Gambardella I, et al. Contemporary outcomes of open repair of acute complicated type B aortic dissection. J Vasc Surg. 2023;78(3):593–601.e4.
30. Durham CA, Cambria RP, Wang LJ, Ergul EA, Aranson NJ, Patel VI, et al. The natural history of medically managed acute type B aortic dissection. J Vasc Surg. 2015;61(5):1192–8.
31. Ray HM, Durham CA, Ocazionez D, Charlton-Ouw KM, Estrera AL, Miller CC 3rd, et al. Predictors of intervention and mortality in patients with uncomplicated acute type B aortic dissection. J Vasc Surg. 2016;64(6):1560–8.
32. Lou X, Duwayri YM, Chen EP, Jordan WD Jr, Forcillo J, Zehner CA, et al. Predictors of failure of medical management in uncomplicated type B aortic dissection. Ann Thorac Surg. 2019;107(2):493–8.
33. Codner JA, Lou X, Duwayri YM, Chen EP, Binongo JN, Moon R, et al. The distance of the primary intimal tear from the left subclavian artery predicts aortic growth in uncomplicated type B aortic dissection. J Vasc Surg. 2019;69(3):692–700.
34. Nienaber CA, Kische S, Rousseau H, Eggebrecht H, Rehders TC, Kundt G, et al. Endovascular repair of type B aortic dissection: long-term results of the randomized investigation of stent grafts in aortic dissection trial. Circ Cardiovasc Interv. 2013;6(4):407–16.

35. Brunkwall J, Kasprzak P, Verhoeven E, Heijmen R, Taylor P, Trialists A, et al. Endovascular repair of acute uncomplicated aortic type B dissection promotes aortic remodelling: 1 year results of the ADSORB trial. Eur J Vasc Endovasc Surg. 2014;48(3):285–91.
36. Hughes GC. Management of acute type B aortic dissection. ADSORB trial. J Thorac Cardiovasc Surg. 2015;149(2 Suppl):S158–62.
37. Iannuzzi JC, Stapleton SM, Bababekov YJ, Chang D, Lancaster RT, Conrad MF, et al. Favorable impact of thoracic endovascular aortic repair on survival of patients with acute uncomplicated type B aortic dissection. J Vasc Surg. 2018;68(6):1649–55.
38. Lou X, Chen EP, Duwayri YM, Jordan WD, Keeling WB, Leshnower BG. Early results of thoracic endovascular aortic repair for the management of acute uncomplicated type B aortic dissection. Semin Thorac Cardiovasc Surg. 2023;35(2):289–97.
39. National Heart L, and Blood Institute. IMPROVE-AD (IMPRoving Outcomes in Vascular DisEase—Aortic Dissection). Available from: https://improvead.org
40. Hughes GC, Ganapathi AM, Keenan JE, Englum BR, Hanna JM, Schechter MA, et al. Thoracic endovascular aortic repair for chronic DeBakey IIIb aortic dissection. Ann Thorac Surg. 2014;98(6):2092–7; discussion 8.
41. Kang WC, Greenberg RK, Mastracci TM, Eagleton MJ, Hernandez AV, Pujara AC, et al. Endovascular repair of complicated chronic distal aortic dissections: intermediate outcomes and complications. J Thorac Cardiovasc Surg. 2011;142(5):1074–83.
42. Leshnower BG, Szeto WY, Pochettino A, Desai ND, Moeller PJ, Nathan DP, et al. Thoracic endografting reduces morbidity and remodels the thoracic aorta in DeBakey III aneurysms. Ann Thorac Surg. 2013;95(3):914–21.
43. Kitagawa A, Greenberg RK, Eagleton MJ, Mastracci TM, Roselli EE. Fenestrated and branched endovascular aortic repair for chronic type B aortic dissection with thoracoabdominal aneurysms. J Vasc Surg. 2013;58(3):625–34.
44. Oderich GS, Ribeiro M, Reis de Souza L, Hofer J, Wigham J, Cha S. Endovascular repair of thoracoabdominal aortic aneurysms using fenestrated and branched endografts. J Thorac Cardiovasc Surg. 2017;153(2):S32–S41.e7.
45. Tenorio ER, Dias-Neto MF, Lima GBB, Estrera AL, Oderich GS. Endovascular repair for thoracoabdominal aortic aneurysms: current status and future challenges. Ann Cardiothorac Surg. 2021;10(6):744–67.
46. Kolbel T, Lohrenz C, Kieback A, Diener H, Debus ES, Larena-Avellaneda A. Distal false lumen occlusion in aortic dissection with a homemade extra large vascular plug: the candy-plug technique. J Endovasc Ther. 2013;20(4):484–9.
47. Miletic KG, Kindzelski BA, Hodges KE, Beach J, Tong MZ, Bakaeen F, et al. Impact of endovascular false lumen embolization on thoracic aortic remodeling in chronic dissection. Ann Thorac Surg. 2021;111(2):495–501
48. Rohlffs F, Spanos K, Tsilimparis N, Debus ES, Kolbel T. Techniques and outcomes of false lumen embolization in chronic type B aortic dissection. J Cardiovasc Surg. 2018;59(6):784–8.
49. Sweet MP. Candy-plug: failure to launch. J Vasc Surg Cases Innov Tech. 2023;9(2):101089.
50. Kolbel T, Carpenter SW, Lohrenz C, Tsilimparis N, Larena-Avellaneda A, Debus ES. Addressing persistent false lumen flow in chronic aortic dissection: the knickerbocker technique. J Endovasc Ther. 2014;21(1):117–22.
51. Hofferberth SC, Nixon IK, Boston RC, McLachlan CS, Mossop PJ. Stent-assisted balloon-induced intimal disruption and relamination in aortic dissection repair: the STABILISE concept. J Thorac Cardiovasc Surg. 2014;147(4):1240–5.
52. Levack MM, Kindzelski BA, Miletic KG, Vargo PR, Bakaeen FG, Johnston DR, et al. Adjunctive endovascular balloon fracture fenestration for chronic aortic dissection. J Thorac Cardiovasc Surg. 2022;164(1):2–10.e5.
53. Barshes NR, Gravereaux EC, Semel M, Bolman RM 3rd, Belkin M. Endovascular longitudinal fenestration and stent graft placement for treatment of aneurysms developing after chronic type B aortic dissection. J Vasc Surg. 2015;61(5):1366–9.

54. Fukuhara S, Khaja MS, Williams DM, Marko X, Yang B, Patel HJ, et al. Aortic septotomy to optimize landing zones during thoracic endovascular aortic repair for chronic type B aortic dissection. J Thorac Cardiovasc Surg. 2021;165(5):1776–1786.e5.
55. Nissen AP, Duwayri Y, Jordan WD, Babaliaros V, Lederman RJ, Leshnowe BG. Transcatheter electrosurgical aortic septostomy optimizes distal landing zone in chronic dissection. JTCVS Tech. 2024;27:19–28.
56. Svensson LG, Crawford ES, Hess KR, Coselli JS, Safi HJ. Experience with 1509 patients undergoing thoracoabdominal aortic operations. J Vasc Surg. 1993;17(2):357–68; discussion 68–70.
57. Estrera AL, Sandhu HK, Charlton-Ouw KM, Afifi RO, Azizzadeh A, Miller CC 3rd, et al. A quarter century of organ protection in open thoracoabdominal repair. Ann Surg. 2015;262(4):660–8.
58. Coselli JS, LeMaire SA, Preventza O, de la Cruz KI, Cooley DA, Price MD, et al. Outcomes of 3309 thoracoabdominal aortic aneurysm repairs. J Thorac Cardiovasc Surg. 2016;151(5):1323–37.

Chapter 13
Management of Thoracic Aortic Infections

Irbaz Hameed and Prashanth Vallabhajosyula

Introduction

Thoracic aortic infections are rare clinical entities associated with high morbidity and mortality [1]. Patients present with a variety of non-specific symptoms including fever, pain, elevated acute phase reactants, vascular insufficiency, and other systemic symptoms [1]. Consequently, these infections risk being misdiagnosed during initial work-up and a high index of suspicion must be maintained [2].

In recent years, the incidence of thoracic aortic infections has increased. This is partly attributable to improved imaging modalities including arteriography and intra-arterial invasive procedures which have improved diagnosis [3]. There has also been a rise in immunocompromised patients and the incidence of drug-related infective endocarditis [3].

Infections vary based on the location of the infection, the presence of aortic graft material, the causative organism, and history of previous surgical interventions [2]. Infective endocarditis due to streptococcal infection has been the most common cause of the majority of thoracic aortic infections [2]. Currently, however, the majority are associated with gram-positive cocci, particularly staphylococci [2]. Other less common causes include gram-negative bacilli with pseudomonas and salmonella being more prevalent [2]. Aggressive management starting with timely diagnosis is critical.

I. Hameed · P. Vallabhajosyula (✉)
Division of Cardiac Surgery, Department of Surgery, Yale School of Medicine, New Haven, CT, USA
e-mail: irbaz.hameed@yale.edu; Prashanth.vallabhajosyula@yale.edu

G. J. Arnaoutakis et al. (eds.), *Aortic Aneurysms*, Contemporary Cardiology,
https://doi.org/10.1007/978-3-032-13134-8_13

Valvular Endocarditis

Valvular endocarditis is a highly morbid complication related to prosthetic valves or reconstructed native valves [4].

Epidemiology

The overall incidence is 0.3–1.2% per patient each year. The incidence is approximately 10–30% in patients who have infective endocarditis [5] and about 69% of patients with valvular endocarditis have some valvular prosthesis [6]. The major risk factors associated with native valve endocarditis include diabetes mellitus, cancer, congenital heart disease, degenerative valve disease, and intravenous drug use [7].

Incidence can be early or late. Early valvular endocarditis occurs within the first 2 months postoperatively. The most common pathogens associated with early valvular endocarditis are *Staphylococcus aureus*, coagulase-negative staphylococci, gram-negative bacilli, and Candida species accounting [8]. Coagulase-negative *Staphylococcus*, *Staphylococcus aureus*, *Streptococcus*, and *Enterococcus* become more prevalent at around 2–12 months after surgical intervention postoperatively [9].

Late valvular endocarditis is more commonly due to community-acquired infection with streptococci, *Staphylococcus aureus*, coagulase-negative staphylococci, and enterococci [10]. Nosocomial infective endocarditis accounts for about 35% of valvular endocarditis cases [11]. This is associated with prolonged and increased use of long-term intravenous line, indwelling cardiac devices, and invasive procedures [11].

Pathogenesis

In early valvular endocarditis, there is invasion of the prosthetic valve intraoperatively by contamination. After valve insertion, the organisms have direct access to the interface of the prosthesis annulus and the tissue along the suture in the paravalvular area. The organisms are able to adhere to the fibrinogen and fibronectin in the paravalvular area resulting in the formation of abscesses in both the bioprosthetic and mechanical valves [12].

In late valvular endocarditis, the prosthesis restricts the organisms from adhering to the leaflets. After a few months of valvular implantation, the sewing ring and sutures become endothelialized. Alterations in the paravalvular surface and the valve result in the formation of microthrombi in which the bacterial organisms can adhere and cause infection [12, 13].

Diagnosis

Patients with valvular endocarditis may present with the following symptoms: shortness of breath, pleuritic chest pain, anorexia, weight loss, fever and chills, malaise, headache, myalgia, arthralgia, night sweats, abdominal pain, and coughing [14]. Left bundle blocks, embolic events, new heart murmurs, and heart failure are also suggestive of valvular endocarditis. Janeway lesions, Osler's nodes, and Roth spots are less frequently seen signs in these patients [14].

Besides the clinical presentations, the diagnosis of valvular endocarditis is based on positive blood cultures. This is part of an accepted criterion to establish the diagnosis of valvular endocarditis known as the modified Duke criteria [14]. Diagnosis can be made following three blood cultures from different sites, echocardiographic findings of vegetation, and presence of a paravalvular abscess or valve dehiscence [14].

Transesophageal echocardiography (TEE) is critical for confirming diagnosis in suspected cases of valvular endocarditis. It is performed for incidentally detected vegetation, abscess, and fistula as well as for valvular hemodynamic assessment [15]. It is also helpful in determining the stability of the ring and estimating the mobility of the leaflets [15]. Transthoracic echocardiography (TTE) can also be used but detection of vegetation may be difficult due to artifacts from the valves. It cannot, therefore, be considered as the gold standard [15]. 18 F-Fluorodeoxyglucose (18-FDG) positron emission tomography (PET)/computed tomography (CT) are also alternative diagnostic modalities in suspected cases of valvular endocarditis with PET being highly sensitive in the detection of inflammatory activity within the focus of infection [15]. When a septic emboli to the brain is suspected, head CT and magnetic resonance imaging (MRI) of the brain should be considered. CT angiography of the chest and abdomen are also helpful in ruling out other concomitant aortic pathology [15].

Management

The causative microorganism should be identified when starting treatment for patients with valvular endocarditis. After an initial period of broad-spectrum empiric antibiotic coverage, at least 6 weeks of antibiotics treatment is recommended by the American Heart Association(AHA) when the valvular endocarditis is as a result of staphylococcus. Methicillin should be considered in the selection of the combination therapy [16]. A triple antibiotic regimen is recommended which can include oxacillin or nafcillin (for 6 weeks) combined with gentamicin (which is administered only for the first 2 weeks) and rifampin (bringing it to a total of 6 weeks of treatment) [16].

Certain situations require early surgical intervention for aortic valvular endocarditis. These include destructive penetrating lesions or evidence of a heart block, development of an abscess (annular) or aortitis, high resistant bacterial organisms or fungi as the causative agent of the valvular endocarditis, a patient with the presence of severe prosthetic valve dysfunction, relapsing valvular endocarditis, large mobile vegetations >10 mm, recurrent emboli despite appropriate antibiotic treatment, development of heart failure due to aortic insufficiency, valve dehiscence or development of intracardiac fistula, and the presence of persistent bacteremia for 5–7 days after the adequate antibiotic regimen [17].

In patients with symptomatic left ventricular dysfunction and aortic regurgitation (ejection fraction less than 60%) who are at risk of septic embolization and have uncontrolled infection or dilatation (left ventricular end-systolic dimension >40 mm), emergency surgery should be offered [18]. Emergency surgery should also be considered for asymptomatic patients without left ventricular dysfunction or dilatation but with large vegetations(>20 mm), particularly in the mitral valve consequence due to the increased risk of neurological complications [18]. Elective surgical correction of valvular endocarditis should be considered in asymptomatic patients with small lesions with mild or no aortic regurgitation when symptoms develop or when there is aorto-mitral regurgitation [18].

Surgical intervention is required if medical therapy fails. Eradication of the infected valvular tissue with consequent valve repair or replacement is the basic therapy for native valve endocarditis [19]. Cryopreserved homografts were previously utilized and proved to have good outcomes in the past but their use has been limited due to risk of recalcification and complexity of surgical implantation [19]. Currently, the use of stentless biological valves is preferred for managing aortic valve endocarditis [19].

Following discharge, adequate follow-up and monitoring for a period of 6–8 weeks are mandatory [20]. Similarly, close collaboration with addiction medicine is critical to ensure long-term follow-up and prevent relapse, especially in patients with a history of intravenous drug use. During follow-up, drug levels must be monitored to ensure therapeutic levels and strict [20]. IV lines should also be monitored by visiting nurses, be checked for any adverse reactions, correct intravenous administration of antibiotics and track patients for any clinical signs and symptoms of valvular endocarditis-related complications [20]. When medication compliance is an issue, both the nurses and pharmacists should inform the clinician and conjunctly create a plan tailored to the patient [20].

Infectious Aortitis

Infectious aortitis is a rare entity in the antibiotic era and has been described in literature as microbial, bacterial, cytogenetic, or mycotic aortitis [21]. This typically presents in patients with infective endocarditis, prior atherosclerotic aortic disease, cystic medial necrosis, and/or valvular endocarditis [21, 22]. Infectious aortitis is associated with both gram-positive bacteria and gram-negative bacilli [21]. Other causative organisms include: *Mycobacterium tuberculosis*, *Clostridium,* human immunodeficiency virus, *Bacteroides fragilis*, and *Treponema pallidum* [21]. Other etiologic factors include vascular malformations, uncontrolled hypertension or diabetes mellitus, iatrogenic inoculation as a result of surgical intervention or the use of medical equipment or devices in and around the aorta, atherosclerotic diseases and cancer [21].

Epidemiology

Incidence is higher in males with a male to female ratio of 3:1 and mean age of presentation of 65 years [22].

Pathogenesis

The pathogenesis of infectious aortitis involves hematogenous seeding of an existing intimal injury, formation of septic emboli, direct spread from the infectious site, and bacterial inoculation [22].

Diagnosis

Clinical manifestations are non-specific and initial symptoms usually result from the expansion or rupture of an aneurysm. Symptoms of infectious aortitis include fever, chills, nausea, vomiting, abdominal, thoracic, and back pain [22].

In 50–85% of patients, blood cultures are positive and in 76% of the patients, microorganisms can be isolated from the excised aortic tissue [14]. In 65–83% of cases, neutrophilia and leukocytosis are present. C-reactive proteins and erythrocyte sedimentation rate are elevated in the majority of the patients [21].

TTE is the first imaging modality and is very effective in ruling out infective endocarditis. TTE can distinguish aneurysms, pseudoaneurysms, intramural hematomas, and dissection of the thoracic aorta, which are complications of infectious aortitis [21, 22].

A CT scan with contrast enhancement is another imaging technique of choice. It excludes other aortic pathologies that resemble acute aortitis such as penetrating atherosclerotic ulcer, aortic dissection, and intramural hematoma. The limitations to using CT, however, include renal dysfunction precluding contrast administration, and small vegetations or milder degrees of inflammation or wall edema may be missed [21].

MRI gives a full image of the aorta with good resolution and without radiation/contrast exposure and can be a reasonable alternative option. MRI, however, should not be used in patients who are unstable or have certain implanted devices because most resuscitation equipment cannot enter the scanning room [21].

Management

Postoperative intravenous broad-spectrum antibiotics following blood cultures should be administered immediately if infectious aortitis is suspected. These can be modified gradually based on the blood culture findings and microbial speciation/sensitivities to reduce inflammation and improve the patient's surgical outcome [23]. Antibiotics should be administered for 2–4 weeks prior to surgery only if surgery is not emergent [23].

Surgical repair is important in patients with thoracic aortic aneurysms larger than 5 cm in diameter, aortic root dilatation leading to significant aortic regurgitation, cerebral ischemia, myocardial ischemia secondary to coronary artery involvement, and significant hypertension due to renal vascular stenosis [23]. Surgery involves resection and reconstruction of the infected aortic segment with in-situ prosthetic graft reconstruction or angioplasty. In unstable patients at high risk for open surgical repair, or patients with aortic rupture, endovascular treatment can be considered [24]. Following surgical excision and clearance of blood cultures, antimicrobial therapy should be continued for at least 6–12 weeks [23].

Close medical follow-up with serial blood cultures and CT scans are recommended by some while clinical surveillance is recommended by others [25].

Pyogenic Aortitis

Pyogenic aortitis commonly affects the ascending and descending aorta and may progress to mycotic aneurysm if left untreated [21].

Epidemiology

There is limited data on the incidence of pyogenic aortitis [21].

Pathogenesis

Pathogenesis is related to hematogenous seeding of the atherosclerotic aortic lesion due to bacteremia from a distant focus of infection, commonly, phlebitis of the arm [27]. The causative organisms are commonly *Enterococcus* and *S. pneumoniae* [26].

Diagnosis

Immunocompromised or elderly patients should be suspected of having pyogenic aortitis if they develop high-grade bacteremia with prolonged fever and pain in the chest, back, or abdomen after an acute episode of gastroenteritis [21].

The initial imaging modalities in many hospitals or centers are CT or MR aortography [27] but CT is preferred because it is more readily available and has shorter acquisition time more often. 18F-FDG PET/CT is also useful for detecting infection and inflammation along the aorta [27].

Management

A high index of suspicion must be maintained and antibiotics such as cloxacillin, daptomycin, and rifampin should be promptly started. In most cases, surgery which involves resection of infected tissue with subsequent restoration of distal flow will be necessary [21].

Mycotic Aneurysm

Mycotic aneurysms develop anywhere in the aorta and about 50% are located above the renal arteries. It is rare with an incidence rate of 0.7–3% [29]. Prevalence is higher in males and older patients >65 years and associated with atherosclerosis, smoking, and diabetes mellitus [28].

Mycotic aneurysms are a common complication of bacterial endocarditis [26]. Other predisposing factors include pre-existing vasculitis, trauma, intravenous drug abuse, and iatrogenic causes such as percutaneous intervention [30].

Epidemiology

Mycotic aneurysms are more common in men because of the increased incidence of atherosclerosis in this population. The median age noted for this condition is 65 years old. Higher incidences have been noted in smokers and diabetics. The arteries that are most commonly involved include the femoral arteries, the aorta, the superior mesenteric, hepatic and splenic arteries, and finally, the cerebral arteries. Reports of coronary mycotic aneurysms after the placement of a stent have been made [31].

Pathogenesis

Pathogenesis involves inflammation of the vascular wall by infective endocarditis along with emboli in vasa vasorum [29]. Infection of the intima results from the combination of bacterial seeding and arterial injury. Following infection of the aortic wall, the deeper layers are quickly degraded by these microorganisms resulting in the formation of an aneurysm [30].

The most common pathogens implicated in mycotic aneurysms include *Staphylococcus aureus* and *Salmonella* [29]. Others include: *Treponema pallidum*, *Mycobacterium* spp., *Klebsiella*, *Clostridium*, and *Pseudomonas aeruginosa* [29].

Diagnosis

The clinical presentation of mycotic aneurysm includes local pain, fever, a pulsatile mass, and inflammation at the arterial site which may be associated with back/chest pain and headaches [32]. Mycotic aneurysms are also suspected when there is history of a rapidly growing, painful aneurysm which ruptured at the time of surgery. A combination of laboratory findings along with clinical signs and symptoms, imagery, and intraoperative findings could guide the diagnosis of mycotic aneurysms [32].

Contrast-enhanced CT scan is the imaging modality of choice for aortic aneurysms. Another suitable alternative is contrast-enhanced MR angiography [33]. Digital subtraction angiography can be useful but is more invasive [33].

Management

Medical therapy for 6–8 weeks is recommended, although duration can be prolonged if infection persists [34]. For effective Salmonella coverage, vancomycin is combined with agents that have activity against gram-negative organisms such as piperacillin-tazobactam or ceftriaxone. The use of fluoroquinolones and ciprofloxacin must be avoided due to their association with aneurysm growth [35]. Serial leukocyte counts and resolution of fever and inflammation markers can be used to monitor therapeutic response [34].

Due to its high perioperative mortality, surgery is high-risk and must be carefully planned [28]. Removal of all infected tissue through surgical intervention is the definitive management for mycotic aneurysms [33]. Surgical strategies include resection and ligation, bypass with an extra-anatomic bypass, in-situ graft insertion, or debridement with or without endovascular revascularization [33]. Aortic tissue with minimal infection is managed by reconstructing with an in-situ graft following which an omental pedicle can be used to cover the conduit to reduce persistent risk of infection. Other options include cryopreserved aortic grafts, rifampin-soaked Dacron graft, and femoral vein graft [33].

The need for extra-anatomic bypass can be considered if purulence is persistent and if there are systemic signs of inflammation [33]. It can also be considered when there is extensive paraaortic or aortic purulence [33]. If emergent surgery is performed requiring graft placement in the infected surgical field, long-term antimicrobial suppression therapy should be considered. Infections occurring after endovascular or open repair should be treated with systemic antibiotics [33].

The complications of extra-anatomic bypass procedures include reinfection, aortic stump disruption, and amputation [33]. Complications of in-situ surgical repair include cerebrovascular accidents, ischemic bowel, myocardial infarctions, or acute kidney injuries. Late complications of in-situ grafts include paraaortic leaks due to anastomotic failure or fistula formation, graft failure, and reinfection [33].

In patients undergoing medical therapy post-operatively, risk factor modification such as smoking cessation, integration of medications such as aspirin, and healthy diet are recommended [34]. Strict postoperative precautions to minimize surgical site infection must be ensured [34].

Tuberculous Aortitis

It predominantly affects the descending thoracic aorta and the distal aortic arch where it presents as a pseudoaneurysm caused by caseous-necrosis of the aortic wall [36]. Due to the high risk of aortic rupture, mortality linked with tuberculous aortitis is as high as 60% [2].

Tuberculous aortitis is precipitated by underlying conditions such as atherosclerosis, diabetes mellitus, cystic medial necrosis, trauma, and vascular malformations [37]. The pathogen is multi-drug-resistant mycobacterium tuberculosis, and other etiologic factors include immunosuppression, especially acquired immunodeficiency syndrome [36].

Epidemiology

Tuberculous aortitis is rare and caused by *Mycobacterium tuberculosis* infection of the thoracic aortic wall [36]. It is a rare complication of disseminated tuberculosis with an incidence of less than 1% in patients with latent tuberculosis [37].

Pathogenesis

The formation of the aortic pseudoaneurysm results from a direct extension from the contagious infection and tuberculous lymphadenitis [38].

Diagnosis

Tuberculous aortitis is diagnosed with clinical symptoms and imaging such as CT scans, angiography, chest radiography, and cardiovascular MRI [39].

The clinical symptoms include: chest pain, dysphagia, bleeding, shock, hoarseness, pulsatile or palpable mass, abdominal pain, back pain, or frank rupture of the aorta [39]. CT angiography and contrast-enhanced CT are the preferred imaging modalities for tuberculous aortitis. They allow for the characterization of the aortic wall and luminal anatomy [39].

Management

In the absence of any concerning aneurysms, intravenous broad-spectrum antibiotic coverage followed by complete surgical excision is recommended. In the event of steroid resistance, high-dose corticosteroids and immunosuppressive agents are recommended. The most frequent medications are anti-tuberculous drugs, prophylactic antibiotics, and antiplatelet therapy [2].

Complete surgical excision of the infected region is performed if an aneurysm is present. Long-term antibiotic therapy is maintained for months after surgery to ensure continued coverage for prophylactic stent purposes [40]. Stent grafts combined with anti-tuberculous drugs are recommended for patients who are unsuitable for open chest surgery such as patients with severe organ failure, age, and weakness [40].

Following surgery and anti-mycobacterial microbial therapy, continuous follow-up for at least 6–24 months is required for close monitoring of recurrent infection [41].

Syphilitic Aortitis

Tertiary syphilis manifests 15–30 years following initial infection as gummas, neurological and cardiovascular complications [2]. Cardiovascular involvement results from endarteritis of the vasa vasorum and can manifest as aortitis, aortic regurgitation, coronary artery stenosis, or aortic aneurysms [2]. The region of aorta most commonly affected is the ascending thoracic aorta followed by the aortic arch [2].

Epidemiology

The incidence of syphillic aortitis following primary infection is about 70–80% in untreated patients, and in about 10% of these patients, other cardiovascular complications such as coronary ostial stenosis, aortic aneurysms, and aortic regurgitation may also occur [42].

Pathogenesis

The pathogenesis involves inflammatory response to the invasion of the aortic wall by *Treponema pallidum* which results in obliterative endarteritis of the vasa vasorum and causes necrosis of connective tissue and elastic fibers in the aortic media [43]. This can progress into late vascular manifestations of syphilis such as aortic aneurysm resulting from weakening of the aortic wall [43].

Diagnosis

Most patients are asymptomatic. Symptomatic patients often present with cough, hoarseness, superior vena cava compression syndrome, dysphagia, and dysphonia due to compression of the surrounding structures by the aneurysm [44]. Syphilitic aortitis is commonly diagnosed by combining laboratory and histologic data although cases with negative laboratory testing have been reported [45]. Non-treponemal testing such as venereal disease research laboratory test and rapid plasma reagin may also be negative in the late stages of syphilis due to low titer of circulatory antibodies [45]. Serologic confirmation of late stages of syphilis is required in patients with aortic aneurysms with treponemal-specific testing such as micro hemagglutination assays, fluorescent treponemal antibody absorption tests, or *Treponema pallidum* particle agglutination assay (TP-PA).

Chest radiographs may identify an aortic aneurysm in asymptomatic patients. Echocardiography and perioperative coronary angiogram are useful to identify accompanying aortic insufficiency and wall limitations of coronary flow [44]. 18-Fluorodeoxyglucose positron emission tomography (18-FDG PET-CT) can also be helpful in detecting aortic involvement in the early stages [44].

Management

Three doses of intramuscular benzathine penicillin at one-week intervals are given to treat late stages of syphilis of unknown duration [46]. Definitive treatment involves surgical repair by resection of dilated segments of the aortic aneurysm and implantation of a prosthetic vascular graft [46].

Although there is limited data on follow-up strategy for syphilitic aortitis, patients must be offered long-term follow-up with repeat imaging to monitor disease progression [46].

Aortic Graft Infections

Aortic graft infection involves infection of the primary prosthesis used for aortic repair/replacement [47]. This could include an endovascular stent used for endovascular aortic repair or a graft used in open surgery [47]. Vascular prostheses are used to treat life-threatening aortic dissection, vascular disease, and aortic aneurysms [47].

Epidemiology

The insertion of these devices can be complicated by infection in 0.5–4% of cases [47] with mortality ranging from 25% to 88% [48]. Compared to open surgery, the incidence of infection associated with endovascular graft repairs is lower with an incidence rate of approximately 1% [48].

Pathogenesis

Staphylococcus aureus is the common microorganism detected in early infection (within the first 3 months) following an open repair while in late infections, coagulase-negative infection is more likely [49].

Diagnosis

The symptoms of aortic graft infections are non-specific including back or chest pain, swelling, fever and chills, weight loss, anorexia, lethargy, and erythema [50]. Culture of microorganisms from surgically explanted grafts or other intraoperative pathological specimens may be diagnostic [50].

Aortic graft infection is diagnosed if there is direct communication between vascular prostheses and a non-sterile field such as exposed grafts in deep open wounds or deployment of an endovascular stent-grafts into previously infected field and fistulae [50]. Computed tomography is the initial imaging modality for the assessment of aortic graft infections although MRI can also be used [51]. 18F-DF PET/CT is used to overcome the limitations of CT and MRI and helpful in diagnosing low-grade aortic graft infections. Careful interpretation is needed because prosthetic grafts can provoke chronic low-grade inflammation for several years following surgery which is associated with diffuse tracer uptake [51].

Management

The treatment of thoracic graft infections involves the removal of the entire prosthetic material, extensive debridement, and orthotropic vascular reconstruction using self-made xeno-pericardial tube grafts as neoaortic segments [52].

To prevent recurrent graft infections, antiseptic solutions, particularly povidone-iodine, or antibiotics should be included in the irrigation. Suture and reinforcement of materials that are likely to harbor bacteria should be avoided [53]. Monofilament sutures should be used instead of braided sutures. Viable tissue material must be used to obliterate dead space and to provide vascularized coverage of the graft. This can be achieved by mobilizing local tissues such as pericardial fat pads and the thymus, or oftentimes with a muscle flap or omental pedicle [53].

There should be a period of intravenous antibiotic administration followed by long-term oral antibiotic therapy. There is limited data, however, on the optimal treatment strategy and the efficacy of long-term antibiotics therapy [53]. Topical cephalosporin or vancomycin powder should be applied to the graft and intravenous antibiotics should be continued postoperatively until all central venous lines and chest drains are removed [53].

The average follow-up period is 24 months. There should be continued antibiotic treatment for about 6 months. Follow-up imaging studies at regular intervals are necessary to monitor for recurrence [52].

Conclusion

In conclusion, thoracic aortic infections are highly morbid infections with non-specific clinical presentations which makes diagnosis challenging. A high index of suspicion must be maintained to ensure timely diagnosis and treatment. Depending on pathogenesis, management may include either antibiotic therapy, surgical intervention, or both, depending on the extent of infection and the duration of the time of infection. Surgical intervention involves either salvaging the original graft or replacing it with synthetic or tissue graft. Strict follow-up protocol is mandatory to optimize outcomes.

References

1. Tresson P, Quiquandon S, Long A. Comment and questions on "European Society For Vascular Surgery (ESVS) 2020 clinical practice guidelines on the management of vascular graft and endograft infections." Eur J Vasc Endovasc Surg [Internet]. 2021 [cited 2022 Apr 14];61(1):162–3. Available from: https://linkinghub.elsevier.com/retrieve/pii/S1078588420306961
2. Restrepo CS, Ocazionez D, Suri R, Vargas D. Aortitis: imaging spectrum of the infectious and inflammatory conditions of the aorta. RadioGraphics [Internet]. 2011 [cited 2022 Apr 14];31(2):435–51. Available from: http://pubs.rsna.org/doi/10.1148/rg.312105069
3. Murie JA. Vascular surgery. 5th ed., Rutherford RB, edirors, 285 × 222 mm. Pp. 2266. Illustrated. 1999. Philadelphia, Pennsylvania: W. B. Saunders. £199.00. Br J Surg [Internet]. 2002 [cited 2022 Apr 14];87(7):972–3. Available from: https://academic.oup.com/bjs/article/87/7/972/6268956
4. Piper C. Valve disease: prosthetic valve endocarditis. Heart [Internet]. 2001 [cited 2022 Apr 14];85(5):590–3. Available from: https://heart.bmj.com/lookup/doi/10.1136/heart.85.5.590
5. Alonso-Valle H, Fariñas-Álvarez C, García-Palomo JD, Bernal JM, Martín-Durán R, Gutiérrez Díez JF, et al. Clinical course and predictors of death in prosthetic valve endocarditis over a 20-year period. J Thorac Cardiovasc Surg [Internet]. 2010 [cited 2022 Apr 14];139(4):887–93. Available from: https://linkinghub.elsevier.com/retrieve/pii/S0022522309008198
6. Habib G, Thuny F, Avierinos J-F. Prosthetic valve endocarditis: current approach and therapeutic options. Prog Cardiovasc Dis [Internet]. 2008 [cited 2022 Apr 14];50(4):274–81. Available from: https://linkinghub.elsevier.com/retrieve/pii/S0033062007001065
7. Cahill TJ, Prendergast BD. Infective endocarditis. Lancet [Internet]. 2016 [cited 2022 Apr 14];387(10021):882–93. Available from: https://linkinghub.elsevier.com/retrieve/pii/S0140673615000677
8. Kahn F, Resman F, Bergmark S, Filiptsev P, Nilson B, Gilje P, et al. Time to blood culture positivity in *Staphylococcus aureus* bacteraemia to determine risk of infective endocarditis. Clin Microbiol Infect [Internet]. 2021 [cited 2022 Apr 14];27(9):1345.e7–1345.e12. Available from: https://linkinghub.elsevier.com/retrieve/pii/S1198743X2030700X
9. Cahill TJ, Baddour LM, Habib G, Hoen B, Salaun E, Pettersson GB, et al. Challenges in infective endocarditis. J Am Coll Cardiol [Internet]. 2017 [cited 2022 Apr 14];69(3):325–44. Available from: https://linkinghub.elsevier.com/retrieve/pii/S0735109716371121
10. Rivas P, Alonso J, Moya J, de Górgolas M, Martinell J, Fernández Guerrero ML. The impact of hospital-acquired infections on the microbial etiology and prognosis of late-onset prosthetic valve endocarditis. Chest [Internet]. 2005 [cited 2022 Apr 14];128(2):764–71. Available from: https://linkinghub.elsevier.com/retrieve/pii/S0012369215504236
11. Murdoch DR. Clinical presentation, etiology, and outcome of infective endocarditis in the 21st century: the international collaboration on endocarditis–prospective cohort study. Arch Intern Med [Internet]. 2009 [cited 2022 Apr 14];169(5):463. Available from: http://archinte.jamanetwork.com/article.aspx?doi=10.1001/archinternmed.2008.603
12. Werdan K, Dietz S, Löffler B, Niemann S, Bushnaq H, Silber R-E, et al. Mechanisms of infective endocarditis: pathogen–host interaction and risk states. Nat Rev Cardiol [Internet]. 2014 [cited 2022 Apr 14];11(1):35–50. Available from: http://www.nature.com/articles/nrcardio.2013.174
13. Grover FL, Cohen DJ, Oprian C, Henderson WG, Sethi G, Hammermeister KE. Determinants of the occurrence of and survival from prosthetic valve endocarditis. J Thorac Cardiovasc

Surg [Internet]. 1994 [cited 2022 Apr 14];108(2):207–14. Available from: https://linkinghub.elsevier.com/retrieve/pii/S0022522394700028
14. Sohail MR, Martin KR, Wilson WR, Baddour LM, Harmsen WS, Steckelberg JM. Medical versus surgical management of *Staphylococcus aureus* prosthetic valve endocarditis. Am J Med [Internet]. 2006 [cited 2022 Apr 14];119(2):147–54. Available from: https://linkinghub.elsevier.com/retrieve/pii/S0002934305008971
15. Vered Z, Mossinson D, Peleg E, Kaplinsky E, Motro M, Beker B. Echocardiographic assessment of prosthetic valve endocarditis. Eur Heart J [Internet]. 1995 [cited 2022 Apr 14];16(suppl B):63–7. Available from: https://academic.oup.com/eurheartj/article-lookup/doi/10.1093/eurheartj/16.suppl_B.63
16. Rice LB, Calderwood SB, Eliopoulos GM, Farber BF, Karchmer AW. Enterococcal endocarditis: a comparison of prosthetic and native valve disease. Clin Infect Dis [Internet]. 1991 [cited 2022 Apr 14];13(1):1–7. Available from: https://academic.oup.com/cid/article/13/1/1/303620
17. Durack DT, Lukes AS, Bright DK, Duke Endocarditis Service. New criteria for diagnosis of infective endocarditis: utilization of specific echocardiographic findings. Am J Med [Internet]. 1994 [cited 2022 Apr 14];96(3):200–9. Available from: https://linkinghub.elsevier.com/retrieve/pii/0002934394901430
18. Pettersson GB, Coselli JS, Pettersson GB, Coselli JS, Hussain ST, Griffin B, et al. 2016 the American Association for Thoracic Surgery (AATS) consensus guidelines: surgical treatment of infective endocarditis: executive summary. J Thorac Cardiovasc Surg [Internet]. 2017 [cited 2022 Apr 14];153(6):1241–1258.e29. Available from: https://linkinghub.elsevier.com/retrieve/pii/S0022522317301162
19. Wang A, Gaca JG, Chu VH. Management considerations in infective endocarditis: a review. JAMA [Internet]. 2018 [cited 2022 Apr 14];320(1):72. Available from: http://jama.jamanetwork.com/article.aspx?doi=10.1001/jama.2018.7596
20. Nguyen Q, White A, Lam W, Wang W, Wang S. Valve-in-valve using perceval prostheses for prosthetic valve endocarditis. Ann Thorac Surg [Internet]. 2022 [cited 2022 Apr 14];S0003497522003010. Available from: https://linkinghub.elsevier.com/retrieve/pii/S0003497522003010
21. Gornik HL, Creager MA. Aortitis. Circulation [Internet]. 2008 [cited 2022 Apr 14];117(23):3039–51. Available from: https://www.ahajournals.org/doi/10.1161/CIRCULATIONAHA.107.760686
22. Revest M, Decaux O, Cazalets C, Verohye J-P, Jégo P, Grosbois B. Aortites thoraciques infectieuses: implications microbiologiques, physiopathologiques et thérapeutiques. Rev Med Interne [Internet]. 2007 [cited 2022 Apr 14];28(2):108–15. Available from: https://linkinghub.elsevier.com/retrieve/pii/S0248866306003262
23. Wein M, Bartel T, Kabatnik M, Sadony V, Dirsch O, Erbel R. Rapid progression of bacterial aortitis to an ascending aortic mycotic aneurysm documented by transesophageal echocardiography. J Am Soc Echocardiogr [Internet]. 2001 [cited 2022 Apr 14];14(6):646–9. Available from: https://linkinghub.elsevier.com/retrieve/pii/S0894731701839481
24. Oderich GS, Panneton JM, Bower TC, Cherry KJ, Rowland CM, Noel AA, et al. Infected aortic aneurysms: aggressive presentation, complicated early outcome, but durable results. J Vasc Surg [Internet]. 2001 [cited 2022 Apr 14];34(5):900–8. Available from: https://linkinghub.elsevier.com/retrieve/pii/S0741521401875224
25. Foote EA, Postier RG, Greenfield RA, Bronze MS. Infectious aortitis. Curr Treat Options Cardio Med [Internet]. 2005 [cited 2022 Apr 14];7(2):89–97. Available from: http://link.springer.com/10.1007/s11936-005-0010-6
26. Castaneda-Zuniga WR, Nath PH, Zollikofer C, Velasquez G, Valdez-Davila O, Edwards E. Mycotic aneurysm of the aorta. Cardiovasc Intervent Radiol [Internet]. 1980 [cited 2022 Apr 14];3(3):144–9. Available from: http://link.springer.com/10.1007/BF02551976
27. Lopes RJ, Almeida J, Dias PJ, Pinho P, Maciel MJ. Infectious thoracic aortitis: a literature review. Clin Cardiol [Internet]. 2009 [cited 2022 Apr 14];32(9):488–90. Available from: https://onlinelibrary.wiley.com/doi/10.1002/clc.20578

28. Reddy DJ. Management of infected aortoiliac aneurysms. Arch Surg [Internet]. 1991 [cited 2022 Apr 14];126(7):873. Available from: http://archsurg.jamanetwork.com/article.aspx?doi=10.1001/archsurg.1991.01410310083012
29. Huang Y-K, Chen C-L, Lu M-S, Tsai F-C, Lin P-L, Wu C-H, et al. Clinical, microbiologic, and outcome analysis of mycotic aortic aneurysm: the role of endovascular repair. Surg Infect [Internet]. 2014 [cited 2022 Apr 14];15(3):290–8. Available from: https://www.liebertpub.com/doi/10.1089/sur.2013.011
30. McCready RA, Bryant MA, Divelbiss JL, Chess BA, Chitwood RW, Paget DS. Arterial infections in the new millenium: an old problem revisited. Ann Vasc Surg [Internet]. 2006 [cited 2022 Apr 14];20(5):590–5. Available from: https://linkinghub.elsevier.com/retrieve/pii/S0890509607601721
31. Majeed H, Ahmad F. Mycotic aneurysm. StatPearls [Internet]. 2022 [cited 2022 Jul 5]. Available from: https://www.ncbi.nlm.nih.gov/books/NBK560736/
32. Wyatt MG. Vascular and endovascular surgical techniques. 4th ed. R. M. Greenhalgh (Ed.) 280 × 222 mm. Pp 548. Illustrated. 2001. Philadelphia, Pennsylvania: WB Saunders. Br J Surg [Internet]. 2002 [cited 2022 Apr 14];89(4):503–503. Available from: https://academic.oup.com/bjs/article/89/4/503/6143902
33. Stenson KM, Grima MJ, Loftus IM, Tripathi RK. Recommendations for management of infected aortic pathology based on current evidence. Semin Vasc Surg [Internet]. 2019 [cited 2022 Apr 14];32(1–2):68–72. Available from: https://linkinghub.elsevier.com/retrieve/pii/S0895796719300456
34. Hollier LH, Money SR, Creely B, Bower TC, Kazmier FJ. Direct replacement of mycotic thoracoabdominal aneurysms. J Vasc Surg [Internet]. 1993 [cited 2022 Apr 14];18(3):477–85. Available from: https://linkinghub.elsevier.com/retrieve/pii/074152149390266O
35. LeMaire SA, Zhang L, Luo W, Ren P, Azares AR, Wang Y, et al. Effect of ciprofloxacin on susceptibility to aortic dissection and rupture in mice. JAMA Surg [Internet]. 2018 [cited 2022 Jul 5];153(9):e181804. Available from: https://jamanetwork.com/journals/jamasurgery/fullarticle/2689031
36. Lin M-M, Cheng H-M. Images in cardiovascular medicine: tuberculous aortitis. Intern Med [Internet]. 2012 [cited 2022 Apr 14];51(15):1983–5. Available from: https://www.jstage.jst.go.jp/article/internalmedicine/51/15/51_51.7690/_article
37. Pierret C, Tourtier J-P, Grand B, Boddaert G, Laurian C, de Kerangal X. Multiple tuberculous aneurysms of the aorta. J Vasc Surg [Internet]. 2011 [cited 2022 Apr 14];53(6):1720–2. Available from: https://linkinghub.elsevier.com/retrieve/pii/S0741521411002291
38. Long R, Guzman R, Greenberg H, Safneck J, Hershfield E. Tuberculous mycotic aneurysm of the aorta. Chest [Internet]. 1999 [cited 2022 Apr 14];115(2):522–31. Available from: https://linkinghub.elsevier.com/retrieve/pii/S0012369215505990
39. Park S-C, Moon I-S, Koh Y-B. Tuberculous pseudoaneurysm of the descending thoracic aorta. Ann Vasc Surg [Internet]. 2010 [cited 2022 Apr 14];24(3):417.e11–417.e13. Available from: https://linkinghub.elsevier.com/retrieve/pii/S0890509609003124
40. Jordan WD, Alcocer F, Wirthlin DJ, Westfall AO, Whitley D. Abdominal aortic aneurysms in "high-risk" surgical patients: comparison of open and endovascular repair. Ann Surg [Internet]. 2003 [cited 2022 Apr 14];237(5):623–30. Available from: https://journals.lww.com/00000658-200305000-00004
41. Huang S, Liu X, Sun Z. Quadricuspid aortic valve with ruptured sinus of valsalva aneurysm: a case report. Braz J Cardiovasc Surg [Internet]. 2022 [cited 2022 Apr 14]. Available from: https://cdn.publisher.gn1.link/bjcvs.org/pdf/AOP-2020-0735.R1.pdf
42. Adachi O, Saiki Y, Akasaka J, Oda K, Iguchi A, Tabayashi K. Surgical management of aortic regurgitation associated with takayasu arteritis and other forms of aortitis. Ann Thorac Surg [Internet]. 2007 [cited 2022 Apr 14];84(6):1950–3. Available from: https://linkinghub.elsevier.com/retrieve/pii/S0003497507015482

43. Heggtveit HA. Syphilitic aortitis: a clinicopathologic autopsy study of 100 cases, 1950 to 1960. Circulation [Internet]. 1964 [cited 2022 Apr 14];29(3):346–55. Available from: https://www.ahajournals.org/doi/10.1161/01.CIR.29.3.346
44. Jackman JD, Radolf JD. Cardiovascular syphilis. Am J Med [Internet]. 1989 [cited 2022 Apr 14];87(4):425–33. Available from: https://linkinghub.elsevier.com/retrieve/pii/S0002934389808265
45. Joseph Davey D, Acosta L del RC, Gupta P, Konda KA, Caceres CF, Klausner JD. Probable syphilitic aortitis documented by positron emission tomography. Sex Transm Dis [Internet]. 2016 [cited 2022 Apr 14];43(3):199–200. Available from: http://journals.lww.com/00007435-201603000-00009
46. Cooley LE, McNamara FP. Syphilitic aortitis with aneurysm of the innominate artery and occlusion of the left common carotid artery. Am Heart J [Internet]. 1934 [cited 2022 Apr 14];9(5):686–9. Available from: https://linkinghub.elsevier.com/retrieve/pii/S000287033490449X
47. A Report of the American College of Cardiology/American Heart Association Task Force on Practice Guidelines (Committee on the Management of Patients With Unstable Angina). ACC/AHA guidelines for the management of patients with unstable angina and non-ST segment elevation myocardial infarction: executive summary and recommendations. Cathet Cardiovasc Intervent [Internet]. 2000 [cited 2022 Apr 14];51(4):505–21. Available from: https://onlinelibrary.wiley.com/doi/10.1002/1522-726X(200012)51:4<505::AID-CCD29>3.0.CO;2-L
48. Zerizer I, Tan K, Khan S, Barwick T, Marzola MC, Rubello D, et al. Role of fdg-pet and pet/ct in the diagnosis and management of vasculitis. Eur J Radiol [Internet]. 2010 [cited 2022 Apr 14];73(3):504–9. Available from: https://linkinghub.elsevier.com/retrieve/pii/S0720048X10000525
49. Chambers S. Diagnosis and management of staphylococcal infections of vascular grafts and stents. Intern Med J [Internet]. 2005 [cited 2022 Apr 14];35(s2):S72–8. Available from: https://onlinelibrary.wiley.com/doi/10.1111/j.1444-0903.2005.00981.x
50. Perera GB, Fujitani RM, Kubaska SM. Aortic graft infection: update on management and treatment options. Vasc Endovascular Surg [Internet]. 2006 [cited 2022 Apr 14];40(1):1–10. Available from: http://journals.sagepub.com/doi/10.1177/153857440604000101
51. Keidar Z, Engel A, Hoffman A, Israel O, Nitecki S. Prosthetic vascular graft infection: the role of 18f-fdg pet/ct. J Nucl Med [Internet]. 2007 [cited 2022 Apr 14];48(8):1230–6. Available from: http://jnm.snmjournals.org/cgi/doi/10.2967/jnumed.107.040253
52. Akowuah E, Narayan P, Angelini G, Bryan AJ. Management of prosthetic graft infection after surgery of the thoracic aorta: removal of the prosthetic graft is not necessary. J Thorac Cardiovasc Surg [Internet]. 2007 [cited 2022 Apr 14];134(4):1051–2. Available from: https://linkinghub.elsevier.com/retrieve/pii/S0022522307010793
53. Luciani N, Lapenna E, De Bonis M, Possati GF. Mediastinitis following graft replacement of the ascending aorta: conservative approach by omental transposition. Eur J Cardio-Thorac Surg [Internet]. 2001 [cited 2022 Apr 14];20(2):418–20. Available from: https://academic.oup.com/ejcts/article-lookup/doi/10.1016/S1010-7940(01)00789-8

Chapter 14
Open Operative Therapy for the Descending and Thoracoabdominal Aorta

Davut Cekmecelioglu and Ourania Preventza

Introduction

Conditions that threaten the integrity of the thoracic aorta, such as aortic dissection, aortic aneurysm, and traumatic injury, can have life-threatening outcomes. Despite the notable morbidity and mortality linked to surgical intervention for these conditions, the frequency of thoracic aortic procedures continues to rise annually. Providing these patients with a sustainable aortic repair necessitates a multifaceted approach. This approach includes a comprehensive preoperative assessment and meticulous intraoperative protection of critical organs (e.g., the brain, heart, spinal cord, kidneys, and other abdominal viscera) against ischemia. Often, this protection is achieved by using cardiopulmonary bypass (CPB) or left heart bypass (LHB).

The aorta is broadly divided into 2 significant segments: the proximal aorta, which comprises the aortic root, ascending aorta, and transverse aortic arch; and the distal aorta, which encompasses the descending thoracic aorta, thoracoabdominal aorta, and abdominal aorta (Fig. 14.1). Segments of the aorta can also be described in terms of their position relative to the diaphragm. The thoracic aorta is located above the diaphragm, and the abdominal aorta is found below it.

These distinctive anatomical aspects of the aorta's segments directly influence the presentation and treatment of associated diseases. The most prevalent system for categorizing thoracoabdominal aortic aneurysms (TAAAs) was presented by

D. Cekmecelioglu
Department of Cardiothoracic Surgery, Heart, Vascular and Thoracic Institute, Cleveland Clinic, Cleveland, OH, USA

Heart Surgeons of San Antonio, San Antonio, TX, USA

O. Preventza (✉)
Heart Surgeons of San Antonio, San Antonio, TX, USA

G. J. Arnaoutakis et al. (eds.), *Aortic Aneurysms*, Contemporary Cardiology,
https://doi.org/10.1007/978-3-032-13134-8_14

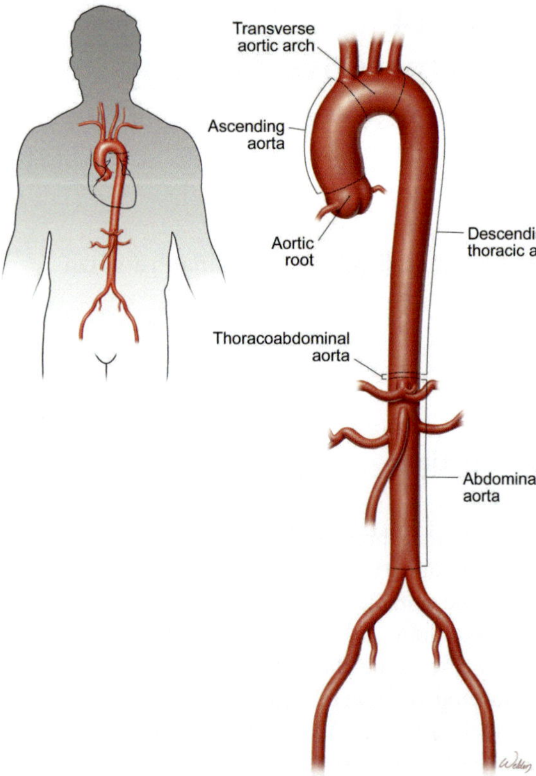

Fig. 14.1 Aortic segments encompass various sections of the aorta, including the ascending thoracic aorta, aortic arch, descending thoracic aorta, suprarenal aorta, and infrarenal aorta. The border between the thoracic and abdominal aorta is at the level of the diaphragm

Crawford and his team [1] in 1986. Their classification, based on the extent of repair required, subdivides TAAA into 4 extents (Fig. 14.2): Extent I involves a significant portion of the descending thoracic aorta (usually initiating near the left subclavian artery) and extends to the suprarenal abdominal aorta; extent II encompasses most of the descending thoracic aorta, similar to extent I, but includes a larger section of the abdominal aorta; extent III involves the middle to lower portion of the descending thoracic aorta (distal to the 6th intercostal space) and various parts of the abdominal aorta; and extent IV originates at the diaphragmatic hiatus and extends into the abdominal aorta. All TAAA repairs involve the 4 visceral branching arteries: the celiac axis, the superior mesenteric artery, and the left and right renal arteries. For extent II to IV aneurysm, repairs often extend to the aortoiliac bifurcation, and on occasion, replacement of the iliac arteries is also necessary.

Open surgical intervention continues to be recognized as the gold-standard treatment for TAAA, which affects both the descending thoracic and abdominal segments of the aorta. Such aneurysms can result from aortic dissection or progressive medial degeneration. Modern surgical strategies aim to strike a balance between maximizing long-term benefits—achieved by replacing as much of the diseased aorta as possible—and minimizing the risk of ischemia-related complications to the spinal cord and other organs.

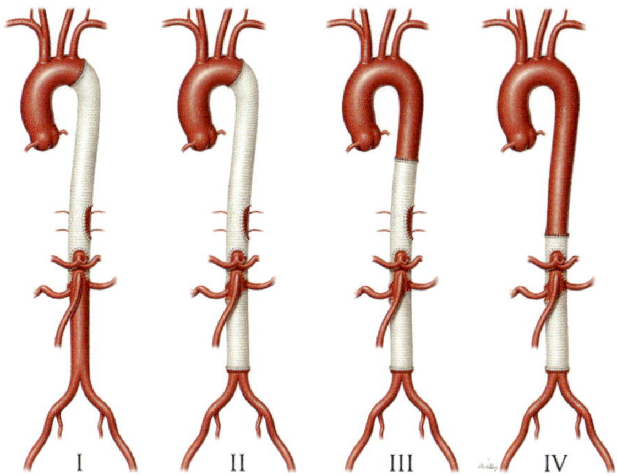

Fig. 14.2 Crawford extents of thoracoabdominal aortic aneurysm repair. Extent I involves the segment starting from the vicinity of the left subclavian artery and extending to the suprarenal abdominal aorta. Extent II encompasses a larger portion of the descending thoracic aorta, extending all the way to the infrarenal abdominal aorta. Extent III involves the mid- to lower descending thoracic aorta and extends into the aortoiliac bifurcation. Extent IV begins at the diaphragmatic hiatus and extends into the aortoiliac bifurcation. Of these, the most extensive repairs are Crawford Extents I and II

Despite the formidable challenges presented by extensive aortic replacement, outcomes—both early and late—after these operations are highly satisfactory. In a recent series of 3309 open TAAA repairs [2], we found an early mortality rate of 7.5% coupled with low rates of persistent paraplegia or paraparesis (5.4%), stroke (2.2%), and renal failure necessitating permanent dialysis (5.7%).

Crawford extent II repairs, which are the most extensive operations, involve replacing the entire descending thoracic and abdominal aorta. The perfusion strategies employed during the repair of descending thoracic aortic aneurysm (DTAA) and TAAA are both described in this chapter because they have much in common.

Indications and Contraindications for Open Surgery

The crucial role of patient selection in determining the course of treatment for TAAA cannot be overstated. Certain categories of patients, such as those of advanced age (80 years or older), those with a life expectancy of less than 2 years, younger patients with significant comorbidities, and those with a contained ruptured aneurysm that has precipitated a critical condition, might derive more benefit from a less invasive hybrid or totally endovascular approach as a stepping stone to definitive aortic repair.

Undeniably, an endovascular approach presents a less invasive alternative to open repair and subjects patients to less physiological stress. It eliminates the need for a thoracoabdominal incision, single-lung ventilation, and aortic cross-clamping, consequently reducing the hemodynamic impact of the intervention and minimizing the risk of end-organ ischemia. However, these therapeutic advantages come at the cost of higher rates of reintervention and substantially poorer durability [3, 4]. As of the time of writing, no device for endovascular TAAA repair has yet received approval from the US Food and Drug Administration. Consequently, endovascular TAAA is currently confined to sites participating in clinical trials and is discussed in a separate chapter.

The guidelines from the American College of Cardiology and the American Heart Association recommend open distal aortic repair for patients with thoracic aortic disease when the aortic diameter surpasses 6 cm (a class I recommendation with a level of evidence B). A lower diameter threshold is suggested for patients whose aneurysm has a rapid growth rate (>0.5 cm/y) or heritable thoracic aortic disease [5]. Symptoms related to the compression of nearby structures by the aneurysm may portend impending rupture, so these aneurysms should be repaired, irrespective of their size [5]. Other predictors of rupture include advanced age, a history of hypertension, tobacco use, and chronic obstructive pulmonary disease. Intervention is indicated for acute type B aortic dissection with rupture or malperfusion syndrome. Endovascular stent grafting, when anatomically feasible, is preferable to open repair as first-line treatment.

The European Society for Vascular Surgery also suggests considering open or endovascular repair at 6.0 cm for asymptomatic patients with TAAA who are at low to moderate surgical risk. In addition, for patients diagnosed with rapidly expanding TAAA (>1.0 cm/y), repair should be considered irrespective of the aortic diameter [6]. For TAAA patients for whom open repair is not recommended, endovascular repair should be contemplated unless the patient's anatomy is unfavorable. In such cases, a hybrid approach should be considered. Both sets of guidelines concur that patients with heritable thoracic aortic disease are not ideal candidates for endovascular repair. For patients with symptomatic TAAA, diameter-based guidelines are not applicable, and an urgent evaluation for prompt repair is warranted. Irrespective of the indication, urgent or emergency open repair of TAAA is associated with a significantly higher risk of morbidity and mortality than elective repair.

Preoperative Planning and Evaluation

In our preoperative evaluation, we assess a patient's age and physiological reserve, stratify their risk levels, discontinue antiplatelet and anticoagulant medications, advocate for tobacco cessation, and optimize any major neurological, cardiovascular, respiratory, and renal comorbidities. Each of the principal surgical risks—mortality, paraplegia, renal failure, stroke, respiratory failure, bleeding, and myocardial infarction—is thoroughly discussed with both the patient and their family.

The timing of the surgery is influenced by various factors, including the aneurysm's size and growth rate, the presence of leak, rupture, or acute dissection, and the patient's symptomatology [7, 8]. This careful and comprehensive approach to preoperative planning helps ensure optimal patient outcomes and is an integral part of the treatment process.

Beyond assessing the patient's cardiopulmonary risk and acuity of presentation as previously detailed, a thorough preoperative examination of the patient's computed tomographic angiograms is vital. This allows precise measurement of the diameter of the thoracoabdominal aorta across the aneurysmal and non-aneurysmal segments.

We also pay particular attention to our clamping and cannulation strategies. Although full CPB with deep hypothermic circulatory arrest is not commonly used at our institution, it may be necessary under specific circumstances. These can include cases in which a proximal clamp cannot be applied because of rupture or a large aneurysm, and redo operations in patients without a preexisting elephant trunk. Similarly, if the arch tissue and synthetic graft are tightly adherent to the recurrent laryngeal nerve, trachea, or pulmonary artery such that safe dissection cannot be performed, CPB with deep hypothermic circulatory arrest may be required. If LHB is the plan, the chosen cannulation site should ideally be devoid of extensive luminal thrombus, atheroma, and heavy calcification of the aorta. These strategies are crucial to ensuring a successful surgical outcome and minimizing potential complications.

Moreover, we are cautious about anatomic variants such as a retroaortic renal vein, and we note the location of any unusually large segmental arteries. We carefully assess potential clamping and cannulation sites for dissection and mural thrombus. In addition, the visceral and renal arteries are meticulously evaluated for stenotic origins. We also study their spatial relationship to each other. In cases of chronic dissection, we determine whether it is the true lumen, false lumen, or both that supply these arteries. This comprehensive assessment allows us to accurately understand the patient's unique anatomy and vascular condition, helping to inform the choice of surgical strategy and improve outcomes.

For a typical elective procedure, antiplatelet medications and warfarin are suspended at least 5 days before surgery. Commonly, patients are bridged with enoxaparin, which is discontinued the day before the operation. We alert the blood bank and hematopathologist if the patient has had prior transfusions and has developed antibodies, because obtaining compatible blood might require additional time. Testing the patient's baseline platelet function before surgery is useful. We establish the patient's blood type and ensure matching for a minimum of 6 units each of packed red blood cells and fresh frozen plasma, as well as 6 doses of platelets and cryoprecipitate.

The patient is instructed not to consume anything by mouth for at least 6 h before the scheduled operation. For hospitalized patients, intravenous fluids are maintained at a rate of 30–75 mL/h during this period, with adjustments made based on the patient's fluid balance and cardiac status. We advise patients to shower with chlorhexidine soap twice before surgery, ideally 12–16 h prior and again 2–4 h before the procedure. One hour before the surgical incision, broad-spectrum intravenous antibiotics (commonly vancomycin and cefepime) are prescribed and administered prophylactically. For patients with allergies, aztreonam can be substituted for cefepime, and linezolid can replace vancomycin. This comprehensive preparatory approach helps to mitigate potential complications and optimize surgical outcomes.

Techniques in Open Operative Therapy

Each procedure commences with a discussion involving the anesthesia and perfusion teams. The perfusion team prepares a cell saver and the LHB circuit or, less frequently, a full CPB circuit in case hypothermic circulatory arrest becomes necessary. The anesthesia team routinely establishes intravenous access via a large-bore peripheral intravenous line and a central venous catheter. Hemodynamic monitoring necessitates the use of a Swan-Ganz catheter, and an arterial line is placed in the right radial or brachial artery. A femoral arterial catheter is also useful for monitoring distal and proximal perfusion simultaneously during the period of aortic cross-clamping. To guide the process of permissive hypothermia and rewarming, a temperature probe is inserted into the nasopharynx. To monitor kidney function and manage fluid balance, a Foley catheter is used. Single-lung ventilation is achieved by intubating patients with a double-lumen endobronchial tube during the procedure. Alternatively, the anesthesiologist can place a bronchial blocker; this obviates endobronchial tube exchange at the end of the procedure but must be done with great care. This meticulous setup allows careful monitoring and management of the patient's physiological status throughout the operation.

Aortic repair requires focused measures to protect the viscera, kidneys, and spinal cord. This sequence of steps is primarily determined by the Crawford extent of TAAA repair (Table 14.1), with extent II repair typically requiring the most extensive use of protective adjuncts. For most TAAA repairs, the use of a cell-saver system for autotransfusion via a rapid-infusion circuit (Fig. 14.3) is indispensable. We

Table 14.1 The use of adjuncts for organ protection during open repair of thoracoabdominal aortic pathologies

		Crawford extent			
Adjunct	DTAA	I	II	III	IV
Left heart bypass	±	+	+	±	–
Selective visceral perfusion	–	±	+	±	–
Cold renal perfusion	–	±	+	+	+
CSF drainage	±	+	+	±	–
Reattachment of intercostals	–	±	+	±	–
Moderate heparinization	+	+	+	+	+
Mild hypothermia	±	+	+	+	+

DTAA descending thoracic aortic aneurysm, *CSF* cerebrospinal fluid
+, generally use, –, generally do not use, ±, may use depending on patient characteristics and intraoperative findings

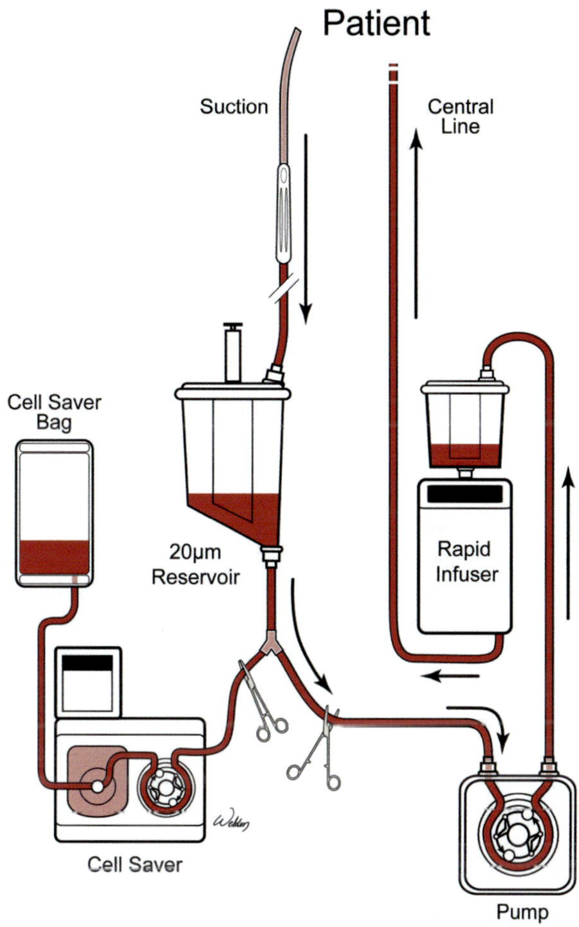

Fig. 14.3 Diagram depicting the rapid-infusion circuit as a component of a cell salvage device. The process involves suctioning moderately heparinized whole blood from the surgical field into a reservoir. The blood is then directed through a roller pump and into a rapid infuser. The rapid infuser returns unwashed whole blood, which has not had plasma or platelets removed, back to the patient through the central line. This circuit enables the rapid and controlled administration of salvaged blood during surgical procedures

consistently use passive mild hypothermia, sequential cross-clamping, and assertive reimplantation of intercostal or lumbar arteries, regardless of the extent of repair. In extent I and II repairs, we routinely use cerebrospinal fluid (CSF) drainage and provide LHB during repair. Furthermore, we use isothermic blood from the redirected LHB circuit to perfuse the celiac axis and superior mesenteric artery (SMA) [9]. If circumstances allow, cold renal solution is infused to safeguard the kidneys [10, 11]. These measures aim to reduce the risk of ischemic complications that might arise from aortic cross-clamping.

To minimize potential damage to the spinal cord [12], a CSF drainage catheter is positioned by the anesthesia team at the L3-L4, L4-L5, or L5-S1 level. It is worth noting that this procedure carries its own risk of complications [13]. This adjunct is predominantly reserved for patients undergoing extensive repair (i.e., Crawford extent I or II TAAA repair), although it can be used during less extensive repairs if deemed necessary. The primary goal of the drainage is to maintain a CSF pressure below 15 mmHg. If drainage is needed, it is done at a rate of 10 mL/h or 25 mL over 4 h. In our practice, we do not routinely use motor-evoked potential monitoring or near-infrared spectroscopy monitoring, as there are no data from randomized trials to support the use of neuromonitoring in open repair. Nonetheless, neuromonitoring is used at many other centers.

Positioning, Incision, and Aortic Exposure

The patient is positioned on a beanbag in a right lateral decubitus position, with the upper body tilted at a 60° angle and the hips at a 30° angle to the operating table (Fig. 14.4). The left arm is supported above the shoulders on an elevated arm board in a freestyle swimming-stroke position. This specific position optimizes exposure of the TAAA and ensures easy access to the groin and femoral vessels, which is crucial in cases requiring a shift to full CPB or the implementation of LHB. After the sterile preparation of the left chest, abdomen, and pelvis, an adhesive antimicrobial drape is applied over all exposed skin.

A sigmoid skin incision is made, starting from the left scapula, running along the seventh rib, and extending across the costal margin to the left of the umbilicus. The ribs are counted, and the 6th intercostal space is accessed while the patient is under single-lung ventilation. This intercostal space is typically used for repairing extent I and II aneurysms. For extent III aneurysms, the 7th intercostal space is accessed, while the 9th is used for extent IV aneurysms. In patients with Marfan syndrome, the ribs have a more vertical orientation, and careful review of the preoperative computed tomography scan can further inform the choice of the intercostal level

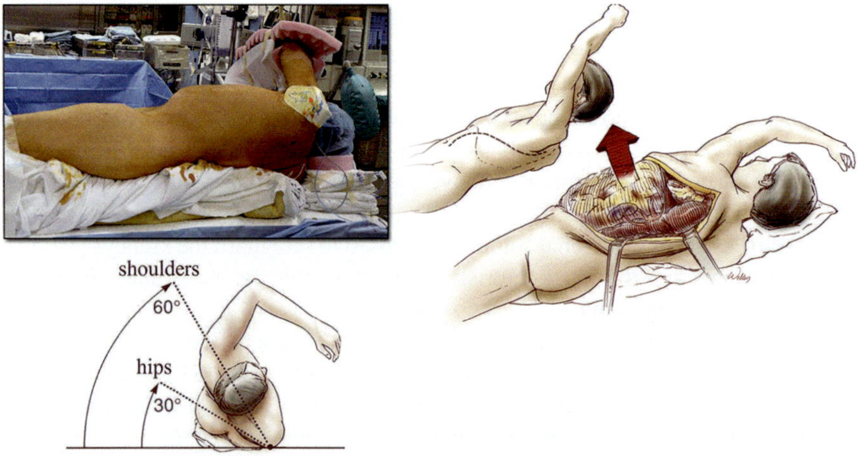

Fig. 14.4 Patient positioning and the incision and exposure during repair of a Crawford extent II thoracoabdominal aortic aneurysm

used to access the thoracic cavity. To maintain adequate and stable exposure throughout the operation, table-mounted retractors should be used.

Once both the chest and abdomen are open, a left medial visceral rotation is performed via a transperitoneal approach along the line of Toldt. The entire thoracoabdominal aorta can also be exposed by a completely retroperitoneal approach. The diaphragm is circumferentially divided, leaving a 3- to 4-cm rim of diaphragm attached to the lateral and posterior chest walls. The spleen is carefully inspected for any injury, and if a significant tear is found, the spleen is removed. However, preserving the spleen is encouraged; we have associated incidental splenectomy with a greater risk of operative mortality, although not late mortality [14].

The stomach and colon are also inspected, and any injuries are promptly repaired. The entire thoracoabdominal aorta, from the left subclavian artery to the aortic bifurcation, is then exposed with electrocautery. A space for the proximal cross-clamp is carefully crafted, ensuring the preservation of both the vagus nerve and the recurrent laryngeal nerve. The emphasis on meticulous hemostasis and surgical technique is especially critical for patients with lung adhesions resulting from a previous type I aortic dissection or prior repair. Damage to the lung can cause pulmonary contusions, leading to oxygenation issues and air leaks, which can be challenging to seal in patients with pulmonary parenchymal disease.

While exposing the distal aorta, the surgeon must take care to identify the origin of the left renal artery and keep the incision posterior to the left ureter and gonadal vein. An epiaortic ultrasonogram can guide the selection of the distal cannulation site, ensuring that it is free of thrombus or locating a free-floating elephant trunk that can be later used for the construction of the proximal anastomosis.

Left Heart Bypass

The use of LHB is an integral part of the surgical strategy for TAAA repair, enhancing patient safety and outcomes, particularly patients with Crawford extent I and II TAAAs. LHB provides vital perfusion to the downstream aorta, thereby reducing the risk of ischemic complications, particularly in patients with acute aortic dissection, prior infrarenal aortic replacement, or other risk factors.

LHB involves withdrawing isothermic, self-oxygenated blood from the left side of the heart and returning this blood via a cannula placed in the distal downstream aorta or, in some cases, the femoral artery. This process creates a closed circuit with a centrifugal pump.

While the LHB circuit does not have a reservoir or heat exchanger and thus cannot be used to cool the patient, it is used during the construction of the proximal anastomosis and offers several significant benefits:

1. Controlled blood flow: The flow of blood in the circuit can be readily managed, ensuring that both upper- and lower-body aortic pressures remain within a desired physiological range.

2. Prevention of heart distention and injury: LHB offloads the heart, thereby reducing the risk of distention and subsequent injury to the myocardium. This aspect of LHB is particularly beneficial for patients with poor cardiac reserve.
3. Continued organ perfusion: During the majority of the repair, the distal organs receive necessary blood flow.
4. Prevention of hypovolemic shock: Ensuring continuous circulation minimizes the risk of hypovolemic shock due to aortic unclamping.

LHB has been a well-established technique in distal thoracic aortic repair for more than six decades [15]. When used in combination with other adjuncts, such as CSF drainage, the beneficial aspects of LHB can be further enhanced [16].

However, it is important to acknowledge certain limitations associated with the LHB technique. Shed blood cannot be directly suctioned into the LHB circuit, necessitating the use of 1 or 2 cell-savers. While cell-savers can be effective in managing blood loss, they are not always adequate in patients with significant unanticipated bleeding, potentially leading to rapid exsanguination.

Some experts have suggested adding a reservoir and aspirators to the LHB circuit, or else performing the reconstruction by using full CPB, which is mandatory when deep hypothermic circulatory arrest is required. However, this modification would require complete heparinization, negating one of the key advantages of LHB and rendering it comparable to standard CPB. In our practice, intravenous heparin is not strictly necessary when a centrifugal pump is used for LHB. Nonetheless, to maintain an activated clotting time (ACT) greater than 200 s, we routinely administer low levels of systemic heparin (1.0–1.5 mg/kg) to prevent thrombosis of the small intercostal arteries, including those that supply the spinal cord. It is worth noting that the centrifugal pumps used in LHB are designed to operate at lower pressures than the roller pumps used in CPB, so the LHB pumps are generally considered safer to use.

The drainage (outflow) cannula is typically inserted into the left atrium for the LHB circuit. This can be done via the left inferior pulmonary vein, left superior pulmonary vein, left atrial appendage, or, in rare cases, the aorta itself (above the proximal aortic clamp) or the femoral vein. The specific approach depends on the surgeon's preference and the patient's anatomy.

The return (inflow) cannula is directly inserted into the descending thoracic aorta, approximately 3 cm above the celiac axis. Alternatively, it can be placed in the infrarenal aorta or the femoral or iliac artery by direct cannulation or via a side-branch graft. This choice is also influenced by individual patient factors and surgeon preference (Fig. 14.5). The flow rate is initially set at 0.5 L/min and subsequently increased to 3.0–3.5 L/min once the aortic cross-clamp is applied. This adjustment helps maintain the patient's mean arterial pressure within the target range of 70–90 mmHg.

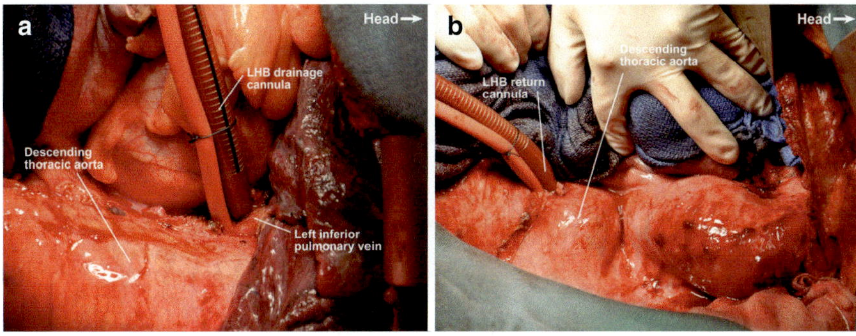

Fig. 14.5 Left heart bypass (LHB) drainage and return cannulation. An intraoperative photograph shows the cannulation sites being prepared for left heart bypass. (**a**) A 24-F angled-tip drainage cannula is placed in the left atrium via the left inferior pulmonary vein. (**b**) A 20-F angled-tip return cannula is placed in the distal aorta, a few centimeters cranial to the origin of the celiac axis

Construction of the Proximal Anastomosis

Once LHB is initiated at a flow rate of 500 mL/min, a straight, padded aortic cross-clamp is typically applied just distal to the left subclavian artery. Manual compression of the proximal descending thoracic aorta with a laparotomy pad helps displace blood distally. Subsequently, a Crafoord clamp is applied distally, usually at the T6-T7 vertebral level, which corresponds to the junction of the proximal and middle thirds of the descending thoracic aorta. Placing the distal aortic clamp at this specific level is crucial to preserving blood flow to the T7-L1 segments, which is where the artery of Adamkiewicz commonly arises. Maintaining blood flow to these levels during the proximal anastomosis provides a measure of protection against spinal cord ischemia. If the aortic segment between the 2 clamps remains pressurized, the proximal clamp may not have been applied completely. In such cases, it may be necessary to readjust the proximal clamp or place a second clamp to achieve proper proximal control.

After the aorta is clamped, the LHB flow is gradually increased to 3.5 L/min to maintain the patient's mean arterial pressure (MAP) around 70–90 mmHg, as measured from the right radial or right brachial artery. The aortic segment between the 2 clamps is opened longitudinally with electrocautery (Fig. 14.6), and the edges are retracted laterally with 0 silk stay sutures.

In cases involving aortic dissection, the dissecting membrane is excised. To manage small, briskly back-bleeding intercostal arteries, 2-0 silk sutures are placed in a figure-of-eight fashion. This technique improves visualization, minimizes overall blood loss, and reduces the risk of shunting blood away from critical spinal circulation. The aorta is transected just distal to the proximal clamp, leaving a cuff of approximately 2–3 cm in the length of the proximal descending thoracic aorta. With electrocautery, the aorta is carefully dissected free from the posterior aspect of the esophagus.

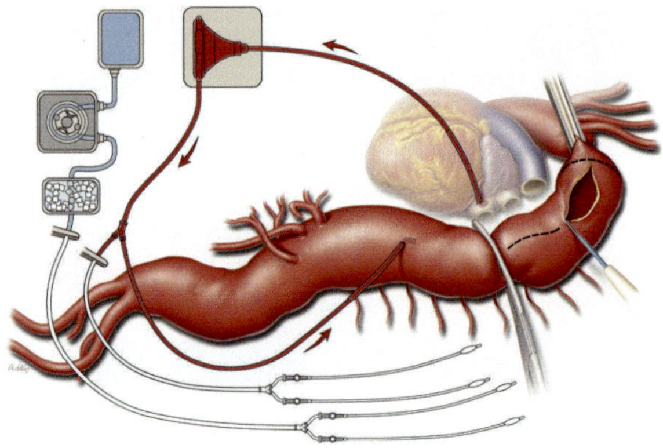

Fig. 14.6 Left heart bypass, placement of aortic clamps, and opening of the proximal aorta with electrocautery

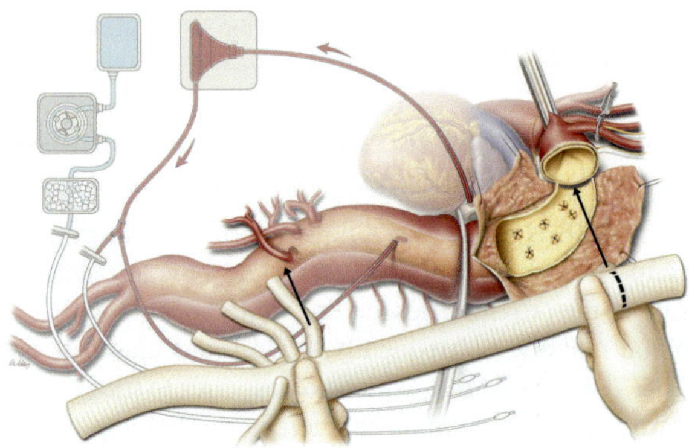

Fig. 14.7 Sizing of a branched aortic graft with respect to the visceral and renal branches

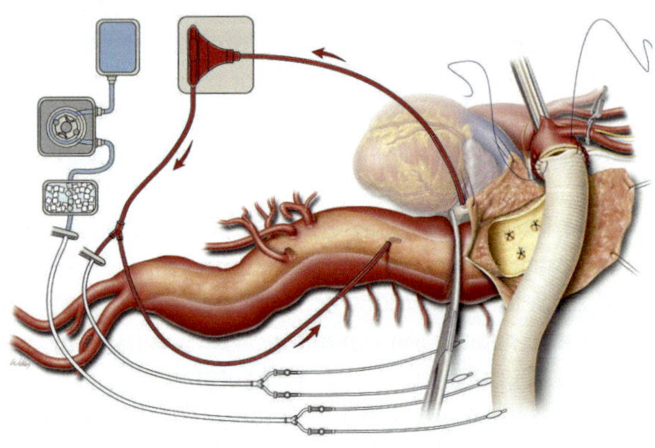

Fig. 14.8 Construction of the proximal anastomosis. Left heart bypass is used

To replace the excised segment of aorta, a gelatin-impregnated Dacron graft of an appropriate size is selected. Typically, a 24- to 28-mm rifampin-soaked Dacron graft is chosen; these grafts are available in both straight and 4-branched configurations. After the graft is sized, the desired length is determined by measuring the distance from the proximal anastomosis to the visceral branches. The surgeon trims the graft to this length by gently stretching the graft and cutting it accordingly (Fig. 14.7).

An end-to-end anastomosis is performed between the graft and the cuff of the proximal descending thoracic aorta with continuous 3-0 polypropylene suture (Fig. 14.8). However, in patients with heritable thoracic aortic disorders, a 4-0 or

5-0 suture may be used. Once the primary suture line is completed, the graft is cautiously retracted and thoroughly inspected for any gaps, overlapping sutures, or tears in the aorta. Pledgeted mattress sutures are liberally applied to ensure that the anastomosis will be secure, even under the higher MAPs that are desirable during the postoperative period. Subsequently, the proximal cross-clamp is moved onto the graft, completing this step of the procedure.

Renal and Visceral Protection

Once the proximal anastomosis is completed, LHB is gradually weaned and discontinued. The distal aortic clamp is removed, and the thoracoabdominal aorta is opened longitudinally with electrocautery until the aortic bifurcation is reached (Fig. 14.9). Shed blood is collected and processed by a cell-saver system, allowing rapid autotransfusion back into the patient.

Attention is then directed toward preparing the distal aortic segment. Any significant pieces of thrombus are removed, and in cases of chronic dissection, the dissecting membrane is excised (Fig. 14.10). The focus now shifts to protecting the abdominal organs. Isothermic blood from the LHB outflow line is used to perfuse the celiac artery and SMA, ensuring their preservation. Additionally, cold crystalloid perfusion is delivered to the left and right renal arteries via four 9-French Pruitt catheters (Fig. 14.11). Cold renal perfusate is delivered into the renal arteries approximately every 6 min at a rate of 300 mL/min for 1–2 min. The perfusion rate is adjusted if the patient becomes excessively cool. Nasopharyngeal temperature is closely monitored to prevent hypothermia-induced arrhythmias.

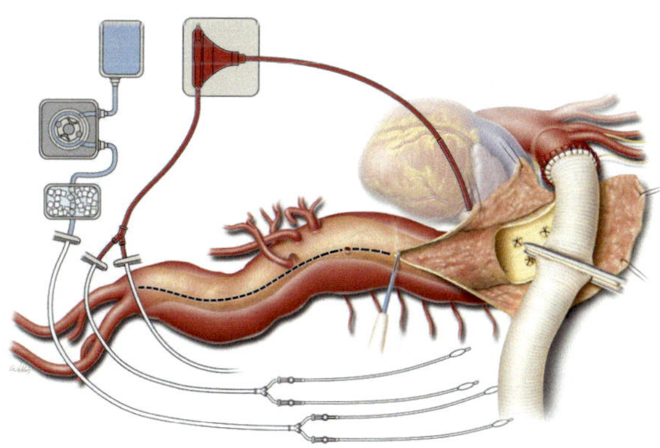

Fig. 14.9 Extension of the aortic incision after the aortic cross-clamp is moved down onto the graft

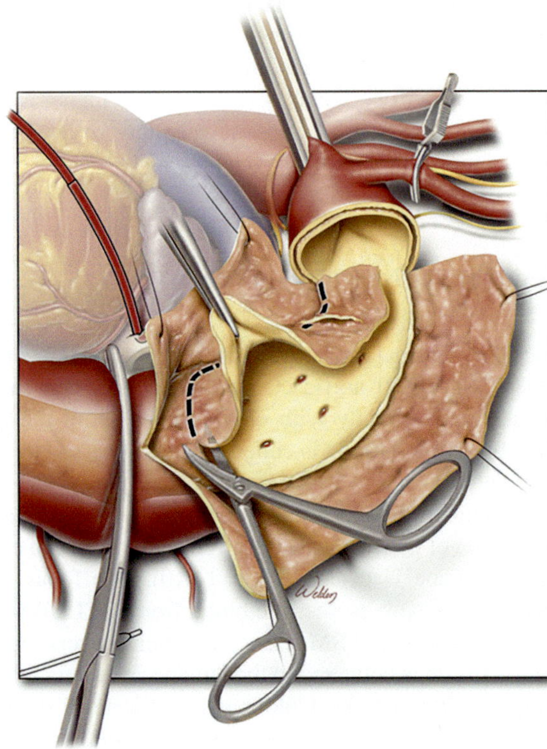

Fig. 14.10 In repairs involving chronic aortic dissection, the dividing septum is removed

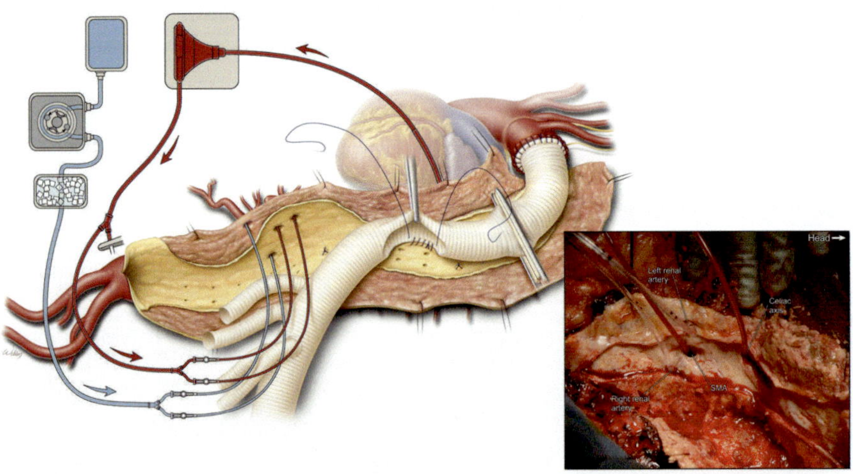

Fig. 14.11 Drawing and intraoperative photograph showing the initiation of visceral perfusion and the intercostal patch anastomosis. Isothermic blood is used to perfuse the celiac axis and the superior mesenteric artery (SMA); cold renal solution is used to perfuse the renal arteries

Reimplantation of Intercostal or Lumbar Arteries

In the reattachment of intercostal arteries, a set of suitable large intercostal arteries between T7 and T12 is typically chosen. The goal is to select arteries with minimal or no back-bleeding. To prevent a steal phenomenon in which blood is diverted away from the spinal cord, vigorously back-bleeding intercostal and lumbar arteries are suture-ligated in a figure-of-eight fashion with 2-0 silk sutures. If the decision whether to reattach a given artery has not yet been made, a small Fogarty catheter can be inserted into the ostium to prevent bleeding and shunting.

Whenever possible, the selected intercostal arteries are attached as an island patch. If the lumbar arteries are separate or if a particular intercostal artery persistently back-bleeds after the release of the proximal clamp, an 8-mm interposition graft is used. Once the reattachment of the intercostal arteries is completed, the proximal clamp is reapplied just distal to the intercostal patch anastomosis. This allows adequate perfusion of the spinal cord during the remainder of the procedure.

Visceral Patch Reimplantation Versus Four-Branched Graft Anastomosis

In older patients with chronic dissection, when the celiac axis, SMA, and renal arteries are in close proximity, it is often feasible to reattach all 4 arteries with a single patch. This patch allows the simultaneous reattachment of these arteries to ensure adequate blood flow to the respective organs. Additionally, the left renal artery is frequently anastomosed to the aortic graft after the construction of the distal anastomosis. This can be done either directly or by using an 8-mm graft.

After these anastomoses are completed, the clamp is moved distally to the visceral patch. This repositioning allows the establishment of perfusion to the visceral segments, ensuring optimal blood supply to these vital areas. The distal aorta is then prepared for an end-to-end anastomosis.

Conversely, in younger patients, especially those with heritable aortopathy or whose arterial origins are significantly displaced, we use a graft with 4 branches to reattach each artery separately. This approach is designed to prevent the development of subsequent visceral patch aneurysms. Typically, we perform the distal aortic anastomosis before reattaching the visceral branches, which ensures continuous perfusion to the branches throughout the construction process (Fig. 14.12).

The graft is carefully cut and trimmed to the appropriate length and then sutured to the aortic bifurcation or iliac vessels, with the aim of preserving blood flow to at least 1 of the hypogastric arteries. This approach effectively restores blood flow to the lower body and provides collateral perfusion to the spinal cord via the internal iliac arteries. Subsequently, each of the graft branches is trimmed to the required length and anastomosed end-to-end to its corresponding artery.

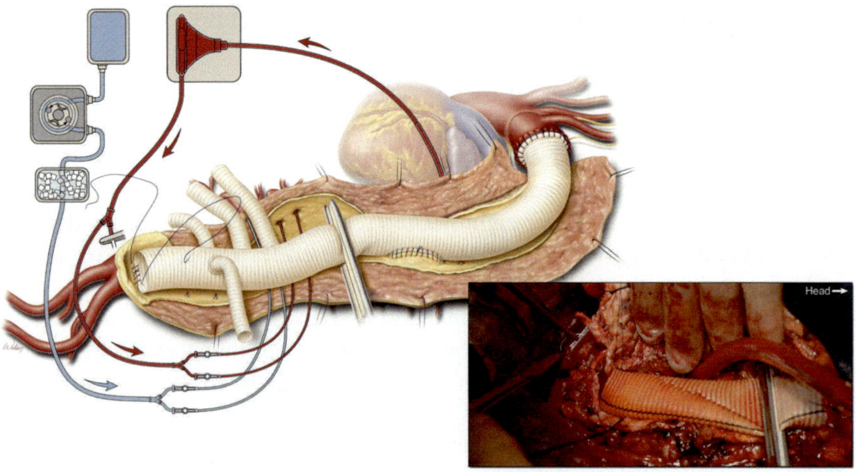

Fig. 14.12 Drawing and intraoperative photograph showing the distal anastomosis being performed. When a 4-branched graft is used, the distal anastomosis is typically performed before the visceral arteries are reattached. Visceral perfusion is continued

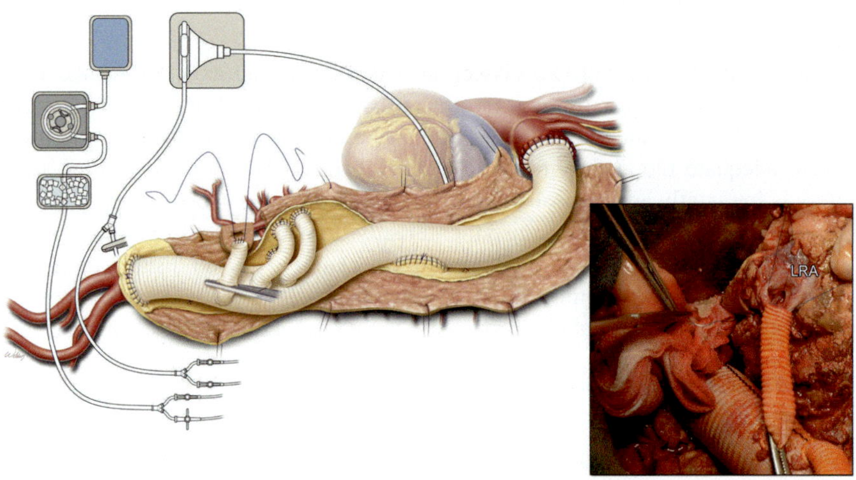

Fig. 14.13 (**a**) Drawing of a left renal artery (LRA) anastomosis with a 4-branched aortic graft. (**b**) Intraoperative photograph of the branch being anastomosed to the LRA

Typically, we begin by reattaching the right renal artery to the right-sided 8-mm branch of the graft. Next, we complete the anastomoses of the SMA and celiac axis to the 10-mm branches. During the celiac axis anastomosis, the SMA graft anastomosis remains clamped to prevent back-bleeding and ensure optimal visualization. Finally, we perform the anastomosis of the left renal artery to the remaining 8-mm graft branch (Fig. 14.13). In certain cases, such as when there are bilateral hypogastric artery occlusions, previous colectomy, or a diseased SMA, we also implant the inferior mesenteric artery.

Distal Aortic Anastomosis

The location of the distal anastomosis is determined by the extent of aneurysmal dilation in the distal aorta and the involvement of the iliac and femoral vessels. If the proximal aorta is of sufficient quality and size, an end-to-end anastomosis is created at that level. However, if the vessels beyond the bifurcation are affected, we perform an end-to-end anastomosis to a bifurcated abdominal aortic graft with 4-0 polypropylene sutures. Each of this graft's 2 limbs is connected to the left or right common iliac, external iliac, or common femoral artery, depending on which one is most proximal and is of adequate quality and size. Whenever possible, blood flow into the internal iliac arteries is preserved. Of note, one advantage of using a multi-branched graft is the flexibility it provides the operator in performing the distal aortic anastomosis before reattaching the 4 visceral branches. This sequencing allows efficient and controlled construction of the distal anastomosis, followed by the reattachment of the visceral branches.

Closure

Once the aortic replacement is completed, intravenous protamine and indigo carmine are administered to reverse the effects of heparin and assess renal perfusion, respectively. Each anastomosis is carefully inspected for any signs of bleeding and repaired as necessary; reinforcing sutures with felt strips or pledgets are used to ensure secure hemostasis. The left atrial cannula is removed, and the venotomy is repaired. The surgical field is irrigated with warm water, and blood products are administered as needed to optimize the patient's hemodynamic status.

During the period between warming and achieving hemostasis, we take the opportunity to perform cryoablation of the intercostal nerves both above and below the thoracotomy incision. This is achieved with a cryoablation probe (AtriCure, Inc., Mason, OH, USA) set to a temperature of −60 °C for a duration of 2 min. We have found that this approach contributes to effective pain management and reduces reliance on narcotic medications in the postoperative period [17]. However, we exercise caution and avoid ablating below the T10 intercostal nerve to preserve sensation in a significant area of the abdominal wall.

After confirming satisfactory perfusion to the abdominal organs and the iliac and femoral arteries, we carefully assess the spleen to ensure there are no capsular tears or subcapsular hematomas. To facilitate drainage, a 19-French closed-suction abdominal drain is placed in the upper left retroperitoneal space. The diaphragm is reapproximated with a continuous #1 polypropylene suture. To facilitate postoperative chest drainage, 2 straight 36-French chest tubes are positioned in anteroapical and posterobasal locations within the left chest cavity. The chest is closed with pericostal sutures and 2 surgical-steel wires. The abdominal fascia, serratus anterior, and latissimus dorsi are each closed separately with continuous #1 polypropylene sutures.

Postoperative Management

In our current postoperative strategy [18], upon arrival in the intensive care unit (ICU), detailed handoff documentation is provided to the nursing and ICU teams to ensure a smooth transition of care and minimize complications related to spinal cord deficit, acute kidney injury, and respiratory failure. Vital signs are closely monitored, with specific attention to core temperature, MAP, central venous pressure, pulmonary arterial pressures, and cardiac output. Patients are kept intubated overnight, and their neurological status is assessed hourly.

The CSF pressure should be kept within the range of 15–20 mmHg. CSF drainage is managed carefully, with a maximum rate of 10 mL/h and a limit of 25 mL over a 4-h period. Exceeding these limits can lead to intracranial hemorrhage or herniation. If there are no complications related to the spinal cord, the CSF drain can be removed 24–48 h postoperatively. If symptoms of spinal cord deficit appear, the target CSF pressure is lowered to 10 mmHg, the goal MAP is increased to 90–110 mmHg, and the target hemoglobin level is raised to above 10 g/dL. Intravenous mannitol (12.5 g/L) and dexamethasone (10 mg/L) are administered every 12 h for 24–48 h. If the CSF drain was removed before the onset of paraparesis or paraplegia, it should be quickly reinserted by the anesthesia team.

Once the patient is extubated, the recovery pathway focuses on early mobilization, physical therapy, and the use of an incentive spirometer to encourage deep breathing and prevent respiratory complications. The introduction of a solid diet is gradual, typically starting around the fourth day after surgery, accompanied by the use of stool softeners and laxatives to promote regular bowel movements.

If the patient has normal renal function, a computed tomography scan with intravenous contrast of the chest, abdomen, and pelvis is requested to establish baseline measurements. This helps in monitoring the patient's progress and detecting any potential complications.

During the early postoperative period, the systolic blood pressure is kept elevated, usually between 140 and 150 mmHg, to prevent late neurological complications, such as delayed paraplegia. After 4–6 weeks, the patient's medication is adjusted to maintain a normal systolic blood pressure below 120 mmHg. In ideal circumstances, patients can be discharged from the hospital within 7–10 days after surgery, provided their recovery is progressing well and there are no significant complications.

Conclusion

Open repair is considered the gold-standard treatment for TAAA because of its established durability. However, it is important to recognize that open repair is a highly invasive procedure and carries inherent risks related to aortic clamping, which can lead to ischemia-related complications. These risks can result in major morbidity and mortality for patients undergoing the procedure [19, 20].

Additionally, patients who have undergone open repair for TAAA require lifelong imaging surveillance. This is necessary because the distal aorta, even after repair, can continue to expand. Residual aortic dissection is also common after repair, and in some cases, it may require further intervention or repair.

Thoracic aortic surgery represents a challenging undertaking, and our approach to these procedures has undergone continuous evolution over the past three decades. The contribution of translational and clinical studies to our understanding of the pathophysiology of organ ischemia cannot be overstated, having significant implications specifically for thoracic aortic surgery. The advancement of cannulation methods, neurologic protection strategies, and repair-specific protective adjuncts has played a pivotal role in modernizing and improving the feasibility of aortic procedures. Concurrently, increased awareness surrounding meticulous preoperative and postoperative management has further enhanced outcomes. Without a doubt, the linchpin for achieving favorable results in patients with thoracic aortic aneurysm and dissection lies in the effective communication and seamless collaboration of a proficient surgical team.

References

1. Crawford ES, Crawford JL, Safi HJ, et al. Thoracoabdominal aortic aneurysms: preoperative and intraoperative factors determining immediate and long-term results of operations in 605 patients. J Vasc Surg. 1986;3:389–404.
2. Coselli JS, LeMaire SA, Preventza O, et al. Outcomes of 3309 thoracoabdominal aortic aneurysm repairs. J Thorac Cardiovasc Surg. 2016;151:1323–37.
3. Cekmecelioglu D, Orozco-Sevilla V, Coselli JS. Open vs. endovascular thoracoabdominal aortic aneurysm repair: tale of the tape. Asian Cardiovasc Thorac Ann. 2021;29:643–53.
4. Kuzniar MK, Wanhainen A, Tegler G, et al. Endovascular treatment of chronic aortic dissection with fenestrated and branched stent grafts. J Vasc Surg. 2021;73:1573–1582.e1.
5. Isselbacher EM, Preventza O, Hamilton Black J 3rd, et al. 2022 ACC/AHA guideline for the diagnosis and management of aortic disease: a report of the American Heart Association/American College of Cardiology Joint Committee on Clinical Practice Guidelines. Circulation. 2022;146:e334–482.
6. Riambau V, Bockler D, Brunkwall J, et al. Editor's choice—management of descending thoracic aorta diseases: clinical practice guidelines of the European Society for Vascular Surgery (ESVS). Eur J Vasc Endovasc Surg. 2017;53:4–52.
7. Chatterjee S, Casar JG, LeMaire SA, et al. Perioperative care after thoracoabdominal aortic aneurysm repair: the Baylor College of Medicine experience. Part 1: preoperative considerations. J Thorac Cardiovasc Surg. 2021;161:693–8.

8. Coselli JS, de la Cruz KI, Preventza O, et al. Extent II thoracoabdominal aortic aneurysm repair: how I do it. Semin Thorac Cardiovasc Surg. 2016;28:221–37.
9. Coselli JS, LeMaire SA. Left heart bypass reduces paraplegia rates after thoracoabdominal aortic aneurysm repair. Ann Thorac Surg. 1999;67:1931–4; discussion 1953–1958.
10. Koksoy C, LeMaire SA, Curling PE, et al. Renal perfusion during thoracoabdominal aortic operations: cold crystalloid is superior to normothermic blood. Ann Thorac Surg. 2002;73:730–8.
11. LeMaire SA, Jones MM, Conklin LD, et al. Randomized comparison of cold blood and cold crystalloid renal perfusion for renal protection during thoracoabdominal aortic aneurysm repair. J Vasc Surg. 2009;49:11–9; discussion 19.
12. Coselli JS, LeMaire SA, Koksoy C, et al. Cerebrospinal fluid drainage reduces paraplegia after thoracoabdominal aortic aneurysm repair: results of a randomized clinical trial. J Vasc Surg. 2002;35:631–9.
13. Youngblood SC, Tolpin DA, LeMaire SA, et al. Complications of cerebrospinal fluid drainage after thoracic aortic surgery: a review of 504 patients over 5 years. J Thorac Cardiovasc Surg. 2013;146:166–71.
14. Chatterjee S, LeMaire SA, Green SY, et al. Is incidental splenectomy during thoracoabdominal aortic aneurysm repair associated with reduced survival? J Thorac Cardiovasc Surg. 2020;160:641–652.e2.
15. Gerbode F, Braimbridge M, Osborn JJ, et al. Traumatic thoracic aneurysms: treatment by resection and grafting with the use of an extracorporeal bypass. Surgery. 1957;42:975–85.
16. Safi HJ, Campbell MP, Miller CC 3rd, et al. Cerebral spinal fluid drainage and distal aortic perfusion decrease the incidence of neurological deficit: the results of 343 descending and thoracoabdominal aortic aneurysm repairs. Eur J Vasc Endovasc Surg. 1997;14:118–24.
17. Clemence J Jr, Malik A, Farhat L, et al. Cryoablation of intercostal nerves decreased narcotic usage after thoracic or thoracoabdominal aortic aneurysm repair. Semin Thorac Cardiovasc Surg. 2020;32:404–12.
18. Chatterjee S, Casar JG, LeMaire SA, et al. Perioperative care after thoracoabdominal aortic aneurysm repair: the Baylor College of Medicine experience. Part 2: postoperative management. J Thorac Cardiovasc Surg. 2021;161:699–705.
19. Çekmecelioğlu D, Kibler K, Orozco-Sevilla V, et al. Chapter 24—cardiopulmonary bypass in thoracic aortic surgery. In: Kırali K, Coselli JS, Kalangos A, editors. Cardiopulmonary bypass. Academic; 2023. p. 395–419.
20. Preventza O, Price MD, Amarasekara HS, et al. Chronic type I and type III aortic dissections: a propensity analysis of outcomes after open distal repair. Eur J Cardiothorac Surg. 2018;54:510–6.

Chapter 15
Endovascular Repair of Thoracic Aortic Aneurysms

Farhang Yazdchi and Shinichi Fukuhara

Descending thoracic aortic aneurysms (DTAAs) with maximum diameter of greater than 6 cm is associated with rupture-associated complications. Aneurysm repair is recommended at 5.5 cm in normal-risk patients and higher diameters if the patient is medically or anatomically at higher risk [1]. The Society of Vascular Surgery guidelines recommend Thoracic Endovascular Aortic Repair (TEVAR) as the preferred approach to DTAAs when anatomy is suitable. Although there is no clinical trial to compare endovascular repair with open surgical repair, endovascular technique has significantly lower morbidity, mortality, and hospital length of stay. Current indications for TEVAR include thoracic aortic aneurysm, traumatic aortic transection, type B aortic dissection, penetrating aortic ulcer [2], intramural hematoma, and thoracoabdominal aortic aneurysm. Unfavorable anatomy such as inadequate proximal and distal landing zone distances or extreme dilations at these sites, aortic tortuosity, or small or diseased iliofemoral vessels are contraindications to TEVAR. Patients with connective tissue disorders initially were not felt to be candidates for TEVAR, but there has been significant worldwide experience in these patients and TEVAR is now considered a reliable option.

The first commercially available endograft, the GORE TAG device, was released in 2005. There are currently 4 commercially available device platforms in the United States as of 2024 (Table 15.1) [1].

F. Yazdchi · S. Fukuhara (✉)
Department of Cardiac Surgery, University of Michigan, Ann Arbor, MI, USA
e-mail: farhangy@med.umich.edu; fukuhara@med.umich.edu

G. J. Arnaoutakis et al. (eds.), *Aortic Aneurysms*, Contemporary Cardiology,
https://doi.org/10.1007/978-3-032-13134-8_15

Table 15.1 Instructions for use of current thoracic devices

Manufacturer	Name	Delivery system diameter, Fr	Intended landing zone aortic diameter, mm	Sheath requirement for delivery	Graft material
W. L. Gore & Associates	Conformable Thoracic Aortic Graft with Active Control System	18–24 (ID) (20.1–26.4 [OD] sheath compatibility)	16–42	Yes	ePTFE
Medtronic	Valiant Captivia	22–25 (OD)	18–42	No	Woven polyester
Cook Medical	Zenith Alpha Thoracic	18–23.1 (OD)	20–42	No	Woven polyester
Terumo Aortic	Relay Pro	19–22 (OD)	20–42	No	Woven polyester

ID inner diameter, *OD* outer diameter, *ePTFE* expanded polytetrafluoroethylene

Preoperative and Intraoperative Imaging

Preoperative measurements and planning are critical for the correct sizing of thoracic endografts and success of the operation. Computed tomography angiography (CTA) with three-dimensional reformatting uploaded in desired application software with capability of adjusted centerline measurements is used to obtain information about the seal zones, coverage length, tortuosity, angulation, and potential wall calcification of the aorta. Magnetic resonance angiography (MRA) can be used for preoperative planning for patients with severe allergy to iodinated contrast material or marginal renal function without dialysis. Intravascular ultrasound (IVUS) has become an important adjunct in the aortic endovascular treatment. IVUS allows for real-time intraoperative measurement of distances and diameters during systole, identification of origins of arch and visceral vessels, and identification of true and false lumen in case of dissection [3]. It also helps to minimize use of contrast and radiation during the procedure.

Arterial Access

Endovascular repair of thoracic aneurysm was originally performed through open femoral access because of large device diameters. However, there are now closure devices that permit a percutaneous approach with minimal morbidity and mortality with excellent success rate if femoral arteries have suitable size and anatomy without previous interventions or significant calcifications [4]. In patients in which femoral and iliac artery sizes or disease precludes the introduction of a stentgraft delivery system, options such as angioplasty and use of dilators, direct common iliac and infrarenal aortic access with primary closure, and creation of iliac conduit by retroperitoneal exposure can be used as the delivery route. Endovascular option includes placing adequate size stent grafts inside the small or diseased iliac vessel and intentional rupture of the vessel to expand it to the needed diameter for graft introduction (internal endoconduit). However, the frequency of difficulty device delivery has come down significantly with the newer generation lower profile endografts.

Thoracic Endovascular Aortic Repair Adjuncts

For most devices, a landing zone of 2–3 cm is adequate to establish seal and prevent occurrence of endoleak. Apposition of the TEVAR device against the aortic wall can be challenging where there is angulation, typically in zones 2 and 3. The landing zone should be determined based on the length of the seal along the inner curve. If there is not enough landing zone in this area, multiple adjunctive procedures can be considered to create an adequate landing zone.

Proximal Debranching

Greater than 40% of patients requiring TEVAR may need left subclavian coverage to obtain adequate proximal landing in zone 2 aortic arch [5]. In emergencies, such as aortic ruptures, the left subclavian artery can be covered without revascularization. However, the risk of combined stroke, paraplegia, and death is reported up to 28% [6]. Perioperative left subclavian artery revascularization, either left carotid-subclavian bypass or subclavian-carotid transposition, can be performed when the left subclavian artery is covered by the stent graft (Fig. 15.1) [7]. Society

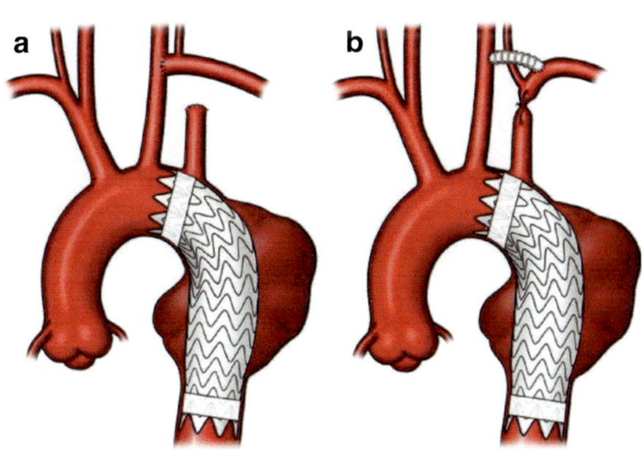

Fig. 15.1 Options for left subclavian artery revascularization. (**a**) Transposition of the left subclavian artery to the left common carotid artery. (**b**) Bypass of the left common carotid artery to the left subclavian artery

of Vascular Surgery (SVS) guidelines suggest routine revascularization in elective repairs and expectant individualized revascularization in emergent repairs. There are situations that left subclavian artery and/or left vertebral artery revascularization is necessary such as presence of patent left internal mammary artery bypass graft, dominant left vertebral artery, left vertebral artery with terminal posterior inferior cerebellar artery without basilar connection, aortic arch origin of dominant left vertebral artery, hypoplastic or stenotic right vertebral artery, and left arm arteriovenous fistula in dialysis patients unless needs to be compromised in emergent cases. If the graft needs to land in zone 1, then right-to-left carotid-carotid bypass or right-to-left axillo-axillary artery bypass in combination with a left carotid-subclavian bypass or subclavian transposition can be performed (Fig. 15.2) [7, 8]. Alternatively, hybrid procedures such as debranching of innominate and left common carotid can be performed through a sternotomy with a side biting clamp without the need for cardiopulmonary bypass along with left subclavian artery revascularization via supraclavicular approach followed by TEVAR and subclavian artery embolization for aneurysm exclusion (Fig. 15.3) [8]. Extraanatomical left axillary artery to ascending aortic graft using an interposition Dacron graft, and ligation of the left subclavian artery stump is another approach to debranch the left subclavian artery.

The hybrid approach to aortic arch aneurysms or other pathologies such as dissection and penetrating ulcers can safely be done. This entails open great vessel debranching with interval TEVAR for stenting the aortic arch. Tackling the arch pathologies has been classified into types I to III hybrid arch repair (Fig. 15.4) [9].

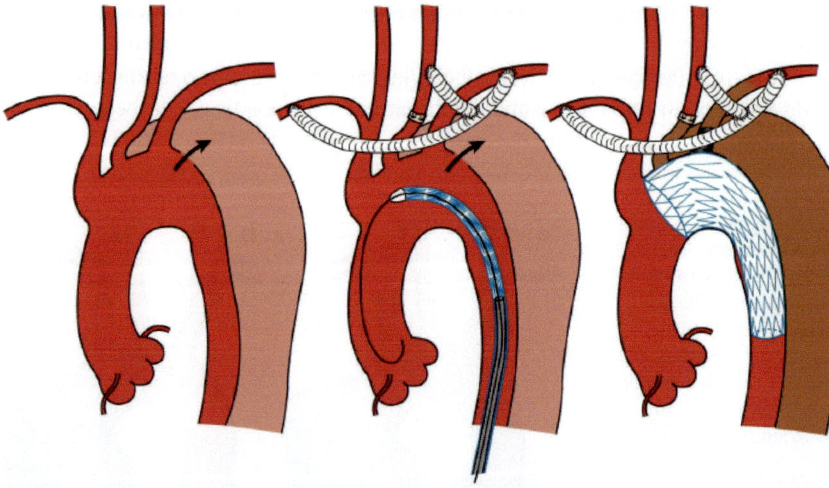

Fig. 15.2 Diagram illustrating aortic repair in three stages. The left panel shows a normal aorta with an arrow indicating the site of intervention. The middle panel depicts a catheter being inserted into the aorta with cervical debranching. The right panel shows a stent graft placed within the aorta, with a synthetic graft attached to the surrounding vessels. The sequence demonstrates the process of endovascular aortic repair with zone 1 deployment

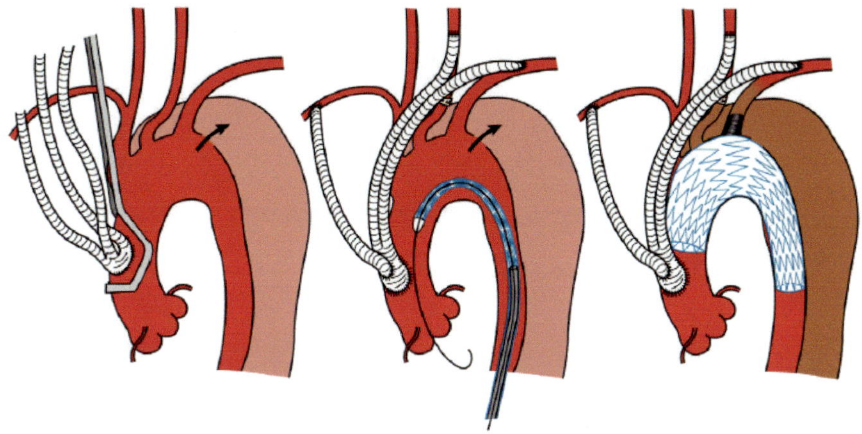

Fig. 15.3 Diagram illustrating aortic surgical procedures in three panels. The left panel shows aortic debranching with bypass originating off ascending aorta. The middle panel depicts a catheter being introduced through the aorta. The right panel displays a stent graft deployed within the aorta, with zone 0 deployment. Arrows indicate site of dissection entry tear

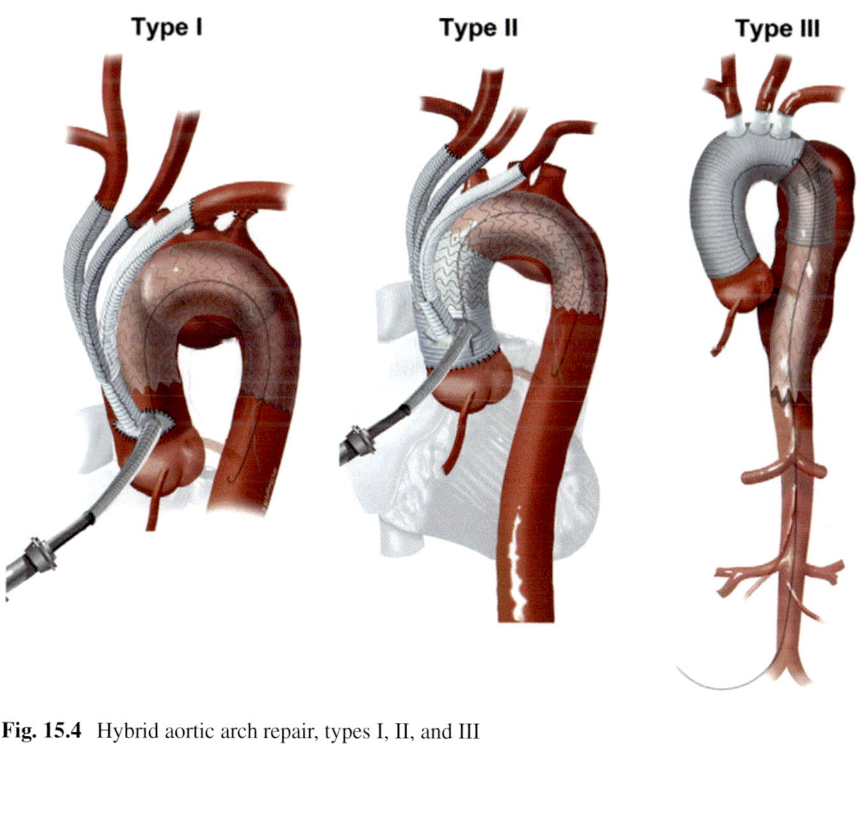

Fig. 15.4 Hybrid aortic arch repair, types I, II, and III

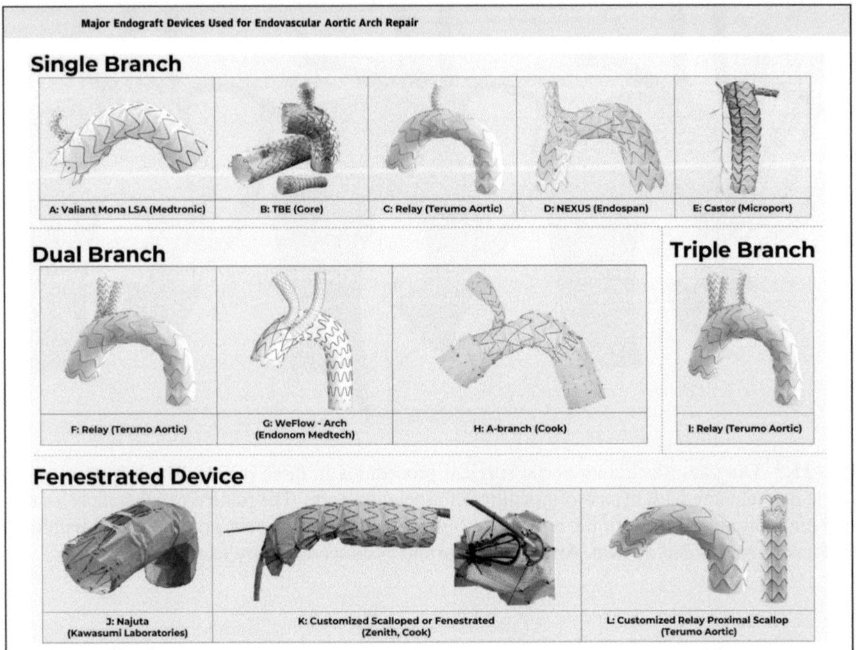

A to I illustrate branched arch endografts ranging from single to triple branch. **J to L** illustrate fenestrated arch endografts. **A, B, D, H, and J** are reproduced with permission from Hauck SR, Kern M, Dachs TM, et al. Applicability of endovascular branched and fenestrated aortic arch repair devices to treat residual type A dissection after ascending replacement. *J Vasc Surg*. 2022;76:1440-1448. (Creative Commons Attribution License). **C, F, I, and L** are courtesy of Terumo Aortic. **E and K** are reprinted with permission from Jing et al[13] and Tsilimparis et al.[25]

Fig. 15.5 Branched endovascular devices

With advancement in technology, branched arch endograft, and fenestrated arch and descending aorta endograft devices are under development and investigational phase at this time [10–13] (Fig. 15.4) except for the first commercially available branched endograft, the GORE Thoracic Branch Endoprosthesis (TBE) device for zone 2 landing with favorable midterm results [12, 14]. Discussion of the detailed procedural steps of deployment of these devices is beyond the scope of this chapter (Fig. 15.5).

Distal Debranching

Coverage of the celiac artery can add up to 2.5 cm of additional distal seal and can be necessary in about 4–6% of the cases. Complications such as bowel and gall bladder ischemia, paraplegia, and death are more common in those who do not undergo celiac artery revascularization [15]. Distal debranching of the celiac artery can be performed through multiple techniques including hepatorenal bypass, splenorenal bypass, and retrograde ilio-celiac bypass.

Procedural Detail

The procedure is performed in hybrid operating room in supine position and under general anesthesia to be able to control respiration and provide more precise imaging. The decision to place the lumbar drain depends on each patient's anatomy, length of coverage, or surgeon's preference. If a percutaneous approach is chosen, ultrasound-guided femoral arterial access is obtained using micropuncture technique under fluoroscopy with Perclose Proglide (Abbott Vascular, CA, USA) suture-mediated closure technique in preclose fashion over a guide wire. Surgical groin cutdown and direct arterial access is another approach. Occasionally retroperitoneal cutdown to access iliac artery directly is necessary because of small or diseased femoral arteries. Additional femoral or arm access is obtained for pigtail placement and angiography. Alternatively, an appropriate size DrySeal Flex Introducer Sheath (W. L. Gore & Associates, Flagstaff, AZ, USA) can be used only on one side for both purposes of device delivery and angiography. C-arm is positioned in left anterior oblique position to splay out the aortic arch. The wire is exchanged for an Extra-Stiff Lunderquist (Cook medical, Bloomington, IN) wire passed into the arch to allow tracking of the device. The patient is heparinized to achieve the goal activated clotting time (ACT). Then the appropriate size graft based on preoperative planning and/or intraoperative IVUS is introduced through the sheath and deployed in stages once the desired position is confirmed. Post-implantation ballooning (not in acute dissections, or traumatic aortic injury) at the seal zones and at any overlap zones may be necessary to ensure full stent-graft sealing to the aortic wall or eliminating a bird beak, kink, or infoldings. Ballooning at landing zones should be avoided in acute aortic dissection cases where there is a significant risk of creating stent-induced new entry tear or causing aortic rupture. If two different size grafts are planned for the operation, the smaller diameter graft is deployed first with larger diameter graft deployed inside the smaller one with appropriate overlap distance. Completion angiography with or without IVUS is then performed to assess for exclusion of the aortic lesion, endoleak, inadvertent branch vessel occlusions, and newly created aortic dissection. The device delivery system and catheters are removed, and the arteriotomy is closed.

Parallel Stenting and In-Situ Endograft Fenestration/Stenting

Other than the surgical revascularization methods described above, alternative revascularization methods for the left subclavian artery and celiac artery, including parallel stenting (chimney, periscope, snorkel stenting) and in-situ fenestration of standard endograft and branch stenting, may be considered in carefully selected patients. Although these options are relatively simple and reproducible methods of revascularization, these are still unproven strategies, particularly the endograft fenestration that entails endograft modification. Therefore, these procedures are considered only in special circumstances such as urgent setting and not currently approved by the Food and Drug Administration (FDA).

Complications

Stroke The incidence of stroke after TEVAR is reported between 2.8% and 8.2% in different series [16–20]. Eighty-nine percent of strokes occurred within 24 h of operation in a Penn series with 33% in-hospital mortality rate. Risk factors are the extent of arch involvement, severity of atherosclerosis, presence of mobile atheromatous disease, coverage of proximal descending thoracic aorta or entire descending thoracic aorta, prior stroke, coverage of the left subclavian artery especially without revascularization, more proximal landing zone (zone 0 > 1 > 2), and severe aortic tortuosity. The mechanisms of stroke include embolism of atheromatous material, thrombus, or air embolism, and cerebral hypoperfusion. However, optimum preventive strategies have not been established yet.

Paraplegia The incidence is lower with TEVAR compared with open repair and ranges from 1% to 4% [21]. Paraplegia is a devastating complication with only 38% of patients who experience it returning to their normal baseline function [22] and 1-year mortality of 70% for those with no functional improvement [23]. Measures such as maintaining patency of left subclavian artery, staging repairs for long segment (>20 cm) aortic coverage, prophylactic cerebrospinal fluid drainage, permissive hypertension, steroid, and Naloxone therapy can mitigate the risk of paraplegia [24–26]. Some centers use cerebrospinal fluid drainage routinely and others only in high-risk patients or do not use it [1].

Other complications of endovascular aortic repair include visceral ischemia [27], device migration, access site complications, and endoleaks [28–30]. Endoleaks are reviewed in detail elsewhere, however type I endoleaks are classified as leaks at the proximal or distal stent attachment sites with early filling of the aneurysm sac. If an endoleak is associated with junctional separation of two stent-graft devices, it is a type III endoleak (Fig. 15.6). Prompt treatment is necessary for Type I and III endoleaks. Type II endoleaks are not communicating with proximal or distal landing zones and are mostly monitored without intervention [31]. Retrograde type A dissection after TEVAR for type B dissection may be more common if TEVAR was performed in acute-early phase, which was defined within 48 h of dissection occurrence [32]. However, its pathogenesis is considered multifactorial such as degree of endograft oversizing, pre-existing ascending aortic dilatation, proximity of landing zones, presence of bare-metal stent, connective tissue disorders, and intraoperative blood pressure management [33].

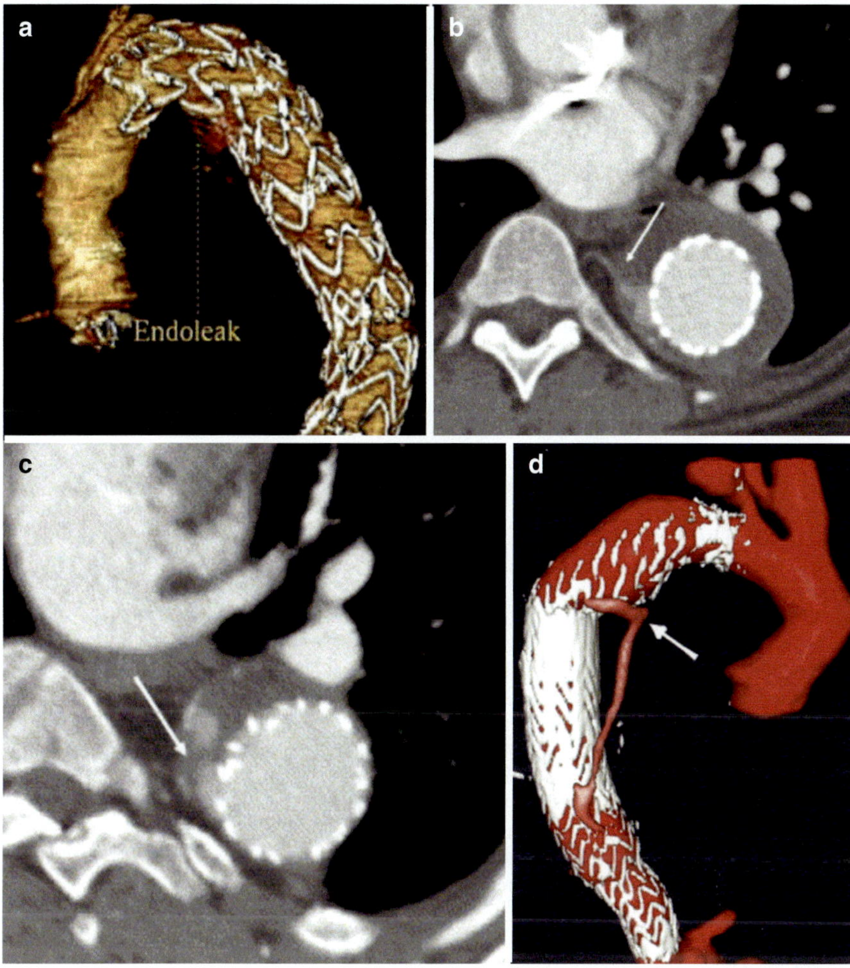

Fig. 15.6 Radiographic appearance of endoleaks. (**a**) Three-dimensional reconstruction of a proximal type I endoleak. (**b**) a type II endoleak filling the aneurysm sac and in communication with an intercostal artery (arrow). (**c**) a type III endoleak between endograft components (arrow) is demonstrated on computed tomographic angiography. (**d**) three-dimensional reconstruction of the type III endoleak depicted in **c**

Surveillance

Most TEVAR patients can be discharged on the first or second postoperative day. Patients will need to be followed with serial imaging for evaluation of complications including aneurysm expansion, stent migration, endoleak, device failure, stenosis, occlusion, and graft infection [1]. Recommendation is CTA at 1 and 12 months after TEVAR and then yearly for life. More aggressive imaging and follow-up may be warranted when detecting an endoleak or if concerned about stability of the repair and potential for complications.

References

1. Upchurch GR Jr, Escobar GA, Azizzadeh A, et al. Society for Vascular Surgery clinical practice guidelines of thoracic endovascular aortic repair for descending thoracic aortic aneurysms. J Vasc Surg. 2021;73:55S–83S.
2. Szeto WY, Vallabhajosyula P, Matsuda H, et al. One-year results with a low-profile endograft in subjects with thoracic aortic aneurysm and ulcer pathologies. J Thorac Cardiovasc Surg. 2022;163:1739–1750.e4.
3. Han SM, Elsayed RS, Ham SW, et al. Comparison of intravascular ultrasound- and centerline computed tomography-determined aortic diameters during thoracic endovascular aortic repair. J Vasc Surg. 2017;66:1184–91.
4. Jaffan AA, Prince EA, Hampson CO, Murphy TP. The preclose technique in percutaneous endovascular aortic repair: a systematic literature review and meta-analysis. Cardiovasc Intervent Radiol. 2013;36:567–77.
5. Matsumura JS, Rizvi AZ. Society for Vascular S. Left subclavian artery revascularization: Society for Vascular Surgery Practice Guidelines. J Vasc Surg. 2010;52:65S–70S.
6. Holt PJ, Johnson C, Hinchliffe RJ, et al. Outcomes of the endovascular management of aortic arch aneurysm: implications for management of the left subclavian artery. J Vasc Surg. 2010;51:1329–38.
7. Riesenman PJ, Farber MA, Mendes RR, Marston WA, Fulton JJ, Keagy BA. Coverage of the left subclavian artery during thoracic endovascular aortic repair. J Vasc Surg. 2007;45:90–4; discussion 94–5.
8. Kuratani T. Best surgical option for arch extension of type B dissection: the endovascular approach. Ann Cardiothorac Surg. 2014;3:292–9.
9. Bavaria J, Vallabhajosyula P, Moeller P, Szeto W, Desai N, Pochettino A. Hybrid approaches in the treatment of aortic arch aneurysms: postoperative and midterm outcomes. J Thorac Cardiovasc Surg. 2013;145:S85–90.
10. Planer D, Elbaz-Greener G, Mangialardi N, et al. NEXUS arch: a multicenter study evaluating the initial experience with a novel aortic arch stent graft system. Ann Surg. 2023;277:e460–6.
11. Roselli EE, Arko FR 3rd, Thompson MM, Valiant Mona LSATI. Results of the Valiant Mona LSA early feasibility study for descending thoracic aneurysms. J Vasc Surg. 2015;62:1465–71.e3.
12. Liang NL, Dake MD, Fischbein MP, et al. Midterm outcomes of endovascular repair of aortic arch aneurysms with the gore thoracic branch endoprosthesis. Eur J Vasc Endovasc Surg. 2022;64:639–45.
13. Kitagawa A, Greenberg RK, Eagleton MJ, Mastracci TM, Roselli EE. Fenestrated and branched endovascular aortic repair for chronic type B aortic dissection with thoracoabdominal aneurysms. J Vasc Surg. 2013;58:625–34.
14. Dake MD, Bavaria JE, Singh MJ, et al. Management of arch aneurysms with a single-branch thoracic endograft in zone 0. JTCVS Tech. 2021;7:1–6.
15. Leon LR Jr, Mills JL Sr, Jordan W, et al. The risks of celiac artery coverage during endoluminal repair of thoracic and thoracoabdominal aortic aneurysms. Vasc Endovasc Surg. 2009;43:51–60.
16. Gutsche JT, Cheung AT, McGarvey ML, et al. Risk factors for perioperative stroke after thoracic endovascular aortic repair. Ann Thorac Surg. 2007;84:1195–200; discussion 1200.
17. Melissano G, Tshomba Y, Bertoglio L, Rinaldi E, Chiesa R. Analysis of stroke after TEVAR involving the aortic arch. Eur J Vasc Endovasc Surg. 2012;43:269–75.
18. Leurs LJ, Bell R, Degrieck Y, et al. Endovascular treatment of thoracic aortic diseases: combined experience from the EUROSTAR and United Kingdom Thoracic Endograft registries. J Vasc Surg. 2004;40:670–9; discussion 679–80.

19. Patel HJ, Williams DM, Upchurch GR Jr, et al. Long-term results from a 12-year experience with endovascular therapy for thoracic aortic disease. Ann Thorac Surg. 2006;82:2147–53.
20. Cao L, Zhang H, Ge Y, Guo W. Avoiding stroke in patients undergoing endovascular aortic arch repair: JACC review topic of the week. J Am Coll Cardiol. 2023;82:265–77.
21. Abraha I, Romagnoli C, Montedori A, Cirocchi R. Thoracic stent graft versus surgery for thoracic aneurysm. Cochrane Database Syst Rev. 2016;2016:CD006796.
22. DeSart K, Scali ST, Feezor RJ, et al. Fate of patients with spinal cord ischemia complicating thoracic endovascular aortic repair. J Vasc Surg. 2013;58:635–42.e2.
23. Buth J, Harris PL, Hobo R, et al. Neurologic complications associated with endovascular repair of thoracic aortic pathology: incidence and risk factors. A study from the European Collaborators on Stent/Graft Techniques for Aortic Aneurysm Repair (EUROSTAR) registry. J Vasc Surg. 2007;46:1103–10; discussion 1110–1.
24. Eagleton MJ, Shah S, Petkosevek D, Mastracci TM, Greenberg RK. Hypogastric and subclavian artery patency affects onset and recovery of spinal cord ischemia associated with aortic endografting. J Vasc Surg. 2014;59:89–94.
25. O'Callaghan A, Mastracci TM, Eagleton MJ. Staged endovascular repair of thoracoabdominal aortic aneurysms limits incidence and severity of spinal cord ischemia. J Vasc Surg. 2015;61:347–354.e1.
26. Acher CW, Wynn MM, Hoch JR, Popic P, Archibald J, Turnipseed WD. Combined use of cerebral spinal fluid drainage and naloxone reduces the risk of paraplegia in thoracoabdominal aneurysm repair. J Vasc Surg. 1994;19:236–46; discussion 247–8.
27. Vaddineni SK, Taylor SM, Patterson MA, Jordan WD Jr. Outcome after celiac artery coverage during endovascular thoracic aortic aneurysm repair: preliminary results. J Vasc Surg. 2007;45:467–71.
28. Matsumura JS, Cambria RP, Dake MD, et al. International controlled clinical trial of thoracic endovascular aneurysm repair with the Zenith TX2 endovascular graft: 1-year results. J Vasc Surg. 2008;47:247–57; discussion 257.
29. Bavaria JE, Appoo JJ, Makaroun MS, et al. Endovascular stent grafting versus open surgical repair of descending thoracic aortic aneurysms in low-risk patients: a multicenter comparative trial. J Thorac Cardiovasc Surg. 2007;133:369–77.
30. Makaroun MS, Dillavou ED, Wheatley GH, Cambria RP, Gore TAGI. Five-year results of endovascular treatment with the Gore TAG device compared with open repair of thoracic aortic aneurysms. J Vasc Surg. 2008;47:912–8.
31. Parmer SS, Carpenter JP, Stavropoulos SW, et al. Endoleaks after endovascular repair of thoracic aortic aneurysms. J Vasc Surg. 2006;44:447–52.
32. Desai ND, Gottret JP, Szeto WY, et al. Impact of timing on major complications after thoracic endovascular aortic repair for acute type B aortic dissection. J Thorac Cardiovasc Surg. 2015;149:S151–6.
33. Chen Y, Zhang S, Liu L, Lu Q, Zhang T, Jing Z. Retrograde type A aortic dissection after thoracic endovascular aortic repair: a systematic review and meta-analysis. J Am Heart Assoc. 2017;6(9):e004649.

Chapter 16
Surgical Treatment of Non-ruptured Infrarenal Abdominal Aortic Aneurysms

C. Adam Banks and Adam W. Beck

Definition

Most medical dictionaries define an aneurysm as a dilation of an artery to greater than 50% of the normal caliber [1]. The most common location for arterial aneurysm is in the intracranial circulation, and the most common location of an extracranial aneurysm is the infrarenal abdominal aorta. Although normal aortic diameters vary with age, sex, and body habitus, using the above definition, an average-sized aorta with a dilation greater than 3 cm can be considered aneurysmal. Histologically, an abdominal aortic aneurysm (AAA) is characterized by macrophage degradation of the medial elastin lamellar architecture by metalloproteinases [2–5].

Historical Perspectives

Aneurysms have been recognized for thousands of years. In fact, the Ebers Papyrus in 2000 BC discusses traumatic aneurysms of the peripheral arteries [6]. In the second century AD, Antyllus wrote of the first elective procedure to treat an aneurysm by proximal and distal ligation of the artery feeding the aneurysm, along with opening the sac and evacuation of its contents [7]. Andreas Vesalius, the sixteenth-century Flemish anatomist, was the first to describe an AAA [8]. Antyllus's technique remained the principal treatment method for at least the next fifteen hundred years until Rudolph Matas, in 1923, performed the successful ligation of a ruptured syphilitic infrarenal AAA [9]. Because of the high mortality associated

C. A. Banks · A. W. Beck (✉)
Division of Vascular Surgery and Endovascular Therapy, University of Alabama at Birmingham, Birmingham, AL, USA
e-mail: cabanks@uabmc.edu; awbeck@uabmc.edu

G. J. Arnaoutakis et al. (eds.), *Aortic Aneurysms*, Contemporary Cardiology,
https://doi.org/10.1007/978-3-032-13134-8_16

with aneurysm ligation, surgeons devised other therapies such as inducing thrombosis of the aneurysm with wires, not surprisingly also with poor results [10]. In the early 1940s, surgeons utilized wrapping of the aneurysm with various materials such as fascia lata, skin grafts, polyvinyl sponge, and even cellophane, in an attempt to prevent aneurysmal rupture [11–13]. The results of this method were poor, and the mortality and rupture rate of aneurysms remained quite high. The current technique for AAA repair was conceptually devised in the early twentieth century by the 1912 Nobel laureate Alexis Carrel [14–17]. His method, which he performed only in animals, consisted of replacing a segment of aorta with a segment from another artery or vein. In 1951, Charles DuBost reported use of a retroperitoneal approach to replace the aneurysmal infrarenal aorta with an aortic homograft [18]. In 1953, Michael DeBakey and Denton Cooley reported success using a similar technique [19]. In the same year, Henry Bahnson described the technique described by DuBost to repair a ruptured AAA [20]. The use of homografts was short-lived due to graft degeneration and subsequent graft rupture. The next major breakthrough for AAA repair was the use of arterial prosthetics made of Vinyon-N, which originated in the work of Arthur Voorhees [21]. Blakemore placed the first Vinyon-N graft in a patient with a ruptured AAA [22]. In 1954, Voorhees and Blakemore described their results in 16 patients with AAA repaired using Vinyon-N grafts with a 56% survival [23, 24]. These advances stimulated industry to evaluate and develop arterial conduits. In 1958, Michael DeBakey's group in Houston reported excellent results on a large group of patients undergoing AAA repair with knitted Dacron grafts [25]. Over the next two decades, many series were reported with operative mortalities in the 10–15% range, using polyester grafts.

Prevalence and Incidence

AAA is most common in elderly males, with increasing prevalence after the sixth decade of life. AAA is two to six times more common in men than women, and two to three times more common in White patients compared to the African-American population. The incidence of AAA varies from 3 to 117 per one hundred thousand person-years [26–29]. Lederle et al. [30] reported that 2.6% of screened patients with a normal ultrasound 4 years prior developed an AAA. They also reported an incidence of AAA of 6.5 per thousand person-years. In men, AAAs typically appear after age 50 and reach a peak incidence at age 80. In women, it is usually later, around age 60, with a steady increase after that [31–33]. Although AAAs fail to demonstrate a clear genetic predisposition or transmission pattern, numerous reports suggest that 15–20% of first-order relatives of patients with AAAs will also have an aneurysm [34–36].

Aortic aneurysm rupture is the tenth leading cause of death in elderly males. Most AAAs are found incidentally and only rarely cause symptoms such as abdominal or back pain. In fact, rupture may be the initial form of presentation of AAAs. Treatment of ruptured AAAs is very costly to healthcare systems. A study from

Great Britain found that about 2000 lives and nearly $50 million dollars could be saved if AAAs were repaired prior to rupture [37]. Breckwoldt et al. suggested that emergent interventions for patients with ruptured AAAs led to hospital losses of $24,655 per patient [38]. Another study from the United Kingdom found that the total cost of emergency AAA repair was 96,700 pounds, with a cost per life saved of 24,175 pounds. The total cost of elective AAA repair was 76,583 pounds with a cost per life saved of 5470 pounds. The cost of emergency intervention was found to be fivefold that of elective repair, per life saved, per year [39].

Diagnosis and Risk of Rupture

Since most AAAs are asymptomatic and patients may not present until their AAA has ruptured, targeted screening of high-risk populations is recommended. A study by Schermerhorn et al. showed that ultrasound screening for AAA was cost-effective and beneficial for men 65–74 years of age with known risk factors such as coronary artery disease (CAD), smoking, or a family history of AAA [40]. A report by Derubertis et al. suggested a high incidence of AAA among women older than 65, with a history of smoking or heart disease. Women with such risk factors, therefore, should also be considered for AAA screening [41]. Aneurysm screening programs have been introduced in some countries [42–50]. A large randomized trial in the United Kingdom demonstrated an early mortality benefit of screening ultrasonography for AAA [51]. Since January 2007, Medicare has offered coverage of a one-time ultrasound screening for senior males with a smoking history of at least 100 cigarettes in their lifetime and for individuals with a family history of AAA. In the Multicentre Aneurysm Screening Study, 70,495 men aged 65–74 were randomized to ultrasound screening versus no screening for AAA. Of the 33,839 patients randomized to ultrasound screening, 80% were screened and 5% had AAAs greater than 3 cm. At 4 years, there were 113 AAA-related deaths in the non-screened control group compared with 65 in the screened group. This trial suggested a 32% reduction in AAA-related mortality in the screened group [50]. One randomized control trial investigating the mortality benefit of aortic aneurysm screening in women demonstrated no mortality benefit at 5–10 years [46]. Importantly, women diagnosed with aortic aneurysms have increased risk of rupture at smaller aortic diameters when compared to men [52]. Therefore, the Society for Vascular Surgery currently recommends ultrasound-guided AAA screening in males and females between 65 and 75 years in age with smoking history or family history of AAA [53]. Additionally, the National Institute for Health and Care Excellence (NICE) guidelines recommend screening of all women over 70 years of age who have any risk factors including hypertension, smoking history, family history of AAA, or COPD [54]. Patients who have an AAA 5.5 cm or larger at time of screening should be referred to regional vascular specialist within 2 weeks. Those found to have aortic diameter of 3.0–5.4 cm should be referred within 12 weeks [54].

Currently, AAAs are more commonly found incidentally than on screening studies, when patients are imaged with ultrasound, CT scan, or MRI for other diseases or symptomatology. The Department of Veterans Affairs Aneurysm Detection and Management (ADAM) study was designed to compare long-term AAA survival following either surveillance or surgical treatment when aneurysm reached 5.5 cm versus immediate open surgical repair for managing AAAs less than 5.5 cm. A total of 1136 patients were enrolled and followed for a mean time of 4.8 years. No significant difference was found between the two groups in terms of long-term mortality, and the study concluded that there was no long-term survival advantage by repairing AAA smaller than 5.5 cm. They thus recommended surveillance of small AAAs until they reach a 5.5 cm diameter [55]. The UK Small Aneurysm Trial followed over 1000 patients for 10 years. This study found no long-term survival benefit for early elective open repair of small aneurysm between 4 and 5.4 cm of maximal diameter [56].

These findings were reiterated in patients undergoing EVAR for small AAAs in the Positive Impact of Endovascular Options for Treating Aneurysms Early (PIVOTAL) and the Comparison of Surveillance versus Aortic Endografting for Small Aneurysm Repair (CAESAR) trials. Overall, these trials demonstrated similar survival in patients treated with aneurysms ranging from 4.0 to 5.4 cm when compared to patients undergoing routine surveillance imaging per guidelines [57–59].

The risk of rupture of an AAA is estimated based on its maximal diameter. Aneurysms between 3 and 5 cm have less than 1% per year risk of rupture. A progressive risk of aneurysm rupture occurs with increasing aneurysm diameter. An aneurysm growth rate greater than 0.5 cm in a 6-month period also appears to increase the risk of rupture. Therefore, it is generally accepted that aneurysms less than 5.5 cm can be safely followed with routine surveillance imaging. Given the increased risk of AAA rupture at any size in women when compared to men, repair is indicated at AAA size of ≥5.0 cm.

Most aneurysms, especially smaller ones, tend to grow at a rate of 0.3–0.5 cm per year [60–62]. Therefore, continued surveillance of aortic aneurysms should be performed if index ultrasound screening reveals aortic diameter >2.5 cm with follow-up at 10 years [53]. As AAAs enlarge, surveillance intervals become more frequent due to increased expansion with larger AAA size (Table 16.1). Patients should undergo Duplex Ultrasound imaging at 6-month intervals with AAA between 5.0

Table 16.1 Society for Vascular Surgery Surveillance Imaging Guidelines for Asymptomatic AAA

Aneurysm size	SVS imaging surveillance recommendation
2.5–2.9 cm	10-years from index ultrasound
3.0–3.9 cm	3-year intervals
4.0–4.9 cm	12-month intervals
5.0–5.4 cm	6-month intervals

and 5.5 cm. Meta-regression demonstrating increased AAA expansion with larger AAA diameter is shown in Fig. 16.1.

Original guidelines regarding risk of AAA rupture were obtained from large-scale autopsy studies demonstrating increased proportion of AAA rupture when >5.0 cm. Many studies have explored different avenues to further understand AAA expansion in order to better predict risk of rupture. Fillinger et al. have reported that aortic wall stress is a key predictor of rupture risk for AAA. A mathematical analysis of AAA geometry, known as finite element analysis, has been suggested to be a better way to estimate wall stress and the risk of rupture. Using this model, Fillinger's group looked at three groups of patients: those who presented with a ruptured AAA, those who were symptomatic and required urgent surgery, and those who underwent elective AAA repair. They found that peak wall stress was significantly higher in ruptured AAA and symptomatic groups compared with that of the elective repair group for diameter-matched subjects. They also found that the location of maximal wall stress in their series was not at the site of maximal AAA diameter but rather in the posterolateral location where most ruptures do occur [64, 65]. Some studies

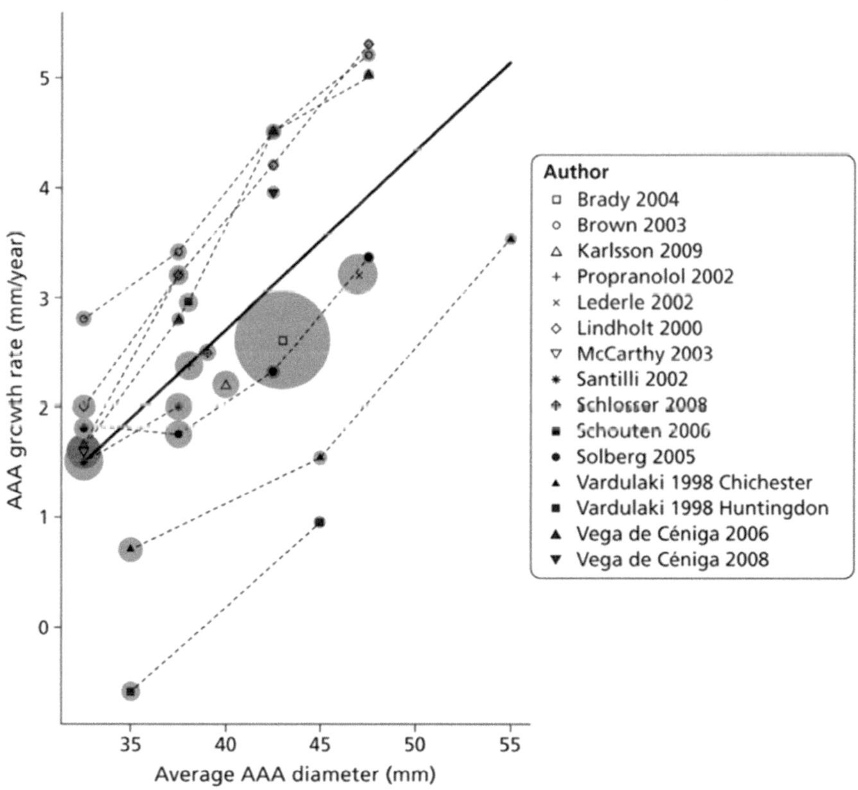

Fig. 16.1 Meta-regression of abdominal aortic aneurysm growth rate estimates by aneurysm diameter. (Adapted from Thompson et al. [63])

have focused on utilizing other imaging modalities such as 3D ultrasound to determine wall stress, define aortic size and shape, and better understand hemodynamics [66]. Others have focused on positron emission tomography and molecular imaging to identify those at risk of rupture [53]. Lastly, studies have introduced models such as finite element analysis, which functions as a model combining aortic geometry with biomechanical properties as a predictive measure [67]. No model is currently endorsed by the SVS or the NICE guidelines for care of patients with AAAs. Maximum aortic diameter remains the mainstay of clinical decision making in managing AAAs.

Modifiable Risk Factors and Medical Optimization

Patients with AAAs typically suffer from multiple comorbidities including uncontrolled hypertension, chronic obstructive pulmonary disease (COPD), female gender, severe CAD, a large volume of luminal thrombus, and advanced age. These factors as well as female gender, luminal thrombus, and advanced age are associated with increased AAA expansion or rupture rate. The primary goal of medical therapy in these patients is to decrease risk of expansion and rupture as well as optimizing cardiovascular status. In accordance with the NICE and SVS guidelines, patients should be offered smoking cessation programs, appropriate hypertensive management, diabetes management, cholesterol reduction, and nutritional counselling [53, 54]. There are currently no specific medications that are advocated for decreasing aortic expansion rate [53]. However, a meta-analysis consisting of over 80,000 patients investigating Statin medication use on AAA expansion demonstrated that Statin use is associated with decreased AAA expansion rates, rupture, and improved survival after elective AAA repair [68]. Routine utilization of Beta blockade in patients being considered for AAA repair should be avoided due to increased mortality in patients undergoing non-cardiac surgery [69].

Additional considerations include patients' functional status and cardiopulmonary reserve prior to repair. Patients should be evaluated utilizing frailty scores and exercise testing to determine METs and physical fitness. Studies have demonstrated that patients undergoing aortic aneurysm repair experience a significant increase in mortality at 30 days if preoperative functional status is poor [70]. Optimizing functional status has been demonstrated to provide benefit in patients undergoing major vascular surgery. Several studies including one randomized controlled trial revealed decreased hospital length of stay and lower rates of cardiopulmonary complications in patients who underwent preoperative fitness program [71, 72]. This process is known as prehabilitation. Recently, Enhanced Recovery Pathways (ERP) have been introduced to standardize and optimize pre- and postoperative care of patients undergoing aortic surgery [69]. Multiple studies have devised different exercise programs with variable postoperative benefit. The current ERP for aortic surgery advocates for a 6-week supervised fitness program consisting of aerobic and resistance training [69]. This program also aims to address other aspects of preoperative

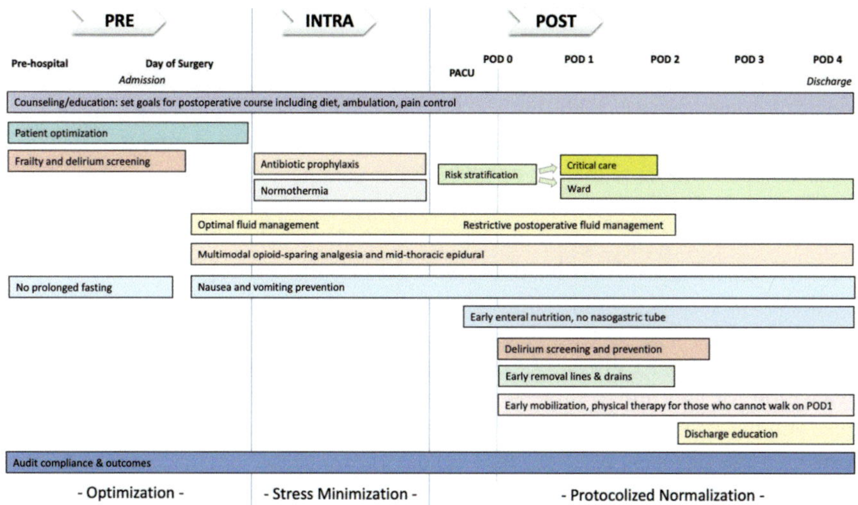

Fig. 16.2 Enhanced recovery pathway after surgery diagram. (Adapted from [73]

patient care including delirium screening, addressing nutritional deficiencies, and providing educational materials [69]. A flow diagram describing ERP is presented in Fig. 16.2.

Preoperative Risk Assessment

If a patient is discovered to have a symptomatic AAA (i.e., back or abdominal pain or hypotension), urgent or expedient surgical intervention is indicated. Stable patients can undergo laboratory testing and cross-sectional imaging to assess their potential for an endoluminal approach. If the patient is unstable, then the patient should be taken to the operating room for repair.

Asymptomatic male patients who are otherwise reasonably healthy with aneurysms greater than 5.5 cm or asymptomatic otherwise healthy female patients with aneurysms greater than 5.0 cm should undergo aneurysm repair. Based on preoperative assessments such as aneurysm anatomy, along with the patient's age and other comorbidities, the treatment strategy is selected. The most important factors that increase the risk of open aneurysm repair are renal dysfunction with a creatinine level greater than 1.8 mg, congestive heart failure, jugular venous distention, ischemic electrocardiographic changes with ST depression greater than 2 mm, history of a prior myocardial infarction, pulmonary dysfunction including COPD, dyspnea on exertion or prior lung surgery, advanced age, and female gender. In the absence of risk factors, elective open AAA carries an operative mortality of 3–5%, but the risk rises as high as 40% if several of the aforementioned risk factors are present [74]. Renal failure alone is the strongest predictor of mortality with a four- to ninefold increase in risk, whereas CAD carries a 2.5- to 5-fold increase in mortality [75].

Mortality is also affected by the given surgeon or hospital experience with AAA repair. Larger centers with higher volumes have better outcomes than less-experienced surgeons or small-volume centers [76]. Dimick et al. reported that hospitals that perform more than 35 open AAA per year have a 30-day mortality of 3%, as compared with lower volume centers that have a 30-day mortality of 5.5%. In general, they found that high-volume surgeons with vascular surgery specialty training working at high-volume hospitals have the best outcomes [77].

To reduce overall operative mortality, perioperative cardiac optimization is vital, especially since CAD is the principal cause of early and late mortality after AAA [78]. The American College of Cardiology has standardized preoperative cardiac evaluation for noncardiac surgery, and created categories for the risk of the procedure and the clinical risk to the patient. Patients with unstable coronary syndromes such as acute or recent MI (less than 30 days) or unstable angina, decompensated CHF, significant arrhythmias such as high-grade AV block or symptomatic ventricular arrhythmias, or severe valvular disease are considered to have major cardiac risks. Intermediate-risk patients are those with stable angina, prior MI by history or the presence of Q waves on an ECG, compensated CHF, insulin-dependent diabetes mellitus, or renal insufficiency. Patients with minor risk include those of advanced age, who have an abnormal ECG (left ventricular hypertrophy, left bundle branch block), have a history of a prior stroke, or have uncontrolled hypertension [79]. Van Damme et al. found that in patients without clinical markers of CAD, non-invasive cardiac testing did not predict cardiac complications. In patients with definite clinical or ECG evidence of CAD, a negative stress test had a high negative predictive value [80].

The indications for cardiac testing and treatment prior to AAA repair are the same as in the nonoperative setting, but the timing of such evaluations is dependent upon the urgency of the surgery, patient risk factors, and surgery-specific considerations. The preoperative evaluation aims at cardiac risk stratification and treatment strategies to reduce the patient's risk of cardiac events [81].

Consideration for coronary revascularization prior to elective AAA repair is largely based on anatomical distribution of disease and patients experiencing acute coronary syndrome. Patients should be considered for coronary revascularization if there is unstable angina, acute coronary syndrome, stable angina with involvement of the left main coronary artery or three-vessel disease, two-vessel disease with left anterior descending artery involvement, and decreased ventricular function on non-invasive studies. Overall, in patients undergoing percutaneous coronary intervention with drug-eluting stent placement, open AAA repair should be delayed at least 6 months while dual antiplatelet therapy is continued. If patients require open repair, dual antiplatelet therapy should be discontinued 10 days prior to repair with resumption of therapy postoperatively. Current recommendations also advocate for consideration of elective EVAR with continued dual antiplatelet therapy under local anesthesia, if the patient has suitable anatomy [53].

Patients with a history of pulmonary insufficiency require preoperative pulmonary function testing, and those who smoke should be encouraged to stop smoking before surgery. Some patients with severe bronchospastic pulmonary disease should be optimized with bronchodilator therapy or steroids prior to open AAA repair.

In patients with a history of stroke or transient ischemic attack or in the presence of a carotid bruit, a carotid duplex scan should be performed. If a high-grade stenosis is found in the internal carotid artery, carotid revascularization should precede elective AAA repair.

Procedural Considerations

Juan Parodi reported the first endoluminal repair of an AAA in 1991 [81]. Since then, numerous endoluminal devices have been tested in clinical trials [82–85]. Endovascular repair of AAA has been shown to reduce operative morbidity, mortality, length of hospital stay, and post-procedure disability. Two European randomized trials, EVAR-1 and DREAM trials, demonstrated a significantly lower mortality for EVAR when compared to open repair, but a higher reintervention requirement for EVAR [86, 87]. However, the mortality benefit observed in patients treated by EVAR dissipates at approximately 3 years [88–90]. Furthermore, analysis of the EVAR-1 and DREAM trials at 15 years revealed higher mortality with EVAR when compared to the open repair [88–90]. An additional randomized control trial by Lederle and colleagues (2019) revealed no difference in secondary reinterventions or mortality between open repair and EVAR at 15 years postoperatively. Differences in the randomized controlled trials investigating EVAR versus open repair have primarily been attributed to timing of patient selection. The DREAM and EVAR-1 trials were conducted closer to the advent of endovascular aortic surgery at which time endovascular devices and techniques were rapidly evolving [88]. To date, open repair has proven to be more durable and requires less follow-up than endoluminal repair. Conrad et al. reported a large series of patients undergoing open AAA repair, with an excellent 10-year survival for patients less than 75 years of age. In addition, the freedom from graft-related reintervention is superior to EVAR [91]. A large series published by Hertzer et al. also showed a low 30-day mortality and excellent long-term survival with open AAA repair [92]. Current NICE guidelines advocate for open surgical repair of AAAs as first-line operative therapy in patients meeting anatomic parameters for repair. EVAR is the preferred option in patients with suitable anatomy who have intrabdominal pathology creating difficult operative exposure or if comorbidities are precluding open repair or general anaesthesia [53, 54].

One issue for today's vascular surgeons in training is the fact that with likely better endovascular devices, fewer open infrarenal AAAs are being performed each year. From 2004 to 2015, the percentage of AAAs being repaired by elective EVAR increased by nearly 100% (Fig. 16.3) [93]. This in turn has led to a large increase in EVARs being performed by vascular surgical residents and subsequent decrease in open aortic cases. During the same period, the percentage of ruptured AAAs being

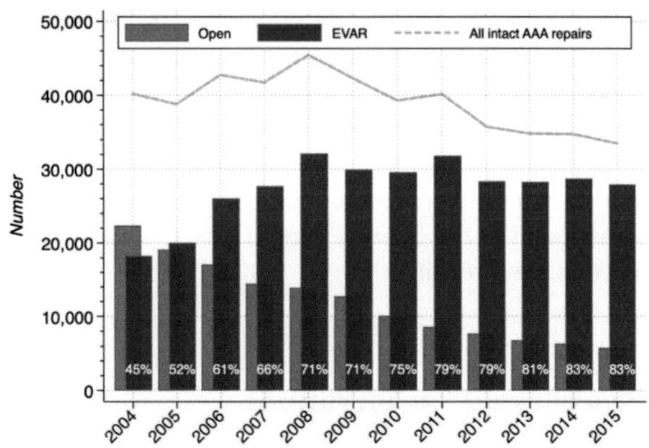

Fig. 16.3 Graphical demonstration of increasing EVAR AAA repair and decreasing open AAA repair. (Adapted from Dansey et al. [93])

repaired by open technique has also decreased with 55% being repaired by EVAR [93]. This has created some concern for vascular surgery residents and fellows obtaining adequate exposure to complex open aortic surgery.

Preoperative Considerations

As discussed previously, ERP for aortic surgery has been introduced by the SVS as guidance for managing patients undergoing AAA repair. Given the novelty of this strategy, the recommendations have been extrapolated from studies in other specialties focusing on major abdominal surgeries. Along with prehabilitation discussed in the previous section, several other preoperative recommendations have been proposed. These include preoperative carbohydrate loading, venous thromboembolism prophylaxis, epidural analgesia, and prophylactic intravenous antibiotic use continued 24 h postoperatively. Carbohydrate loading the evening prior to surgery and 2 h before surgery has been associated with multiple perioperative benefits. These include decreased insulin resistance, decreased myocardial injury, and decreased ICU length of stay [69]. Epidural analgesia in patients undergoing AAA repair has been recommended by the SVS as well as the NICE guidelines in patients in an effort to reduce postoperative opioid use [54, 69]. Other studies demonstrated lower incidence of myocardial events, improved pulmonary outcomes, and decreased ICU length of stay [69].

Technical Considerations

Once a patient has been deemed medically suitable for open surgery, the specific approach and operation is individualized based on several factors. The most critical is the CT scan evaluation of the shape and configuration of the aneurysm. The infrarenal neck, the portion of the aorta immediately below the renal arteries, along with the iliac arteries, must be assessed. If the iliac arteries have significant occlusive disease, the graft may have to be anastomosed to the femoral arteries. The presence of severe COPD is important because a laparotomy may not be well tolerated in these patients. The history of previous abdominal surgeries will also determine which approach is utilized. The two most frequently used approaches for AAA repair are the left retroperitoneal and the midline transperitoneal. A transverse incision has also been described, especially for patients with multiple upper abdominal surgeries (Fig. 16.4).

For a transperitoneal exposure, the patient is placed in a supine position and prepped and draped from the nipples down. A sufficient midline incision is made to provide exposure for an infrarenal repair, titrated to the need for suprarenal and iliac exposure. After entering the abdominal cavity, a full exploration of the abdominal contents should occur to rule out other intra-abdominal pathology that might have not been visible in the CT scan. If an unexpected lesion is discovered, it must be evaluated and a surgeon must make a judgment as to how best to proceed.

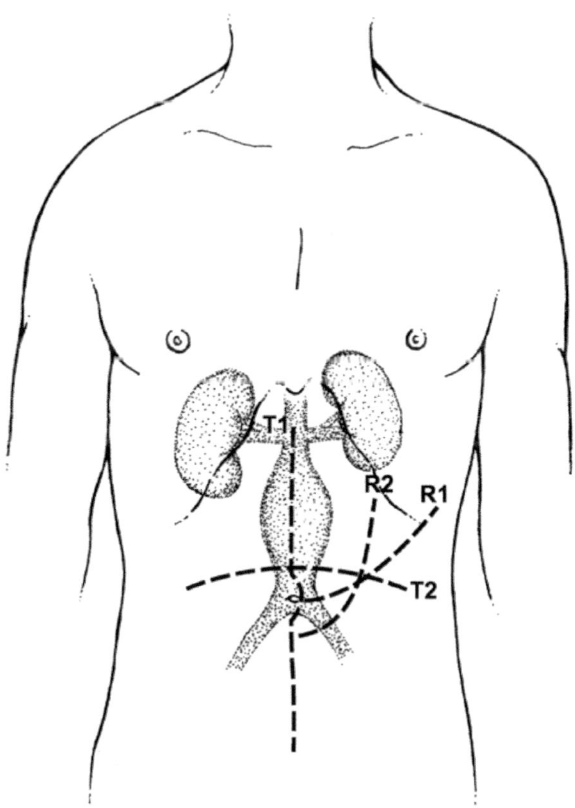

Fig. 16.4 Three most commonly used incisions for open repair of infrarenal abdominal aortic aneurysm: transabdominal midline (T1), transabdominal transverse (T2), and retroperitoneal (R1)

The next step is to retract superiorly the greater omentum and transverse colon. The small bowel is eviscerated to the right side of the abdomen. This exposes the base of the mesenteries of the left colon and the small intestine (Fig. 16.5).

The posterior peritoneum is then incised from the ligament of Treitz to the aortic bifurcation, thus exposing the infrarenal aorta (Fig. 16.5). The posterior peritoneum should be incised just to the right of the inferior mesenteric vein until the left renal vein crossing over the neck of the AAA is identified (Fig. 16.6a). The left renal vein can be divided close to the IVC and ligated or re-anastomosed if indicated, but this is rarely necessary in the author's experience. If the left renal vein is divided, it is important to preserve the left gonadal and adrenal vein to preserve left renal function. In cases in which the CT scan demonstrates a wide infrarenal neck, or aneurysmal disease above the renal arteries, our group prefers the left retroperitoneal approach with elevation of the left kidney which provides excellent exposure of the juxta- and suprarenal aorta for appropriate cross-clamping (Fig. 16.7). The use of self-retaining retractors should be employed to aid in the exposure of the operative field. Distally, the iliac arteries must be exposed for cross-clamping. If the aneurysm involves one or both iliacs, the dissection must be extended to the bifurcation of the common iliac(s), assuring identification of ureters. Usually circumferential aortic or iliac dissection is not necessary, and avoiding this can help avoid venous injuries.

Throughout the operation, active communication should take place between the surgical and anesthesia teams. Once the dissection is complete, the anesthesia team should give 80–100 U/kg of intravenous heparin and then be notified that aortic and iliac clamps will be applied shortly. Clamp placement should begin with the distal vessels and then the aorta, to prevent or reduce the risk of distal embolization. The aneurysm sac is then opened longitudinally and the mural thrombus should be removed. Any back bleeding from lumbar arteries or the IMA can be controlled with silk suture ligatures from within the aneurysm sac (Fig. 16.6b, c). If

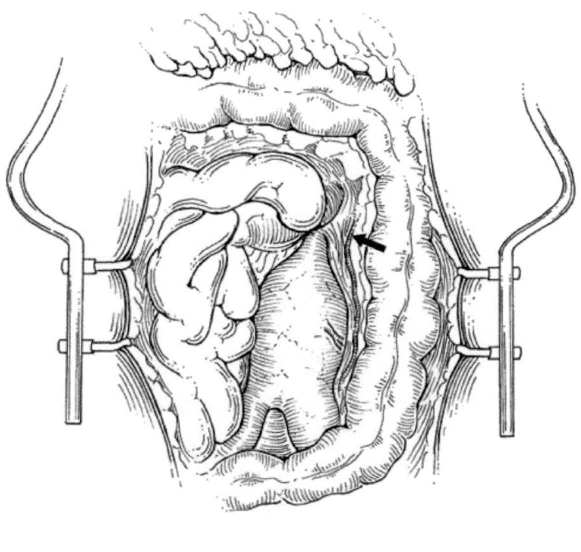

Fig. 16.5 Midline transabdominal exposure of infrarenal abdominal aortic aneurysm (*AAA*). Note inferior mesenteric vein (*arrow*)

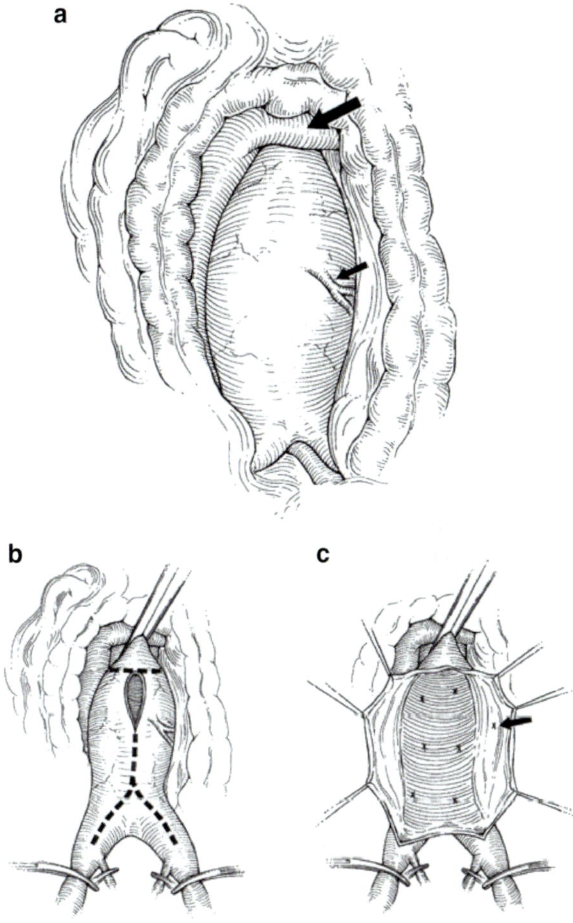

Fig. 16.6 Midline transabdominal exposure of infrarenal abdominal aortic aneurysm (*AAA*); (**a**) note left renal vein (*large arrow*) and inferior mesenteric artery (*small arrow*), (**b**) opening aortic aneurysm sac postdistal and proximal clamp, (**c**) endoluminal oversewing of bleeding lumbar arteries and inferior mesenteric artery (*arrow*)

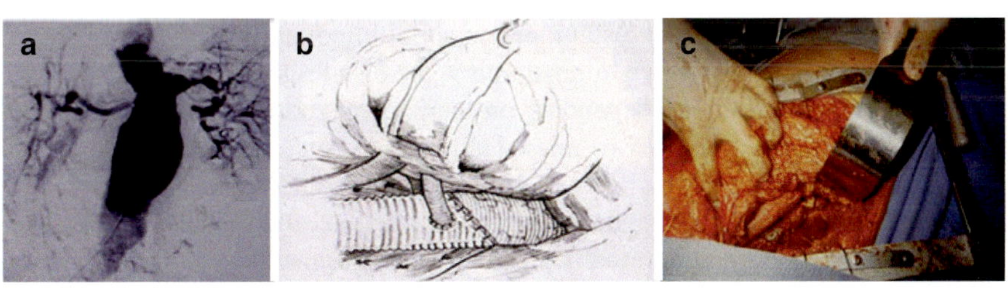

Fig. 16.7 (**a**) Abdominal aortic aneurysm (*AAA*) involving left renal artery treated via retroperitoneal approach. (**b**) Retroperitoneal exposure with superior displacement, left kidney, and renal artery reimplantation. (**c**) Intraoperative picture demonstrating retroperitoneal exposure with completed aortic graft and reimplantation of left renal artery (*See Color Plates*)

extraluminal control of the IMA is attempted, inadvertent ligation of marginal or sacral branches should be avoided to prevent decreasing sigmoid perfusion.

If the aneurysm has an adequate infrarenal neck and no involvement of the iliac vessels, a tube graft can be used. However, if the iliac arteries are aneurysmal, a bifurcated graft should be used and the distal limbs should be anastomosed end-to-end to the distal common iliac arteries preserving hypogastric flow. If more extensive iliac disease is present, the distal reconstruction should ideally be performed in a manner that allows preservation of flow to at least one hypogastric artery. If severe bilateral iliac disease is present, the limbs of the graft can be sewn to the common femoral arteries with oversewing of the distal common iliac arteries allowing retrograde hypogastric flow through the external iliac arteries.

Prior to removing all the clamps, it is important to back bleed the iliac system and flush any residual or remaining debris out of the graft. After hemostasis is achieved, pedal Doppler signal/pulses should be assessed prior to beginning the closure.

Typically, the aneurysm sac and the posterior peritoneum are closed over the graft in an effort to prevent visceral contact with the prosthetic graft. An omental flap can be created to cover the graft in the event that adequate retroperitoneal tissue is not available to separate the aortic graft from the duodenum. The abdominal wall is then closed in the standard fashion.

The transperitoneal approach affords the most flexibility for exposure of the aneurysm, the renal arteries, both iliac arteries, and both femoral arteries. This approach can be challenging in a patient who has undergone multiple prior abdominal surgeries due to adhesive disease. In addition, juxta- or suprarenal extension, the presence of ascites, or inflammatory aneurysm can be challenging with the transabdominal approach.

Some surgeons prefer a retroperitoneal approach for repairing all infrarenal AAAs. The aorta is a retroperitoneal structure and avoiding the intraperitoneal contents is preferable in certain circumstances. A left-sided retroperitoneal incision from lateral rectus margin through the 11th or 12th intercostal space provides excellent exposure to the infrarenal aorta, with progressively higher exposure to optimize access to the paravisceral and distal thoracic aorta. Importantly, the retroperitoneal exposure limits access to the right renal artery, the distal right common iliac artery, and the right femoral artery, depending on the patient's body habitus. In addition, intra-abdominal pathology may be missed although the preoperative evaluation and imaging should detect the majority of significant intra-abdominal pathology. The relative indications for a retroperitoneal multiple previous abdominal surgeries, previous radiation therapy, abdominal wall stoma, a horseshoe kidney, or the suprarenal repair.

For a retroperitoneal incision, a vacuum-assisted beanbag is placed on the operating room table. After induction of general anesthesia and placement of all of required monitors, the patient is positioned in the right lateral decubitus position with the fold of the bed between the top of the iliac crest and the costal margin. The patient is then placed in approximately 45° of right lateral decubitus with the left arm padded on an arm support. Slightly more tilt of the upper portion of the patient and slightly less rotation of the hips allow for easier access to the right groin if it is needed. The kidney rest is elevated, the bed is flexed, and the suction is applied to the beanbag to maintain this desired position. Positioning is key, and improper positioning will lead to less than ideal exposure.

The precise location of the incision depends on the planned procedure. For an infrarenal or aortoiliac exposure, the surgeon should make an incision medial but at the level on the umbilicus just lateral to the medial border of the rectus abdominus muscle. Based on the patient's size and body habitus, the incision should be extended in a curvilinear fashion superiorly and posteriorly to either the 12th rib or the interspace between the 11th and 12th ribs for an infrarenal/juxtarenal aneurysm. If exposure of the supraceliac or distal thoracic aorta is necessary, incision at a higher intercostal space may be preferred.

The abdominal wall muscles can be divided using electrocautery, although every effort should be made to preserve the left rectus. The retroperitoneal space is entered at the junction of the left rectus abdominus muscle and the lateral abdominal wall muscles by dividing the transversalis fascia and mobilizing the peritoneum medially and superiorly. These maneuvers allow for the exposure of the aorta from the renal arteries to the left external iliac artery and the right common iliac artery (Fig. 16.8).

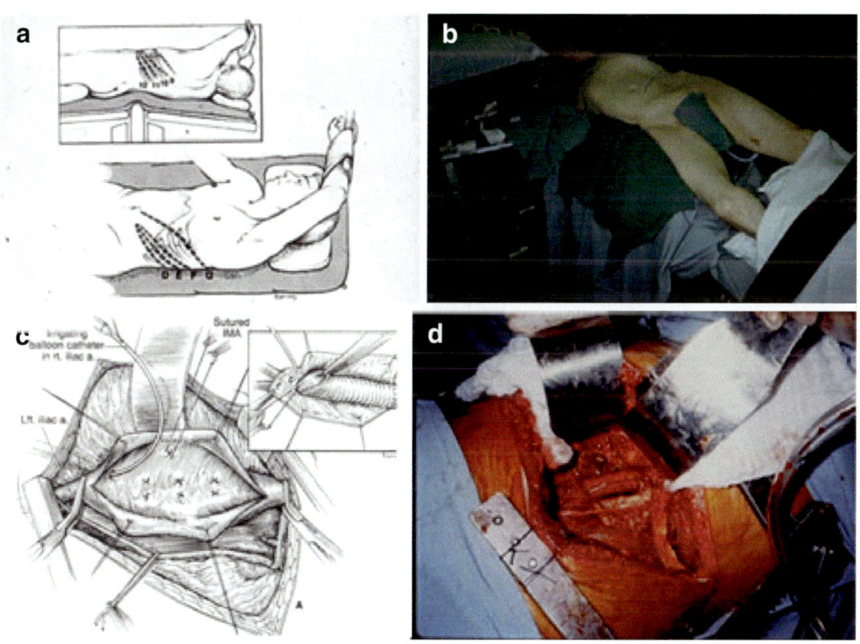

Fig. 16.8 Retroperitoneal approach to aortic pathology. (**a**) Various incisions based on body habitus and proximal extent of aortic pathology. (**b**) Patient position for retroperitoneal aortic exposure. (**c**) Drawing of retroperitoneal exposure for infrarenal AAA repair. (**d**) Intraoperative view of infrarenal AAA repair with tube graft (*See Color Plates*)

The peritoneum is mobilized further anteriorly until the left ureter and left gonadal vein are identified. The left ureter is then dissected and mobilized from the level of the renal pelvis down to the iliac artery bifurcation, looped with a vessel loop, and gently retracted medially to avoid an avulsion or traction injury. Care must also be taken not to devascularize the ureter, which can lead to an ischemic injury. The gonadal vein is then dissected up to its insertion into the left renal vein. The gonadal vein is ligated and divided at the level of the left renal vein to allow for needed infrarenal exposure of the neck of the AAA (Fig. 16.9).

In most cases, both common iliac arteries can be dissected to allow for clamp placement. If the right common iliac artery is difficult to clamp, intraluminal control of the right iliac system can be accomplished (Fig. 16.10).

The use of self-retaining retractors facilitates exposure and avoids unnecessary trauma to intra-abdominal organs, especially the spleen that may occur with hand retraction.

The clamping sequence is the same as for a transperitoneal approach. The iliac arteries are clamped first for distal control followed by the proximal aortic clamp to avoid distal embolization. The aneurysm sac is opened and the intramural thrombus is removed. Any back-bleeding lumbar vessels, along with the IMA, are ligated. If

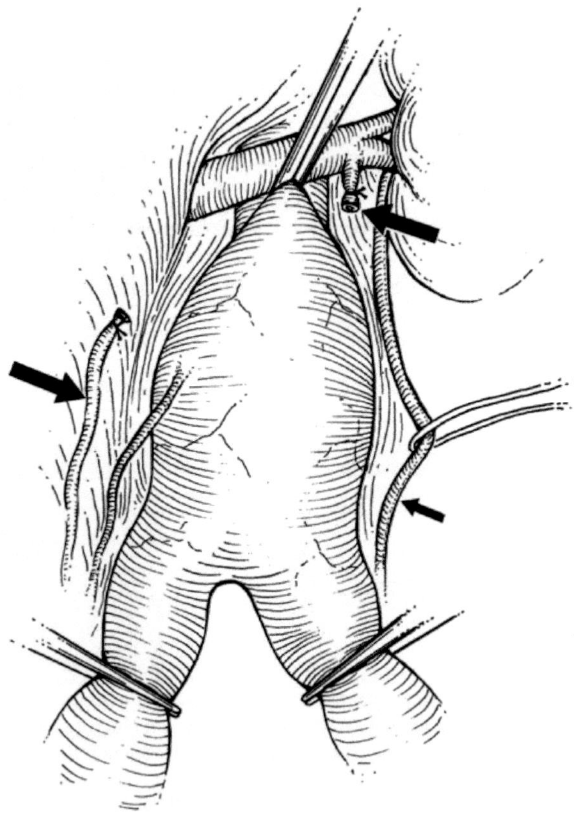

Fig. 16.9 Drawing of retroperitoneal exposure of large infrarenal abdominal aortic aneu-rysm (*AAA*). Note lateral mobilization of left ureter (*small arrow*) and ligation of left gonadal vein (*large arrow*)

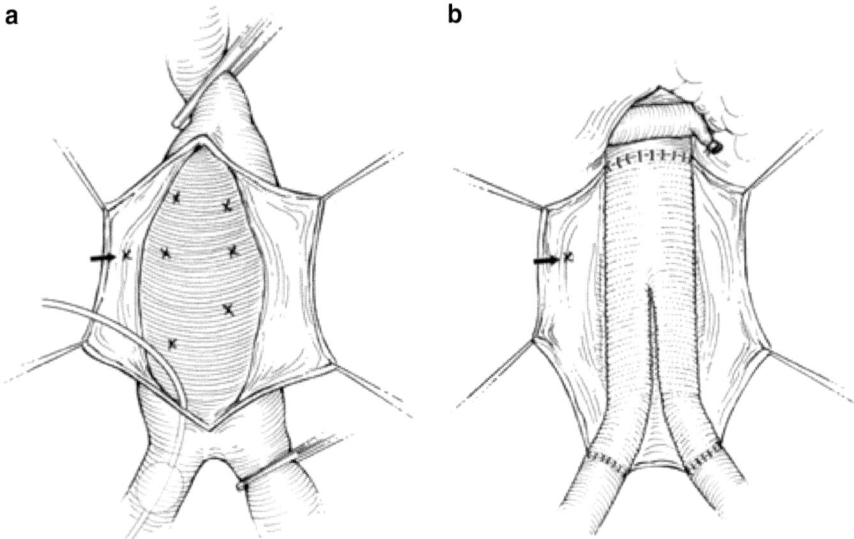

Fig. 16.10 Retroperitoneal exposure of abdominal aortic aneurysm (*AAA*) with balloon occlusion of right iliac artery. Note inferior mesenteric artery sutured from within the AAA sac (*arrow*)

the right iliac system cannot be controlled with a clamp, a number 6 or 9 Pruitt-type balloon occlusion irrigation catheter can be inserted into the right common iliac orifice. Based on the anatomy, either a tube graft or a bifurcated aortobi-iliac graft can be sewn into place. If an aortobifemoral bypass is required, we prefer to suture-ligate the common iliac arteries from within the aneurysm sac. We complete the aortic anastomosis and then rotate the table to provide better access to both groins. A careful tunnel is made with blunt finger dissection right on top of the iliac arteries and ureters from within the abdomen and on top of the femoral arteries from the groin incision. It is critical to ensure that both femoral limbs are passed posterior to the patient's ureters to avoid ureteral injury or compression (Fig. 16.11). The femoral anastomoses are usually performed in a standard end-to-side fashion. Once hemostasis has been achieved, the aneurysm sac is closed over the graft, if possible, and the abdominal lateral wall muscle and fascia are closed in two layers.

The two principal complications from this approach are abdominal wall laxity or true hernias and chronic incisional pain. La Croix, et al. reported a large series and found that only 5% had an incisional hernia, but 28% had a 2 cm or larger incision bulge [94]. Of 1000 patients who underwent retroperitoneal approaches for AAA, many described some level of incisional pain that ultimately resolved after 12–24 months, but fewer than 1% required nerve blocks to relieve the pain [95].

Retroperitoneal exposure of the abdominal aorta has traditionally been reserved for proximal AAAs or thoracoabdominal aneurysms that may require suprarenal control or visceral revascularization. Studies comparing these techniques have produced inconsistent results [96]. However, in elective AAA repair, a retroperitoneal exposure may be advantageous in patients with a gastrointestinal, urological stoma,

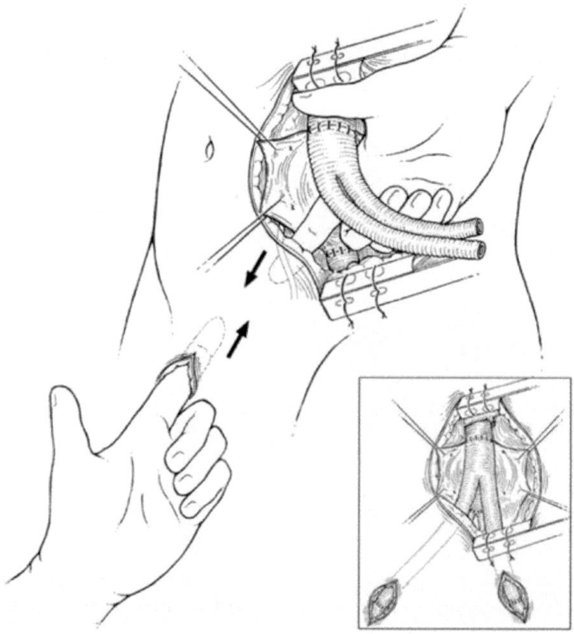

Fig. 16.11 Retroperitoneal exposure for AAA repair requiring aortobifemoral bypass. Tunnel to pass right limb must be posterior to ureter (*arrows*)

or hostile abdomen. There have also been studies that have shown that ileus, pulmonary complications, and fluid requirements are decreased with this approach [95]. A meta-analysis conducted in 2016 appraising five randomized control trials revealed no significant difference in mortality, wound complications, aortic cross clamp time, or total operative time when comparing transperitoneal and retroperitoneal exposures [97]. However, patients undergoing retroperitoneal exposure experienced shorter ICU length of stay, shorter hospital stay, and lower blood loss when compared to transperitoneal approach. The authors indicated heterogeneity among the studies and a relatively low quality of evidence favoring either approach [97]. A large study utilizing NSQIP data revealed overall similarity between the two methods of operative exposure in multivariate analysis with retroperitoneal approach associated with more frequent reintubations, pneumonia, and transfusion requirement [96]. A study by Sieunarine et al. found no difference in operative time, cross-clamp time, blood loss, fluid replacement, analgesia requirement, gastrointestinal function, intensive care, or hospital stay between either exposure. In their long-term follow-up, however, there were significantly more wound problems such as hernias or pain in the retroperitoneal group [98]. One randomized control trial found no statistical difference in pulmonary complications, fluid or blood requirements, or other postoperative complications, except a slightly prolonged return to oral intake after the transperitoneal approach [99]. Overall, operative approach should be selected based upon specific patient factors and at the surgeon's preference.

Postoperative Management

Most patients are followed immediately postoperatively in a surgical intensive care unit. Some patients will require some period of continued mechanical ventilation while they are rewarmed and associated coagulopathies are corrected. Close monitoring is also vital to monitor hemodynamic responses, fluid shifts, and pain control. Patients should have full laboratory values checked immediately postoperatively. In our center, we check patient lab values every 4–6 h for the first 24-h with relaxation of lab draws thereafter. Primary focus should be to correct coagulopathies, trending coagulation factors and thromboelastographs, goal-directed fluid resuscitation, and blood product administration as indicated. We attempt to maintain platelet count >100 and INR <1.5 in the immediate post-operative period. In addition, they should have a chest x-ray and an ECG performed, and the patients should be maintained on their β-blockers.

Postoperative, ERP programs attempt to return patients to normalcy and preserve homeostasis perioperatively. Current ERP recommendations regarding postoperative management in elective AAA repair advocate for the judicious use of crystalloid fluids (<1.5 L/day). However, fluid resuscitation should remain goal-directed utilizing laboratory values, base deficit, hemodynamics, and urinary output as guidance. Additionally, routine long-term use of nasogastric drainage and urinary catheter should be avoided due to delayed return of bowel function and risk of urinary tract infection, respectively [69]. Early initiation of oral diet and nutritional supplementation should be considered. Additionally, utilization of epidural pain block assists with decreased postoperative opioid use and decreases pulmonary complications [100]. Lastly, early mobilization and involvement of physical and occupational therapy is critical in decreasing length of stay and risk of delirium [69].

Postoperative Complications

As with all major abdominal operations, there is risk of iatrogenic injury to adjacent organs and structures. Ureteral injury occurs in less than 1% of elective open AAA repairs. When injury occurs, prompt recognition and repair is imperative due to an increased risk of urinary leak and potential prosthetic graft infection [101]. Splenic injury can also occur typically due to excessive retraction. Splenic injury is rare occurring in approximately 0.6% of aortoiliac or thoracoabdominal aneurysm repairs. These injuries have mostly been reported during retroperitoneal approach. Approximately 0.7% of patients experience significant splenic injury requiring splenectomy. Patients requiring splenectomy have a three-fold increase in mortality [102]. The treatment for a fractured spleen, especially in the face of an ongoing coagulopathy, is a splenectomy. Inadvertent enterotomies during the initial opening should be repaired and the AAA portion should be aborted.

The large physiological impact of open AAA repair combined with a comorbid patient population leads to largely predictable postoperative complications. Cardiopulmonary complications have remained the most common in the postoperative period. Cardiac complications include arrhythmia, myocardial infarction, and congestive heart failure exacerbation occurring in up to 15–20% [51]. Approximately 47% of patients undergoing elective AAA repair will have elevated troponin levels with roughly 50% of these patients experiencing a true cardiac event [103]. Elkouri et al. reported their large series of elective AAA patients and found cardiac complications in 22% [104]. Patients with an elevated troponin level postoperatively experience an increase in mortality. Some studies have promoted ischemic preconditioning in an effort to reduce myocardial and renal stress during aortic cross-clamping and repair [103]. It remains imperative to screen patients undergoing elective AAA repair for extent of cardiac disease to limit postoperative complications.

Pulmonary complications including pneumonia or respiratory failure requiring prolonged mechanical ventilation have also occurred following elective AAA repair. Vascular patients often suffer from varying degrees of pulmonary disease such as COPD. Patients with oxygen dependence and severe COPD are predisposed to all adverse events, pulmonary complication and mortality [105]. Elkouri et al. reported that 16% of their patients had pulmonary complications [104]. A large series by Hertzer et al. at the Cleveland Clinic reported only 4.2% of their patients developed pulmonary complications, with the majority having pneumonia, although 1% developed adult respiratory distress syndrome [92]. Early extubation and aggressive pulmonary toilet and early ambulation can aid in preventing pulmonary complications [69]. Furthermore, judicious use of crystalloid IV fluids and goal-directed fluid resuscitation of these patients should be considered. Patients undergoing elective open AAA repair have significantly increased risk in cardiopulmonary complications and length of hospital stay if fluid balance remains positive throughout multiple hospital days [106].

Postoperative renal dysfunction following open AAA repair predisposes patients to decreased overall survival, increased hospital length of stay, and increased costs [107]. Although postoperative renal dysfunction is more highly associated with suprarenal repairs, infrarenal clamping can decrease renal perfusion up to 60%. Approximately 5–6% of patients undergoing open infrarenal AAA repair experience renal complications [108, 109]. Open repair and preoperative renal dysfunction (GFR < 60) are independent risk factors for postoperative renal complications [107, 108, 110, 111]. Patients with postoperative renal failure experience a profound increase in 30-day mortality at 35% compared to 4.3% [109]. Other factors associated with postoperative renal complications include transfusion requirements and longer operative times [107]. If suprarenal clamping is required, several maneuvers can be performed intraoperatively for renal protection and to reduce these complications. In preparation for aortic clamp placement above the renal arteries, a solution of 1 L of Lactated Ringers, 250 mL of 20% mannitol, and 500 mg of solumedrol is prepared on the back table and maintained at 4–6 °C. After aortic clamp placement and opening of the aorta, 250 mL of this solution is instilled into each kidney. The authors perform this routinely with suprarenal clamping to preserve renal function.

Bowel ischemia after AAA repair is rare in elective open AAA repair with an incidence of approximately 0.6–12% with clinically significant ischemia ranging from 1% to 3% [112–119]. However, the presence of severe postoperative bowel ischemia necessitates further operative intervention and carries a perioperative mortality risk of approximately 50–90% [119, 120]. Unexplained leukocytosis, fever, and/or left lower quadrant pain and hematochezia or melena should prompt urgent evaluation for colonic ischemia with a flexible sigmoidoscopy or colonoscopy. However, this constellation of symptoms is only present in 30% of cases [113]. A study by Brandt et al. in 1997 reported that flexible sigmoidoscopy reliably predicts full-thickness colonic ischemia for AAA repair. Patients with nonconfluent ischemia limited to the mucosa can be safely followed by serial endoscopic examinations [121]. Boley and colleagues have categorized the degree of colonic ischemia and management based on severity. Mild colonic ischemia is most commonly experienced with ischemia limited to the colonic mucosa and submucosa [122, 123]. Patients may experience abdominal pain, ileus, distention, or hematochezia, but the disease process is self-limited and resolves with adequate resuscitation. Moderate colonic ischemia is a more progressive form that involves the muscularis and may lead to eventual stricture formation. Severe colonic ischemia affects less than 20% of the patients with postoperative colonic ischemia. Endoscopy reveals transmural ischemia with colonic infarction and possible colonic perforation. This mandates a return to the operating room for a washout of the contamination, along with a bowel or colonic resection with colostomy or ileostomy creation. Concern here is also for graft contamination and ultimately infection [122, 123]. Additional abdominal washouts are required to ensure integrity of aortic repair and reduce prosthetic graft contamination.

Colonic ischemia after AAA repair can be secondary to alteration of sigmoid and rectal perfusion after ligation of the IMA or interruption of internal iliac arteries, embolization from aneurysmal sac, prolonged hypotension, or a retractor injury. In patients undergoing an AAA repair, 50% have a patent IMA, which could be reimplanted or bypassed [124]. Most surgeons evaluate collateral colonic circulation by assessing the back bleeding of the IMA. Brisk back bleeding along with a normal appearing colon typically indicates healthy collateral perfusion and suggests that it is safe to ligate the IMA. Several studies have shown that IMA reimplantation did not influence postoperative colonic ischemia but certainly was safe and may be advantageous in selected patients [116, 117, 125, 126]. Preoperative imaging by CT angiography can be useful in assessing the potential need to reimplant the IMA, especially if evidence of chronic mesenteric arterial obstruction is present. This demonstrates the importance of preserving in-line blood flow to the pelvic viscera and colon whenever possible.

Due to the thrombus burden of the AAA sac, there is concern for possible lower extremity ischemia secondary to thromboembolic event intraoperatively. Several intraoperative techniques such as systemic heparinization, back-bleeding prior to completing distal anastomosis, and compression of the femoral artery during initial reperfusion to drive flow into the hypogastric vessels before opening flow to the leg can help to reduce this occurrence. Overall, approximately 2% of patients will experience lower extremity ischemia after elective AAA repair [127]. One study utilizing data from NSQIP demonstrated significant increased hospital length of stay, overall complication rate, and 30-day mortality. As with most complications, lower extremity ischemia is more commonly associated with ruptured AAA repair.

Sexual dysfunction and impotence have also been described as late complications after open AAA repair as a result of injury to the autonomic nerves during the distal aortic and iliac dissection. It usually presents as erectile dysfunction or more frequently as retrograde ejaculation. Most men undergoing elective AAA repair have some component of this preoperatively. In the ADAM trial, 40% of men had impotence before AAA repair [128]. Being cautious when dissecting around the distal left side of the aorta, especially around the region of the IMA and the left common iliac artery, has been shown to reduce this complication substantially, which has been reported as high as 25% [129, 130]. Another important component to preserved sexual function is preservation of at least one internal iliac artery with antegrade blood flow.

One other dreaded complication with a very high postoperative morbidity and mortality is spinal cord ischemia and paralysis. This is much more common after thoracoabdominal repairs, because the accessory spinal artery emerges proximal to the abdominal aorta, although it has been reported in rare cases. These reports have stressed the importance of preserving pelvic collaterals and internal iliac arteries if at all possible. Occlusion or division of these vessels combined with periods of severe hypotension can lead to spinal cord ischemia and paralysis [131].

Conclusion

Open infrarenal AAA repairs have been performed for over 60 years with significant improvement in clinical outcomes. This operation has proven to be extremely durable and safe, especially in high-volume institutions. Although endovascular repair of AAAs is rapidly evolving, open repair remains a primary modality of operative therapy for young, healthy patients due to long-term durability. The knowledge and skill to perform an open infrarenal AAA remains vital for today's vascular surgeon, regardless of the operative approach utilized. Moreover, a comprehensive preoperative evaluation of patients undergoing elective open AAA repair allows for patient optimization and reveals predictive factors for adverse outcomes postoperatively.

References

1. Johnston KW, Rutherford RB, Tilson MD, Shah DM, Hollier L, Stanley JC. Suggested standards for reporting on arterial aneurysms. Subcommittee on Reporting Standards for Arterial Aneurysms, Ad Hoc Committee on Reporting Standards, Society for Vascular Surgery and North American Chapter, International Society for Cardiovascular Surgery. J Vasc Surg. 1991;13(3):452–8.

2. Thompson RW, Holmes DR, Mertens RA, et al. Production and localization of 92-kilodalton gelatinase in abdominal aortic aneurysms. An elastolytic metalloproteinase expressed by aneurysm-infiltrating macrophages. J Clin Invest. 1995;96(1):318–26.
3. Thompson RW. Basic science of abdominal aortic aneurysms: emerging therapeutic strategies for an unresolved clinical problem. Curr Opin Cardiol. 1996;11(5):504–18.
4. Thompson RW, Parks WC. Role of matrix metalloproteinases in abdominal aortic aneurysms. Ann N Y Acad Sci. 1996;800:157–74.
5. Curci JA, Liao S, Huffman MD, Shapiro SD, Thompson RW. Expression and localization of macrophage elastase (matrix metalloproteinase-12) in abdominal aortic aneurysms. J Clin Invest. 1998;102(11):1900–10.
6. Osler W. Aneurysm of the abdominal aorta. Lancet. 1905;2(94):1089.
7. Osler W. Remarks on arterio-venous aneurysm. Lancet. 1915;2:949.
8. Leonardo R. History of surgery. New York: Froben Press; 1943.
9. Matas R. Aneurysm of the abdominal aorta at its bifurcation into the common iliac arteries: a pictorial supplement of illustrating the history of corinne D. Previously reported as the first recorded instance of cure of an aneurysm of the abdominal aorta by ligation. Ann Surg. 1940;112(5):909–22.
10. Power D. The palliative treatment of aneurysms by wiring with Colt's appartus. Br J Surg. 1921;9(27):27–36.
11. Pearse HE. Experimental studies on the gradual occlusion of large arteries. Ann Surg. 1940;112(5):923–7.
12. Harrison PW, Chandy J. A subclavian aneurysm cured by cellophane fibrosis. Ann Surg. 1943;118(3):478–81.
13. Abbott OA. Clinical experiences with the application of polythene cellophane upon the aneurysms of thoracic vessels. J Thorac Surg. 1949;18(4):453–61.
14. Dente CJ, Feliciano DV. Alexis Carrel (1874-1944): Nobel Laureate, 1912. Arch Surg. 2005;140(6):609–10.
15. Edwards W. Alexis carrel 1873-1944. Contemp Surg. 1979;14:65–79.
16. Carrel A. La technique operatoire des anastomoses vascularies et la transplation de viscere. Lyon Med. 1902;98:859.
17. Carrel A. Suture of blood vessels and transplantation of organs. In: Nobel lecture 1912. Amsterdam: Elsevier; 1967.
18. Dubost CMA, Oeconomos N. Resection of an aneurysm of the abdominal aorta: reestablishment of the continuity by a preserved human arterial graft, with result after five months. Arch Surg. 1952;64(3):405–8.
19. De Bakey ME, Cooley DA. Surgical treatment of aneurysm of abdominal aorta by resection and restoration of continuity with homograft. Surg Gynecol Obstet. 1953;97:257–66.
20. Brock RC, Rob CG, Forty F. Discussion on reconstructive arterial surgery. Proc R Soc Med. 1952;46(2):115–30.
21. Voorhees ABJ, Jaretzki A 3rd, Blakemore AH. The use of tubes constructed from vinyon "N" cloth in bridging arterial defects. Ann Surg. 1952;135(3):332–6.
22. Friedman SG. A history of vascular surgery. Mt Kisco: Futura; 1989.
23. Levin SM. Reminiscences and ruminations: vascular surgery then and now. Am J Surg. 1987;154(2):158–62.
24. Blakemore AH, Voorhees AB. The use of tubes constructed from vinyon N cloth in bridging arterial defects; experimental and clinical. Ann Surg. 1954;140(3):324–34.
25. de Bakey ME. Clinical application of a new flexible knitted dacron arterial substitute. AMA Arch Surg. 1958;77(5):713–24.
26. Katz DJ, Stanely JC, Zelenock GB. Operative mortality rates for intact and ruptured abdominal aortic aneurysms in Michigan: an eleven-year statewide experience. J Vasc Surg. 1994;19(5):804–15.
27. LaMorte WW, Scott TE, Menzoian JO. Racial differences in the incidence of femoral bypass and abdominal aortic aneurysmectomy in Massachusetts: relationship to cardiovascular risk factors. J Vasc Surg. 1995;21(3):422–31.

28. Blanchard JF. Epidemiology of abdominal aortic aneurysms. Epidemiol Rev. 1999;21(2):207–21.
29. Wilmink AB, Hubbard CS, Day NE, Quick CR. The incidence of small abdominal aortic aneurysms and the change in normal infrarenal aortic diameter: implications for screening. Eur J Vasc Endovasc Surg. 2001;21(2):165–70.
30. Lederle FA, Johnson GR, Wilson SE, et al. Yield of repeated screening for abdominal aortic aneurysm after a 4-year interval. Aneurysm Detection and Management Veterans Affairs Cooperative Study Investigators. Arch Intern Med. 2000;160(8):1117–21.
31. Melton LJ 3rd, Bickerstaff LK, Hollier LH, et al. Changing incidence of abdominal aortic aneurysms: a population-based study. Am J Epidemiol. 1984;120(3):379–86.
32. McFarlane MJ. The epidemiologic necropsy for abdominal aortic aneurysm. JAMA. 1991;265(16):2085–8.
33. Bengtsson H, Bergqvist D, Sternby NH. Increasing prevalence of abdominal aortic aneurysms. A necropsy study. Eur J Surg. 1992;158(1):19–23.
34. Verloes A, Sakalihasan N, Koulischer L, Limet R. Aneurysms of the abdominal aorta: familial and genetic aspects in three hundred thirteen pedigrees. J Vasc Surg. 1995;21(4):646–55.
35. Johansen K, Koepsell T. Familial tendency for abdominal aortic aneurysms. JAMA. 1986;256(14):1934–6.
36. Darling RC 3rd, Brewster DC, Darling RC, et al. Are familial abdominal aortic aneurysms different? J Vasc Surg. 1989;10(1):39–43.
37. Pasch AR, Ricotta JJ, May AG, Green RM, DeWeese JE. Abdominal aortic aneurysm: the case for elective resection. Circulation. 1984;70(3 Pt 2):I1–4.
38. Breckwoldt WL, Mackey WC, O'Donnell TF Jr. The economic implications of high-risk abdominal aortic aneurysms. J Vasc Surg. 1991;13(6):798–803; discussion 803–794.
39. Cota AM, Omer AA, Jaipersad AS, Wilson NV. Elective versus ruptured abdominal aortic aneurysm repair: a 1-year cost-effectiveness analysis. Ann Vasc Surg. 2005;19(6):858–61.
40. Schermerhorn M, Zwolak R, Velazquez O, Makaroun M, Fairman R, Cronenwett J. Ultrasound screening for abdominal aortic aneurysm in medicare beneficiaries. Ann Vasc Surg. 2008;22(1):16–24.
41. Derubertis BG, Trocciola SM, Ryer EJ, et al. Abdominal aortic aneurysm in women: prevalence, risk factors, and implications for screening. J Vasc Surg. 2007;46(4):630–5.
42. Bengtsson H, Bergqvist D, Ekberg O, Janzon L. A population based screening of abdominal aortic aneurysms (AAA). Eur J Vasc Surg. 1991;5(1):53–7.
43. Lindholt JS, Henneberg EW, Fasting H, Juul S. Mass or high-risk screening for abdominal aortic aneurysm. Br J Surg. 1997;84(1):40–2.
44. Morris GE, Hubbard CS, Quick CR. An abdominal aortic aneurysm screening program for all males over the age of 50 years. Eur J Vasc Surg. 1994;8(2):156–60.
45. Scott RA, Ashton HA, Kay DN. Abdominal aortic aneurysm in 4237 screened patients: prevalence, development and management over 6 years. Br J Surg. 1991;78(9):1122–5.
46. Scott RA, Bridgewater SG, Ashton HA. Randomized clinical trial of screening for abdominal aortic aneurysm in women. Br J Surg. 2002;89(3):283–5.
47. Vardulaki KA, Walker NM, Couto E, et al. Late results concerning feasibility and compliance from a randomized trial of ultrasonographic screening for abdominal aortic aneurysm. Br J Surg. 2002;89(7):861–4.
48. Lindholt JS, Juul S, Fasting H, Henneberg EW. Hospital costs and benefits of screening for abdominal aortic aneurysms. Results from a randomised population screening trial. Eur J Vasc Endovasc Surg. 2002;23(1):55–60.
49. Heather BP, Poskitt KR, Earnshaw JJ, Whyman M, Shaw E. Population screening reduces mortality rate from aortic aneurysm in men. Br J Surg. 2000;87(6):750–3.
50. Ashton HA, Buxton MJ, Day NE, et al. The Multicentre Aneurysm Screening Study (MASS) into the effect of abdominal aortic aneurysm screening on mortality in men: a randomised controlled trial. Lancet. 2002;360(9345):1531–9.
51. Kim LG, Scott RAP, Ashton HA, Thompson SG, Multicentre Aneurysm Screening Study G. A sustained mortality benefit from screening for abdominal aortic aneurysm. Ann Intern Med. 2007;146(10):699–706.

52. Lo RC, Schermerhorn ML. Abdominal aortic aneurysms in women. J Vasc Surg. 2016;63(3):839–44.
53. Chaikof EL, Dalman RL, Eskandari MK, et al. The Society for Vascular Surgery practice guidelines on the care of patients with an abdominal aortic aneurysm. J Vasc Surg. 2018;67(1):2–77.e72.
54. Excellence NIfHaC. Abdominal aortic aneurysm: diagnosis and management (NICE Guidelines). Excellence NIfHaC; 2020. p. 1–57.
55. Lederle FA, Wilson SE, Johnson GR, et al. Immediate repair compared with surveillance of small abdominal aortic aneurysms. N Engl J Med. 2002;346(19):1437–44.
56. Powell JT, Brown LC, Forbes JF, et al. Final 12-year follow-up of surgery versus surveillance in the UK Small Aneurysm Trial. Br J Surg. 2007;94(6):702–8.
57. Cao P, De Rango P, Verzini F, et al. Comparison of surveillance versus aortic endografting for small aneurysm repair (CAESAR): results from a randomised trial. Eur J Vasc Endovasc Surg. 2011;41(1):13–25.
58. Ouriel KCD, Kent KC, Zarins CK. Impact of Endovascular Options for treating Aneurysms Early (PIVOTAL) Investigators. Endovascular repair compared with surveillance for patients with small abdominal aortic aneurysms. J Vasc Surg. 2010;51:1081–7.
59. Filardo G, Powell JT, Martinez MA, Ballard DJ. Surgery for small asymptomatic abdominal aortic aneurysms. Cochrane Database Syst Rev. 2015;2015(2):CD001835.
60. Hirose Y, Hamada S, Takamiya M. Predicting the growth of aortic aneurysms: a comparison of linear vs exponential models. Angiology. 1995;46(5):413–9.
61. Englund R, Hudson P, Hanel K, Stanton A. Expansion rates of small abdominal aortic aneurysms. Aust N Z J Surg. 1998;68(1):21–4.
62. Bengtsson H, Ekberg O, Aspelin P, Kallero S, Bergqvist D. Ultrasound screening of the abdominal aorta in patients with intermittent claudication. Eur J Vasc Surg. 1989;3(6):497–502.
63. Thompson SG, et al. Systematic review and meta-analysis of the growth and rupture rates of small abdominal aortic aneurysms: implications for surveillance intervals and their cost-effectiveness. Health Technol Assess. 2013;17:1–118.
64. Fillinger MF, Raghavan ML, Marra SP, Cronenwett JL, Kennedy FE. In vivo analysis of mechanical wall stress and abdominal aortic aneurysm rupture risk. J Vasc Surg. 2002;36(3):589–97.
65. Fillinger MF, Marra SP, Raghavan ML, Kennedy FE. Prediction of rupture risk in abdominal aortic aneurysm during observation: wall stress versus diameter. J Vasc Surg. 2003;37(4):724–32.
66. Kok AM, Nguyen VL, Speelman L, et al. Feasibility of wall stress analysis of abdominal aortic aneurysms using three-dimensional ultrasound. J Vasc Surg. 2015;61(5):1175–84.
67. Larsson E, Labruto F, Gasser TC, Swedenborg J, Hultgren R. Analysis of aortic wall stress and rupture risk in patients with abdominal aortic aneurysm with a gender perspective. J Vasc Surg. 2011;54(2):295–9.
68. Salata K, Syed M, Hussain MA, et al. Statins reduce abdominal aortic aneurysm growth, rupture, and perioperative mortality: a systematic review and meta-analysis. J Am Heart Assoc. 2018;7(19):e008657.
69. McGinigle KL, Spangler EL, Pichel AC, et al. Perioperative care in open aortic vascular surgery: a consensus statement by the Enhanced Recovery After Surgery (ERAS) Society and Society for Vascular Surgery. J Vasc Surg. 2022;75(6):1796–820.
70. Harris DG, Bulatao I, Oates CP, et al. Functional status predicts major complications and death after endovascular repair of abdominal aortic aneurysms. J Vasc Surg. 2017;66(3):743–50.
71. Hughes MJ, Hackney RJ, Lamb PJ, Wigmore SJ, Deans C, Skipworth RJE. Prehabilitation before major abdominal surgery: a systematic review and meta-analysis. World J Surg. 2019;43(7):1661–8.
72. Barakat HM, Shahin Y, Khan JA, McCollum PT, Chetter IC. Preoperative supervised exercise improves outcomes after elective abdominal aortic aneurysm repair: a randomized controlled trial. Ann Surg. 2016;264(1):47–53.

73. McGinigle KL, Eldrup-Jorgensen J, McCall R, et al. A systematic review of enhanced recovery after surgery for vascular operations. J Vasc Surg. 2019;70(2):629–640 e1. https://doi.org/10.1016/j.jvs.2019.01.050.
74. Steyerberg EW, Kievit J, de Mol Van Otterloo JC, van Bockel JH, Eijkemans MJ, Habbema JD. Perioperative mortality of elective abdominal aortic aneurysm surgery. A clinical prediction rule based on literature and individual patient data. Arch Intern Med. 1995;155(18):1998–2004.
75. Hallin A, Bergqvist D, Holmberg L. Literature review of surgical management of abdominal aortic aneurysm. Eur J Vasc Endovasc Surg. 2001;22(3):197–204.
76. Dardik A, Lin JW, Gordon TA, Williams GM, Perler BA. Results of elective abdominal aortic aneurysm repair in the 1990s: a population-based analysis of 2335 cases. J Vasc Surg. 1999;30(6):985–95.
77. Dimick JB, Cowan JA Jr, Stanley JC, Henke PK, Pronovost PJ, Upchurch GR Jr. Surgeon specialty and provider volumes are related to outcome of intact abdominal aortic aneurysm repair in the United States. J Vasc Surg. 2003;38(4):739–44.
78. Roger VL, Ballard DJ, Hallett JW Jr, Osmundson PJ, Puetz PA, Gersh BJ. Influence of coronary artery disease on morbidity and mortality after abdominal aortic aneurysmectomy: a population-based study, 1971-1987. J Am Coll Cardiol. 1989;14(5):1245–52.
79. Fleisher LA, Beckman JA, Brown KA, et al. ACC/AHA 2007 Guidelines on Perioperative Cardiovascular Evaluation and Care for Noncardiac Surgery: executive summary: a report of the American College of Cardiology/American Heart Association Task Force on Practice Guidelines (Writing Committee to Revise the 2002 Guidelines on Perioperative Cardiovascular Evaluation for Noncardiac Surgery) Developed in Collaboration With the American Society of Echocardiography, American Society of Nuclear Cardiology, Heart Rhythm Society, Society of Cardiovascular Anesthesiologists, Society for Cardiovascular Angiography and Interventions, Society for Vascular Medicine and Biology, and Society for Vascular Surgery. J Am Coll Cardiol. 2007;50(17):1707–32.
80. Van Damme H, et al. Cardiac risk assessment before vascular surgery: a prospective study comparing clinical evaluation, dobutamine stress echocardiography, and dobutamine Tc-99m sestamibi tomoscintigraphy. Cardiovasc Surg. 1997;5(1):54–64.
81. Parodi JC, Palmaz JC, Barone HD. Transfemoral intraluminal graft implantation for abdominal aortic aneurysms. Ann Vasc Surg. 1991;5(6):491–9.
82. Zarins CK, White RA, Schwarten D, et al. AneuRx stent graft versus open surgical repair of abdominal aortic aneurysms: multicenter prospective clinical trial. J Vasc Surg. 1999;29(2):292–305; discussion 306–298.
83. participants Et. Endovascular aneurysm repair and outcome in patients unfit for open repair of abdominal aortic aneurysm (EVAR trial 2): randomised controlled trial. Lancet. 2005;365(9478):2187–92.
84. Lifeline registry of EVAR Publications Committee. Endovascular aneurysm repair: long-term primary outcome measures. J Vasc Surg. 2005;42(1):1–10.
85. Brewster DC, Geller SC, Kaufman JA, et al. Initial experience with endovascular aneurysm repair: comparison of early results with outcome of conventional open repair. J Vasc Surg. 27(6):992–1003; discussion 1004–1005.
86. Blankensteijn JD, de Jong SE, Prinssen M, et al. Two-year outcomes after conventional or endovascular repair of abdominal aortic aneurysms. N Engl J Med. 2005;352(23):2398–405.
87. Greenhalgh RM, Brown LC, Kwong GP, Powell JT, Thompson SG, participants Et. Comparison of endovascular aneurysm repair with open repair in patients with abdominal aortic aneurysm (EVAR trial 1), 30-day operative mortality results: randomised controlled trial. Lancet. 2004;364(9437):843–8.
88. Lederle FA, Kyriakides TC, Stroupe KT, et al. Open versus endovascular repair of abdominal aortic aneurysm. N Engl J Med. 2019;380(22):2126–35.
89. Patel RSM, Powell JT, Greenhalgh RM. Endovascular versus open repair of abdominal aortic aneurysm in 15-years' follow-up of the UK endovascular aneurysm repair trial 1 (EVAR trial 1): a randomised controlled trial. Lancet. 2016;388:2366–74.

90. van Schaik TG, Yeung KK, Verhagen HJ, et al. Long-term survival and secondary procedures after open or endovascular repair of abdominal aortic aneurysms. J Vasc Surg. 2017;66(5):1379–89.
91. Conrad MF, Crawford RS, Pedraza JD, et al. Long-term durability of open abdominal aortic aneurysm repair. J Vasc Surg. 2007;46(4):669–75.
92. Hertzer NR, Mascha EJ, Karafa MT, O'Hara PJ, Krajewski LP, Beven EG. Open infrarenal abdominal aortic aneurysm repair: the Cleveland Clinic experience from 1989 to 1998. J Vasc Surg. 2002;35(6):1145–54.
93. Dansey KD, Varkevisser RRB, Swerdlow NJ, et al. Epidemiology of endovascular and open repair for abdominal aortic aneurysms in the United States from 2004 to 2015 and implications for screening. J Vasc Surg. 2021;74(2):414–24.
94. LaCroix H. The optimal surgical approach for elective reconstruction of the infra. ACTA Biomed Lovaniensia. 1997;157:1–131.
95. Sicard GA, Reilly JM, Rubin BG, et al. Transabdominal versus retroperitoneal incision for abdominal aortic surgery: report of a prospective randomized trial. J Vasc Surg. 1995;21(2):174–81; discussion 181–173.
96. Buck DB, Ultee KHT, Zettervall SL, et al. Transperitoneal vs. retroperitoneal approach for open abdominal aortic aneurysm repair in the targeted vascular NSQIP. J Vasc Surg. 2016;64(3):585–91.
97. Mei F, Hu K, Zhao B, et al. Retroperitoneal versus transperitoneal approach for elective open abdominal aortic aneurysm repair. Cochrane Database Syst Rev. 2021;6:CD010373.
98. Sieunarine K, Lawrence-Brown MM, Goodman MA. Comparison of transperitoneal and retroperitoneal approaches for infrarenal aortic surgery: early and late results. Cardiovasc Surg. 1997;5(1):71–6.
99. Cambria RP, Brewster DC, Abbott WM, et al. Transperitoneal versus retroperitoneal approach for aortic reconstruction: a randomized prospective study. J Vasc Surg. 1990;11(2):314–24; discussion 324–315.
100. Bardia A, Sood A, Mahmood F, et al. Combined epidural-general anesthesia vs general anesthesia alone for elective abdominal aortic aneurysm repair. JAMA Surg. 2016;151(12):1116–23.
101. York JW, Money SR. Prevention and management of ureteral injuries during aortic surgery. Semin Vasc Surg. 2001;14(4):266–74.
102. Wirth G, Moccia R, Clement Darling R 3rd, et al. Aortoiliac reconstruction: the retroperitoneal approach and splenic injury. Ann Vasc Surg. 2003;17(6):604–7.
103. Ali ZA, Callaghan CJ, Ali AA, et al. Perioperative myocardial injury after elective open abdominal aortic aneurysm repair predicts outcome. Eur J Vasc Endovasc Surg. 2008;35(4):413–9.
104. Elkouri S, Gloviczki P, McKusick MA, et al. Perioperative complications and early outcome after endovascular and open surgical repair of abdominal aortic aneurysms. J Vasc Surg. 2004;39(3):497–505.
105. Stone DH, Goodney PP, Kalish J, et al. Severity of chronic obstructive pulmonary disease is associated with adverse outcomes in patients undergoing elective abdominal aortic aneurysm repair. J Vasc Surg. 2013;57(6):1531–6.
106. McArdle GT, Price G, Lewis A, et al. Positive fluid balance is associated with complications after elective open infrarenal abdominal aortic aneurysm repair. Eur J Vasc Endovasc Surg. 2007;34(5):522–7.
107. Zettervall SL, Ultee KHJ, Soden PA, et al. Predictors of renal dysfunction after endovascular and open repair of abdominal aortic aneurysms. J Vasc Surg. 2017;65(4):991–6.
108. Hobson C, Ozrazgat-Baslanti T, Kuxhausen A, et al. Cost and mortality associated with postoperative acute kidney injury. Ann Surg. 2015;261(6):1207–14.
109. Grant SWGA, Grant MJ, Purkayastha D, McCollum CN. What are the risk factors for renal failure following open elective abdominal aortic aneurysm repair? Eur J Vasc Endovasc Surg. 2012;43(2):182–7.
110. Miller DC, Myers BD. Pathophysiology and prevention of acute renal failure associated with thoracoabdominal or abdominal aortic surgery. J Vasc Surg. 1987;5(3):518–23.

111. West CA, Noel AA, Bower TC, et al. Factors affecting outcomes of open surgical repair of pararenal aortic aneurysms: a 10-year experience. J Vasc Surg. 2006;43(5):921–7; discussion 927–928.
112. Brewster DC, Franklin DP, Cambria RP, et al. Intestinal ischemia complicating abdominal aortic surgery. Surgery. 1991;109(4):447–54.
113. Bjorck M, Bergqvist D, Troeng T. Incidence and clinical presentation of bowel ischaemia after aortoiliac surgery—2930 operations from a population-based registry in Sweden. Eur J Vasc Endovasc Surg. 1996;12(2):139–44.
114. Longo WE, Lee TC, Barnett MG, et al. Ischemic colitis complicating abdominal aortic aneurysm surgery in the U.S. veteran. J Surg Res. 1996;60(2):351–4.
115. Levison JA, Halpern VJ, Kline RG, Faust GR, Cohen JR. Perioperative predictors of colonic ischemia after ruptured abdominal aortic aneurysm. J Vasc Surg. 1999;29(1):40–5; discussion 45–47.
116. Pittaluga P, Batt M, Hassen-Khodja R, Declemy S, Le Bas P. Revascularization of internal iliac arteries during aortoiliac surgery: a multicenter study. Ann Vasc Surg. 1998;12(6):537–43.
117. Van Damme H, Creemers E, Limet R. Ischaemic colitis following aortoiliac surgery. Acta Chir Belg. 2000;100(1):21–7.
118. Bast TJ, van der Biezen JJ, Scherpenisse J, Eikelboom BC. Ischaemic disease of the colon and rectum after surgery for abdominal aortic aneurysm: a prospective study of the incidence and risk factors. Eur J Vasc Surg. 1990;4(3):253–7.
119. Ultee KH, Zettervall SL, Soden PA, et al. Incidence of and risk factors for bowel ischemia after abdominal aortic aneurysm repair. J Vasc Surg. 2016;64(5):1384–91.
120. Kudo T. Surgical complications after open abdominal aortic aneurysm repair: intestinal ischemia, buttock claudication and sexual dysfunction. Ann Vasc Dis. 2019;12(2):157–62.
121. Brandt CP, Piotrowski JJ, Alexander JJ. Flexible sigmoidoscopy. A reliable determinant of colonic ischemia following ruptured abdominal aortic aneurysm. Surg Endosc. 1997;11(2):113–5.
122. Boley SJ, Brandt LJ, Veith FJ. Ischemic disorders of the intestines. Curr Probl Surg. 1978;15(4):1–85.
123. Boley SJ. 1989 David H. Sun lecture. Colonic ischemia—25 years later. Am J Gastroenterol. 1990;85(8):931–4.
124. Batt M, Ricco JB, Staccini P. Do internal iliac arteries contribute to vascularization of the descending colon during abdominal aortic aneurysm surgery? Ann Vasc Surg. 2001;15(2):171–4.
125. Kuttila K, Perttila J, Vanttinen E, Niinikoski J. Tonometric assessment of sigmoid perfusion during aortobifemoral reconstruction for arteriosclerosis. Eur J Surg. 1994;160(9):491–5.
126. Schiedler MG, Cutler BS, Fiddian-Green RG. Sigmoid intramural pH for prediction of ischemic colitis during aortic surgery. A comparison with risk factors and inferior mesenteric artery stump pressures. Arch Surg. 1987;122(8):881–6.
127. Behrendt CA, Dayama A, Debus ES, et al. Lower extremity ischemia after abdominal aortic aneurysm repair. Ann Vasc Surg. 2017;45:206–12.
128. Lederle FA, Johnson GR, Wilson SE, et al. Quality of life, impotence, and activity level in a randomized trial of immediate repair versus surveillance of small abdominal aortic aneurysm. J Vasc Surg. 2003;38(4):745–52.
129. Flanigan DP, Schuler JJ, Keifer T, Schwartz JA, Lim LT. Elimination of iatrogenic impotence and improvement of sexual function after aortoiliac revascularization. Arch Surg. 1982;117(5):544–50.
130. Weinstein MH, Machleder HI. Sexual function after aorto-lliac surgery. Ann Surg. 1975;181(6):787–90.
131. Rosenthal D. Spinal cord ischemia after abdominal aortic operation: is it preventable? J Vasc Surg. 1999;30(3):391–7.

Chapter 17
Endovascular Aneurysm Repair

James H. Black III

Introduction

The treatment of abdominal aortic aneurysms (AAA) has been transformed since the first endovascular abdominal aortic aneurysm repair (EVAR) in 1991 [1]. EVAR offers shorter hospitalizations and improved short-term morbidity and mortality rates than traditional open surgical repair (OSR), particularly in the elderly [2]. EVAR has also been shown to decrease aneurysm-related mortality compared to no intervention in patients deemed too ill to undergo OSR [3]. Despite some of the advantages, however, EVAR does have a number of known complications, some that are particular to the endovascular approach and some that are shared with OSR, especially in a patient population frequently afflicted with a heavy comorbidity burden. These complications encompass the entire spectrum, from transient, minor problems to those that threaten life and limb. To identify such complications, it is mandatory that EVAR patients have regular postoperative surveillance.

Selection for AAA Repair

Most patients with abdominal aortic aneurysms are asymptomatic at the time of their diagnosis. For these patients, surveillance of their aneurysm is appropriate. The most common modality for AAA surveillance is ultrasound of the aorta (Fig. 17.1), and this modality is recommended for all male patients >65 years of age with a history of tobacco abuse, during their "Welcome to Medicare Examination."

J. H. Black III (✉)
Division of Vascular Surgery and Endovascular Therapy, Johns Hopkins Hospital, Baltimore, MD, USA
e-mail: jhblack@jhmi.edu

G. J. Arnaoutakis et al. (eds.), *Aortic Aneurysms*, Contemporary Cardiology, https://doi.org/10.1007/978-3-032-13134-8_17

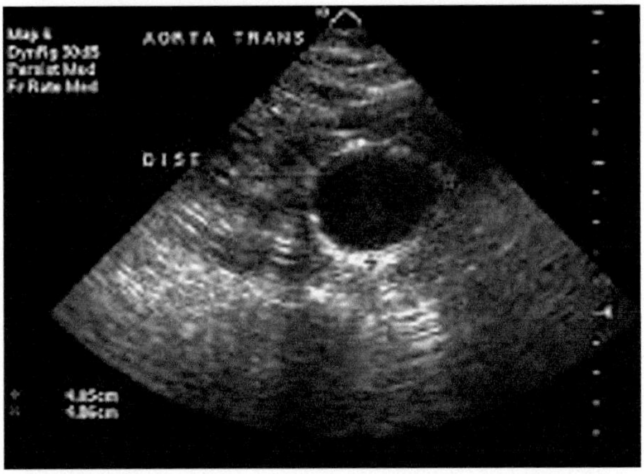

Fig. 17.1 Ultrasound duplex image of AAA. The diameter assessment requires the ultrasonographer to ensure the window is orthogonal for a correct measurement. If the anterior wall of the AAA is very calcified, this may shadow the posterior wall, but a lateral-lateral measurement is usually possible

Screening of women has not been recommended, based on lack of available evidence. For patients whose aorta measures between 3 and 4 cm in size, surveillance duplex every 2–3 years is appropriate. When the aneurysm is between 4 and 5 cm in diameter, duplex evaluation annually is appropriate. Once the aneurysm is greater than 5 cm in size, endovascular aneurysm can be considered, particularly if the aneurysm anatomy is suitable for such devices. OSR is considered when the aneurysm diameter is 5.5 cm or greater. Although many published series for endovascular AAA repair include patients with small AAA, findings of randomized clinical trials showed that, compared with surveillance by CT or ultrasonography, a strategy of immediate repair did not improve survival among patients who had AAA of 4–5.4 cm in diameter [4, 5]. Preoperative risk assessment is informed by a number or risk calculators from the Vascular Quality Initiative (https://www.vqi.org/resources/vqi-risk-calculators-2/). These calculators can be used to inform patients in the process of shared decision-making in EVAR timing. Optimization of patients for EVAR is generally accepted however, aggressive cardiac interventions before aneurysm repair have not proven more effective than medical management for most patients [6].

Symptomatic AAA usually requires urgent treatment. The most common misdiagnosis of a AAA that is symptomatic is that of renal colic [7]. Since the pain constellation is similar with a throbbing and pulsing pain in the back, flanks, and abdomen, unfortunately this misdiagnosis is common for this condition. Indeed, other gastrointestinal diagnoses such as diverticulitis and appendicitis may also engender a CT scan in which the aneurysm is then identified. For patients who are symptomatic yet not ruptured, hospitalization for blood pressure control, stabilization, and device selection is best. For patients who present with a ruptured abdominal aortic aneurysm, urgent endovascular or open surgery is appropriate, and strategies to expedite care of these patients have been shown helpful at providing excellent overall survival. Preoperative variables that indicate mortality risk for ruptured AAA EVAR are validated and include age >76, serum creatinine >2.0, pH <7.2, and blood pressure <70 mmHg at any time [8].

Anatomic Evaluation

The feasibility of endovascular repair is determined by the diameter and length of the proximal neck of the aneurysm, the tortuosity of the aorta, and the anatomy of the iliac arteries, with a goal to eliminate pressurization of the sac (Fig. 17.2). If the angle between the neck of the aneurysm and the aorta is excessive, the graft may be displaced from its intended position with a subsequent leak at the attachment site. If the common iliac arteries are too large, the limb of the stent may not be well apposed to the wall of the artery, and a leak at the attachment site will result. However, the recent approval of the Gore Iliac Branch Endoprosthesis has allowed dilated common iliac arteries, once too large for EVAR to now be encompassed with the EVAR. Thus, relative anatomic contraindications for EVAR include proximal neck <15 mm, infrarenal aortic neck diameter >32 mm, external iliac diameter <6 mm or >16 mm, and bilateral internal and external iliac aneurysms that preclude secure distal fixation or usage of the iliac branch devices.

Patients considered for EVAR must undergo preoperative imaging to assess anatomy. CT with thin cuts of the abdomen and pelvis and subsequent multiplanar reconstruction is used for operative planning including device selection and sizing (Fig. 17.3). Anatomic and technical criteria must be fulfilled to enable EVAR to be

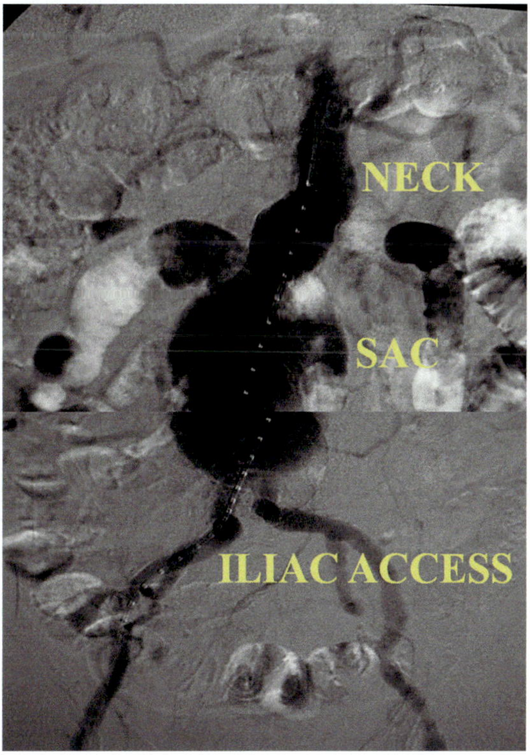

Fig. 17.2 The key areas for assessment are the neck diameter, the sac diameter, and the iliac vessels for access issues with the 16-22F arterial sheaths for EVAR

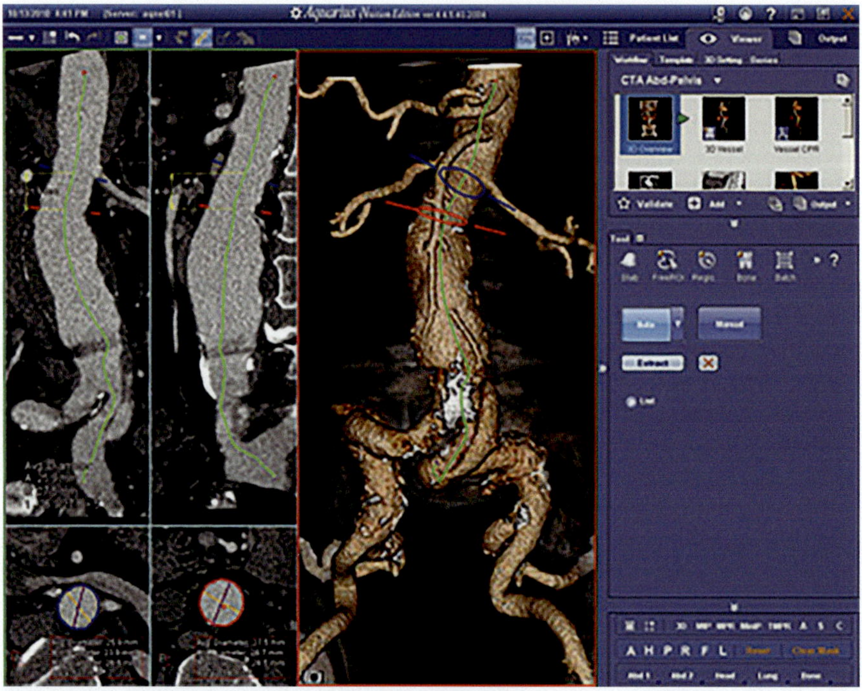

Fig. 17.3 Multiplanar and three-dimensional imaging can assess in determination of device suitability for EVAR. Such reconstructions are not mandatory, but may aid the assessment of vessel tortuosity

performed successfully. Inadequate proximal neck anatomy is one of the most common reasons why patients are found unsuitable for EVAR. Ideally, an infrarenal neck length of at least 10–15 mm from the lowest renal artery is required for adequate proximal device fixation. Graft diameter is usually oversized by approximately 10–15% to ensure adequate radial forces to prevent migration and allow good apposition to the aortic wall. Current commercially available devices range up to 36 mm in diameter, therefore an aortic neck diameter <32 mm is necessary for adequate fixation. An ideal neck should have minimal thrombus and calcification so that proximal fixation is easier and decrease the risk for migration or type I endoleaks (blood surging around stent into the AAA). Aortic neck angulation greater than 60 degrees can lead to imprecise proximal placement with kinking and poor fixation and is considered a relative contraindication to EVAR. Treatment of aneurysms with neck angle greater than 60 degrees is determined by the conformability of the specific device or fenestrated/branched endovascular technology may be considered.

Approach to EVAR Performance

A percutaneous approach to insertion of the endovascular devices is preferred by our team. Percutaneous approach to EVAR is associated with improved time to hemostasis, earlier ambulation of the patient, and has yielded a reduction in length of stay of 1–2 days since implementation [9]. Percutaneous access is obtained with ultrasound guidance to ensure that the entry point is directly anterior on a suitable diameter common femoral vessel. Bulky plaque posteriorly, or even plaque present on the anterior femoral wall may be a contraindication to considering a percutaneous approach. Once access is obtained, percutaneous sutures are placed in 2 locations, in a crisscross pattern, to facilitate later hemostasis. Thereafter, a large diameter sheath is inserted over a Lunderquist wire or a similarly stiff wire to the approximate level of the renal arteries and an angiogram is performed (Fig. 17.4).

Once the proximal fixation zone is confirmed by angiography, the device is deployed to the level of the contralateral gate. The cannulation of the endovascular gate is performed from the contralateral access, using a catheter and wire combination. It is critical to confirm the catheter has passed into the main body of the device, otherwise the iliac limb endograft will be deployed outside the main body of the device. Methods to confirm proper cannulation into the main body include angiography (Fig. 17.5) or inflation of a balloon in the gate and examination in several projections. Insertion of the contralateral iliac endograft is performed next. Since most devices have multiple device length options, an angiogram to identify the hypogastric artery and the proximal gate is performed. This angiogram should also include a marker catheter, so the length from the proximal endograft to the

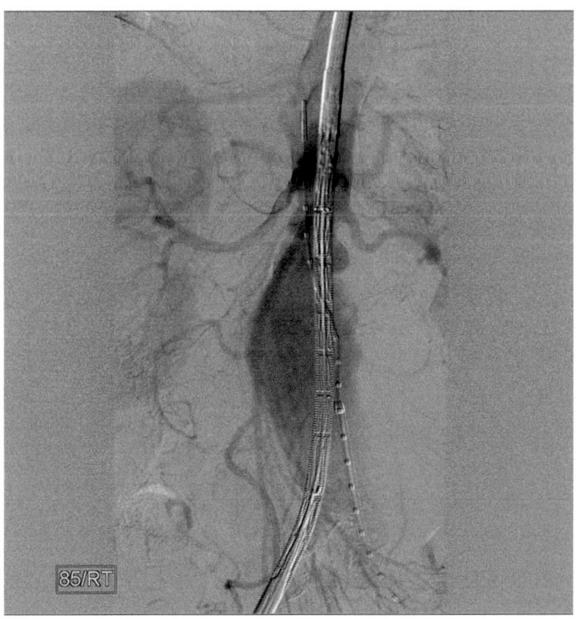

Fig. 17.4 The endograft delivery system is located in the area of the AAA neck, with the intention to land the device deployment at the lower edge of the lowest renal artery

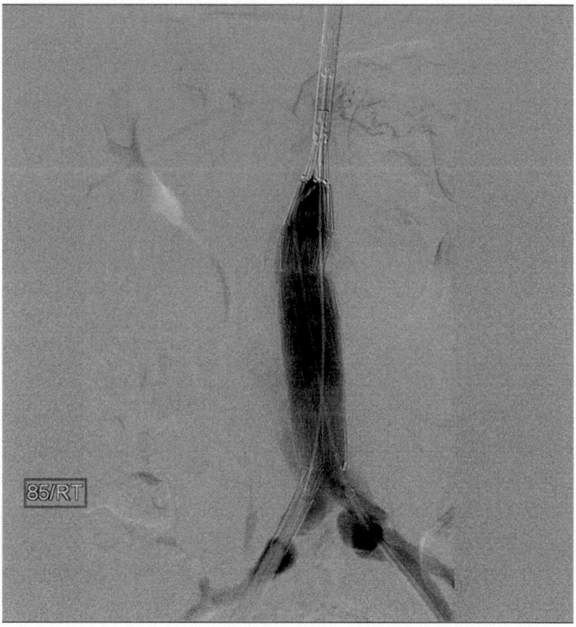

Fig. 17.5 The main body of the endograft is deployed to allow partial opening and access to the contralateral gate of the device. Thereafter, the gate is cannulated from the other femoral access, and proper passage into the main body is confirmed

hypogastric artery can be measured easily (Fig. 17.6). A similar series of steps is performed to complete the ipsilateral deployment and additional iliac extension deployment as needed. Once the endovascular components are completely deployed,

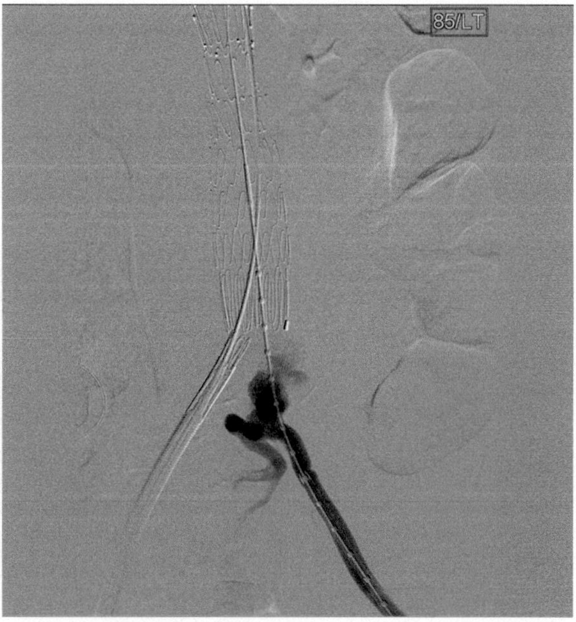

Fig. 17.6 The contralateral iliac endograft is planned by sizing the length of the device with a retrograde angiogram from the femoral sheath. The iliac endograft diameter is chosen by assessment

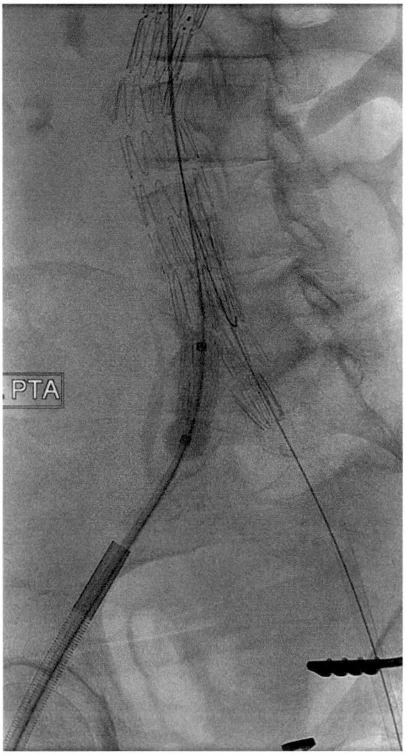

Fig. 17.7 Once the endograft components are completely deployed, the areas of proximal fixation, device overlaps, and the iliac fixation are gently dilated with a compliant balloon. The shoulders of the balloon should not extend beyond the stent-graft edges, to avoid damaging the vessel or embolizing neighboring atheroma

gentle dilation using a compliant balloon is performed to mold the endograft into the proximal aortic neck and the distal iliac fixation zones (Fig. 17.7). Additionally, the overlap of the iliac devices with main aortic device should also be dilated with compliant balloons to reduce their risk of migration apart. A final angiogram of the device and its components is performed via catheter angiography; this step serves to confirm the device is located close to lowest renal artery and the hypogastric origins. The more delayed phases of the final angiogram can also identify endoleaks, particularly type 2 endoleaks where the lumbar arteries are noted to fill the AAA sac (Fig. 17.8).

Endoleak

Endoleak, a complication unique to endovascular aneurysm repair, is defined as persistent blood entry into the aneurysm sac following EVAR, and is discussed in detail in a separate chapter. This all-too-common complication results in continued pressurization of the aneurysm sac, placing the patient at risk for continued aneurysm growth and rupture. Endoleaks are classified into five categories (Fig. 17.9) types I through IV and endotension (sometimes referred to as type V endoleak), and

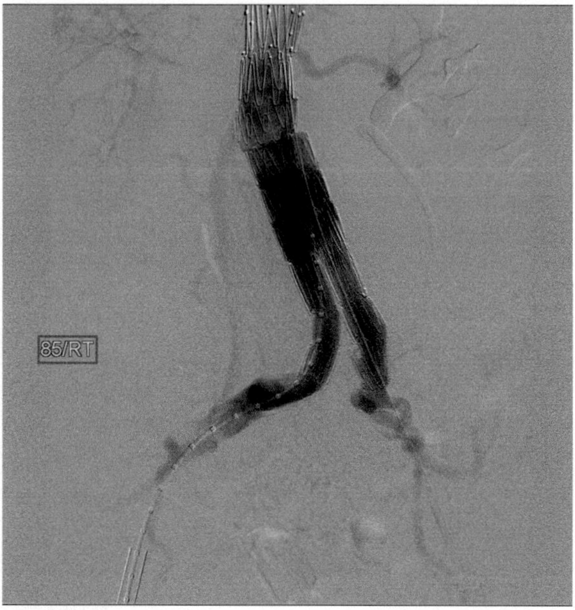

Fig. 17.8 Final angiography during EVAR is chiefly performed to rule out major endoleaks (type 1 and type 3), confirm no impingement on renal artery or hypogastric origins, and to confirm the AAA sac is excluded. Type 2 endoleaks do not require intervention during the initial EVAR procedure

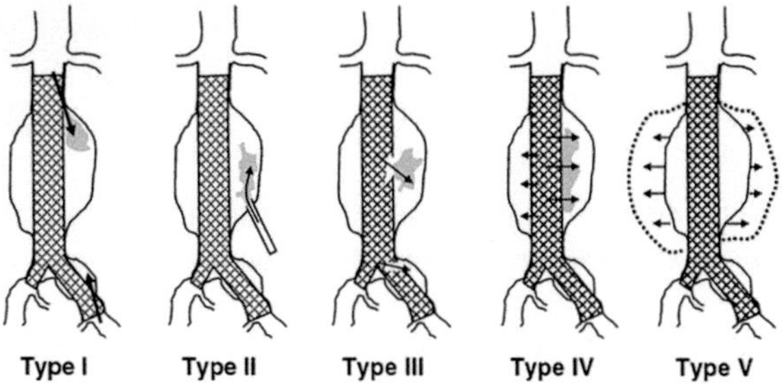

Fig. 17.9 Figure of endoleaks Types 1–5

the categories aid in determining the appropriate treatment and its urgency. Endoleaks can be seen at the time of device delivery and at any time thereafter. Endoleak rates as high as 50% at 2 years have been reported [10]. Because of these concerns, patients do require routine surveillance. While the optimal surveillance regimen is still debated, there is mounting evidence that ultrasonography may be able to supplant to some degree computerized tomography (CT), the current gold standard, to minimize intravenous contrast and radiation exposures. A meta-analysis of studies comparing the imaging modalities found that duplex ultrasound is only 77% sensitive and 94% specific compared to CT, but that non-nephrotoxic contrast-enhanced ultrasound is 98% sensitive and 88% specific in detecting endoleak [11].

Type I Endoleak

Type I endoleak occurs when there is an incomplete seal between the stent graft device and the native vessel, either at the proximal (type Ia) or distal (type Ib) attachment site, resulting in continued blood flow into the aneurysm sac and concomitant sac growth. Type I endoleaks typically are encountered at the time of EVAR placement and in the early post-procedure period, though they can develop later. They represent a continued risk for aneurysm rupture and treatment is generally mandated. Initial treatment of either type Ia or Ib endoleaks usually consists of balloon angioplasty to approximate more fully the device to the vessel in an attempt to exclude the aneurysm from blood flow. If that fails, type Ia endoleaks can be treated with a Palmaz stent placement (Cordis Corporation; Miami Lakes, FL) and Ib endoleaks can be remedied by deploying an extension aortic cuff or iliac limb.

Type II Endoleak

Type II endoleak results from persistent retrograde blood flow into the aneurysm sac secondary to collateral vessels, usually the inferior mesenteric artery or patent lumbar arteries. These can present at any point after EVAR, and the optimal management remains controversial. Steinmetz and colleagues have advocated a conservative approach to the management as over 60% of these endoleaks will resolve spontaneously, only 1% are associated with aneurysm sac enlargement, and the presence of a type II endoleak does not alter survival at 48 months [11]. For those type II endoleaks that are apparent immediately at the time of the procedure, the discontinuation of anticoagulation at the end of the procedure will frequently cause a spontaneous resolution of the leak. Treatment is indicated for symptoms (abdominal or back pain) or in the setting of continued aneurysm growth. Interventions range from embolization to surgical ligation of the culprit vessel.

Type III Endoleak

Blood flow through a tear or rupture in the fabric of the graft or flow between separated components of the graft is a type III endoleak. The natural history of continued aneurysm sac growth and increased risk of rupture is similar to that of type I endoleak, necessitating an intervention. Treatment entails the placement of a cuff or redeployment of a stent within the stent to cover the tear in the fabric. Component separation is best appreciated using multiple plain-view radiographs.

Type IV Endoleak

Type IV endoleak, a rather rare finding, especially in contemporary stent graft devices, is the passage of blood through the graft fabric and is related to the graft's porosity. It is most apparent in fully anticoagulated patients and, as with type II endoleak, will often resolve once the anticoagulation has been discontinued. Type IV endoleak was mostly seen in the high-porosity Excluder device (W. L. Gore and Associates, Flagstaff, AZ) which has since been redesigned to eliminate this issue.

Type V Endoleak (Endotension)

Type V endoleak, more commonly called endotension, refers to persistently elevated intra-aneurysmal sac pressure in the absence of an endoleak on delayed contrast CT scan. A number of theories exist to explain the etiology of endotension, which underscores the uncertainty surrounding this phenomenon and the appropriate methods of diagnosing and treating it. For example, it has been proposed that endotension results from endoleak that is so slow in nature as to be invisible to current radiographic techniques. Others advocate that the aneurysm growth results from pressure transmitted across thrombus, whether the thrombus is within occluded vessels that communicate with the sac or clot that sits between the aortic wall and the stent graft. Endotension affects 5.4% of EVAR patients [12], and is usually asymptomatic, though it can occasionally present with symptoms of mass effect, such as abdominal pain and constipation. While rupture is rare, rapid aneurysm growth and/or symptoms attributable to the enlarged sac are indications for intervention. A variety of repair methods have been described, including OSR and relining the stent graft with another stent graft via an endovascular approach.

Results of Randomized Trials

Randomized trials successfully showed the perioperative advantages of EVAR over open repair, but there is still debate regarding the long-term advantages of EVAR. The midterm data from the DREAM (Dutch Randomized Endovascular Aneurysm Trial) trial obtained at the 2-year follow-up appear to suggest that the initial perioperative advantages of EVAR may not be maintained over time [13]. The overall survival rate 2 years after randomization was 89.7% for patients undergoing EVAR compared with 89.6% for those undergoing open repair. Quality of life improved initially for EVAR, but after 6 months, it was equivalent for both groups. The authors concluded that the initial mortality advantage of EVAR over open was lost by 1 year because of nonaneurysm-related deaths. The midterm data from EVAR 1ctrial drew similar conclusions [14]. All-cause mortality 4 years after randomization was similar between patients undergoing EVAR and patients undergoing open repair at approximately 28%. Additionally, both studies showed significantly higher rates of reintervention after EVAR compared with open repair (20% vs 6% in EVAR 1 and a nearly three times higher rate in the DREAM trial). Given the short-term and mid-term data produced by these trials, a question remains with regard to the long-term advantages of EVAR over open surgery. In particular, the questions of whether survival will be different over the long term compared with patients undergoing open repair and if EVAR will prove to be cost-effective given the higher rates of reintervention.

The OVER Trial (Open Versus Endovascular Aneurysm Repair Trial) has the advantage of being more modern than DREAM and EVAR-1 trials. Thus, OVER did not include first-generation endografts that were known to have high rates of mechanical issues. In the last analysis of OVER [15], similar to other trials, endovascular repair conferred a perioperative survival advantage that continued for several years and then disappeared because of increased deaths in the endovascular-repair groups. The important questions are, what caused these later deaths in the endovascular-repair groups, and would the trend continue, with the result that endovascular repair would become the inferior strategy? The first question remains unanswered, but the most widely accepted explanation is that the perioperative deaths after open repair most likely occurred in the frailest patients, so the curves converged as later deaths occurred in the frailest patients in the endovascular-repair groups.

Conclusion

The treatment of aneurysmal disease of the aorta has been revolutionized with the advent of endovascular technologies; however, certain complications of EVAR remain problematic, such as endoleaks and concerns of device durability. There is clinical equipoise as to how best to treat type 2 endoleaks, but other device issues may require open surgical conversion in the long-term timeframe. Surveillance and treatment algorithms emphasize the critical need for long-term imaging to improve outcomes for patients after EVAR.

References

1. Parodi JC, Palmaz JC, Barone HD. Transfemoral intraluminal graft implantation for abdominal aortic aneurysms. Ann Vasc Surg. 1991;5(6):491–9.
2. Schermerhorn ML, O'Malley AJ, Jhaveri A, Cotterill P, Pomposelli F, Landon BE. Endovascular vs. open repair of abdominal aortic aneurysms in the Medicare population. N Engl J Med. 2008;358(5):464–74.

3. Greenhalgh RM, Brown LC, Powell JT, Thompson SG, Epstein D. Endovascular repair of aortic aneurysm in patients physically ineligible for open repair. N Engl J Med. 2010;362(20):1872–80.
4. Mortality results for randomised controlled trial of early elective surgery or ultra-sonographic surveillance for small abdominal aortic aneurysms. The UK Small Aneurysm Trial Participants. Lancet. 1998;352(9141):1649–55.
5. Lederle FA, et al. Immediate repair compared with surveillance of small abdominal aortic aneurysms. N Engl J Med. 2002;346(19):1437–44.
6. McFalls EO, Ward HB, Moritz TE, Goldman S, Krupski WC, Littooy F, Pierpont G, Santilli S, Rapp J, Hattler B, Shunk K, Jaenicke C, Thottapurathu L, Ellis N, Reda DJ, Henderson WG. Coronary-artery revascularization before elective major vascular surgery. N Engl J Med. 2004;351(27):2795–804. https://doi.org/10.1056/NEJMoa041905. PMID: 15625331.
7. Marston WA, Ahlquist R, Johnson J. Misdiagnosis of ruptured abdominal aortic aneurysms. J Vasc Surg. 1992;16:17–22.
8. Garland BT, Danaher PJ, Desikan S, Tran NT, Quiroga E, Singh N, Starnes BW. Preoperative risk score for the prediction of mortality after repair of ruptured abdominal aortic aneurysms. J Vasc Surg. 2018;68(4):991–7. https://doi.org/10.1016/j.jvs.2017.12.075. Epub 2018 May 9. Erratum in: J Vasc Surg. 2018;68(5):1623. PMID: 29753581.
9. Nelson PR, Kracjer Z, Kansal N, Rao V, Bianchi C, Hashemi H, Jones P, Bacharach JM. A multicenter, randomized, controlled trial of totally percutaneous access versus open femoral exposure for endovascular aortic aneurysm repair (the PEVAR trial). J Vasc Surg. 2014;59(5):1181–93. https://doi.org/10.1016/j.jvs.2013.10.101. Epub 2014 Jan 17. PMID: 24440678.
10. Parent FN, Meier GH, Godziachvili V, LeSar CJ, Parker FM, Carter KA, et al. The incidence and natural history of type I and II endoleak: a 5-year follow-up assessment with color duplex ultrasound scan. J Vasc Surg. 2002;35(3):474–81.
11. Steinmetz E, Rubin BG, Sanchez LA, Choi ET, Geraghty PJ, Baty J, et al. Type II endoleak after endovascular abdominal aortic aneurysm repair: a conservative approach with selective intervention is safe and cost-effective. J Vasc Surg. 2004;39(2):306–13.
12. Toya N, Fujita T, Kanaoka Y, Ohki T. Endotension following endovascular aneurysm repair. Vasc Med. 2008;13(4):305–11.
13. Prinssen M, Verhoeven EL, Buth J, Cuypers PW, van Sambeek MR, Balm R, Aneurysm Management (DREAM)Trial Group. A randomized trial comparing conventional and endovascular repair of abdominal aortic aneurysms. N Engl J Med. 2004;351(16):1607–18.
14. EVAR trial participants. Endovascular aneurysm repair versus open repair in patients with abdominal aortic aneurysm (EVAR trial 1): randomised controlled trial. Lancet. 2005;365(9478):2179–86.
15. Lederle FA, Kyriakides TC, Stroupe KT, Freischlag JA, Padberg FT Jr, Matsumura JS, Huo Z, Johnson GR. OVER Veterans Affairs Cooperative Study Group. Open versus endovascular repair of abdominal aortic aneurysm. N Engl J Med. 2019;380(22):2126–35. https://doi.org/10.1056/NEJMoa1715955. PMID: 31141634.

Chapter 18
Complications and Secondary Interventions After Elective Endovascular Aneurysm Repair

Michael J. Singh and Nathan L. Liang

Introduction

Device-related complications after endovascular aneurysm may originate from a variety of sources including failure of sealing or aneurysm exclusion, problems with the actual device itself, disruption in the flow through the graft from stenosis or occlusion, or from external factors such as infection. Identification of these complications and recognizing the need for operative intervention is a critical skill in the toolbox of the aortic interventionalist.

Endoleaks and Failure of Endograft Sealing

The most often studied or anticipated modality of device failure is the loss of seal and failure of endograft exclusion of blood flow. As the endograft works by excluding pressurized arterial flow from entering the aneurysm through the proximal and distal sealing zones, disruption of these seals and repressurization of the aneurysm represents a regression back to an unrepaired state with similar risks of aneurysm growth and rupture.

Any flow of arterial blood into the aneurysm sac, including those causing repressurization of the aneurysm, is termed an "endoleak." Endoleaks present from a variety of sources but may not always lead to immediate sac repressurization. Endoleaks

M. J. Singh (✉)
UPMC Presbytarian/Shadyside, UPMC Heart and Vascular Institute, Pittsburgh, PA, USA
e-mail: singhmj@upmc.edu

N. L. Liang
UPMC Presbyterian/Shadyside, Pittsburgh, PA, USA
e-mail: Liangnl@upmc.edu

G. J. Arnaoutakis et al. (eds.), *Aortic Aneurysms*, Contemporary Cardiology,
https://doi.org/10.1007/978-3-032-13134-8_18

Table 18.1 Types of endoleak

	Description
Type 1	Flow from disruption of proximal or distal seal zone
Type 1a	Proximal seal
Type 1b	Distal seal
Type 2	Retrograde flow from aneurysm side branches including lumbar and inferior mesenteric arteries
Type 3	Flow through a graft defect due to fabric failure or component separation
Type 4	Graft wall porosity

are currently classified into four major categories (Table 18.1) [1, 2]. Three of these (Types 1–3) have the potential to cause further complications requiring reintervention and will be discussed here.

Diagnostic Modalities for Endoleak

Endoleaks are best visualized using contrasted studies. Intraprocedural angiography with digital subtraction (DSA) and power injection can demonstrate endoleaks as contrast filling the aneurysm sac outside of the endograft. This also allows for visualization of very delayed filling if a prolonged exposure is taken. However, due to the two-dimensional nature of traditional angiography, an endoleak may be missed if subtle and overlying the area of contrast already filling the endograft. The standard modalities for evaluation of endoleaks in the postoperative period are computed tomographic angiography (CTA) and duplex ultrasound (DUS) [1, 2].

Endoleaks are often evaluated using CTA as part of routine follow-up. CTA allows for noticeably clear visualization of contrast in the aneurysm sac. A delayed imaging series is critical as filling of endoleaks that depend on collaterals may fill slowly, limiting visualization on the initial arterial phase. The location of contrast can be used to estimate the type and source of arterial flow feeding this endoleak nidus. Although CTA allows for more accurate detection of contrast inside the aneurysm sac, the static nature of CT imaging does not allow for visualization of flow and can be nondiagnostic for determining the type of endoleak. For example, a small amount of contrast on CTA near the proximal seal may represent either a proximal Type 1 endoleak, or if a high lumbar is visualized, may also represent a Type 2 endoleak. Nidus locations near the proximal or distal seal zones or overlap zones of the endograft should be investigated closely for the presence of Type 1 or 3 endoleaks.

Duplex ultrasound is a third commonly used modality for evaluating endoleaks [3]. Brightness mode ultrasound is often used for in-office measurement of aneurysm size during follow-up or for surveillance. Spectral Doppler and color flow modes can be used to assess the presence of any flow within the aneurysm sac which may suggest endoleak. In certain situations, flow within the aneurysm sac may be localized, allowing the physician to distinguish between different types of endoleaks. However, duplex ultrasound evaluation of abdominal aortic aneurysms, especially post-EVAR, is highly technologist dependent and visualization is often limited by visceral fat or bowel gas. If available, duplex ultrasound should be utilized as a complementary modality alongside CT for diagnosis and evaluation of endoleaks [4].

Type 1 Endoleak

Type 1 endoleaks result from the disruption of the proximal or distal seal of the endograft. Type 1A endoleaks result from disruption of the proximal seal, whereas Type 1B endoleaks are related to disruption of the distal seal. Type 1 endoleaks are considered critical complications of the endograft as there is failure to exclude aortic blood flow from reentering the aneurysm. Type 1 endoleaks lead to repressurization of the aneurysm, eventual growth, and increased rupture risk. For this reason, the presence of a Type 1 endoleak always requires a detailed evaluation and consideration of reintervention [1, 2].

Immediate Type 1 Endoleak Type 1 endoleaks may be identified immediately following EVAR. These may be due to inadequate length of seal, but also may be due to other graft or anatomic factors leading to inadequate fabric apposition to the aortic wall including oversizing resulting in graft infolding, incomplete expansion due to calcification, or extreme aortic neck angulation. Inadequate fabric apposition to the aortic wall can often be improved by aggressive balloon dilation of the proximal seal zone, whereas inadequate length of seal most often requires extension with an aortic cuff if there is enough remaining infrarenal aorta. Occasionally, small intraprocedural Type 1 endoleaks remain due to residual anticoagulation during the procedure and may resolve once the anticoagulation has been reversed. However, all other causes of endoleak must be thoroughly investigated prior to this determination to avoid missing any correctable causes.

The introduction of endoanchors (Medtronic, Minneapolis, MN, USA) has allowed for salvage of proximal Type 1 endoleaks which may be caused by inadequate seal length. Placement of endoanchors fixes the fabric at the proximal seal zone to the aortic wall to improve permanent fabric apposition and has been utilized successfully in aneurysms with short necks up to 4 mm or hostile neck anatomy [5, 6]. However, the use of endoanchors in secondary procedures to treat proximal endoleak may carry a lower technical success rate compared to planned use during the primary procedure [7]. Although this may constitute selection bias in those who are chosen a priori to have endoanchors compared to the use of endoanchors for salvage, we recommend that hostile seal zone characteristics be accounted for in the planning stage as much as possible to avoid salvage situations.

Delayed Type 1 Endoleak Any factor causing a loss of proximal or distal seal during the follow-up period is categorized as a delayed Type 1 endoleak. The most common cause of delayed Type 1 endoleak formation is continued progression of the aneurysm to include the proximal or distal seal zones. As aneurysm formation is a degenerative condition, previously uninvolved areas of the aorta may continue to degenerate over time and eventually lead to loss of seal and a Type 1 endoleak.

Certain endograft and anatomic characteristics have been shown to increase the likelihood of aneurysmal degeneration. Most publications have focused on the identification of a "hostile neck" using multiple preoperative anatomic characteristics. These hostile neck characteristics, including large or diseased aortic necks with thrombus or calcification, are hypothesized to be representative of a diseased aneurysm neck or early aneurysmal degeneration which may continue to degenerate over time and compromise the proximal or distal seal. Multiple published studies have identified short aneurysm neck (<10 mm) as a factor associated with eventual aneurysmal degeneration [8, 9]. Similarly, a large diameter aneurysm neck has been shown to also carry an association with eventual failure of the proximal seal [9–11].

Due to the wide variation of severity and presentation of Type 1 endoleaks, difficult-to-visualize Type 1 endoleak may often be misdiagnosed as Type 2. These are often termed "occult Type 1 endoleaks", appearing benign on imaging studies but continuing to cause sac growth despite multiple attempts at treatment before being recognized as a Type 1 endoleak [12]. In our practice, suspected Type 2 endoleaks that cause significant growth or continual growth despite treatment all undergo thorough evaluation for occult Type 1 endoleak.

Treatment of delayed Type 1 endoleak depends heavily on the reason for failure of the proximal or distal seal. Extension of the graft proximally or distally may be enough to resolve the endoleak if there is sufficient landing zone. However, more complex endovascular interventions including extension with iliac branch devices, coiling of the internal iliac artery and extension to the external iliac artery, or proximal extension with parallel or fenestrated grafts may be required to obtain an adequate seal zone. Open conversion with graft explantation as a definitive repair should also be considered and discussed with the patient and family if the patient is of suitable medical risk and the durability of an endovascular repair is unclear [13].

Type 2 Endoleak Type 2 endoleaks develop due to retrograde flow of blood through aortic branches in the aneurysm. This back bleeding develops because of the altered pressure dynamics after exclusion of aortic inflow by the endograft. The most common sources of Type 2 endoleaks are the inferior mesenteric artery (IMA) and lumbar arteries. Type 2 endoleaks have been suggested in some studies to exist on postoperative imaging in up to 44% of patients after EVAR [14].

The significance of most Type 2 endoleaks is unclear. The majority appear to be small and low flow with no clear effect on the aneurysm sac. However, some may develop into high flow high-pressure arterial systems causing repressurization of the aneurysm sac and leading to sac expansion. This rarely leads to rupture, but continued aneurysm expansion may eventually cause disruption of the proximal or distal seals and development of a Type 1 endoleak.

The treatment of Type 2 endoleaks causing sac expansion is currently recommended by all societal guidelines including those from the Society for Vascular Surgery and the European Society of Vascular Surgery [1, 2]. However, treatment of Type 2 endoleaks in the absence of sac growth remains controversial. Judging the success of endoleak treatment is also controversial, with published outcome measures ranging from lack of flow on postoperative imaging to sac stability or shrinkage [14, 15].

Our approach to suspected Type 2 endoleaks causing sac expansion begins with a CT angiogram and duplex ultrasound. An angiogram is then performed to evaluate the graft and collateral pathways. A slow, high-volume power injection of contrast at the level of the superior mesenteric artery (SMA) allows for visualization of collateral pathways to the inferior mesenteric artery (IMA) and evaluation of the proximal seal. Further selective injections into the SMA and internal iliac arteries identify collateral networks feeding the IMA or low pairs of lumbar arteries that may be sources of Type 2 endoleak. If a clear Type 2 endoleak with flow into the aneurysm sac is identified, transarterial selective catheterization of the feeding vessel via collaterals with a microcatheter may be attempted (Fig. 18.1). Once the feeding vessel is successfully catheterized, selective injection is used to confirm placement of the microcatheter in the nidus of flow within the aneurysm sac. If the feeding vessel is a low lumbar, an attempt is usually made to catheterize the paired contralateral lumbar artery through the aneurysm sac, but

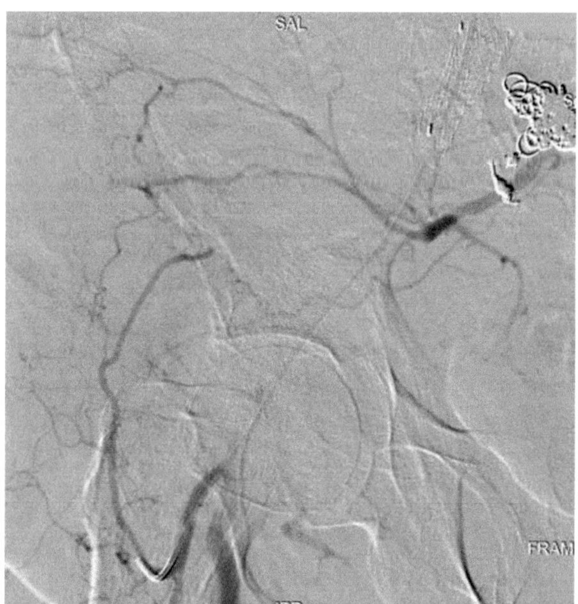

Fig. 18.1 Transarterial embolization of Type 2 endoleak. Selective catheterization of the aneurysm sac through a feeding lumbar via internal iliac artery collaterals and embolization with detachable coils

this is often not possible as maneuverability within the aneurysm sac is limited. The nidus of flow within the aneurysm sac is embolized with coils with or without other adjuncts such as liquid embolic agents or gelfoam slurry. The feeding artery is then embolized before the microcatheter is withdrawn. The transarterial approach to IMA and lumbar endoleaks has demonstrated a favorable success rate of 84% in a pooled analysis of case series [14].

IMA and low lumbar endoleaks arising from the L4 level can consistently be treated using this transarterial approach via collateral pathways. However, higher lumbar endoleaks at the L3 and occasionally L2 levels may not be reachable through collaterals and require a separate approach to access the aneurysm sac directly. If the nidus of flow within the aneurysm sac is immediately adjacent to the vena cava, a transcaval approach can provide direct sac access for embolization. In this approach, a directional sheath is brought from the common femoral vein and positioned in the inferior vena cava using bony landmarks and angled toward the aneurysm sac at the endoleak nidus as determined preoperatively by CT imaging. An endovascular needle is used to simultaneously puncture both the vena cava wall and the aneurysm sac. A catheter is then placed over a wire into the nidus, allowing for microcatheter insertion and embolization (Fig. 18.2).

Percutaneous fluoroscopy-guided direct puncture of the sac from a posterior approach is another well-established method for access to higher lumbar endoleaks. The patient is positioned supine. Bony and endograft landmarks (or fusion imaging

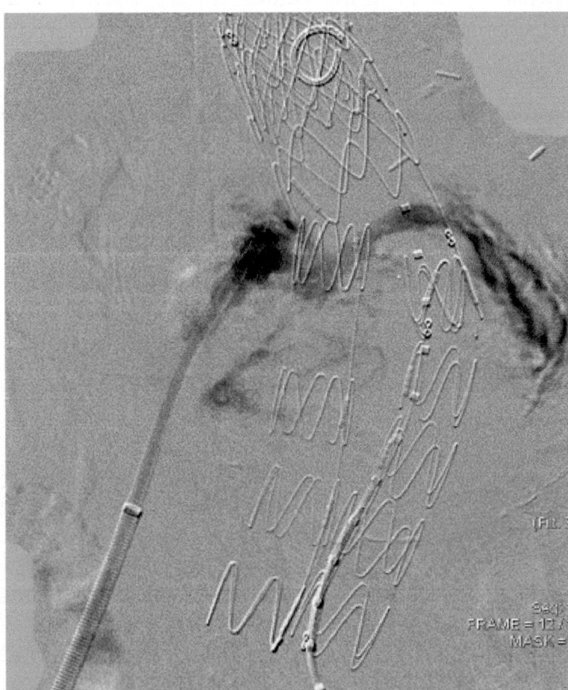

Fig. 18.2 Transcaval embolization of Type 2 endoleak. Transcaval access to endoleak nidus within the aneurysm sac using endovascular needle and embolization with detachable coils and gelfoam slurry

if available) are used to orient the direction of travel of the needle to avoid major structures based on preoperative CT imaging. A long needle is inserted percutaneously into the aneurysm sac. When using fluoroscopic guidance, we prefer to use a "gunsight" technique with the fluoroscopic c-arm gantry angle at the anticipated angle of entry, aiming toward a bony or endograft landmark visible on x-ray. Entry into the nidus is confirmed by removing the trocar of the access needle and visualizing blood return. We prefer to use a long (15–20 cm) 21-gauge needle allowing passage of an 0.018″ wire and subsequent placement of a long 4F introducer. A microcatheter is then directed into the aneurysm sac for embolization.

With either direct sac puncture method, directional manipulation of catheters inside the aneurysm sac is limited and selective catheterization and embolization of feeding vessels is often difficult. Injectable liquid embolic agents such as Onyx (Medtronic, Minneapolis, MN, USA) and n-butyl-cyanoacrylate polymerize on contact with blood and can fill the feeding vessels before setting which may improve the chances of successful embolization compared to coiling of the nidus alone [16].

Embolization for treatment of Type 2 endoleaks has demonstrated some success in arresting sac growth with pooled estimates of 78% for postoperative sac stabilization or regression. However, recurrent sac growth remains significant and has been shown to be as high as 66% on long-term follow-up [16]. Failure of endovascular treatment methods for Type 2 endoleak with continued sac growth may eventually require an open surgical approach such as laparoscopic or open ligation of lumbar arteries from within the sac or full explantation of the endograft and open reconstruction [13]. A full understanding of the significance of Type 2 endoleaks and treatment strategies remains incomplete and presents an ongoing field of study, but long-term follow-up after any intervention is critical.

Type 3 Endoleak Type 3 endoleaks result from a separation of the mechanical components of the graft in vivo. This most often happens at the overlapping portions of the different endograft components, such as separation of the contralateral iliac limb from the gate of the main body. Occasionally, failure of the graft material itself may lead to a Type 3 endoleak. This fabric fatigue and eventual failure have been demonstrated most clearly with the Endologix AFX graft. The first generation of the AFX was prone to delayed failure of the graft material even years after implantation, resulting in fabric tears in the structure of the main body leading to repressurization of the sac [17].

Type 3 endoleaks are often repaired by relining the failed or separated component with another limb or, in the case of proximal Type 3 endoleaks, relining of the entire graft with another endograft. In instances where there is no adequate seal below the renal arteries or if the separated components cannot be selectively cannulated due to wide anatomic separation, open conversion is the definitive solution (Fig. 18.3).

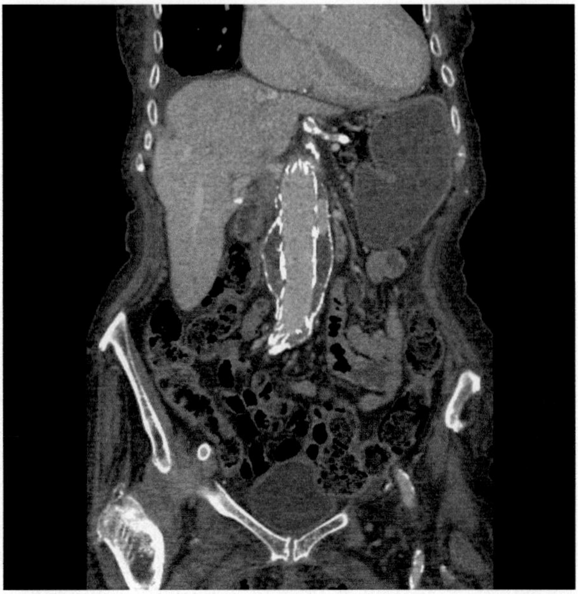

Fig. 18.3 Presence of a Type 3 endoleak from the left lateral endograft wall

Endograft Iliac Limb Complications

Barring any anatomic constriction or maldeployment, the endograft main body rarely develops significant stenosis or occlusion. However, complications of the iliac limbs are more common and are a major source of endograft failure with an incidence rate of 5.6% in a 2018 systematic review [18]. Evaluation of pooled data in this review showed that the incidence of iliac limb complications is identified early, with over half of limb occlusions occurring within the first 30 days. This study also demonstrated that the rate of iliac limb complications has decreased over time, potentially because of improvements in endograft design in recent generations. Common reasons identified for iliac limb complications include kinking of the graft, small diameter of the native iliac system, and poor outflow or residual distal disease-causing stenosis.

Kinking of the iliac limbs may happen with tortuous iliac anatomy, especially if the distal end of the limb is placed at a bend (Fig. 18.4). Stenosis may also be caused by external compression from highly calcified arteries, such as compression of both iliac limbs by a small calcified aortic bifurcation. Small-diameter native iliac systems are thought to cause limb complications due to the smaller size of the stent grafts required. This has been demonstrated in studies of low-profile devices designed for use specifically in patients with small diseased iliac arteries. Studies of these low-profile devices have consistently demonstrated higher rates of limb occlusion and complication compared to standard endograft trials [19, 20].

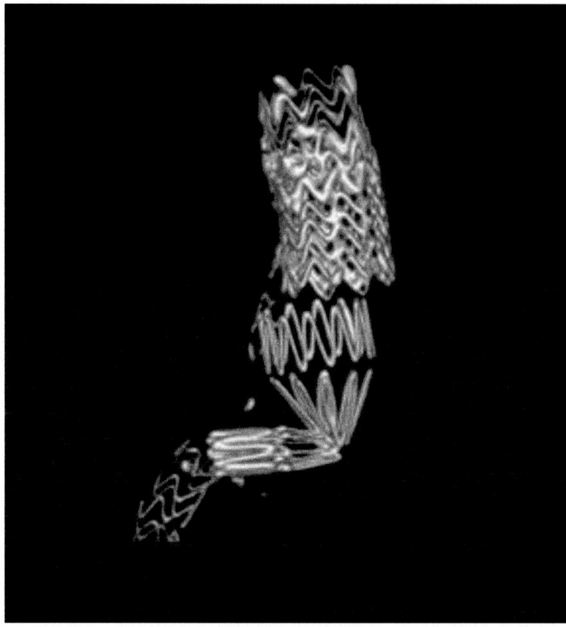

Fig. 18.4 CT scan with 3D reconstruction of aorto-uni-iliac endograft migration, separation from proximal aortic cuff, and kinking of iliac limb

Most limb complications causing stenosis can be addressed by fixing the cause of the lesion. This may be accomplished by extension of the iliac limb past any tortuous areas and landing in a straighter segment with a flexible limb extension or by aggressive balloon dilation of any calcified lesions preventing full expansion of the graft. Limb occlusions may be approached via percutaneous or open mechanical thrombectomy if acute and via percutaneous endovascular recanalization and stent relining if chronic, but the precipitating source of the occlusion must be identified and addressed, or recurrent occlusion is likely. Failure of thrombectomy or chronically occluded limbs that fail endovascular recanalization should be addressed by an extra anatomic bypass or more definitively by explantation of the endograft and direct aortofemoral reconstruction.

Endograft Infection

Aortic endograft infection is an uncommon complication after EVAR, and reports in the published literature are limited. Unlike surgical grafts placed during open aortic aneurysm repair, which result in disrupted retroperitoneal tissue planes and opening of the aneurysm sac near bowel, endovascular grafts are shielded by an intact aneurysm sac and do not often encounter bowel or other sources of visceral contamination during implantation. Potential sources of seeding for endograft infection include external contamination during implantation and bacteremia from sources such as urinary tract infections and less commonly native aortoenteric fistulas. Onset may be insidious, and symptoms may range widely from persistent abdominal pain to sepsis and even aneurysm rupture.

Aortic endograft infections may be suspected based on an atypical symptom distribution but are primarily diagnosed on imaging. Periaortic inflammation/collections or air in the aneurysm sac, especially in combination with bacteremia or other clinical symptoms, is the most common finding in this population. CT is the most commonly used diagnostic modality but can be supplemented with leukocyte scan or confirmatory positron emission tomography to identify metabolically active periaortic areas suggestive of infection (Fig. 18.5).

There are few published reports in the literature on repair and outcomes of aortic endograft infection. A 2018 systematic review by Li and colleagues identified only eleven studies with 402 patients with infected aortic endografts [21]. The pooled in-hospital mortality rate was 17%. Almost one-quarter had aorto-enteric fistula identified as a primary source, while the rest were unknown. The most common organisms were staphylococcus species in 30%, followed by streptococcus species and fungus. Gram-negative organisms were uncommon, with *E. coli* species making up 7.7% of infections and pseudomonas 4%. The vast majority (90%) of patients underwent surgical treatment with explantation of the infected endograft. Extra-anatomic reconstruction was performed in only 16%, with in-situ reconstruction using a variety of infection-resistant conduits in the remainder. The pooled cohort was too heterogeneous to make clear determinations, but the 10% undergoing non-surgical treatment with antibiotics only had worse survival rates in both the immediate and follow-up periods.

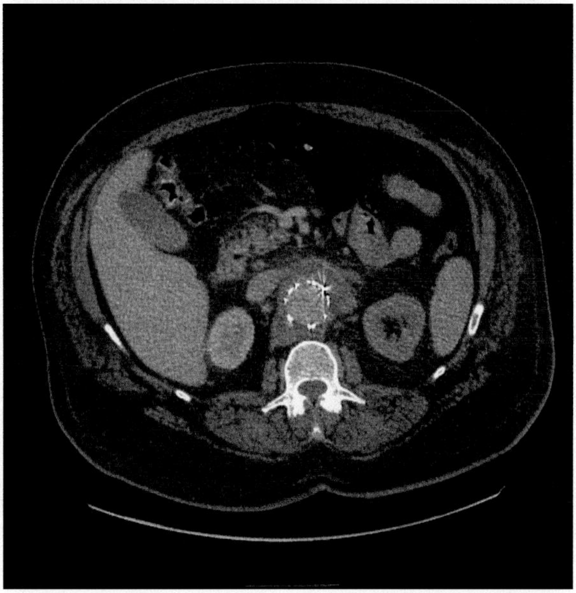

Fig. 18.5 CTA showing periaortic rind and inflammation from an infected EVAR

If there is suspicion of an aortic infection, rapid identification, antibiotic treatment, and surgical intervention with wide debridement and either extra-anatomic or in-situ reconstruction with an infection-resistant graft is critical if the patient can tolerate such an operation.

Endograft Migration

Caudal migration of the endograft may cause loss of proximal seal and creation of a Type Ia endoleak. Factors that may compromise proximal fixation include large proximal neck diameter, short proximal neck length, angulated necks >60 degrees, reverse conical necks, and placing the endograft in a diseased neck. Adhering to device-specific instructions for use (IFU) is critically important to minimize the migration risk as devices placed outside of the IFU tend to have a higher rate of failure. Following device implant aortic neck dilation or shrinkage of the aortic sac can cause device migration. Predictors of aortic neck dilation are large diameter AAA, large diameter aortic neck, and mural thrombus lining the proximal neck. Advancing the proximal seal zone or open repair are alternative options for managing challenging anatomy (Fig. 18.6).

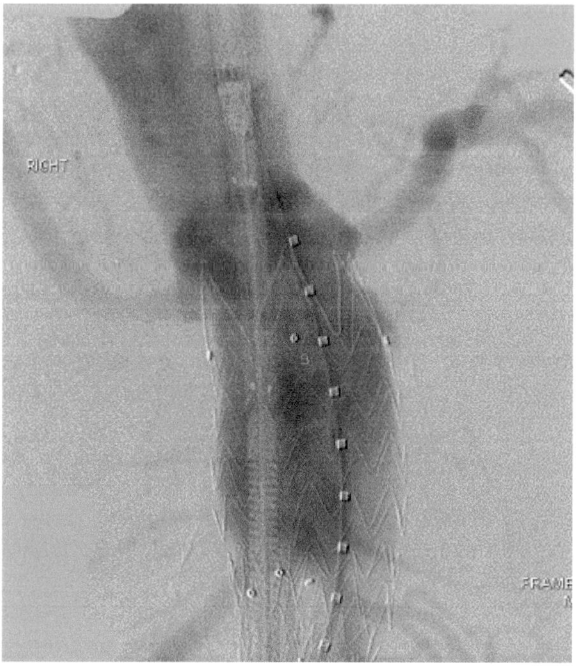

Fig. 18.6 Angiogram showing EVAR migration, suprarenal fixation resides at the level of the renal arteries

Endograft Stent Fracture

Stent fracture is a rare complication of EVAR. Most contemporary grafts are constructed with a fabric layered onto a stent, but different graft constructions result in different responses to stent fracture. Much of the initial concern for stent integrity came from the pulsation of the aorta resulting in constant flexion motion of the endograft, but the majority of commercially available endografts have been shown to be exceptionally durable to these stresses. Systematic issues with stent fracture are rare, with most stent fractures asymptomatic and going clinically undetected.

An example of a high-profile systematic stent graft fracture problem came with the voluntary global recall of the Medtronic Navion thoracic endograft device in 2021 [22]. Multiple structural failures were noted in eleven patients on further imaging analysis of pivotal trial subjects. Among these, stent fractures in the body of the device occurred in four patients along the fabric seam resulting in Type 3 endoleaks.

Stent fractures have also been associated with lower-profile devices. The Cordis Incraft device, a low-profile conventional EVAR device, was found to have a 13% fracture rate of the suprarenal stent segment over a 5-year period [20]. However, these fractures did not affect the integrity of the device or the proximal seal and did not require any intervention.

Systemic Complications The incidence of systemic complications after EVAR ranges from 3% to 12%. This includes cardiopulmonary, renal, and ischemic complications. Cardiovascular events occur in 1.8–5.3% of patients and remain a common cause of morbidity and mortality following EVAR [23–25]. Clinical trials have failed to show any significant differences in long-term cardiovascular outcomes between open repair and EVAR [26–28]. The incidence of pulmonary complications ranges from 2.9% to 3.3% and remains the second most common reason of mortality after EVAR. Octogenarians, active smokers, and patients with chronic obstructive pulmonary disease tend to be at higher risk for postoperative adverse events. Percutaneous access using local anesthesia has been shown to lower pulmonary adverse events compared to patients receiving general anesthesia [29–33].

Ischemia Ischemic complications are not infrequent and occur in 9% of cases [34]. Ischemia is often multifactorial and attributed to arterial thrombosis, embolization, or dissection. Vascular territories and organs affected by ischemia include both lower extremities, intestines, pelvis, spinal cord, and kidneys. Lower extremity ischemia is the most frequent form of ischemia following EVAR. As discussed earlier, endograft limb occlusion due to challenging native anatomy, device maldeployment, or malpositioning is often the underlying problem [34]. The management of each was addressed previously.

Renal Ischemia Renal dysfunction may result from contrast-induced nephropathy, suprarenal fixation, microembolic renal artery embolization, vessel dissection, hypotension, ischemia-reperfusion injury, long operative time, preoperative ACE inhibitor use, advanced age and/or inadvertent renal artery coverage/impingement by the endograft. The overall 1-year renal complication rate during EVAR is 18% and the risk increases in patients with existing renal insufficiency. Postoperative acute kidney injury is associated with increased incidence of cardiovascular events and all-cause mortality. Although the data is conflicting, preoperative and intraoperative intravenous hydration may mitigate contrast-induced nephropathy. Clinically relevant accessory renal arteries can perfuse one-third of renal parenchyma and are present in 30% of the general population. Exclusion of accessory renal arteries can lead to renal infarction with decrease in the glomerular filtration rate. Inadvertent renal artery coverage may occur in short aortic necks, angulated aortic necks, and obese patients where imaging may be compromised [26, 27]. If the renal arteries are not visualized or partially covered post-endograft placement bail-out options include renal stenting, "pulling the endograft caudally" and performing an open hepato-renal or spleno-renal bypasses (Fig. 18.7).

Intestinal Ischemia After EVAR, intestinal ischemia most often involves the left colon and occurs in 1–3% of patients [35, 36]. Colonic ischemia is assumed to be related to coverage of the inferior mesenteric artery. If mesenteric collaterals are poorly developed, perfusion to the internal iliac arteries compromised or hypoten-

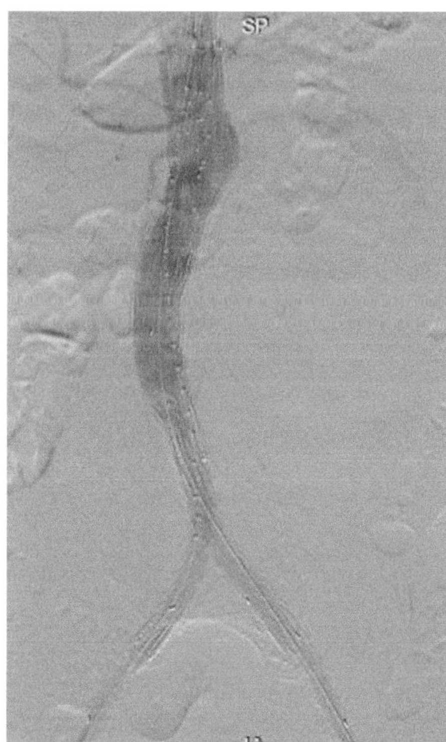

Fig. 18.7 Iatrogenic exclusion of both renal arteries during EVAR

sion occurs, left colonic ischemia may develop in the watershed region. Clinical features may include abdominal pain, early bowel movements, and hematochezia in addition to fluid sequestration. Right colon and small bowel ischemia may occur if perfusion to the superior mesenteric artery is compromised. This event occurs less frequently than left colon ischemia and is associated with superior mesenteric artery thromboembolism from catheter or guidewire manipulations and insertion of the endograft delivery systems which may dislodge atheromatous plaque into the SMA during advancement.

Pelvic Ischemia Pelvic ischemia has been reported after EVAR and is often related to atheromatous embolization and/or disruption of the pelvic collateral circulation. Planned internal iliac artery embolization in patients with complex iliac artery anatomy can be effectively used to extend the iliac artery landing zones (Fig. 18.8). However, it may lead to features of pelvic ischemia including buttock claudication, buttock necrosis, colorectal ischemia, erectile dysfunction, and spinal cord ischemia. Buttock claudication occurs in 30–55% and erectile dysfunction 17–24% of patients [37, 38]. The incidence is greater after bilateral internal iliac artery embolization. Symptoms often improve with time, and at 1 year the incidence of persistent claudication is 9–10%. Colorectal ischemia after EVAR is rare (<1%) and slightly

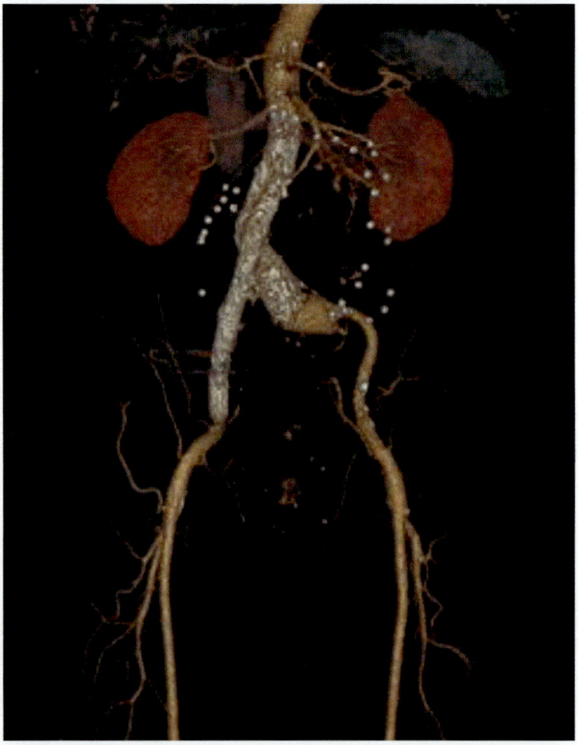

Fig. 18.8 CTA reconstruction showing right iliac limb extension and chronic occlusion of the right internal iliac artery in a patient with bilateral buttock claudication

higher (2.6%) after planned internal iliac artery embolization. Strategies to maintain pelvic perfusion include use of iliac artery branched devices, open surgical revascularization, and use of parallel endografts. Fortunately, spinal cord ischemia (SCI) rarely occurs during standard infrarenal endovascular repair. Risk factors for SCI include extended aortic coverage, prior thoracic aortic repair, compromised pelvic perfusion, coverage of left subclavian artery, intraoperative hypotension, long procedure duration, and chronic kidney disease [34, 37–41].

Post Implantation Syndrome Following EVAR transient post implantation syndrome occurs in 13–60% of cases. It represents an inflammatory state due to release of cytokines that occurs in response to the body's exposure to endograft material and aortic sac thrombosis. Symptoms manifest as a systemic inflammatory response characterized by low-grade fever, leukocytosis, fatigue, lethargy, constipation, and anorexia. Post implant syndrome is defined by fever, leukocytosis, and elevated CRP level in the absence of infection. Additional inflammatory markers (SED, tumor necrosis factor alpha, interleukin 6) are often elevated. There are no factors that predict which patients are at risk to develop this syndrome. Antibiotics are not required, and symptoms typically resolve in 1–2 weeks after EVAR implantation [42, 43].

Allergic Reaction Intravenous contrast allergy is rare and should be considered in patient with prior reactions to iodinated contrast agents. Mild and moderate reactions are best managed with premedicating patients (antihistamines and glucocorticoids) prior to contrast exposure. For patients with a history of severe or anaphylactic reaction to contrast, they should be evaluated by allergy and immunology specialists before proceeding. Alternative imaging options include non-iodinated contrast agents (e.g., gadolinium), carbon dioxide, and intravascular ultrasound. Allergy to the metal components of endografts is exceedingly rare. If suspected, patients should be evaluated by allergy and immunology specialists and skin testing offered to rule out metal allergies. EVAR should be avoided in patients with gold, nickel, titanium, and stainless-steel allergies.

Access-Related Complications Arterial access site complications occur in 9–16% of all cases following EVAR and include vessel dissection, rupture, thrombosis, distal embolization, arteriovenous fistula, pseudoaneurysm formation, and infection [44, 45]. The incidence of access site infection and lymphatic leaks has been reduced by utilization of percutaneous femoral artery access. The PEVAR Trial found percutaneous access was associated with less blood loss, shorter procedures, shorter length of stay, and fewer groin infections. Suture-mediated large-bore closure devices and preclosure techniques are routinely performed with a high degree of success. A learning curve is expected for percutaneous access, improvements of delivery systems and simplifying deployment steps has significantly improved device outcomes for large-bore access (12–25F). Access-related adverse events occur in 4.4% of cases which is lower than the complication rate of open surgical exposure [46–48].

Arterial dissection of the femoral or iliac artery may occur during wire advancement, sheath, or device insertion (Fig. 18.9). Advancing large diameter sheaths (12F–25F) into native ileo-femoral vessels with atherosclerotic plaque, tortuosity, or small diameters has been associated with vessel rupture and dissection. Preoperative imaging with CT angiography is essential for interrogating the access vessels and avoiding these pitfalls. A variety of techniques can be used to minimize the risk to native vessels prior to sheath insertion. This includes insertion of smaller contralateral sheath in the less diseased ipsilateral side, predilation angioplasty of the iliac arteries prior to sheath insertion, use of hydrophilic sheaths, creation of iliac conduits, and selective use of the "crack and pave" technique for calcified vessels. After EVAR implantation, wire access should be maintained, and completion imaging performed with a soft wire or catheter in place evaluating for vessel dissection, angulation, or kinking. If a flow-limiting dissection is present, options for treatment are dependent on the lesion location and extent. In most cases, extending the iliac limb or placing a self-expanding stent in the external iliac artery will sufficiently address the injury.

Rupture of the iliac artery rupture is most likely to occur during sheath insertion, exchanges, or removal. A sudden blood pressure decrease, and angiographic appearance of contrast extravasation should alert the surgeon to this catastrophic event. It is imperative to maintain wire access during sheath exchanges or removal. If an "iliac on a stick" occurs, immediately replace the sheath, insert an occlusion balloon in the iliac limb followed by deploying an iliac extension limb or covered stent (Fig. 18.10). If ipsilateral arterial access is lost, inserting an occlusion balloon through the contralateral sheath will minimize blood loss, provide time to stabilize

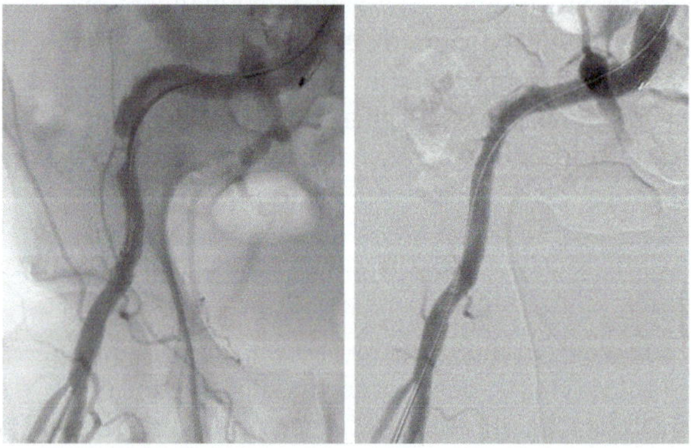

Fig. 18.9 Angiogram following EVAR showing right external iliac artery dissection and stenosis that was successfully treated with covered self-expanding stent placement

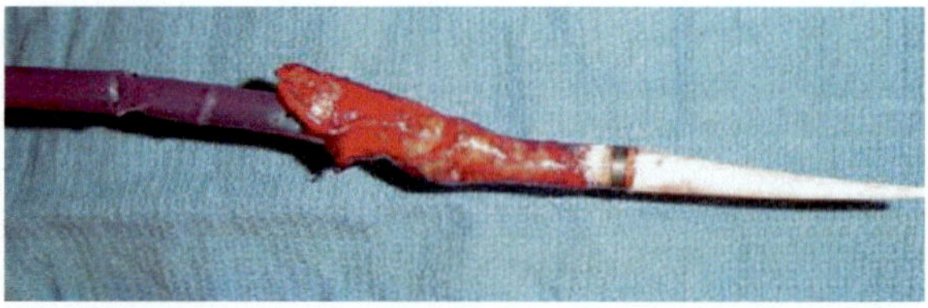

Fig. 18.10 EVAR sheath removal with "Iliac artery on a stick"

the patient, and determine the best treatment. Repair options include endovascular therapy, extra-anatomic bypass, or open iliac artery repair via retroperitoneal exposure.

Distal embolization may occur during or after EVAR insertion. Sheath and wire manipulation in calcified or diseased vessels increases the risk of atheroembolization. Large diameter sheaths induce stagnation of flow and thrombus formation. Aspiration of large-diameter sheaths prior to removal can minimize the embolic event. If an open femoral artery cut down was performed, clamping the outflow vessels, and flushing the inflow prior to sheath removal will minimize the risk of distal embolization. If there is noticeable change in the lower extremity perfusion following EVAR, a diagnostic angiogram should be performed. Treatment of distal embolization can often be successfully managed via femoral artery access.

Thrombosis of the common femoral artery may be associated with subtherapeutic anticoagulation, large sheaths, heavily diseased femoral artery, or access site closure device misadventures. After sheath removal, if the femoral pulse is diminished or absent an intraoperative arterial duplex scan or diagnostic angiogram should be performed. Based on the findings, open repair options include thrombectomy, endarterectomy, or interposition graft for extreme cases (Fig. 18.11).

Increasing use of percutaneous access and closure of large bore access is related to a higher incidence of pseudoaneurysm formation. Data suggests an incidence of 2% [47–49]. Risk factors for closure device failure included obesity, female gender, small native arteries, aberrant femoral access sites, and anticoagulation. The

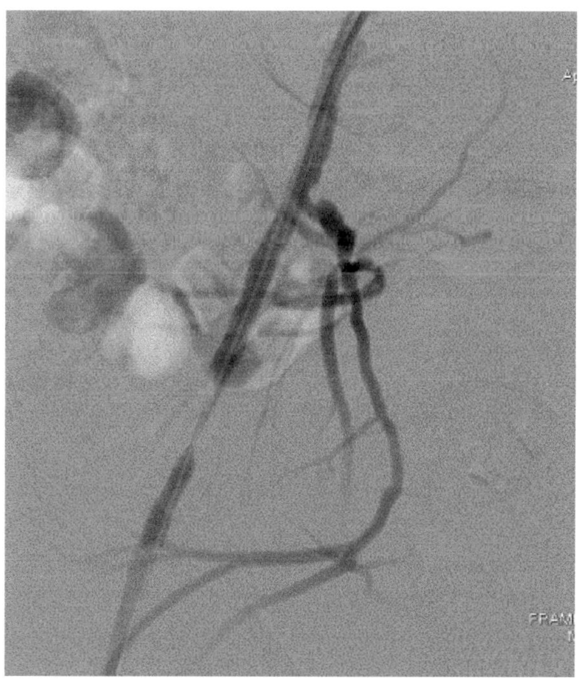

Fig. 18.11 Right external iliac and common femoral artery occlusion following EVAR

diagnosis can effectively be made with duplex imaging or CT angiography. Small (<20 mm) pseudoaneurysms typically thrombose by 30 days. For those that persist or those larger than 20 mm, ultrasound-guided thrombin injection is an effective treatment option in those with suitable anatomy [50–52].

Conclusion In the last two decades, EVAR has increasingly been used for the treatment of AAA and appears to be the standard of care. Technology advancements, percutaneous closure devices, and development of lower profile delivery systems have increased utilization and lowered 30-day morbidity and mortality. One disadvantage of EVAR is procedure-related and postoperative adverse events which necessitate lifelong imaging surveillance for all EVAR patients. Proper patient anatomic selection and closely following device-specific IFU appear to improve outcomes and lower the rate of complications. A modest number of EVAR patients require secondary interventions; the majority are endovascular-based. Based on this, it is imperative for physicians to be familiar with common adverse events and treatment strategies during and after EVAR.

References

1. Chaikof EL, Dalman RL, Eskandari MK, Jackson BM, Lee WA, Mansour MA, et al. The Society for Vascular Surgery practice guidelines on the care of patients with an abdominal aortic aneurysm. J Vasc Surg. 2018;67(1):2–77.e2. https://doi.org/10.1016/j.jvs.2017.10.044.
2. Wanhainen A, Verzini F, van Herzeele I, Allaire E, Bown M, Cohnert T, et al. European Society for Vascular Surgery (ESVS) 2019 clinical practice guidelines on the management of abdominal aorto-iliac artery aneurysms. Eur J Vasc Endovasc Surg. 2019;57(1):8–93. https://doi.org/10.1016/j.ejvs.2018.09.020.
3. Abraha I, Luchetta ML, de Florio R, Cozzolino F, Casazza G, Duca P, et al. Ultrasonography for endoleak detection after endoluminal abdominal aortic aneurysm repair. Cochrane Database Syst Rev. 2017;2017(6):CD010296. https://doi.org/10.1002/14651858.CD010296.PUB2.
4. Smith L, Thomas N, Arnold A, Bell R, Zayed H, Tyrrell M, et al. Editor's choice—a comparison of computed tomography angiography and color duplex ultrasound surveillance post infrarenal endovascular aortic aneurysm repair: financial implications and impact of different international surveillance guidelines. Eur J Vasc Endovasc Surg. 2021;62(2):193–201. https://doi.org/10.1016/j.ejvs.2021.04.005.
5. Jordan WD, Mehta M, Ouriel K, Arko FR, Varnagy D, Joye J, et al. One-year results of the ANCHOR trial of EndoAnchors for the prevention and treatment of aortic neck complications after endovascular aneurysm repair. Vascular. 2016;24(2):177–86. https://doi.org/10.1177/1708538115590727.
6. Jordan WD, de Vries J-PPM, Ouriel K, Mehta M, Varnagy D, Moore WM, et al. Midterm outcome of EndoAnchors for the prevention of endoleak and stent-graft migration in patients with challenging proximal aortic neck anatomy. J Endovasc Ther. 2015;22(2):163–70. https://doi.org/10.1177/1526602815574685.
7. Qamhawi Z, Barge TF, Makris GC, Patel R, Wigham A, Anthony S, et al. Editor's choice—systematic review of the use of endoanchors in endovascular aortic aneurysm repair. Eur J Vasc Endovasc Surg. 2020;59(5):748–56. https://doi.org/10.1016/j.ejvs.2020.02.008.

8. Stokmans RA, Teijink JAW, Forbes TL, Böckler D, Peeters PJ, Riambau V, et al. Early results from the ENGAGE registry: real-world performance of the endurant stent graft for endovascular AAA repair in 1262 patients. Eur J Vasc Endovasc Surg. 2012;44(4):369–75. https://doi.org/10.1016/j.ejvs.2012.07.005.
9. Oliveira NFG, Oliveira-Pinto J, van Rijn MJ, Baart S, ten Raa S, Hoeks SE, et al. Risk factors, dynamics, and clinical consequences of aortic neck dilatation after standard endovascular aneurysm repair. Eur J Vasc Endovasc Surg. 2021;62(1):26–35. https://doi.org/10.1016/j.ejvs.2021.03.020.
10. Kouvelos GN, Oikonomou K, Antoniou GA, Verhoeven ELG, Katsargyris A. A systematic review of proximal neck dilatation after endovascular repair for abdominal aortic aneurysm. J Endovasc Ther. 2017;24(1):59–67. https://doi.org/10.1177/1526602816673325.
11. Oliveira NFG, Gonçalves FB, Ultee K, Pinto JP, Josee van Rijn M, ten Raa S, et al. Patients with large neck diameter have a higher risk of type IA endoleaks and aneurysm rupture after standard endovascular aneurysm repair. J Vasc Surg. 2018:1–9. https://doi.org/10.1016/j.jvs.2018.07.021.
12. Madigan MC, Singh MJ, Chaer RA, Al-Khoury GE, Makaroun MS. Occult type I or III endoleaks are a common cause of failure of type II endoleak treatment after endovascular aortic repair. J Vasc Surg. 2019;69(2):432–9. https://doi.org/10.1016/j.jvs.2018.04.054.
13. Mohapatra A, Robinson D, Malak O, Madigan MC, Avgerinos ED, Chaer RA, et al. Increasing use of open conversion for late complications after endovascular aortic aneurysm repair. J Vasc Surg. 2019;69(6):1766–75. https://doi.org/10.1016/j.jvs.2018.09.049.
14. Ultee KHJ, Büttner S, Huurman R, Bastos Gonçalves F, Hoeks SE, Bramer WM, et al. Editor's choice—systematic review and meta-analysis of the outcome of treatment for type II endoleak following endovascular aneurysm repair. Eur J Vasc Endovasc Surg. 2018;56(6):794–807. https://doi.org/10.1016/j.ejvs.2018.06.009.
15. Sidloff DA, Stather PW, Choke E, Bown MJ, Sayers RD. Type II endoleak after endovascular aneurysm repair. Br J Surg. 2013;100(10):1262–70. https://doi.org/10.1002/bjs.9181.
16. Sarac TP, Gibbons C, Vargas L, Liu J, Srivastava S, Bena J, et al. Long-term follow-up of type II endoleak embolization reveals the need for close surveillance. J Vasc Surg. 2012;55(1):33–40. https://doi.org/10.1016/j.jvs.2011.07.092.
17. Forsyth A, Carlson S, Martin M, Raffetto J, Alfson D, McPhee J. Late type III endoleaks are common in early generation Endologix AFX stent grafts. J Vasc Surg. 2022;76(3):680–7. https://doi.org/10.1016/j.jvs.2022.02.020.
18. Hammond A, Hansrani V, Lowe C, Asghar I, Antoniou SA, Antoniou GA. Meta-analysis, and meta regression analysis of iliac limb occlusion after endovascular aneurysm repair. J Vasc Surg. 2018;68(6):1916–1924.e7. https://doi.org/10.1016/j.jvs.2018.08.153.
19. Uilings TAJ, de Vries AC, de Mol van Otterloo JCA, Eefting D, van der Linden E. Thromboembolic complications after zenith® low profile endovascular graft for infrarenal abdominal aneurysms. Cardiovasc Intervent Radiol. 2015;38(3):600–5. https://doi.org/10.1007/s00270-014-0972-4.
20. Liang NL, Ohki T, Ouriel K, Teigen C, Fry D, Henretta J, et al. Five-year results of the INSPIRATION study for the INCRAFT low-profile endovascular aortic stent graft system. J Vasc Surg. 2021;73(3):867–873.e2. https://doi.org/10.1016/j.jvs.2020.06.128.
21. Li HL, Chan YC, Cheng SW. Current evidence on management of aortic stent-graft infection: a systematic review and meta-analysis. Ann Vasc Surg. 2018;51:306–13. https://doi.org/10.1016/j.avsg.2018.02.038.
22. Verzini F, Cieri E, Kahlberg A, Sternbach Y, Heijmen R, Ouriel K, et al. A preliminary analysis of late structural failures of the Navion stent graft in the treatment of descending thoracic aortic aneurysms. J Vasc Surg. 2021;74(4):1125–1134.e2. https://doi.org/10.1016/j.jvs.2021.04.018.
23. Prinssen M, Verhoeven EL, Buth J, et al. A randomized trial comparing conventional and EVAR. N Engl J Med. 2004;351:1607.

24. Brown LC, Thompson SG, Greenhalgh RM, et al. Incidence of cardiovascular events and death after open or endovascular repair of AAA in the randomized EVAR trial 1. Br J Surg. 2011;98:935.
25. Cuypers PW, Gardien M, Buth J, et al. Randomized study comparing cardiac response in endovascular and open AAA repair. Br J Surg. 2001;88:1059.
26. Lederle FA, Fresichlag JA, Kyriakides TC, et al. Outcomes following endovascular vs open repair of AAA: a randomized trial. JAMA. 2009;302:1535.
27. Karthikesalingam A, Bahia S, Patel S, et al. A systematic review and meta-analysis indicate underreporting of renal dysfunction following EVAR. Kidney Int. 2015;87:442–51.
28. Brown LC, Greenhalgh RM, Thompson SG, et al. Does EVAR alter the rate of cardiovascular events in patients with AAA considered unfit for open repair? Results from the randomized EVAR trial 2. Eur J Vasc Endovasc Surg. 2010;39:396.
29. Varkevisser RRB, O'Donnell TFX, Swerdlow NJ, et al. Factors associated with in-hospital complications and long-term implications of these complications in elderly patients undergoing endovascular aneurysm repair. J Vasc Surg. 2020;71:470.
30. Fonseca R, Rockman C, Pitti A, et al. Intermediate-term EVAR outcomes in octogenarians. J Vasc Surg. 2010;52:556.
31. Oussoren FK, Holewijn S, Claessens N, et al. Pulmonary complications, and survival after elective EVAR in patients with documented COPD. Vascular. 2020;28(5):557–67.
32. Marchetti AA, Citoni G, Foti C, et al. Respiratory rehabilitation in patients with AAA submitted to open and EVAR treatment: predictive factors of postoperative pulmonary complications and clinical implications. J Vasc Med Surg. 2020;8(3):1–5.
33. Van Orden K, Farber A, Schermerhorn ML, et al. Local anesthesia for percutaneous EVAR is associated with few pulmonary complications. J Vasc Surg. 2018;68:1023–9.
34. Maldonado TS, Rockman CB, Riles E, et al. Ischemic complications after EVAR. J Vasc Surg. 2004;40:703–9.
35. Becquemin JP, Majewski M, Fermani N, et al. Colon ischemia following AAA repair in the era of EVAR. J Vasc Surg. 2008;47:258–63.
36. Miller A, Marotta M, Scordi-Bello I, et al. Ischemic colitis after EVAR; a 10-year retrospective study. Arch Surg. 2009;144:900–3.
37. Angiletta D, Marinazzo D, Guido G, et al. Spinal cord, bowel, and buttock ischemia after EVAR. Ann Vasc Surg. 2011;25:980.
38. Freyrie A, Testi G, Gargiulo M, et al. Spinal cord ischemia after EVAR. Case report and literature review. J Cardiovasc Surg. 2011;52:731–4.
39. Setacci F, Sirignano P, De Donato G, et al. Endovascular thoracic aortic repair, and risk of spinal cord ischemia: the role of previous or concomitant treatment for aortic aneurysms. J Cardiovasc Surg. 2010;51:168–76.
40. Alvarez-Tostado JA, Moise MA, Bena JF, et al. The brachial artery: a critical access for endovascular procedures. J Vasc Surg. 2009;49:378–85.
41. Buth J, Harris PL, Hobo R, et al. Neurologic complications associated with TEVAR: incidence and risk factors, a study from the EUROSTAR registry. J Vasc Surg. 2007;46:1103–10.
42. Kakisis JD, Moulakakis KG, Antonopoulos CN, et al. Volume of new-onset thrombus is associated with the development of post implantation syndrome after EVAR. J Vasc Surg. 2014;60:1140.
43. Voute MT, Bastos GFM, van de Luijtgaarden KM, et al. Stent graft composition plays a material role in the pos implantation syndrome. J Vasc Surg. 2012;56:1503.
44. Feezor RJ, Huber TS, Martin TD, et al. Perioperative differences between endovascular repair of thoracic and abdominal aortic diseases. J Vasc Surg. 2007;45:86.
45. Blankensteijn JD, de Jong SE, Prinssen M, et al. Two-year outcomes after conventional or endovascular repair of AAA. N Engl J Med. 2005;352:2398.

46. Krajcer Z, Wood DA, Strickman N, et al. Pivotal clinical study to evaluate the safety and effectiveness of the MANTA vascular closure device during percutaneous EVAR and TEVAR procedures. J Endovasc Ther. 2020;27:414.
47. Krajcer Z, Nelson P, Bianchi C, et al. Percutaneous EVAR: methods and initial outcomes from the first prospective, multicenter trial. J Cardiovasc Surg. 2011;52(5):651–9.
48. Grenon SM, Gagnon J, Hsiang YN, Chen JC. Canadian experience with percutaneous endovascular aneurysm repair: short-term outcomes. Can J Surg. 2009;52(5):E156–60.
49. O'Donnell TFX, Deery SE, Boitano LT, et al. The long-term implications of access complications during endovascular aneurysm repair. J Vasc Surg. 2021;73:1253–60.
50. Vaakencherry G, Molloy C, Sheth N, et al. Percutaneous access planning, techniques, and considerations for EVAR. Cardiovasc Diagn Thor. 2018;8:184–90.
51. Dwivedi, Regi JM, Cleveland TJ, et al. Long-term evaluation of percutaneous groin access for EVAR. Cardiovasc Intervent Radiol. 2019;42:28–33.
52. Lee WA, Brown MP, Nelson PR, et al. Midterm outcomes of femoral arteries after percutaneous endovascular aortic repair using the Preclose technique. J Vasc Surg. 2008;47(5):919–23.

Chapter 19
Fenestrated/Branched Endovascular Stent-Grafts: Current Applications

Trung Nguyen and Dean J. Arnaoutakis

Introduction

The pioneering work of both Nicolai Volodos and Juan Parodi in the late 1980s using stent-grafts transformed the delivery of care for patients with aortic disease [1, 2]. Endovascular aortic aneurysm repair (EVAR) is now the most common approach for treating abdominal aortic aneurysms (AAA) accounting for more than 80% of repairs in the United States [3, 4]. EVAR is associated with improved perioperative mortality and morbidity compared to open AAA repair, although long-term outcomes remain equivocal [5–7]. Despite advances in stent-graft design and endovascular techniques, various anatomical constraints remain fundamental for treatment success. More specifically, the health of the proximal aortic neck is critical for durable aortic aneurysm exclusion. The Eurostar registry has demonstrated that EVAR in proximal necks shorter than 15 mm is associated with a higher risk of complications [8].

When treating more complex aortic aneurysms, such as juxtarenal, suprarenal, or thoracoabdominal aortic aneurysms (TAAA), conventional EVAR devices are not suitable. To help preserve visceral-renal perfusion while obtaining more proximal seal, custom fenestrations were fabricated onto stent-grafts, meant to align with each visceral-renal branch vessel to maintain end-organ perfusion. The first report of a fenestrated endovascular aortic repair (FEVAR) in humans was in 1996 by Park and colleagues, a group of interventional radiologists from South Korea [9]. Their technique and design were further refined by Michael Lawrence-Brown and David Hartley in Australia. Another option for renal-visceral perfusion is the incorporation of short directional branches onto the stent-graft, an approach referred to as branched

T. Nguyen · D. J. Arnaoutakis (✉)
Division of Vascular Surgery, University of South Florida Morsani College of Medicine, Tampa, FL, USA
e-mail: Nguyen77@usf.edu; arnaoutakis@usf.edu

G. J. Arnaoutakis et al. (eds.), *Aortic Aneurysms*, Contemporary Cardiology,
https://doi.org/10.1007/978-3-032-13134-8_19

endovascular aortic aneurysm repair (BEVAR). The first reports of a modular branched endograft were made by Tim Chuter in 2001 [10]. These two techniques have been combined such that some stent-grafts have both fenestrations and branches. The global experience with F/BEVAR has dramatically increased over the past two decades and reached a state of maturity. Although there will always be a role of open repair, F/BEVAR has been shown to have better perioperative outcomes than an open repair that would otherwise require supraceliac cross-clamping [11, 12].

This chapter will discuss the indications for repair, current F/BEVAR devices and design, operative technique, and the limitations of fenestrated repair.

Indications

The primary goal of F/BEVAR repair is to prolong meaningful life by preventing aortic-related mortality. When considering elective repair of a complex aortic aneurysm, the patient's comorbidities in addition to overall life expectancy and goals of care must be balanced with the inherent risks of surgery. Several preoperative risk stratification calculators have been devised for patients who undergo EVAR for intact infrarenal AAA, but no such calculator has been published for FEVAR. Our center has validated an algorithm using national data, which provides an estimate of 1-year survival following FEVAR thereby guiding our preoperative patient selection.

Although more nuanced and individualized criteria are needed, aneurysm diameter remains the standard indicator for repair as it most reliably predicts rupture. Aortic diameters should be measured outer wall to outer wall in an orthogonal view to eliminate parallax. Current size criteria for repair of fusiform AAA, as indicated by the Society for Vascular Surgery, include a diameter ≥5.5 cm in men and ≥5.0 cm in women [13]. Given the increased complexity and therefore risks of surgery with TAAA repair, the size threshold for repair is usually larger than that of AAA. The European Society for Vascular Surgery recommends repair in low to moderate-surgical-risk patients with TAAA ≥6.0 cm (less for patients with connective tissue disorders), rapid growth (>10 mm/year), or with symptoms [14]. It is unknown how, if at all, total endovascular repair of TAAAs will impact this diameter threshold in the future.

Principles and Technique

The fundamentals of F/BEVAR involve the use of custom fenestrations or branches on a stent-graft to allow for perfusion of the renal-visceral branches thereby permitting a larger seal zone in the supraceliac aorta. Bridging covered stents are inserted that extend from the fenestration/branch into the target vessel thereby providing aneurysm exclusion. The decision of when to utilize fenestrations or branches remains provider-specific, but most would agree that directional branches are favorable in anatomy where there will be moderate distance to bridge from the endograft to the target vessel orifice (typically if the aortic lumen is >35 mm). Meticulous preoperative aortic measurements and case planning are essential for technical success.

FEVAR procedures are typically done in a hybrid operating room under general anesthesia with invasive hemodynamic monitoring and central venous access established. Most centers performing F/BEVAR utilize fusion imaging software in order to decrease contrast volume, procedure time, and radiation exposure [15]. The use of a cerebrospinal fluid (CSF) drain is oftentimes placed preoperatively when patients are deemed high risk for spinal cord ischemia (SCI). Risk factors include extensive aortic coverage, chronic hypogastric artery occlusion, left subclavian artery occlusion, and prior aortic surgery. Transfemoral arterial access is always required for F/BEVAR device insertion and deployment. In addition, the contralateral femoral artery or the brachial/axillary artery is required for fenestration/branch cannulation and delivery of bridging stent. Deciding between femoral or brachial/axillary access is dependent upon the preoperative case plan, angulation of target vessels, device selection, and surgeon preference. Brachial/axillary artery access is customary when using devices with downward branches (e.g., Gore "TAMBE" and Cook "t-Branch"); however, improvements in steerable sheaths are changing this paradigm as many will fully implant these devices using retrograde transfemoral access alone [16].

Once inserted, the device is then unsheathed under fluoroscopy taking care to align the fenestrations and/or branches to their target vessels. At this point, the endograft's diameter is partially constrained permitting cannulation of target arteries using a hydrophilic wire and support catheter. Steerable sheaths have greatly refined this technique. Once all target vessels are cannulated, the diameter reduction constraints are released and the device fully expanded. Delivery of bridging stents ensues with about 4–5 mm of the bridging stent extending into the lumen of the aortic endograft. This section is then flared with a 9–12 mm balloon in order to obtain junctional seal between the fenestration and the bridging stent. Of note, several different covered stents have been used as "bridging" stents, none of which has Food and Drug Administration (FDA) approval for this indication. However, most feel that the ideal stent should be low-profile, flexible, accurate, and resistant to mechanical stress. Atrium iCAST (Atrium Medical Corporation, Hudson, New Hampshire) and Gore Viabahn VBX (Gore, Flagstaff, Arizona) are the most commonly used balloon-expandable covered stents in the United States and the Bentley BeGraft (Bentley InnoMed, Hechingen, Germany) is commonly used in Europe. Next, insertion of a bifurcated aortic component along with iliac endoprostheses is done if obtaining distal seal in the iliac arteries. Completion angiography is performed in a standard fashion to assess for aneurysm sac exclusion, presence of endoleak, and patency of bridging stents. Some perform intraoperative cone beam CT at completion in order to assess bridging stent patency and adequate overlap of components.

Current Fenestrated/Branched Endografts

Access to F/BEVAR remains somewhat limited in the United States although a number of different options exist in Europe. In the United States, options include custom-made devices (CMD), manufacturer-made off-the-shelf devices, and physician-modified fenestrated/branched endografts (PM-F/BEVAR).

The only commercially available FEVAR device in the United States is the Zenith fenestrated endovascular stent-graft (Cook Medical, Bloomington, Indiana), which has been available since 2012. It is a custom-made, multicomponent device that is typically configured with two small fenestrations for the renal arteries and either a large fenestration or scallop for the superior mesenteric artery. This device requires ≥4 mm of healthy infrarenal neck and is therefore intended for short-neck infrarenal AAA or juxtarenal AAA. If requiring more than two fenestrations for supraceliac seal zone, then a CMD is required which is limited to select centers with an industry-sponsored clinical trial or a physician-sponsored investigational device exemption (PS-IDE). CMDs can be constructed in a variety of permutations including both fenestrations and/or directional branches, heavily tapered and/or thin polyester fabric design, and pre-loaded catheters. Despite limited access in the United States, thousands of CMDs have been effectively implanted across the nation and worldwide [17].

Off-the-shelf devices are another F/BEVAR option which eliminate the 6–8 week manufacturing period that is required for CMDs. However, in the United States, no such devices are commercially available. Clinical trials using off-the-shelf endografts include the Cook "p-Branch", Cook "t-Branch", and Gore Excluder Thoracoabdominal Branch Endoprosthesis (TAMBE) [18–20]. Despite a pre-specified number and/or spacing of fenestrations or branches, their design offers more degrees of freedom thereby accommodating 50–60% of patient anatomy [21, 22]. The Cook "p-Branch" is configured with three fenestrations (bilateral renal arteries and superior mesenteric artery) and one scallop (for celiac artery) and is therefore designed for pararenal AAA. The renal fenestrations have a pocket of redundant fabric that can "pivot" allowing for increased margin of error for target vessel cannulation (Fig. 19.1). The Cook "t-branch" and Gore TAMBE utilize four downward branches on a thoracic endograft that is then married to a standard infrarenal EVAR device (Fig. 19.2).

Another option is PM-F/BEVAR. During this procedure, a physician fabricates fenestrations and/or branches onto a commercially available endograft on a sterile back-table prior to device implantation (Fig. 19.3). Different methods are used to make the fenestration/branch openings radiopaque. Commonly used endografts include the Cook TX2, Alpha, and Zenith platforms (Cook Medical, Bloomington, Indiana), Gore TAG (W. L. Gore & Associates, Flagstaff, Arizona), Medtronic Endurant system (Medtronic, Santa Rosa, California), and the Terumo Aortic Treo (Bolton Medical, Inc., Sunrise, Florida) [23–25]. Each platform has its advantages and disadvantages. In situ laser fenestration is another physician-modified technique whereby an off-the-shelf endograft can be modified to treat TAAAs [26].

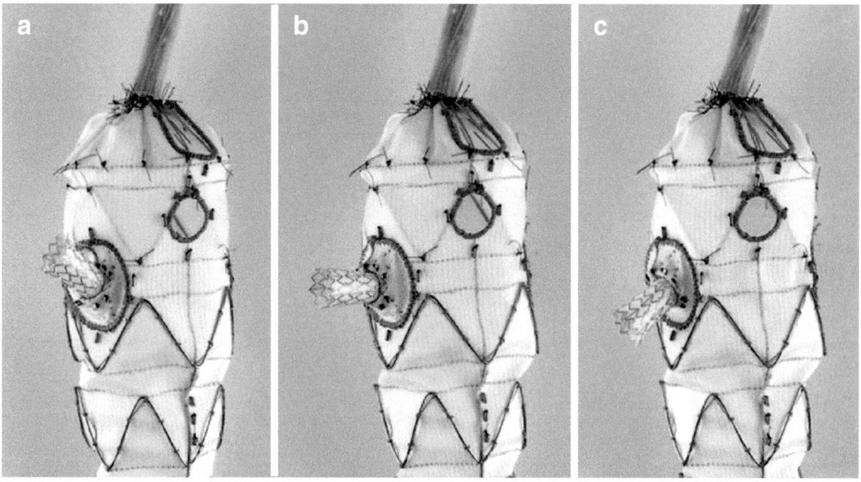

Fig. 19.1 Cook Zenith "p-Branch". Cook "p-Branch" is designed with fenestrations for the renal and superior mesenteric arteries and a scallop of the celiac artery. Redundant fabric at the renal fenestrations permits directional versatility for target vessel cannulation and bridging stent deployment (insets **a**, **b**, and **c**)

With this technique, after deploying the endograft across the visceral-renal segment, a laser catheter is used to make a fenestration in the endograft directed at the target visceral/renal artery origin. The opening is progressively dilated with an angioplasty balloon followed by covered stent placement into the target vessel. Physician-modified techniques are useful for providers who do not have access to CMDs or off-the-shelf devices and for patients who present with symptomatic/urgent pathology, but there is a steep learning curve with such procedures and they should ideally be carried out under the auspices of a PS-IDE clinical trial.

Results

Results with the Cook Zenith Fenestrated endograft have been very favorable when used for short-neck infrarenal or juxtarenal AAA. Final 5-year outcomes from 67 patients enrolled in a prospective, multicenter clinical trial using the device were recently reported. The 30-day mortality was 1.5% and freedom from 5-year all-cause mortality was 88.8 ± 4.2% [16]. Reintervention was required in 30% and primary and secondary renal target patency were 82.7 ± 4.1% and 95.7 ± 2.1% at 5 years, respectively. Retrospective series from single institutions demonstrate similar results with primary target vessel patency at 5 years of 89 ± 2%, reintervention of 39.4%, and 5-year overall survival of 71.0 ± 4.7% [27]. These results compare favorably to that of open repair. A retrospective review using national data comparing the outcomes of open complex AAA repair to that of the Cook Zenith

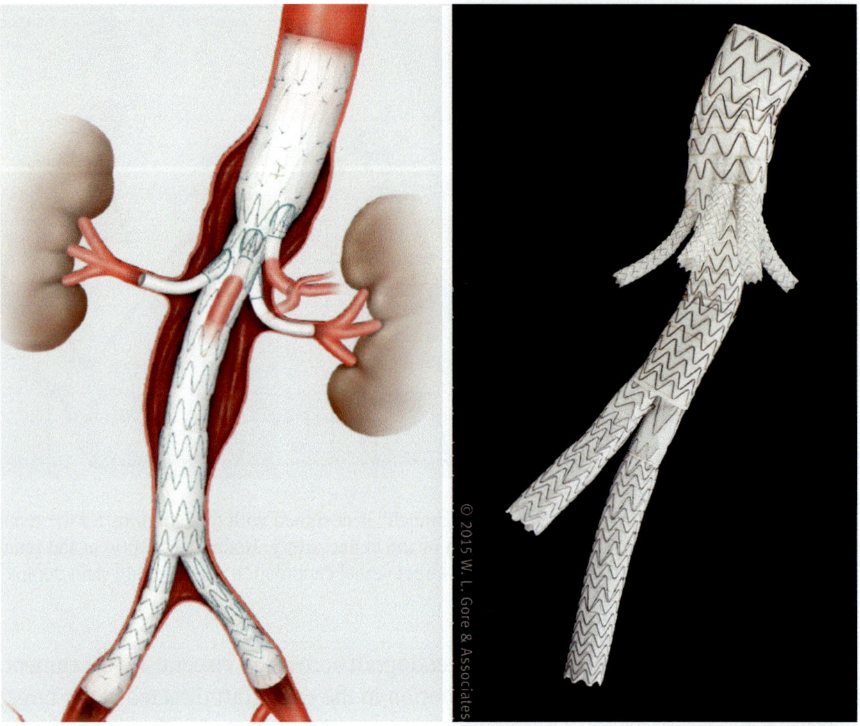

Fig. 19.2 Cook Zenith "t-Branch" and Gore TAMBE. Both off-the-shelf platforms have four downward branches for renal-visceral target artery cannulation to permit treatment of thoracoabdominal aortic aneurysms

fenestrated device found a nearly 5 times increased risk of perioperative death and 4 times increased risk of complications with open repair [28]. Overall, the long-term data encourages the use of FEVAR in complex abdominal aortic disease such that the 2019 European Society for Vascular Surgery aortic guidelines recommend FEVAR as the first-line treatment of juxtarenal aortic aneurysms [29].

Open repair of thoracoabdominal aortic aneurysms is a technically and physiologically demanding operation. In centers of excellence using modern adjunctive measures for end-organ perfusion and spinal cord ischemia protection, rates of spinal cord ischemia (6–13%), renal failure (8%), and 30-day mortality (6–9%) are significant [30, 31]. Short-term outcomes from national datasets are much more sobering with mortality rates approaching 20% [32, 33]. In comparison, results from single centers using F/BEVAR with CMDs for thoracoabdominal aortic aneurysms are much more favorable. In these series, which have more than 500 patients combined, rates of 30-day mortality were 0–5%, permanent spinal cord ischemia were 0–4%, and renal failure requiring dialysis were 1–5% [34–36]. The 3-year primary and secondary bridging stent patency rates were 95% and 98%, respectively. However, reinterventions are common, reported in up to 46% of cases.

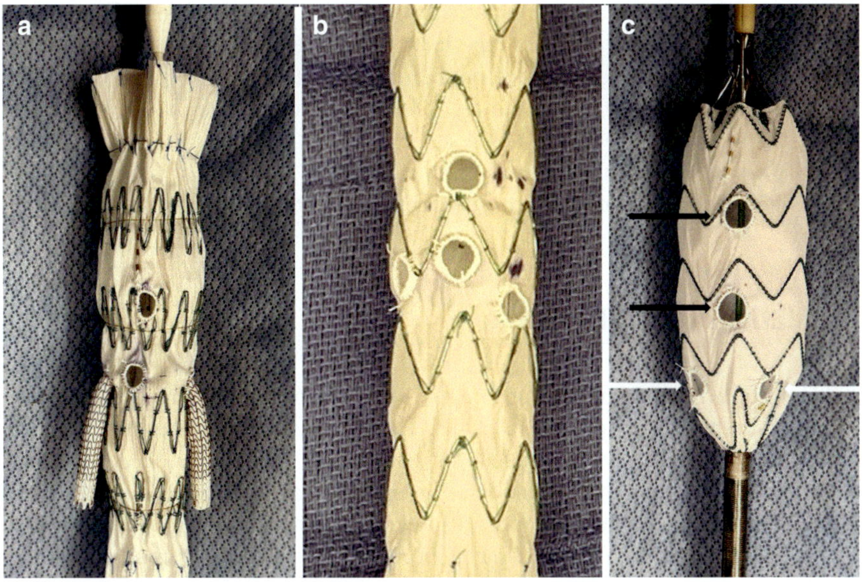

Fig. 19.3 Physician-modified fenestrated/branched endografts. Examples of fenestrated/branched device on a Cook TX2 platform (**a**), Cook Alpha platform (**b**), and Terumo TREO platform (**c**)

Further supporting an endovascular first approach for thoracoabdominal disease, a direct comparison of open, hybrid, and endovascular repair of extent II and III thoracoabdominal aortic aneurysms demonstrated a significantly higher 30-day mortality with open repair compared to F/BEVAR [37].

Results from the Cook "p-Branch" national pivotal trial in the United States are pending. Study accrual was slow as only one-third of patients screened with accepted for enrollment. In the early feasibility trial, the device was implanted in 30 patients with a 93% technical success rate. Secondary interventions, mostly for renal or superior mesenteric artery stenosis or occlusion, were necessary in 32% [18]. The Cook "t-Branch" has not been through a pivotal trial in the United States but rather has been only available through PS-IDE at select centers. In Europe, however, the device has been available since 2012 with mid-term data. A meta-analysis analyzing 197 patients who underwent repair with "t-Branch" from 2014 to 2018 demonstrated technical success of 93%, early endoleak of 10%, and early mortality of 5.8%. A large portion of these patients presented in an urgent/emergent manner. Primary branch vessel patency was 98% at a mean follow-up of 15 months [38]. The Gore TAMBE device is completing its pivotal trial in the United States and has been designated as a breakthrough device by the FDA. In the early feasibility study, the device was implanted in 13 patients with 92% technical success and no type I or III endoleak at 30 days [20].

Even though PM-F/BEVAR are widely implemented, there is minimal large-series data on their outcomes. One of the largest PMEG series evaluated 59 patients with juxtarenal AAA who underwent repair with an average of 2.5 target arteries per patient. In this series, the 30-day mortality was 5.1%, 30-day major adverse event rate was 12%, and there were no type Ia or III endoleaks at 30 days [39]. A more recent single-center series reported on their outcomes on 103 patients who underwent PM-F/BEVAR [40]. Interestingly, 27 (26%) of these cases were done in the setting of prior failed EVAR, which poses additional technical challenges to endovascular repair. Despite this, overall technical success was 99% with no increase in radiation dose, contrast use, or procedure time if a prior EVAR was present.

Limitations of the Technique

Besides limited access to CMD and off-the-shelf devices in the United States, there are several other challenges to F/BEVAR. These procedures, especially if performing a PM-F/BEVAR, have a steep learning curve. Fenestration/branch location must be precisely positioned on the endograft in order to have immediate technical success and a durable result. Intraoperative device deployment ensuring target vessel alignment is also critical for technical success. Performing these procedures in a hybrid operating room with a fusion imaging software system facilitates accurate device deployment and helps decrease contrast volume, procedure time, and radiation exposure [15]. Anatomic challenges such as severe aortic or iliac tortuosity, calcified and/or stenosis access vessels, and prior endograft in place can very much limit the rotational control of the device during deployment. Even if aligned properly, severe angulation can make target vessel cannulation and delivery of bridging stent challenging. Steerable guide sheaths have greatly improved this process.

Although reintervention is not exclusive to endovascular repair, there is a relatively high rate of reintervention following F/BEVAR as mentioned previously. Most reinterventions following F/BEVAR are performed based on findings identified during routine follow-up imaging [27]. Therefore, surveillance imaging is important to assess for endoleak, aneurysm sac diameter, bridging stent patency, and other issues. Typical postoperative protocol includes CT imaging at 1 month, 6 months, 12 months, and annually thereafter. Despite the relatively high rate of reintervention, most of these procedures are minor and percutaneous. In addition, data suggests that reintervention after F/BEVAR does not impact 1-year or 3-year overall survival [41].

Conclusion

F/BEVAR has become a reliable strategy in treating complex aortic pathology in the past decade. The results of currently available devices are very promising with outcomes that are favorable compared to open repair. As FEVAR continues to become more ubiquitous and less regionalized, robust, long-term data will emerge. Although open repair will always have a role in the management of aortic disease, advances in endovascular surgery have allowed a catheter-based approach to become the preferred treatment modality for complex aortic aneurysm in most centers.

References

1. Volodos NL, Karpovich IP, Troyan VI, et al. Clinical experience of the use of self-fixing synthetic prostheses for remote endoprosthetics of the thoracic and the abdominal aorta and iliac arteries through the femoral artery and as intraoperative endoprosthesis for aorta reconstruction. Vasa Suppl. 1991;33:93–5.
2. Parodi JC, Palmaz JC, Barone HD. Transfemoral intraluminal graft implantation for abdominal aortic aneurysms. Ann Vasc Surg. 1991;5(6):491–9.
3. Dua A, Kuy S, Lee CJ, Upchurch GR Jr, Desai SS. Epidemiology of aortic aneurysm repair in the United States from 2000 to 2010. J Vasc Surg. 2014;59(6):1512–7.
4. Dansey KD, Varkevisser RRB, Swerdlow NJ, et al. Epidemiology of endovascular and open repair for abdominal aortic aneurysms in the United States from 2004 to 2015 and implications for screening. J Vasc Surg. 2021;74(2):414–24.
5. Prinssen M, Verhoeven ELG, Buth J, et al. A randomized trial comparing conventional and endovascular repair of abdominal aortic aneurysms. N Engl J Med. 2004;351(16):1607–18.
6. Lederle FA, Freischlag JA, Kyriakides TC, et al. Outcomes following endovascular vs open repair of abdominal aortic aneurysm: a randomized trial. JAMA. 2009;302(14):1535–42.
7. Endovascular aneurysm repair and outcome in patients unfit for open repair of abdominal aortic aneurysm (EVAR trial 2): randomised controlled trial. Lancet. 2005;365(9478):2187–92.
8. Leurs LJ, Stultiëns G, Kievit J, Buth J. Adverse events at the aneurysmal neck identified at follow-up after endovascular abdominal aortic aneursym repair: how do they correlate? Vascular. 2005;13(5):261–7.
9. Park JH, Chung JW, Choo IW, Kim SJ, Lee JY, Han MC. Fenestrated stent-grafts for preserving visceral arterial branches in the treatment of abdominal aortic aneurysms: preliminary experience. J Vasc Interv Radiol. 1996;7(6):819–23.
10. Chuter TA, Gordon RL, Reilly LM, Goodman JD, Messina LM. An endovascular system for thoracoabdominal aortic aneurysm repair. J Endovasc Ther. 2001;8(1):25–33.
11. Tsilimparis N, Perez S, Dayama A, Ricotta JJ. Endovascular repair with fenestrated-branched stent grafts improves 30-day outcomes for complex aortic aneurysms compared with open repair. Ann Vasc Surg. 2013;27(3):267–73.
12. Rao R, Lane TRA, Franklin IJ, Davies AH. Open repair versus fenestrated endovascular aneurysm repair of juxtarenal aneurysms. J Vasc Surg. 2015;61(1):242–55.e5.
13. Chaikof EL, Dalman RL, Eskandari MK, et al. The Society for Vascular Surgery practice guidelines on the care of patients with an abdominal aortic aneurysm. J Vasc Surg. 2018;67(1):2–77.e2.
14. Riambau V, Böckler D, Brunkwall J, et al. Editor's choice—management of descending thoracic aorta diseases: clinical practice guidelines of the European Society for Vascular Surgery (ESVS). Eur J Vasc Endovasc Surg. 2017;53(1):4–52.
15. McNally MM, Scali ST, Feezor RJ, Neal D, Huber TS, Beck AW. Three-dimensional fusion computed tomography decreases radiation exposure, procedure time, and contrast use during fenestrated endovascular aortic repair. J Vasc Surg. 2015;61(2):309–16.
16. Watkins AC, Avramenko A, Soler R, Fabre D, Haulon S. A novel all-retrograde approach for t-Branch implantation in ruptured thoracoabdominal aneurysm. J Vasc Surg Cases Innov Tech. 2018;4(4):301–4.
17. Haulon S. Fenestrated and branched endovascular aortic repair has reached a state of maturity. J Vasc Surg. 2017;65:1247–8.

18. Farber MA, Oderich GS, Timaran C, Sanchez LA, Dawson Z. Results from a prospective multicenter feasibility study of Zenith p-Branch stent graft. J Vasc Surg. 2019;70(5):1409–18.e3.
19. Eleshra A, Oderich GS, Spanos K, et al. Short-term outcomes of the t-Branch off-the-shelf multibranched stent graft for reintervention after previous infrarenal aortic repair. J Vasc Surg. 2020;72(5):1558–66.
20. Oderich GS, Farber MA, Silveira PG, et al. Technical aspects and 30-day outcomes of the prospective early feasibility study of the GORE EXCLUDER Thoracoabdominal Branched Endoprosthesis (TAMBE) to treat pararenal and extent IV thoracoabdominal aortic aneurysms. J Vasc Surg. 2019;70(2):358–68.e6.
21. Bisdas T, Donas KP, Bosiers M, Torsello G, Austermann M. Anatomical suitability of the T-branch stent-graft in patients with thoracoabdominal aortic aneurysms treated using custom-made multibranched endografts. J Endovasc Ther. 2013;20(5):672–7.
22. Cambiaghi T, Grandi A, Bilman V, Melissano G, Chiesa R, Bertoglio L. Anatomic feasibility of the investigational GORE EXCLUDER Thoracoabdominal Branch Endoprosthesis (TAMBE), off-the-shelf multibranched endograft for the treatment of pararenal and thoracoabdominal aortic aneurysms. J Vasc Surg. 2021;73(1):22–30.
23. Starnes BW, Tatum B, Singh N. Procedural and perioperative results in patients treated with fenestrated endovascular aneurysm repair planned by automated software in a physician-sponsored investigational device exemption trial of physician-modified endografts. J Vasc Surg. 2018;68(5):1297–307.
24. Jorgensen BD, Malek M, VandenHull A, et al. A novel physician-assembled endograft for the repair of pararenal, paravisceral, Crawford type IV thoracoabdominal aortic aneurysms, and aneurysms requiring treatment after prior repair. J Vasc Surg. 2020;72(6):1897–905.e2.
25. Dossabhoy SS, Simons JP, Flahive JM, et al. Fenestrated endovascular aortic aneurysm repair using physician-modified endovascular grafts versus company-manufactured devices. J Vasc Surg. 2018;67(6):1673–83.
26. Le Houérou T, Fabre D, Alonso CG, et al. In situ antegrade laser fenestrations during endovascular aortic repair. Eur J Vasc Endovasc Surg. 2018;56(3):356–62.
27. Sveinsson M, Sonesson B, Kristmundsson T, Dias N, Resch T. Long-term outcomes after fenestrated endovascular aortic repair for juxtarenal aortic aneurysms. J Vasc Surg. 2022;75(4):1164–70.
28. Varkevisser RRB, O'Donnell TFX, Swerdlow NJ, et al. Fenestrated endovascular aneurysm repair is associated with lower perioperative morbidity and mortality compared with open repair for complex abdominal aortic aneurysms. J Vasc Surg. 2019;69(6):1670–8.
29. Wanhainen A, Verzini F, Van Herzeele I, et al. Editor's choice—European Society for Vascular Surgery (ESVS) 2019 clinical practice guidelines on the management of abdominal aorto-iliac artery aneurysms. Eur J Vasc Endovasc Surg. 2019;57(1):8–93.
30. Coselli JS, Bozinovski J, LeMaire SA. Open surgical repair of 2286 thoracoabdominal aortic aneurysms. Ann Thorac Surg. 2007;83(2):S862–4; discussion S90–2.
31. Schepens MA, Heijmen RH, Ranschaert W, Sonker U, Morshuis WJ. Thoracoabdominal aortic aneurysm repair: results of conventional open surgery. Eur J Vasc Endovasc Surg. 2009;37(6):640–5.
32. Derrow AE, Seeger JM, Dame DA, et al. The outcome in the United States after thoracoabdominal aortic aneurysm repair, renal artery bypass, and mesenteric revascularization. J Vasc Surg. 2001;34(1):54–61.
33. Cowan JA Jr, Dimick JB, Henke PK, Huber TS, Stanley JC, Upchurch GR Jr. Surgical treatment of intact thoracoabdominal aortic aneurysms in the United States: hospital and surgeon volume-related outcomes. J Vasc Surg. 2003;37(6):1169–74.
34. Oderich GS, Ribeiro M, Hofer J, et al. Prospective, nonrandomized study to evaluate endovascular repair of pararenal and thoracoabdominal aortic aneurysms using fenestrated-branched endografts based on supraceliac sealing zones. J Vasc Surg. 2017;65(5):1249–59.e10.

35. Mastracci TM, Eagleton MJ, Kuramochi Y, Bathurst S, Wolski K. Twelve-year results of fenestrated endografts for juxtarenal and group IV thoracoabdominal aneurysms. J Vasc Surg. 2015;61(2):355–64.
36. Eagleton MJ, Follansbee M, Wolski K, Mastracci T, Kuramochi Y. Fenestrated and branched endovascular aneurysm repair outcomes for type II and III thoracoabdominal aortic aneurysms. J Vasc Surg. 2016;63(4):930–42.
37. Arnaoutakis DJ, Scali ST, Beck AW, et al. Comparative outcomes of open, hybrid, and fenestrated branched endovascular repair of extent II and III thoracoabdominal aortic aneurysms. J Vasc Surg. 2020;71(5):1503–14.
38. Konstantinou N, Antonopoulos CN, Jerkku T, et al. Systematic review and meta-analysis of published studies on endovascular repair of thoracoabdominal aortic aneurysms with the t-Branch off-the-shelf multibranched endograft. J Vasc Surg. 2020;72(2):716–25.e1.
39. Starnes BW, Heneghan RE, Tatum B. Midterm results from a physician-sponsored investigational device exemption clinical trial evaluating physician-modified endovascular grafts for the treatment of juxtarenal aortic aneurysms. J Vasc Surg. 2017;65(2):294–302.
40. Asirwatham M, Konanki V, Lucas SJ, et al. Comparative outcomes of physician-modified fenestrated/branched endovascular aortic aneurysm repair in the setting of prior failed EVAR. J Vasc Surg. 2023;78(5):1153–61.
41. Giles KA, Scali ST, Pearce BJ, et al. Impact of secondary interventions on mortality after fenestrated branched endovascular aortic aneurysm repair. J Vasc Surg. 2019;70(6):1737–46.e1.

Chapter 20
Open Surgical Treatment of Pararenal Abdominal Aortic Aneurysms

Robert J. Beaulieu

Introduction

Pararenal AAAs account for 2–7% of all aortic aneurysms. Despite increased utilization of advanced endovascular techniques such as fenestrated endovascular aortic repairs (fEVAR) and physician-modified endografts (PMEG), open surgical management of these aneurysm remains an important tool in the arsenal of any vascular surgeon endeavoring to treat this pathology. The open surgical treatment of pararenal AAAs is complex and requires a detailed knowledge of the anatomic disease, careful attention to thorough preoperative patient preparation, precise operative intervention, and contemporary intensive care in the early postoperative period.

Pararenal AAAs (pAAAs) are classified as juxtarenal or suprarenal, depending on involvement of the renal artery (Fig. 20.1). An important commonality in both types is that the celiac and superior mesenteric artery remain uninvolved. Juxtarenal AAAs outnumber suprarenal AAAs, 4 to 1. Juxtarenal AAAs extend superiorly to just below the renal arteries such that no normal aorta exists between the aneurysm and the renal arteries. Suprarenal AAAs extend superiorly to include the orifices of the renal arteries to one or both kidneys. As defined by contemporary nomenclature, pAAAs proximally involve zones 8 and 9 but not 7 [1]. Accessory renal arteries may be present in 9–16% of patients and warrant consideration though distinction of pAAA is reliant on the main renal artery. Coexistent renal artery arteriosclerosis is near universal with pararenal AAAs, but it is severe enough in only 10–25% of cases to cause renovascular hypertension or ischemic nephropathy.

R. J. Beaulieu (✉)
Department of Surgery, Section of Vascular Surgery, University of Michigan Cardiovascular Center, Ann Arbor, MI, USA
e-mail: robeauli@med.umich.edu

G. J. Arnaoutakis et al. (eds.), *Aortic Aneurysms*, Contemporary Cardiology,
https://doi.org/10.1007/978-3-032-13134-8_20

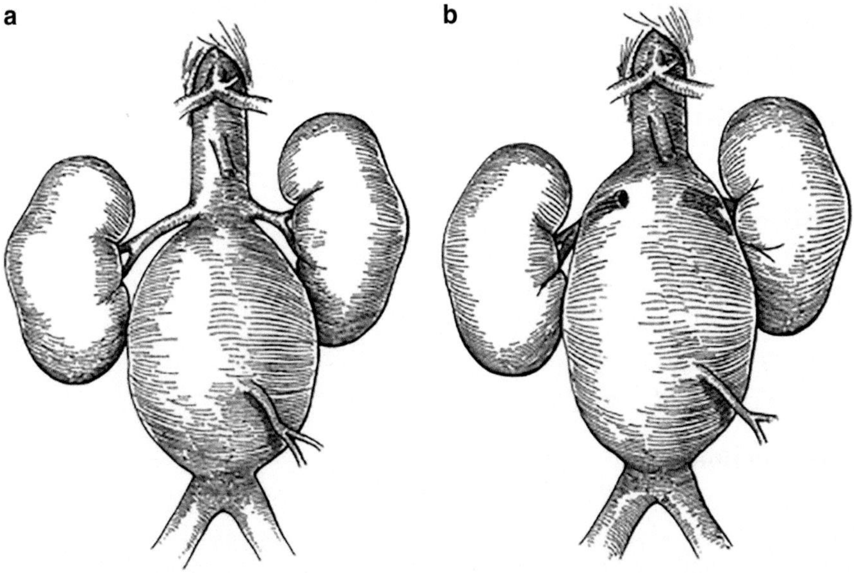

Fig. 20.1 Pararenal aortic aneurysms: Juxtarenal aneurysms (**a**) outnumber suprarenal aneurysms (**b**), 4-to-1. (Reprinted with permission from Henke and Stanley [27, p. 229])

Clinical Presentation

Most pararenal AAAs are asymptomatic. In contemporary times, pararenal AAAs are usually discovered as incidental findings during imaging studies undertaken for other illnesses. The average age at the time of diagnosis is 67 years. Men are twice as likely as women to have pararenal AAAs [2–5]. This gender predilection is not as great as the 3.5- to 4-fold male predominance that exists with infrarenal AAAs. It is conceivable that the increased proportion of women having pararenal AAAs compared to infrarenal AAAs may be due to practice patterns with more common delays in treating women until their AAAs become larger. It is well known that larger AAAs carry a greater likelihood of aneurysmal changes in the more cephalic pararenal aorta. However, it is also possible that following menopause, the loss of reproductive hormones such as estrogen that enhance both elastin and collagen crosslinking may contribute to a more generalized form of aortic dilation, such that when infrarenal AAAs evolve in women, the juxta-renal aorta and suprarenal aorta are also likely to exhibit aneurysmal changes. Considerable anecdotal experience exists to support this contention.

Pararenal AAAs are usually larger than infrarenal AAAs. Nevertheless, their recognition on physical examination is uncommon. A definitive diagnosis of a pararenal AAA requires sophisticated imaging. Computed tomography with thin slices (<1 mm thickness) should be considered standard-of-care for treatment and allows for 3D reconstructions that can aid in case preparation and visualization (Figs. 20.2 and 20.3). Renal artery anatomy must be precisely delineated to plan optimal

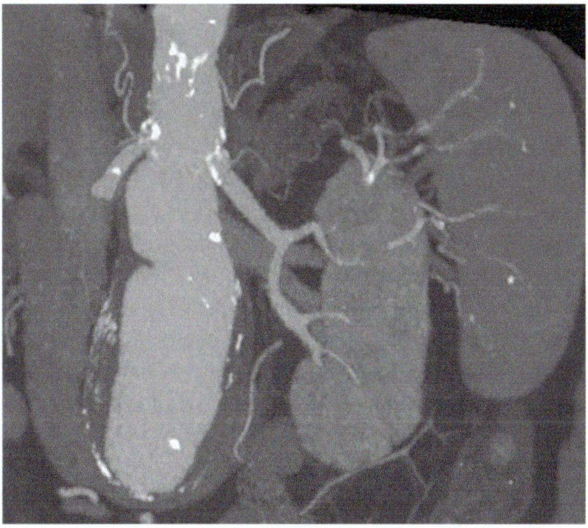

Fig. 20.2 Computed tomogram of a juxtarenal aortic aneurysm

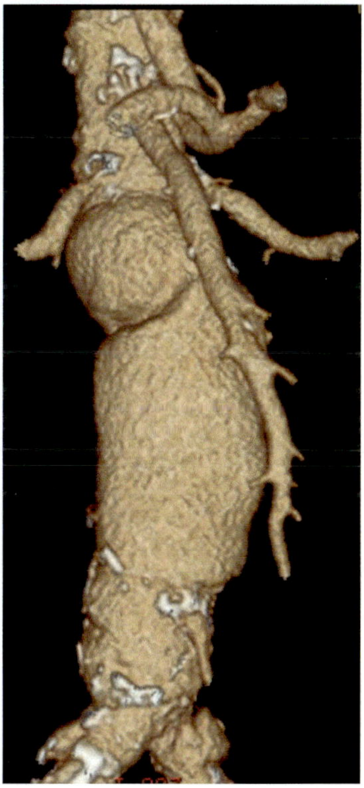

Fig. 20.3 Reformatted 3-D tomographic arteriogram of the juxtarenal aortic aneurysm in Fig. 20.2 (*See Color Plates*)

therapy of these aneurysms, especially identifying ostial disease that may impact the need for concomitant renal revascularization. CT studies require the use of iodinated contrast with its nephrotoxic risks; however, it bears noting that consensus statements from both the American College of Radiology and the National Kidney Foundation have downgraded the threat of contrast-induced nephropathy, even in patients with impaired renal function [6]. Magnetic resonance arteriography (MRA) is a frequent screening study, often obtained because of its noninvasive nature and avoidance of using nephrotoxic agents. However, in the case of pararenal AAAs, aortic branch disease may not be adequately defined by MRA studies because of turbulent flow and phase-dropout phenomenon.

Renal artery stenotic disease should be evaluated in instances in which native renal ostia are to be included in the proximal repair. Disease severe enough to warrant endovascular or open operative therapy complicates the treatment of patients with pararenal AAAs. In some series, renal artery interventions have been undertaken in more than 40% of cases [7]. Aortic spillover arteriosclerosis accounts for 80% of the renal stenoses, and critical narrowings exceeding 70–80% are bilateral in a third of the patients. The surgical therapy in many of these cases is controversial, in part due to the lack of clinical data to conclusively support renal artery reconstruction. Nevertheless, treatment of coexisting renal artery stenotic disease is justified when anatomic or functional studies support a diagnosis of renovascular hypertension. The technique of reconstructing the renal artery in these cases varies, with some favoring an aortorenal bypass [8] and others an aortorenal endarterectomy [5, 9–12].

Surgical risks attending operations for pararenal AAA are greater than for treatment of infrarenal AAAs [13]. Among recent European guidelines, a weak recommendation (Clase IIb) remains for repairing aneurysm >55 mm in men and >50 mm in women though, in practice, larger aneurysm diameters are often tolerated for patients with more complex anatomy or comorbid disease [14]. Indeed, in many series, patients with pAAA are treated with a mean diameter of 60 mm.

Several factors contribute to the increased risk associated with pAAA repair. More extensive aortic dissection, as compared with infrarenal repair, increases operative time and branch vessel manipulation. Pararenal AAA often requires clamps above one or both renal arteries, with resultant intraoperative renal ischemia. Several strategies have been utilized to reduce this physiologic insult during suprarenal clamping and these are outlined in more detail below. Finally, more proximal clamp increases cardiac strain during aortic cross-clamping and may further increase the ischemia-reperfusion response, such as metabolite circulation with unclamping [15].

Whereas most clinicians are selective with cardiac evaluations for infrarenal AAA repair, the magnitude of treating pararenal AAAs supports a more liberal screening of occult coronary artery disease. Indeed, significant variation exists between centers regarding preoperative coronary evaluation. Use of traditional risk calculators has been shown to underestimate cardiovascular risk for patients undergoing aneurysm repair. AHA/ACC guidelines recommend risk stratification based on patients' achievable metabolic equivalents for patients undergoing non-coronary surgery but in practice this is often difficult to accurately determine due to variable comorbid diseases. It is the author's advice that noninvasive pharmacological or exercise cardiac testing be undertaken in all patients with pararenal AAAs. Patients with inducible ischemia may benefit further from evaluation with an interventional cardiologist for coronary angiography. Although by no means direct proof of the validity of such testing, preoperative cardiac studies have become common in most practices, resulting in an acceptable cardiac morbidity in those patients undergoing open surgical treatment of their pararenal AAAs [2–5, 11, 16].

Operative Technique

Certain technical aspects of open surgical treatment, including patients' anatomy, prior surgical history, body habitus, and physician preference, significantly inform the surgical approach for patients with pAAAs. Three basic means of exposing pAAAs for optimal surgical therapy exist: (1) transabdominal, (2) retroperitoneal, and (3) thoracoabdominal. Each has distinct advantages and each carries different risks to the overall procedure.

A direct abdominal approach with a vertical midline or supraumbilical transverse incision is used in treating most pararenal AAAs [5]. This approach allows for adequate visualization of the suprarenal aorta to the level of the SMA, bilateral renal arteries, and bilateral iliac arteries for distal anastomosis. Direct exposure of the pararenal aorta at the base of the mesentery and mesocolon is usually pursued, although indirect aorta exposure following medial visceral rotation may be undertaken as an alternative approach, especially in the case of unusually large pararenal AAAs. While medial visceral rotation yields excellent exposure of the aneurysm neck and renal vessels, pancreatitis is a potential complication [5, 17]. In some patients, such as those with a very acute costophrenic angle, an abdominal approach alone limits the surgical exposure and increases the operative risks. In that setting, a thoracoabdominal incision allows greater visualization of the aorta and its branches.

A retroperitoneal approach through a flank or thoracic incision is preferred by some [4, 7, 18, 19]. This approach is associated with less postoperative fluid requirements and a shorter hospital stay, but no difference in morbidity or mortality has been documented [4]. This approach additionally allows for identification of multiple proximal clamp sites without retractor repositioning, which may be particularly useful in pAAAs with a friable proximal neck. If a right renal artery or iliac artery reconstruction is required, it may be technically very difficult using this approach, and in such circumstances, a second abdominal incision may be required. This approach limits the exposure of the right iliac system as well, though with effort the right iliac system can often be identified up to its bifurcation. Such exposure is more complicated in patients with concomitant iliac aneurysms.

A major factor contributing to operative morbidity relates to the proximal aortic clamp placement at the suprarenal levels, be it between the renal and superior mesenteric arteries as well as above the superior mesenteric artery or celiac artery. The patient's anatomy and disease are often the primary determinants of where clamp placement is to occur.

Supraceliac aortic clamping may be easier in terms of dissection in retroperitoneal or thoracoabdominal approaches but may require retractor repositioning in the midline approach. The aorta at that level is usually less atherosclerotic. This site provides positioning of the clamp away from the renal artery orifices and anastomotic area which may further improve visualization of the proximal anastomosis. Although some have reported no difference in patient morbidity and mortality between any of the potential clamp sites [5], others have presented evidence that supraceliac control increases mortality and postoperative renal failure [20]. As such, the most recent European Guidelines have recommended to avoid supraceliac clamping when possible. In instances where there is not an adequate clamp site below the SMA, supramesenteric cross-clamping may have reduced ischemia-reperfusion effect and myocardial demand by reducing hepatic ischemia, but requires at least 8 mm of distance between celiac and SMA and may be more technically difficult to achieve [21]. The potentially severe coagulopathy accompanying supraceliac clamping in the experimental setting [24] has not been evident in recent clinical series [2, 3, 22].

If the segment of aorta being clamped is not free of extensive atherosclerosis or luminal thrombus, unclamping and repositioning the clamp to a more proximal site may be associated with atheroembolization, visceral infarction, and death [3, 4, 12, 14]. In regard to the latter, once the pararenal aorta has been exposed, isolation and transient occlusion of the renal and mesenteric arteries with microvascular clamps or silastic vessel loops in a Potts fashion before proximal aortic clamping is a very important means of preventing embolization of dislodged aortic debris that might cause irreversible injury to the kidneys and intestines.

The dominant cause of morbidity and a substantial cause of mortality following open pararenal AAA repair is renal failure [12]. Timing of proximal aortic cross-clamping plays a critical role in minimizing renal dysfunction. Limiting the proximal aortic clamp time to less than 25 min may decrease the incidence of postoperative renal insufficiency [3, 10, 15]. It has been noted that the duration of supravisceral clamp time is directly related to morbidity and mortality [4, 22, 23]. The proximal aortic anastomosis may often be completed in a more expeditious manner if adequate preparation of the left renal vein is completed prior to cross-clamping. This can be accomplished in one of two ways: (1) ligation and division of the left renal vein or (2) division of adrenal and gonadal veins while maintaining left renal vein. If division of the left renal vein is performed, care should be taken to maintain renal outflow through adrenal, lumbar, and gonadal vessels. Transecting the left renal vein to gain easier exposure of the pararenal aorta has been associated with greater postoperative renal insufficiency, though this may be due to disruption of collaterals in this setting [24]. Replacing the clamp to the graft below the renal arteries and restoring flow to the kidneys after proximal aortic anastomosis completion will decrease renal ischemia, but caution must be taken to flush any aortic debris loosened by the proximal clamp, before restoring renal blood flow. If flushing is not done, loose material may embolize to the kidneys.

Another adjunctive maneuver to minimize renal ischemic injury is with kidney hypothermia [7]. The author favors infusion of chilled (4 °C) Ringer's lactate, to which is added 1000 U heparin, 12.5 g Mannitol, and 44.6 mEq of sodium bicarbonate/liter. This solution is preferred over chilled blood due to significantly lower rates of renal dysfunction [28]. Approximately 150 ml of this solution is infused through each renal artery orifice, with repeated administration if the occlusion time exceeds 30 min. Continuous infusion can also be completed if a renal vein cannula is left in place with a sufficiently long tubing such that another member of the surgical team may continuously infuse cold solution but not interrupt the operation. This practice may be most efficacious for patients with preoperative renal insufficiency [2–4, 12]. Ice-slurry packing of the kidneys may also lower the core kidney temperature, but such is more cumbersome and less often undertaken in most practices.

In most patients with *juxtarenal* aortic aneurysms, the proximal graft-to-aorta anastomosis occurs at the level of the renal artery orifices (Fig. 20.4). In some patients, the graft must be carried posteriorly above the renal arteries. In other instances, the anastomosis incorporates the proximal aorta and one renal artery with reimplantation of the other renal artery. In the instances of reimplantation of one renal, traditional Carrell patching may be pursued though it may be challenging due to the impact on the proximal aortic anastomosis but can facilitate more facile reimplantation.

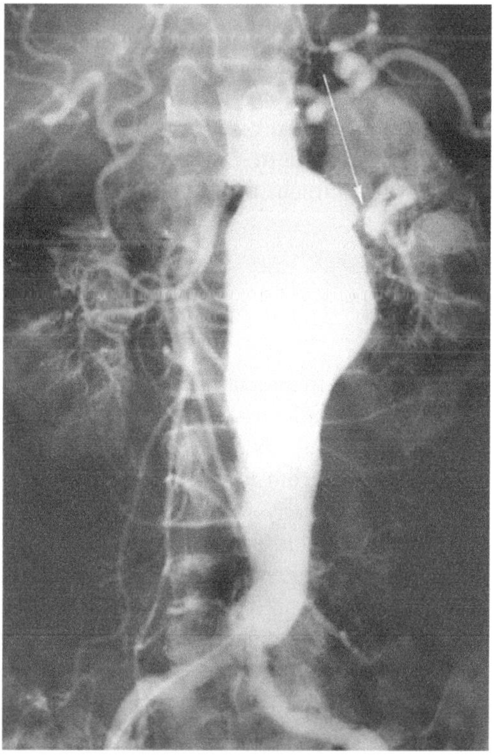

Fig. 20.4 Common open surgical reconstructive options used in treating juxtarenal aortic aneurysms: (**a**) juxtarenal graft placement, abutting the renal arteries and (**b**) tapered graft extending posteriorly above the renal arteries. (Reprinted with permission from Henke and Stanley [27, p. 231])

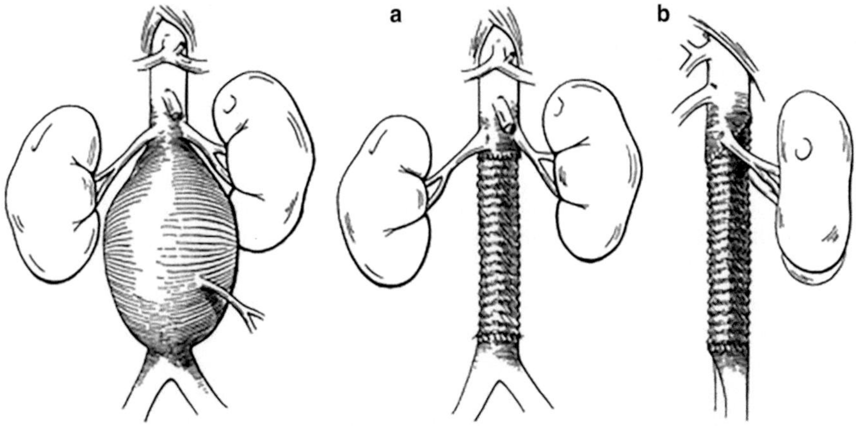

Fig. 20.5 Common open surgical reconstructive options used in treating suprarenal aortic aneurysms: (**a**) suprarenal graft placement with bilateral renal artery implantation and (**b**) suprarenal graft placement with right hepatorenal bypass and left splenorenal bypass. (Reprinted with permission from Henke and Stanley [27, p. 232])

In most *suprarenal* aortic aneurysms, the graft anastomosis will be above the renal vessels with bilateral reimplantation of the renal arteries or some other means of maintaining normal renal blood flow. In instances of inadequate renal artery mobilization, bypass grafting with 6 mm ringed PTFE can be performed, often starting with distal anastomosis to the renal artery and then proximal grafting to the aortic aneurysm graft below the level of the proximal aortic anastomosis. Nonanatomic renal revascularization with grafts to the kidney originating from the supraceliac aorta, or in some instances as hepatorenal or splenorenal bypasses, is of value in these circumstances (Fig. 20.5).

Surgical Outcomes

Open operative treatment of pAAAs in contemporary series has been accompanied by modest morbidity and mortality rates (Table 20.1). Mortality figures from experienced institutions average around 5% [4, 7, 11, 12, 24–26, 28] being slightly greater than that from contemporary series on infrarenal AAAs. Some have reported mortality rates nearly fourfold higher with suprarenal versus juxtarenal aneurysm repair [29]. Blood loss and fluid requirements are typically twice that of infrarenal AAA repairs. While not specific to pAAAs, increased intraoperative blood loss has been associated with higher risk of postoperative myocardial infarction following vascular surgery though not mortality. According to recent meta-analysis, open surgical repair of pAAAs carries higher perioperative mortality than endovascular repair, but this difference is no longer observed at 30 months follow-up [30]. There are multiple large cohort reports of higher mid-term mortality for patients

Table 20.1 Operative outcomes of treating pararenal abdominal aortic aneurysm[a]

Institution	Number of patients	Operative mortality (%)	New onset postoperative dialysis (%)
University of California, San Francisco, California [12]	257	5.8	7.0
Mayo Clinic, Rochester, Minnesota [24]	247	2.8	3.7
H San Raffaele Institute, Milan, Italy [26]	107	4.2	3.4
Methodist Hospital, Houston, Texas [11]	101	7.9	7.9
University of Michigan, Ann Arbor, Michigan[b]	84	3.5	2.4
Washington University, St. Louis, Missouri [7]	65	1.5	3.1
Henry Ford Hospital, Detroit, Michigan [4]	53	3.8	5.7

[a]Reported series composed of differing numbers of juxtarenal and suprarenal aneurysms, as well as differing numbers of patients subjected to concomitant renal revascularization procedures. This invalidates direct comparisons of one series to another

[b]Three-year experience (1996–1999) originally presented in 2000

undergoing endovascular repair, citing higher rates of reintervention among endovascular patients compared with open patients as the likely cause.

Unfortunately, the morbidity associated with the open surgical treatment of pararenal AAAs remains high. The major complication of the operative treatment of pararenal AAAs and often times the cause of death, as previously mentioned, is renal failure. The incidence of postoperative renal failure ranges from 10% to 30%, and is highest among patients with preoperative renal insufficiency and in those requiring concomitant renal artery reconstruction [3, 5, 7, 10, 24, 26, 28, 29]. However, the need for chronic hemodialysis in survivors is low. Intestinal ischemia and infarction is also a recognized cause of death in these patients [9]. Renal failure has accounted for more than half the mortality in several series [2–4, 7, 10]. Treatment of coexisting renal artery disease causing renovascular hypertension may improve blood pressure control but rarely results in cure and there is no evidence-based data supporting the routine reconstruction of the renal arteries in this subgroup of patients.

Overall survival at 5 years following the open surgical therapy of pararenal AAAs has been cited as low as 40% and as high as 75% with most late deaths due to cardiac causes [10, 23, 29], not unlike that observed after infrarenal AAA repairs. In the setting of multiple endovascular options for repair of these aneurysms, it is highly recommended that a surgeon facile in both open and endovascular techniques participate in discussions of operative choices when possible. Endovascular therapy has emerged as a front-line therapy but concerns regarding unproven techniques in patients with unsuitable anatomy and the risk of reintervention with subsequent patient harm loom heavy. It bears mentioning that in certain patients, unsuitable anatomy and severe comorbidities may preclude safe endovascular or open operative repair of their aneurysms, and in these individuals, nonoperative therapy may be quite appropriate [31–33]. Nevertheless, given the lethal nature of aneurysmal expansion with rupture, operative treatment of pararenal AAAs is warranted in all patients who are otherwise acceptable surgical candidates.

References

1. Czerny M, Schmidli J, et al. Current options and recommendations for the treatment of thoracic aortic pathologies involving the aortic arch: an expert consensus document of the European Association for Cardio-Thoracic surgery (EACTS) and the European Society for Vascular Surgery (ESVS). Eur J Cardiothorac Surg. 2019;55(1):133–62.
2. Green RM, Ricotta JJ, Ouriel K, DeWeese JA. Results of supraceliac aortic clamping in the difficult elective resection of infrarenal abdominal aortic aneu rysm. J Vasc Surg. 1989;9:125–34.
3. Nypaver TJ, Shepard AD, Reddy DJ, Elliott JP, Ernst CB. Supraceliac aortic cross clamping: determinants of outcome in elective abdominal aortic reconstructions. J Vasc Surg. 1993;17:868–76.
4. Nypaver TJ, Shepard AD, Reddy DJ, Elliott JP, Smith RF, Ernst CB. Repair of pararenal abdominal aortic aneurysms. An analysis of operative management. Arch Surg. 1993;128:803–13.
5. Qvarfordt PG, Stoney RJ, Reilly LM, Skioldebrand CG, Goldstone J, Ehrenfeld WK. Management of pararenal aneurysms of the abdominal aorta. J Vasc Surg. 1986;3:84–93.
6. Davenport MS, Perazella MA, et al. Use of intravenous iodinated contrast media in patients with kidney disease: consensus statements from the American College of Radiology and the National Kidney Foundation. Kidney Med. 2020;2(1):85–93.
7. Allen BT, Anderson CB, Rubin BG, Flye MW, Baumann DS, Sicard GA. Preservation of renal function in juxtarenal and suprarenal abdominal aortic aneu-rysm repair. J Vasc Surg. 1993;17:948–59.
8. Cambria RP, Brewster DC, L'Italien G, Koustas G, Atamian S, LaMuraglia GM, Gertler JP, Abbott WM. Simultaneous aortic and renal artery reconstruction: evolution of an eighteen-year experience. J Vasc Surg. 1995;21:916–25.
9. Clair DG, Belkin M, Whittemore AD, Mannick JA, Donaldson MC. Safety and efficacy of transaortic renal endarterectomy as an adjunct to aortic surgery. J Vasc Surg. 1995;21:926–34.
10. Crawford ES, Beckett WC, Greer MS. Juxtarenal infrarenal abdominal aortic aneu-rysm. Special diagnostic and therapeutic considerations. Ann Surg. 1986;203:661–70.
11. Jean-Claude J, Reilly LM, Stoney RJ, Messina LM. Pararenal aortic aneu-rysms: the future of open aortic aneurysm repair. J Vasc Surg. 1999;29:902–12.
12. McNeil JW, String ST, Pfeifer RB Jr. Concomitant renal endarterectomy and aortic reconstruction. J Vasc Surg. 1994;20:331–7.
13. Faggioli G, Stella A, Freyrie A, Gargiulo M, Tarantini S, Rodio M, Pilato A, D'Addato M. Early and long-term results in the surgical treatment of juxtarenal and pararenal aortic aneurysms. Eur J Vasc Endovasc Surg. 1998;15:205–11.
14. Wanhainen A, Van Herzeele I, et al. European Society for Vascular Surgery (ESVS) 2024 clinical practice guidelines on the management of abdominal aorto-iliac artery aneurysms. Eur J Vasc Endovasc Surg. 2024;67(2):192–331.
15. Zammert M, Gelman S. The pathophysiology of aortic cross-clamping. Best Pract Res Clin Anaesthesiol. 2016;30(3):257–69.
16. Messina LM. Pararenal aortic aneurysms: the future of open repair. Cardiovasc Surg. 2002;10:424–33.

17. Reilly LM, Ramos TK, Murray SP, Cheng SWK, Stoney RJ. Optimal exposure of the proximal abdominal aorta: a critical appraisal of transabdominal medial visceral rotation. J Vasc Surg. 1994;19:375–90.
18. Illig KA, Green RM. Diagnosis and management of the "difficult" abdominal aortic aneurysm: pararenal aneurysms, inflammatory aneurysms, and horseshoe kidney. Semin Vasc Surg. 2001;14:312–7.
19. Pokrovsky AV, Karimov SI, Yermolyuk RS, Thursunov BZ, Asamov RE. Thoracophrenolumbotomy as an approach of choice in reconstruction of the proximal abdominal aorta and visceral branches. J Vasc Surg. 1991;13:892–6.
20. Varkevisser R, Guerre L, et al. The impact of proximal clamp location on peri-operative outcomes following open surgical repair of juxtarenal abdominal aortic aneurysms. Eur J Vasc Endovasc Surg. 2020;59(3):411–8.
21. Martelli E, Sung Cho J. Merits of and technical tips for supra-mesenteric aortic cross clamping. Vasc Spec Int. 2019;35(2):55–9.
22. Hines GL, Chorost M. Supraceliac aortic occlusion: a safe approach to parea-renal aortic aneurysms. Ann Vasc Surg. 1998;12:335–40.
23. Schneider JR, Gottner RJ, Golan JF. Supraceliac versus infrarenal aortic cross-clamp for repair of non-ruptured infrarenal and juxtarenal abdominal aortic aneurysm. Cardiovasc Surg. 1997;5:279–85.
24. Cohen JR, Angus L, Asher A, Chang JB, Wise L. Disseminated intravascular coagulation as a result of supraceliac clamping: implications for thoracoabdominal aneurysm repair. Ann Vasc Surg. 1987;1:552–7.
25. Back MR, Bandyk M, Bradner M, Cuthbertson D, Johnson BL, Shames ML, Bandyk DF. Critical analysis of outcome determinants affecting repair of intact aneurysms involving the visceral aorta. Ann Vasc Surg. 2005;19:648–56.
26. Poulias GE, Doundoulakis N, Skoutas B, Prombonas E, Haddad H, Papaioannou K, Lymberiades D, Savopoulkos G. Juxtarenal abdominal aneurysmectomy. J Cardiovasc Surg. 1992;33:324–30.
27. West CA, Noel AA, Bower TC, Cherry KJ Jr, Gloviczki P, Sullivan TM, Kalra M, Hoskin TL, Harrington JR. Factors affecting outcomes of open surgical repair of pararenal aortic aneurysms: a 10-year experience. J Vasc Surg. 2006;43:921–8.
28. Lemaire S, Jones M, et al. Randomized comparison of cold blood and cold crystalloid renal perfusion for renal protection during thoracoabdominal aortic aneurysm repair. J Vasc Surg. 2009;49(1):11–9.
29. Chiesa R, Marone EM, Brioschi C, Frigerio S, Tshoma Y, Melissano G. Open repair of pararenal aortic aneurysms: operative management, early results, and risk factor analysis. Ann Vasc Surg. 2006;20:739–46.
30. Patel S, Ormesher D, et al. Comparison of open, standard, and complex endovascular aortic repair treatments for juxtarenal/short neck aneurysms: a systematic review and network meta-analysis. Eur J Vasc Endovasc Surg. 2022;63(5):696–706.
31. Tanquilut EM, Veith FJ, Ohki T, Lipsitz EC, Shaw PM, Suggs WD, Wain RA, Mehta M, Cayne NS, McKay J. Nonoperative management with selective delayed surgery for large abdominal aortic aneurysms in patients at high risk. J Vasc Surg. 2002;36:41–6.
32. Veith FJ, Tanquilut EM, Ohki T, Lipsitz EC, Suggs WD, Wain RA, Gargiulo NJ. Conservative observational management with selective delayed repair for large abdominal aortic aneurysms in high risk patients. J Cardiovasc Surg. 2003;44:459–64.
33. Henke PK, Stanley JC. Surgical treatment of pararenal aortic aneurysm. In: Ernst CB, Stanley JC, editors. Current therapy in vascular surgery. 4th ed. Mosby: St. Louis; 2001.

Chapter 21
Treatment of Ruptured Abdominal Aortic Aneurysm

Brian Fazzone, Gilbert R. Upchurch Jr., and Zain Shahid

Introduction

The contemporary annual estimate of ruptured abdominal aortic aneurysm (RAAA) incidence is 7.9 per one million persons, a decrease of 70% since 1999 [1]. Despite a decreasing incidence, mortality after rupture remains high at 53–77% [2, 3]. RAAA deaths have decreased substantially due to increased rates of elective repair, better screening and risk factor modification, and improvements in perioperative care and endovascular capabilities [1, 4, 5]. However, mortality is near absolute without surgical repair, typically occurring within 8 h of rupture in hemodynamically unstable patients [6].

Risk Factors

Hypertension, active smoking, family history of aneurysm, increasing age, and female sex are well-characterized risk factors for rupture. Though the incidence of rupture is four times greater in men, the rupture risk may be four times greater in women [7–9], perhaps due to a greater growth rate [10]. The mean growth rate for all patients is 2.0–3.0 mm per year, and faster in larger aneurysms [11]. Smoking is the most important modifiable risk factor for rupture as growth rates are up to 25% faster in smokers compared to non-smokers [3].

B. Fazzone · G. R. Upchurch Jr. · Z. Shahid (✉)
Division of Vascular Surgery and Endovascular Therapy, Department of Surgery, University of Florida, Gainesville, FL, USA
e-mail: brian.fazzone@surgery.ufl.edu; gib.upchurch@surgery.ufl.edu; zain.shahid@surgery.ufl.edu

G. J. Arnaoutakis et al. (eds.), *Aortic Aneurysms*, Contemporary Cardiology,
https://doi.org/10.1007/978-3-032-13134-8_21

Aneurysm size, wall thickness, presence of intra-luminal thrombus (ILT), and peak wall stress are important biomechanical risk factors for rupture [2, 12, 13]. Aneurysm size remains the strongest predictor of rupture, with rupture rates exceeding 10% in aortas greater than 6 cm [14]. However, models incorporating aortic geometry, tissue properties, and clinical data may provide greater accuracy for estimating individual-level risks for rupture [15, 16].

Pathophysiology

Aortic rupture occurs when aortic wall stress exceeds wall strength. Increased intraluminal pressure and decreased aortic wall integrity are the primary mechanisms contributing to rupture. Hemodynamic flow patterns may uniquely contribute to increased intraluminal pressure and patients with helical flow within an aneurysmal segment may be at higher risk of rupture [17, 18]. Aortic wall integrity is affected by several factors including the presence of ILT, calcification, and inflammation [2]. ILT itself may cause regional hypoxia across the vessel wall leading to inflammation and wall thinning over time [19, 20]. Evidence of chronic aortic wall inflammation, increased proteolysis, extracellular matrix degradation, and smooth muscle cell dysregulation all underlie the biology of aneurysm formation and have been found in aortic tissue after rupture [2, 21].

Presentation

The classic presentation for RAAA is a triad of severe abdominal or back pain, hypotension, and a pulsatile mass [22, 23]. Unfortunately, this traditional presentation occurs in less than half of the patients. A meta-analysis summarizing the common presenting symptoms of RAAA reports abdominal pain as the most reported symptom (61%), followed by hypotension (46%), a pulsatile mass (45%), back and/or flank pain (42%), syncope (25%), and nausea and/or emesis (22%) [24]. Misdiagnosis rates range from 10% to 50% and negatively influence mortality in the acute setting [24, 25].

Less common presentations include trauma (motor vehicle accident) [23], hiccups [26], gross hematuria [27], renal colic [28], gastrointestinal bleeding [29], crural neuropathy [30, 31], urethral obstruction [32], obstruction of the left colon [33], hip pain [34], altered mental status [35], right testicular pain [36, 37], and even groin hernias and incarcerations [38]. Patients who rupture into their vena cava, iliac vein, or renal vein may present in congestive heart failure with distended neck veins, an abdominal bruit, microscopic or macroscopic hematuria, or an acute left varicocele. Aorto-caval fistulas occur in as many as 2–4% of patients with RAAA [39, 40].

A minority of patients may present with late RAAA after a previous EVAR. One meta-analysis calculated the incidence of late rupture after EVAR at 0.9% with a mean time to rupture of 37 months and primarily driven by graft-related endoleaks [41].

Differentiation between symptomatic and ruptured aneurysms is important as they have different mortality rates. Patients with symptomatic aneurysms may have symptoms of variable severity (ranging from mild tenderness to pain indistinguishable from rupture); however, no blood is identified outside the aortic wall at laparotomy. The etiology of the pain is thought to be related to acute expansion of the aortic wall, intramural hemorrhage, and bleeding into the thrombus. These patients do not have hypotension, and their prognosis is much better than the prognosis of patients with rupture, but worse than with elective repair with an operative mortality five times that of elective AAA repairs [42].

Diagnosis

Plain Films

Plain films of the lumbar region, routinely obtained in patients with back pain, may show a calcified shell of the aorta. In one review of 31 patients with surgically proven ruptured AAAs, 65% had calcification of the aneurysm that was visible on a plain abdominal radiograph [43]. Ruptured aneurysm may appear as a large abdominal soft tissue mass with peripheral calcification on abdominal plain films [44].

Abdominal Ultrasound

Ultrasonography should not be used to diagnose RAAA. Despite having nearly 100% sensitivity in detecting AAAs [45], it is very poor at detecting rupture. Sonographic evaluation of rupture is limited by poor detection of retroperitoneal blood, inferior sensitivity to CT for detection of intra-abdominal free fluid, operator-dependence, and dependence on body habitus [46].

Computed Tomography (CT)

CT is the best imaging technique to diagnose RAAA. Retroperitoneal blood on CT imaging is 77% sensitive and 100% specific for RAAA. The positive predictive value is 100%, and the negative predictive value is 89% [47]. Figure 21.1 shows a ruptured abdominal aortic aneurysm with a large retroperitoneal hematoma.

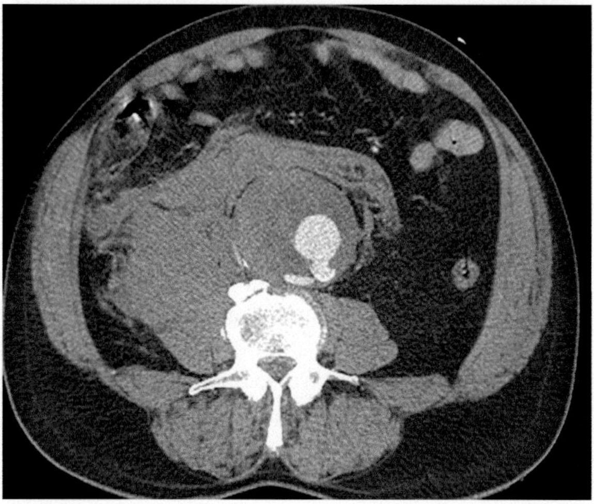

Fig. 21.1 CTA demonstrating a ruptured abdominal aortic aneurysm with a large retroperitoneal hematoma

Some of the signs used to help diagnose RAAA by CT are [48]:

1. A retroperitoneal hematoma adjacent to an abdominal aortic aneurysm.
2. The draped aorta sign. This sign is present when the posterior wall of the aorta either is not identifiable as distinct from adjacent structures or when it closely follows the contour of adjacent vertebral bodies.
3. A focal discontinuity in the calcifications of the circumferential wall around the aorta.
4. A well-defined peripheral crescent of increased attenuation within the thrombus of a large abdominal aortic aneurysm.

CT should be performed in all stable or hemodynamically responsive patients with RAAA to evaluate patient candidacy for endovascular repair, particularly given the potential mortality benefit of endovascular repair in select patients [49]. CT should be obtained using a 3-mm (or smaller) thin-cut protocol with intravenous contrast.

MRI/MRA

Magnetic resonance (MR) imaging requires a much longer acquisition time, and MR imaging is less available and less convenient, therefore rarely used to diagnose RAAA.

Risk Scoring

Multiple risk scoring systems have been devised to identify patients at risk for mortality after attempted repair [50–54]. Prediction of immediate postoperative death allows for consoling the families, especially the elderly patient who may decide to forgo surgery. Generally, advanced age, elevated serum creatinine, anemia, and the presence of myocardial ischemia and hypotension most negatively affect mortality after repair [50–52, 55]. However, no scoring system can predict postoperative mortality with 100% accuracy [56]. Given inconsistent scoring system performance and lack of absolute validity, we maintain that only in the direst of situations (e.g., severe Alzheimer's, widely metastatic cancer, multiple advanced co-morbid conditions, etc.) should operative repair be denied.

Initial Management

Transfer

First and foremost, if there are no personnel who are qualified in the institution, urgent transfer to a center with trained individuals is required. One in six patients transferred will die before receiving operative repair; however, operative mortality is lower in transferred patients [57]. The Western Vascular Society published guidelines for transfer which include rapid transfer to a hospital with appropriate facilities and expertise, expedited physician to physician discussion, and transfer to the facility that allows for the shortest time from diagnosis to treatment [57].

Immediately upon diagnosis, two large-bore intravenous accesses should be established with labs sent and a minimum of 6 units of packed red blood cells should be crossmatched. Transfusion devices that warm and rapidly transfuse blood products are extremely useful. A Foley catheter should be placed to help determine end-organ perfusion. If the patient is hemodynamically stable, a baseline electrocardiogram and chest x-ray are rapidly acquired. An arterial line can be placed if it does not delay transfer to the operative room. Given the widespread use of endovascular surgery for RAAA repair, a CT scan should be obtained in stable or quasi-stable patients to assess suitability for EVAR. This may be obtained at the pre-transfer hospital if CT does not delay diagnosis and that imaging can be readily transferred to the receiving hospital [57].

Resuscitation

The optimal degree of preoperative resuscitation before operative intervention is controversial [58, 59]. Crawford was the first to suggest minimal fluid resuscitation to maintain the systolic blood pressure at 50–70 mm Hg [60]. A normotensive resuscitation strategy (i.e., resuscitation with crystalloids and/or colloids with a target systolic blood pressure > 100 mmHg) may be detrimental to the hemorrhaging hypotensive patient. Dilutional coagulopathy, rapid increases in blood pressure exacerbating hemorrhage, or hypothermia caused by infusion of cold fluids can worsen hemorrhage after large volume resuscitation. Most of these observations are derived from trauma literature. Among patients with penetrating trauma and hypotension (systolic blood pressure < 90 mm Hg), improved survival was observed in patients who received minimal fluid resuscitation therapy until they arrived in the operating room [59].

There are no randomized controlled trials to support the use of a controlled (i.e., permissive) hypotension resuscitation strategy in RAAA patients [61]. Specific to RAAA, normalization or even elevation of the blood pressure may lead to rupture of the temporary aortic seal. Current Society for Vascular Surgery guidelines recommend a permissive hypotensive resuscitation strategy, targeting a systolic blood pressure range of 70–90 mmHg; however, the evidence for this remains poor [62]. One must keep in mind that this may not apply to RAAA patients who are older and have significant cardiovascular co-morbidities.

Balloon Tamponade

Intra-aortic balloon tamponade was first described in the 1950s as a potential method to control refractory hemorrhage in Korean war injuries [63]. In 1961, Hesse and Kletschka further described its use in a RAAA patient. A Foley catheter inserted over a stylet and placed directly into the aorta, and the balloon was inflated with 30 mL of saline facilitating proximal aortic control [64]. This technique remains useful for rapidly achieving proximal aortic control in a hypotensive RAAA patient prior to definitive repair.

There is minimal evidence to support its effect on RAAA outcomes, but the primary indication for its use is hemodynamic instability in a rapidly deteriorating patient [62]. Some institutions routinely use aortic balloon occlusion in all RAAA patients with systolic blood pressures <90 mmHg [65]. Techniques may vary between institutions, but percutaneous or femoral cut-down is the preferred initial approach for access. Once access is obtained a 0.035-inch guidewire can be inserted to the level of the descending thoracic aorta under fluoroscopy. The guidewire is then exchanged for a long extra-stiff guidewire to accommodate a long 12–14 F sheath to the level of the celiac axis. An aortic occlusion balloon is inserted over the guidewire and inflated proximal to the RAAA. The sheath should be about the inflated balloon and the balloon should be secured to the skin to prevent migration [66].

Operative Strategy

Deciding Endovascular vs Open Repair

Improvements in endovascular technology and infrastructure have made endovascular repair of RAAA (i.e., rEVAR) the preferred repair choice in capable centers. Open surgical repair (OSR) is generally reserved for patients anatomically unsuitable for rEVAR or if patients are too unstable to receive a preoperative CT scan for anatomic evaluation. Three randomized controlled trials comparing OSR to rEVAR have been conducted, each showing similar mortality outcomes out to 1 year between repair strategies [67–69]. However, the interpretation of these trial results is inherently flawed given patient selection and randomization challenges, high crossover rates, and even high misdiagnosis rates. Historically, many observational studies have shown a considerable mortality benefit for patients undergoing rEVAR, but are inherently limited by their retrospective nature. We currently support an endovascular first approach for all anatomically suitable patients with favorable anatomy, reserving OSR for patients too unstable to receive a preoperative CT scan or with anatomy not suitable for rEVAR.

Open Repair

Operative Strategy

In the operating room while the patient is being prepped, broad-spectrum antibiotics are administered. An arterial line and a central venous catheter are placed while the patient is awake. However, these procedures should not delay the operation as it is imperative that the bleeding is stopped. The patient is prepped and draped before anesthesia is induced with agents designed to have minimal effect on blood pressure. This practice allows the operation to be started immediately after induction. Hypotension after induction should be anticipated due to loss of sympathetic drive. One should be ready to get rapid control of the aorta if this should happen. Some surgeons routinely deploy an aortic occlusion balloon for rapid proximal aortic control in the event of hypotension after induction. Some have suggested that in moribund patients experiencing severe shock, the surgeon should start even before the induction of anesthesia. Cell saver may be used at the surgeon's discretion, but has been shown to reduce intraoperative transfusion requirements in RAAA patients [70].

Proximal Control

The first goal of this operation is cessation of hemorrhage. Most surgeons prefer a transperitoneal, midline incision because it affords wide exposure to the abdominal aorta and allows rapid supra-celiac control if necessary. This is accomplished initially by manual compression. The supraceliac aorta is exposed at the diaphragm by retracting the left lobe of the liver to the right, opening the gastrohepatic omentum and retracting the esophagus and stomach which are identified by the nasogastric tube to the left. The aorta is identified between the crura of the diaphragm which are divided with electrocautery. After isolating the aorta, the clamp is guided over the surgeon's index and middle fingers and placed on either side of the aorta.

Supraceliac aortic control is beneficial in cases of severe hypotension or uncontrolled bleeding. It also helps avoid renal and gonadal vein injury often associated with blind dissection in a hematoma to identify the infrarenal aortic neck. Supraceliac aortic clamping, however, incurs ischemia time to the viscera and along with its complications, notably postoperative bleeding, and multi-system organ failure. Therefore, supraceliac aortic clamping is usually temporary, until the peri-duodenal aorta is dissected out to see if there is adequate room for infrarenal aortic clamping.

Other options for rapid proximal aortic control include [71]:

1. Direct placement of an aortic balloon (or Foley catheter) through the aneurysm sac. If this approach is used, try to thread the graft through the balloon before deployment. This maneuver facilitates the proximal aortic anastomosis.
2. Brachial or femoral artery puncture or cut down to insert an occlusion balloon into the visceral aorta using fluoroscopic guidance.
3. Thoracotomy with descending aortic clamping. There is some data to support worse outcomes for this approach when compared to transhiatal control [72].

Caution needs to be used with these methods, as the aortic thrombus can be disrupted leading to embolization. Aortic balloons are associated with mal-positioning or movement as the aneurysm sac is opened [73]. Recognize that aortic compression and balloon techniques are blind and may not provide complete control.

In the more stable patient, dissecting out the infra-renal aorta may reward you with a suitable neck where you can avoid a supraceliac aortic clamp. This is our first choice, however, if the patient becomes unstable, if there is a large hematoma around the renal arteries, or if we encounter significant bleeding the supraceliac aorta is promptly clamped. Here, care must be taken to avoid injury to the left renal vein, the lumbar veins, and the IVC. The left renal vein can be ligated and divided granted you preserve the venous collaterals to the left kidney, which include the left adrenal vein, the left gonadal vein, and the lumbar vein.

If a suprarenal AAA is approached anteriorly, medial visceral rotation is required to expose the suprarenal aorta. In this technique, the left colon is mobilized by incising the lateral peritoneal attachments. The colon, pancreas, spleen, and kidney are elevated, allowing access to the diaphragmatic crura, which cover the aorta at this level. Division of the crura allows access to the entire intra-abdominal aorta and the visceral and renal vessels.

After obtaining proximal aortic control, allow anesthesia to fully resuscitate the patient and transfuse to an adequate blood pressure. This is important because after opening the aorta there is additional blood loss from the lumbar arteries.

The use of heparin during RAAA repair remains controversial with no clear guidelines. Many surgeons avoid systemic heparinization because of bleeding complications, although heparinized saline can be given directly into the iliac arteries to try to reduce distal thrombosis. Some authors maintain that heparinization may be beneficial in decreasing the incidence of DIC and maintaining microcirculatory perfusion in patients with RAAA [74]. Contemporary studies further suggest that RAAA itself leads to a pro-coagulable state which may respond to systemic heparinization [75]. A recent large propensity score-matched analysis demonstrated reductions in perioperative transfusion requirements and 30-day all-cause mortality without an increase in bleeding complications in patients who received heparin during RAAA repair compared to those who did not [76]. At our institution, the standard is to give a partial dose of heparin to keep the activating clotting time (ACT) around 200.

Distal Control

This can be achieved with clamps on the iliac arteries or occasionally the distal aorta. Occlusion balloons can also be placed in the iliac arteries after opening the aneurysm sac if there is a large hematoma and dissection is hazardous. Some surgeons open the aneurysm and get distal control by packing the iliac artery orifices under retractors. Iliac aneurysms are left alone if they are not too large (<3 cm) as this ensures a rapid operation with the least amount of cross-clamping.

Description of Operation

After eviscerating the small bowel and carefully mobilizing the duodenum from the aorta, the aneurysm is opened. The lumbar arteries and inferior mesenteric artery are suture ligated from inside the aneurysm. A Dacron or PTFE graft (usually 16–22 mm in diameter) is used and anastomosed proximally with a 3-0 permanent monofilament suture. A strip of felt may be incorporated into the anastomosis in degenerative aortas on the aortic side as a continuous pledget. Blood volume should have been restored by this time, and adequate fresh frozen plasma and platelets should be available. The anastomosis is tested with retrograde heparin flush prior to removing the clamp. Re-perfusing the visceral and renal vessels may result in significant hypotension and requires careful coordination with anesthesia to ensure that the proper fluids are administered and that a presser agent and bicarbonate are prepared for use if required. If there are no significant leaks the clamp is placed on the infrarenal aorta (or graft), packed, and attention turned to the distal anastomosis. A tube graft will suffice for 80–90% of the patients. If the repair involves the iliac arteries, an aorto-biiliac graft is used to maintain flow to at least one hypogastric

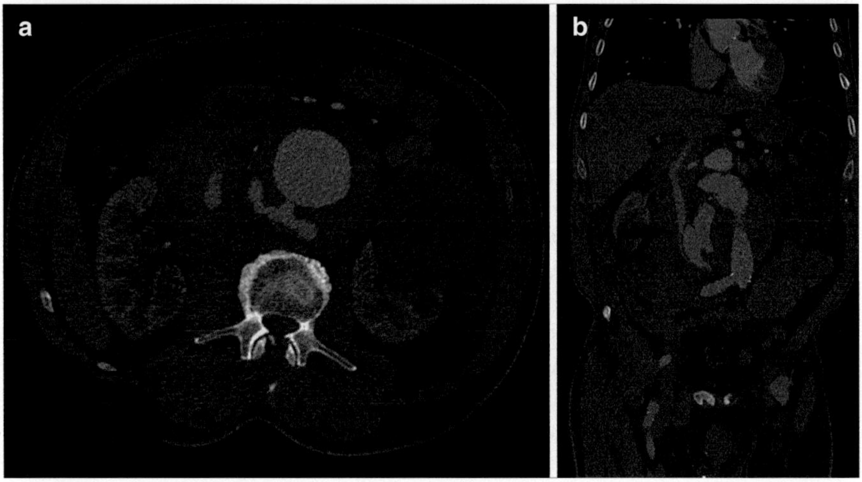

Fig. 21.2 CTA showing ruptured abdominal aortic aneurysm with an aortocaval fistula showing (**a**) axial view of infrarenal aorta, (**b**) coronal view with solid arrow pointing at the fistula

artery to insure perfusion to the pelvis. Rarely is an aorto-bifemoral bypass required for RAAA.

If discovered intraoperatively, treatment of an aorto-caval fistula (Fig. 21.2) is done after opening the aorta and placing pressure via sponge sticks on the cava distally and proximally. The vena cava is repaired by suturing the fistula from within the aneurysm. Care is taken to avoid air, thrombus, or other debris from entering the vena cava while repairing it.

The aneurysm sac is closed over the prosthesis, isolating it from the bowel. No attempt is made to decompress the retroperitoneal hematoma. The abdomen is closed with a heavy monofilament. If the patient has required massive resuscitation and/or there is significant edema in the bowel, then a Vacuum Assisted Closure (VAC) dressing is used to temporarily close the abdomen.

Retroperitoneal Approach

A retroperitoneal (RP) approach may be considered in stable patients or patients with contained rupture, particularly if the patient has a hostile abdomen, enteric stoma, juxtarenal, pararenal, or suprarenal aneurysm. Historically, the RP approach has been associated with decreased pulmonary and gastrointestinal complications, decreased intraoperative fluid requirements and blood loss, and quicker recovery compared to the transperitoneal (TP) approach in patients undergoing elective AAA repair [77, 78]. However, a recent Cochrane review demonstrated no evidence for benefit of either approach with regard to mortality or postoperative complications [79]. The RP approach was associated with shorter ICU admission and less blood loss; however, the certainty of evidence is limited given the low quality of RCTs performed. The benefits of the RP over the TP approach for the repair of RAAA have not been studied. Regardless, surgeons performing open RAAA repair should be familiar with the RP approach to facilitate aortic exposure.

The patient should be in the right lateral decubitus position with their hips elevated approximately 30–45 degrees over a bean bag. The shoulders should be positioned at 60 degrees from the left flank. A curvilinear incision is made starting halfway between the umbilicus and pubic symphysis, extending posteriorly towards the ninth or tenth interspace. The incision should course 5 cm medial to the anterior iliac spine. Once through the subcutaneous tissues, the fibers of the external oblique, internal oblique, transversus abdominus, and serratus anterior are divided with cautery. The retroperitoneal space is entered bluntly at the lateral costal margin. The dissection is extended cephalad dividing the intercoastal muscles and entering the left chest. In patients who are unstable, the distal descending thoracic aorta can be dissected out from the left chest, in an expedited manner, and a clamp can be placed. The abdominal contents are identified and their overlying peritoneal is gently mobilized away from the retroperitoneal space. A Bookwalter (or similar) retractor can be used to facilitate aortic exposure. Further dissection is performed to expose the aorta. The left kidney may be left in the posterior position or mobilized anteriorly depending on the proximal extent of aneurysm and surgeon preference. At our institute, it is standard to mobilize the kidney anteriorly to expose the entire paravisceral aorta. Regardless, the left ureter should be identified and protected. The lumbar veins and lymphatics should be clipped, ligated, and divided as they are identified. Once the dissection is complete, the entire abdominal aorta and the left iliac system should be easily visualized. In most cases, the proximal right common iliac artery is also able to be dissected free. The left crus of the diaphragm may be divided if more proximal exposure is needed in the event of a juxtarenal, pararenal, or suprarenal aneurysm or need for supraceliac clamping. The aorta is then clamped proximally and iliac arteries are controlled distally and the aneurysm is repaired as described in the transperitoneal approach.

In patients with pararenal or suprarenal aneurysms, there is usually no infrarenal sewing ring, and the proximal anastomosis has to be extended proximally. In such situations, the proximal clamp is placed either on the supraceliac aorta or in between the celiac and the superior mesenteric artery. The latter is preferred if possible to allow perfusion of the celiac artery and bowel via collaterals. The proximal anastomosis is beveled and a left renal artery bypass is performed. At our institute, it is standard to pre-sew a 6 mm Dacron graft to the tube or bifurcated graft intended for aortic repair to decrease the renal ischemia time. Of note, this is usually performed in patients who are stable and after dissection is complete and proximal clamp is in position. Premade branched grafts are also available that can be used as a substitute. The proximal anastomosis is performed first, generally using a 3-0 permanent monofilament suture. The clamp is then moved to the graft allowed reperfusion of the celiac, superior mesenteric, and right renal artery. The left renal anastomosis is performed next using a 5-0 permanent monofilament suture. This is followed by distal reconstruction.

Endovascular Repair

Anatomical Considerations

Preoperative CT is critical for evaluating aortoiliac anatomy for rEVAR. Advancements in endograft systems have expanded the suitability of patient anatomy for rEVAR. As many as 85% of patients meet criteria for elective repair based on commercial endograft instructions for use (IFU) [80]. Anatomic eligibility for endograft placement is device and patient-dependent but generally suitable for proximal sealing zones ≥15 mm, infernal neck angulation ≤60 degrees, and aortic neck diameters ≤32 mm. Some contemporary devices may accommodate shorter neck lengths and more severe neck angulation.

In the IMPROVE trial, 36% of patients were anatomically excluded from rEVAR after randomization to the endovascular first approach [69]. Using criteria for suitability defined by a neck length ≥10 mm, diameter ≤32 mm, and angulations ≤75 degrees, Mehta et al. found that 80% of RAAA patients could be anatomically suitable for rEVAR [81]. Surgeons should be facile with intravascular ultrasound (IVUS) for intraoperative anatomic evaluation for any borderline CT findings. Endograft placement in an unsuitable candidate can increase the risk of endoleaks, graft migration, or aneurysm rupture.

Anesthesia

A significant advantage of rEVAR over OSR is the ability to perform under local anesthesia (LA). rEVAR performed under LA is associated with a significant reduction in 30-day mortality compared to rEVAR performed under general anesthesia (GA) [82, 83]. In their large review of VQI data, Fazier et al. found that LA was associated with lower 30-day (15.5% vs. 23.3%) and 1-year (22.5% vs 32.3%) mortality compared to GA, with young and normotensive patients having the greatest benefit [84]. Some institutions may start all rEVARs under LA, converting to open only for secondary procedures (e.g., abdominal exploration) or inability to tolerate LA [85].

Equipment

A standardized approach to rEVAR should be adopted by institutions with hybrid capabilities. This includes multidisciplinary collaboration with emergency department physicians for preoperative resuscitation and minimization of door to CT scanner and OR time, anesthesiologists for intraoperative resuscitation approach and anesthetic approach, and operating room nurses and technologists with the appropriate expertise and equipment [86, 87]. At minimum, an operating suite should have hybrid capabilities, intravascular ultrasound (IVUS), and access to standard sheaths, stents, and balloons for endovascular surgery. The operating room should also include the necessary instruments to perform OSR if rEVAR must be aborted.

Access

The groin may be accessed via percutaneous micro puncture technique or by femoral-cut-down. Once ipsilateral access is obtained, a guide wire is used to access the descending thoracic aorta under fluoroscopic guidance. The wire is exchanged for a super stiff guidewire which can accommodate a long and large sheath (12–14 Fr × 45 cm) and the endograft. An aortic occlusion balloon can be deployed in unstable patients at this time. If an occlusion balloon is used, contralateral femoral access may be attempted in a similar manner to obtain an aortogram. The endograft used will depend on the patient's aortoiliac anatomy, the available of stents grafts, and surgeon preference [81, 87].

Endograft Choice

A unibody or bifurcated endograft may be placed based on patient anatomy, ability to expeditiously access the contralateral gate, and surgeon preference [81]. Significant unilateral occlusive disease or tortuosity generally mandates unibody endograft placement [87]. A unibody endograft may also be preferred in the hemodynamically unstable patient (Fig. 21.3). A graft converting device may be used if a patient becomes unstable during bifurcated endograft placement or if the contralateral gate is not able to be accessed [81]. It is prudent to ensure maintaining pelvic perfusion with at least one patent internal iliac artery should a bifurcated graft be placed.

Technique

Heparin may be administered upon completion of the aortogram. The main body of the endograft is then advanced through the iliac artery over a super-stiff guidewire under fluoroscopy. This may be performed ipsilaterally in stable patients who do not require an occlusion balloon or contralaterally in unstable patients requiring balloon occlusion. The endograft should be advanced to the level of the infrarenal aorta. The graft is then deployed until the contralateral gate is opened if a bifurcated endograft is used. The gate can then be accessed from the contralateral groin. The main body endograft is then fully deployed. The iliac limbs are then inserted from each side and deployed. Ballooning is performed of the proximal and distal seal zones, and

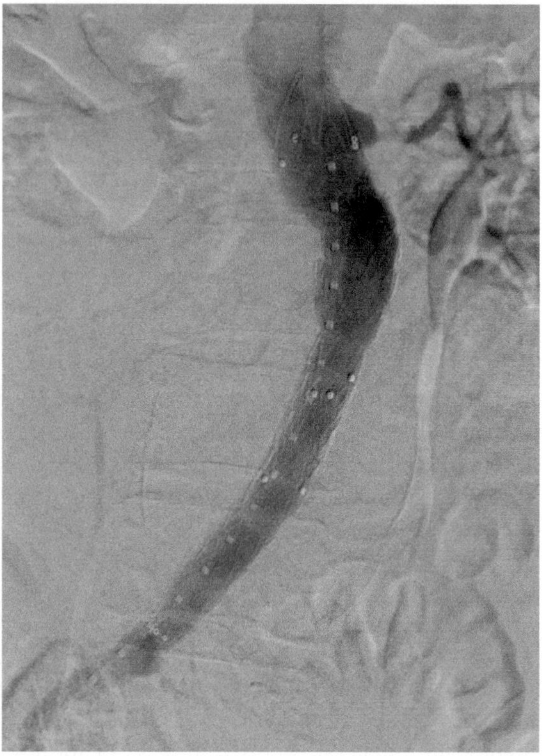

Fig. 21.3 Intraoperative completion angiogram after placement of an aorto-uni-iliac (AUI) endograft showing no evidence of endoleak

the graft overlap zones. Completion angiography (Fig. 21.4) should be performed to evaluate endoleaks and the need for adjunctive procedures such as proximal and/or distal extension or re-ballooning.

The femoral arteries may be closed by patchy angioplasty or with the vascular closure device depending on the surgical approach and surgeon preference.

Other Considerations

Covering the IMA

The IMA is routinely covered during rEVAR and generally does not result in any consequences. However, surgeons must be aware of patients at risk for colonic ischemia after rEVAR, which includes those with a severely stenosed SMA and celiac axis or those with prior left colon surgery. Worsening acidosis, increased abdominal pain and distention, and hematochezia/melena after rEVAR in these patients should raise suspicion and prompt further investigation with CT and bedside flexible sigmoidoscopy.

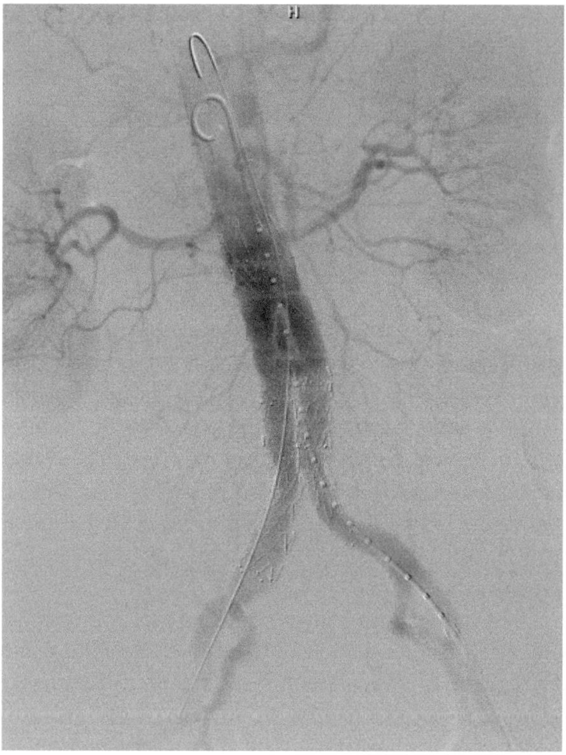

Fig. 21.4 Intraoperative completion angiogram after placement of an aorto-bi-iliac endograft demonstrating aneurysm exclusion with no endoleak and widely patent visceral, renal, and iliac arteries

Abdominal Compartment Syndrome (ACS)

ACS is a feared complication after open surgery and rEVAR secondary to retroperitoneal hematoma, continued bleeding, and generalized multivisceral edema. ACS is defined as an intra-abdominal pressure (IAP) >20 mm Hg with evidence of end-organ dysfunction or as an abdominal perfusion pressure (MAP-IAP) <60 mm Hg with evidence of end-organ dysfunction. Incidence of ACS is generally higher after open repair (34–50%) but remains a significant complication after rEVAR (9–21%). Mortality is ~50% in RAAA patients who develop ACS after repair [88, 89]. Risk factors for ACS in vascular surgery patients include preoperative hypotension, use of an aortic occlusion balloon, and massive blood transfusion (>5 units RBCs) [90].

Any patient at risk or suspected of having ACS should have routine bladder pressure measurements, serial laboratory and clinical monitoring for end-organ malperfusion, and thoughtful regulation of fluid balance and resuscitative strategies. Conservative measures to maintain IAP $\leq$15 mmHg should be initiated in all patients with elevated IAP. These include liberal use of decompressive tubes (e.g., nasogastric and/or rectal tubes), minimizing enteral nutrition, use of prokinetic agents, ensuring adequate analgesia and sedation, and neuro-muscular blockade in select patients. Decompressive laparotomy is the most invasive intervention for ACS and should be rapidly considered in patients with ACS refractory to medical treatments [91, 92].

A temporary vacuum-assisted closure dressing may be used in RAAA patients after open repair, particularly if they require significant intraoperative resuscitation or prolonged ischemic clamp times. This may help prevent ACS and allow for a second-look operation upon return to the operating room within 24–48 h for definitive closure.

Outcomes

Reported 30-day mortality rates vary widely among institutions and between trials but generally range from 20% to 40%. Early results from IMPROVE trial showed similar mortality rates between patients undergoing rEVAR and OSR (36.4% vs 40.6%); however, patients were analyzed on an intention-to-treat basis and there was high crossover between groups. A mortality benefit was found in patients who underwent rEVAR at 3-year follow-up (48% vs 56%) [69, 93]. The 30-day mortality rate in the ECAR trial was much lower at 18% compared to 24% in the OSR group, which seems like other 30-day mortality rates for rEVAR and OSR reported in single institution studies [94, 95].

A recent large propensity-matched analysis comparing outcomes between rEVAR and OSR patients demonstrated a favorable 30-day mortality benefit of rEVAR over OSR (21% vs 34%), which persisted after matching (18% vs 32%). Patients undergoing OSR experienced more major adverse events compared to rEVAR (68% vs 35%), and all-cause 1-year survival was greater in rEVAR patients (73% vs 59%) [96]. Notably, short and long-term mortality may be worse in women after repair, regardless of the repair type [97]; however, the cause for this observation is unknown.

Conclusions

RAAA remains a lethal diagnosis without expeditious surgical repair. rEVAR has evolved as an at least equal alternative to open surgical repair and may be superior in anatomically suitable patients. Hospitals treating RAAA should have hybrid capabilities and a standardized approach to perioperative management of RAAA.

References

1. Abdulameer H, Al Taii H, Al-Kindi SG, Milner R. Epidemiology of fatal ruptured aortic aneurysms in the United States (1999-2016). J Vasc Surg. 2019;69(2) https://doi.org/10.1016/j.jvs.2018.03.435.
2. Schmitz-Rixen T, Keese M, Hakimi M, Peters A, Böckler D, Nelson K, Grundmann RT. Ruptured abdominal aortic aneurysm—epidemiology, predisposing factors, and biology. Langenbeck's Arch Surg. 2016;401(3):275–88. https://doi.org/10.1007/s00423-016-1401-8.

3. Sakalihasan N, Limet R, Defawe O. Abdominal aortic aneurysm. Lancet. 2005;365(9470):1577–89. https://doi.org/10.1016/s0140-6736(05)66459-8.
4. Schermerhorn ML, Bensley RP, Giles KA, Hurks R, O'Malley AJ, Cotterill P, Chaikof E, Landon BE. Changes in abdominal aortic aneurysm rupture and short-term mortality, 1995–2008. Ann Surg. 2012;256(4):651–8. https://doi.org/10.1097/sla.0b013e31826b4f91.
5. Lilja F, Wanhainen A, Mani K. Changes in abdominal aortic aneurysm epidemiology. J Cardiovasc Surg. 2017;58(6) https://doi.org/10.23736/s0021-9509.17.10064-9.
6. van Beek SC, Vahl AC, Wisselink W, Balm R. Fate of patients unwilling or unsuitable to undergo surgical intervention for a ruptured abdominal aortic aneurysm. J Vasc Surg. 2015;61(2):570. https://doi.org/10.1016/j.jvs.2014.12.019.
7. Sweeting MJ, Ulug P, Roy J, Hultgren R, Indrakusuma R, Balm R, Thompson MM, Hinchliffe RJ, Thompson SG, Powell JT, Balm R, Koelemay MJ, Idu MM, Kox C, Legemate DA, Huisman LC, Willems MC, Reekers JA, van Delden OM, et al. Value of risk scores in the decision to palliate patients with ruptured abdominal aortic aneurysm. Br J Surg. 2018;105(9):1135–44. https://doi.org/10.1002/bjs.10820.
8. Talvitie M, Åldstedt-Nyrønning L, Stenman M, Roy J, Cohnert T, Hultgren R. Women with large intact abdominal aortic aneurysms remain untreated. J Vasc Surg. 2023;78(3) https://doi.org/10.1016/j.jvs.2023.05.025.
9. Kessler V, Klopf J, Eilenberg W, Neumayer C, Brostjan C. AAA revisited: a comprehensive review of risk factors, management, and hallmarks of pathogenesis. Biomedicine. 2022;10(1):94. https://doi.org/10.3390/biomedicines10010094.
10. Solberg S, Singh K, Wilsgaard T. Increased growth rate of abdominal aortic aneurysms in women, the Tromso Study. J Vasc Surg. 2005;42(1):178–9. https://doi.org/10.1016/j.jvs.2005.04.008.
11. Moll FL, Powell JT, Fraedrich G, Verzini F, Haulon S, Waltham M, van Herwaarden JA, Holt PJE, van Keulen JW, Rantner B, Schlösser FJV, Setacci F, Ricco J-B. Management of abdominal aortic aneurysms clinical practice guidelines of the European Society for Vascular Surgery. Eur J Vasc Endovasc Surg. 2011;41 https://doi.org/10.1016/j.ejvs.2010.09.011.
12. Landenhed M, Engström G, Gottsäter A, Caulfield MP, Hedblad B, Newton-Cheh C, Melander O, Smith JG. Risk profiles for aortic dissection and ruptured or surgically treated aneurysms: a prospective Cohort Study. J Am Heart Assoc. 2015;4(1) https://doi.org/10.1161/jaha.114.001513.
13. Anagnostakos J, Lal BK. Abdominal aortic aneurysms. Prog Cardiovasc Dis. 2021;65:34–43. https://doi.org/10.1016/j.pcad.2021.03.009.
14. Brown PM, Zelt DT, Sobolev B. The risk of rupture in untreated aneurysms: the impact of size, gender, and expansion rate. J Vasc Surg. 2003;37(2):280–4. https://doi.org/10.1067/mva.2003.119.
15. Leemans EL, Willems TP, van der Laan MJ, Slump CH, Zeebregts CJ. Biomechanical indices for rupture risk estimation in abdominal aortic aneurysms. J Endovasc Ther. 2016;24(2):254–61. https://doi.org/10.1177/1526602816680088.
16. Gasser TC. Biomechanical rupture risk assessment. AORTA. 2016;04(02):42–60. https://doi.org/10.12945/j.aorta.2015.15.030.
17. Qiu Y, Wang J, Zhao J, Wang T, Zheng T, Yuan D. Association between blood flow pattern and rupture risk of abdominal aortic aneurysm based on computational fluid dynamics. J Vasc Surg. 2022;76(5):1424. https://doi.org/10.1016/j.jvs.2022.08.024.
18. Scotti CM, Jimenez J, Muluk SC, Finol EA. Wall stress and flow dynamics in abdominal aortic aneurysms: finite element analysis vs. fluid–structure interaction. Comput Methods Biomech Biomed Engin. 2008;11(3):301–22. https://doi.org/10.1080/10255840701827412.
19. Vorp DA, Geest JP. Biomechanical determinants of abdominal aortic aneurysm rupture. Arterioscler Thromb Vasc Biol. 2005;25(8):1558–66. https://doi.org/10.1161/01.atv.0000174129.77391.55.
20. Kazi M, Thyberg J, Religa P, Roy J, Eriksson P, Hedin U, Swedenborg J. Influence of intraluminal thrombus on structural and cellular composition of abdominal aortic aneurysm wall. J Vasc Surg. 2003;38(6):1283–92. https://doi.org/10.1016/s0741-5214(03)00791-2.

21. Nordon IM, Hinchliffe RJ, Loftus IM, Thompson MM. Pathophysiology and epidemiology of abdominal aortic aneurysms. Nat Rev Cardiol. 2010;8(2):92–102. https://doi.org/10.1038/nrcardio.2010.180.
22. Khaw H, Sottiurai VS, Craighead CC, Batson RC. Ruptured abdominal aortic aneurysm presenting as symptomatic inguinal mass: report of six cases. J Vasc Surg. 1986;4(4):384–9. https://doi.org/10.1067/mva.1986.avs0040384.
23. Marston WA, Ahlquist R, Johnson G, Meyer AA. Misdiagnosis of ruptured abdominal aortic aneurysms. J Vasc Surg. 1992;16(1):17–22. https://doi.org/10.1016/0741-5214(92)90412-2.
24. Azhar B, Patel S, Holt P, Hinchliffe R, Thompson M, Karthikesalingam A. Misdiagnosis of ruptured abdominal aortic aneurysm: systematic review and meta analysis. Int J Surg. 2014;12 https://doi.org/10.1016/j.ijsu.2014.08.336.
25. Smidfelt K, Nordanstig J, Davidsson A, Törngren K, Langenskiöld M. Misdiagnosis of ruptured abdominal aortic aneurysms is common and is associated with increased mortality. J Vasc Surg. 2021;73(2) https://doi.org/10.1016/j.jvs.2020.06.047.
26. Stine RJ, Trued SJ. Hiccups: an unusual manifestation of an abdominal aortic aneurysm. J Am Coll Emerg Physicians. 1979;8(9):368–70. https://doi.org/10.1016/s0361-1124(79)80261-0.
27. Georgopoulos SE, Arvanitis DP, Tekerlekis P, Chronopoulos A, Kostakopoulos A. Rupture of an aortic anastomotic aneurysm into a ureter. Urol Int. 2003;71(3):333–5. https://doi.org/10.1159/000072692.
28. Eckford SD, Gillatt DA. Abdominal aortic aneurysms presenting as renal colic. Br J Urol. 1992;70(5):496–8. https://doi.org/10.1111/bju.1992.70.5.496.
29. Keripe S, Slavik S, Oshodi T. Primary aortoappendicular fistula arising from an infected, chronic, contained, ruptured abdominal aortic aneurysm. Ann Vasc Surg. 2006;20(6):820–4. https://doi.org/10.1007/s10016-006-9084-1.
30. Defraigne J-O, Sakalihasan N, Lavigne J-P, Van Damme H, Limet R. Chronic rupture of abdominal aortic aneurysm manifesting as crural neuropathy. Ann Vasc Surg. 2001;15(3):405–11. https://doi.org/10.1007/s100160010069.
31. Razzuk MA. Femoral neuropathy secondary to ruptured abdominal aortic aneurysms with false aneurysms. JAMA. 1967;201(11):817. https://doi.org/10.1001/jama.1967.03130110043010.
32. Tejada E, Becker GJ, Waller BF. Two unusual manifestations of aortic aneurysms. Clin Cardiol. 1990;13(2):132–5. https://doi.org/10.1002/clc.4960130213.
33. Politoske EJ. Ruptured abdominal aortic aneurysm presenting as an obstruction of the left colon. Am J Gastroenterol. 1990;85(6):745–7.
34. Smith DL, Campbell SM. Unruptured abdominal aortic aneurysm mimicking hip joint disease. J Rheumatol. 1987;14(1):172–3.
35. Garrity BM, Sugarman E, Pulley S. Abdominal aortic aneurysm rupture presenting with focal weakness and altered mental status: a case report. Int J Emerg Med. 2022;15(1) https://doi.org/10.1186/s12245-022-00433-5.
36. Sufi PA. A rare case of leaking abdominal aneurysm presenting as isolated right testicular pain. CJEM. 2007;9(02):124–6. https://doi.org/10.1017/s1481803500014925.
37. Forsythe RO, Lavin V, Fraser SC, McNeill A. Isolated right testicular pain for six days: an unusual presentation of occult abdominal aortic aneurysm leak. Ann R Coll Surg Engl. 2011;93(4) https://doi.org/10.1308/003588411x569406.
38. Grabowski EW, Pilcher DB. Ruptured abdominal aortic aneurysm manifesting as symptomatic inguinal hernia. Am Surg. 1981;47(7):311–2.
39. Duong C, Atkinson N. Review of AORTOILIAC aneurysms with spontaneous large vein fistula. ANZ J Surg. 2001;71(1):52–5. https://doi.org/10.1046/j.1440-1622.2001.02004.x.
40. Woolley DS, Spence RK. Aortocaval fistula treated by aortic exclusion. J Vasc Surg. 1995;22(5):639–42. https://doi.org/10.1016/s0741-5214(95)70053-6.
41. Antoniou GA, Georgiadis GS, Antoniou SA, Neequaye S, Brennan JA, Torella F, Vallabhaneni SR. Late rupture of abdominal aortic aneurysm after previous endovascular repair. J Endovasc Ther. 2015;22(5):734–44. https://doi.org/10.1177/1526602815601405.

42. Valentine RJ, Barth MJ, Myers SI, Clagett GP. Nonvascular emergencies presenting as ruptured abdominal aortic aneurysms. Surgery. 1993;113(3):286–9.
43. Loughran CF. A review of the plain abdominal radiograph in acute rupture of abdominal aortic aneurysms. Clin Radiol. 1986;37(4):383–7. https://doi.org/10.1016/s0009-9260(86)80292-6.
44. Chien D-K, Chang W-H, Yeh Y-H. Radiographic findings of a ruptured abdominal aortic aneurysm. Circulation. 2010;122(18):1880–1. https://doi.org/10.1161/circulationaha.110.972018.
45. LaRoy L, Cormier P, Matalon T, Patel S, Turner D, Silver B. Imaging of abdominal aortic aneurysms. Am J Roentgenol. 1989;152(4):785–92. https://doi.org/10.2214/ajr.152.4.785.
46. Missiroli C, Singh AK. Nontraumatic emergencies of abdominal aorta. Semin Ultrasound CT MRI. 2008;29(5):369–77. https://doi.org/10.1053/j.sult.2008.06.008.
47. Weinbaum FI, Dubner S, Turner JW, Pardes JG. The accuracy of computed tomography in the diagnosis of retroperitoneal blood in the presence of abdominal aortic aneurysm. J Vasc Surg. 1987;6(1):11–6. https://doi.org/10.1067/mva.1987.avs0060011.
48. Rakita D, Newatia A, Hines JJ, Siegel DN, Friedman B. Spectrum of CT findings in rupture and impending rupture of abdominal aortic aneurysms. Radiographics. 2007;27(2):497–507. https://doi.org/10.1148/rg.272065026.
49. Lloyd GM, Bown MJ, Norwood MGA, Deb R, Fishwick G, Bell PRF, Sayers RD. Feasibility of preoperative computer tomography in patients with ruptured abdominal aortic aneurysm: a time-to-death study in patients without operation. J Vasc Surg. 2004;39(4):788–91. https://doi.org/10.1016/j.jvs.2003.11.041.
50. Samy AK, Murray G, MacBain G. Glasgow aneurysm score. Cardiovasc Surg. 1994;2(1):41–4.
51. Hardman DTA, Fisher CM, Patel MI, Neale M, Chambers J, Lane R, Appleberg M. Ruptured abdominal aortic aneurysms: who should be offered surgery? J Vasc Surg. 1996;23(1):123–9. https://doi.org/10.1016/s0741-5214(05)80042-4.
52. Copeland GP, Jones D, Walters M. Possum: a scoring system for surgical audit. Br J Surg. 1991;78(3):355–60. https://doi.org/10.1002/bjs.1800780327.
53. Chen JC, Hildebrand HD, Salvian AJ, Taylor DC, Strandberg S, Myckatyn TM, Hsiang YN. Predictors of death in nonruptured and ruptured abdominal aortic aneurysms. J Vasc Surg. 1996;24(4):614–23. https://doi.org/10.1016/s0741-5214(96)70077-0.
54. Johnston KW. Ruptured abdominal aortic aneurysm: six-year follow-up results of a Multicenter Prospective Study. J Vasc Surg. 1994;19(5):888–900. https://doi.org/10.1016/s0741-5214(94)70015-x.
55. Garland BT, Danaher PJ, Desikan S, Tran NT, Quiroga E, Singh N, Starnes BW. Preoperative risk score for the prediction of mortality after repair of ruptured abdominal aortic aneurysms. J Vasc Surg. 2018;68(4):991–7. https://doi.org/10.1016/j.jvs.2017.12.075.
56. Vos CG, de Vries J-PPM, Werson DAB, van Dongen EPA, Schreve MA, Ünlü Ç. Evaluation of five different aneurysm scoring systems to predict mortality in ruptured abdominal aortic aneurysm patients. J Vasc Surg. 2016;64(6):1609–16. https://doi.org/10.1016/j.jvs.2016.05.099.
57. Mell MW, Wang NE, Morrison DE, Hernandez-Boussard T. Interfacility transfer and mortality for patients with ruptured abdominal aortic aneurysm. J Vasc Surg. 2014;60(3):553–7. https://doi.org/10.1016/j.jvs.2014.02.061.
58. Holmes JF. Effects of delaying fluid resuscitation on an injury to the systemic arterial vasculature. Acad Emerg Med. 2002;9(4):267–74. https://doi.org/10.1197/aemj.9.4.267.
59. Bickell W, Wall M, Pepe P, Martin R, Ginger V, Allen M, Mattox K. Immediate versus delayed fluid resuscitation for hypotensive patients with penetrating torso injuries. Resuscitation. 1995;29(2):183–4. https://doi.org/10.1016/0300-9572(95)90705-m.
60. Crawford ES. Ruptured abdominal aortic aneurysm [editorial]. J Vasc Surg. 1991;13:348–50.
61. Moreno DH, Cacione DG, Baptista-Silva JC. Controlled hypotension versus normotensive resuscitation strategy for people with ruptured abdominal aortic aneurysm. Cochrane Database Syst Rev. 2018; https://doi.org/10.1002/14651858.cd011664.pub3.
62. Chaikof EL, Dalman RL, Eskandari MK, Jackson BM, Lee WA, Mansour MA, Mastracci TM, Mell M, Murad MH, Nguyen LL, Oderich GS, Patel MS, Schermerhorn ML, Starnes BW. The

Society for Vascular Surgery Practice Guidelines on the care of patients with an abdominal aortic aneurysm. J Vasc Surg. 2018;67(1) https://doi.org/10.1016/j.jvs.2017.10.044.
63. Hughes CW. Use of an intra-aortic balloon catheter tamponade for controlling intra-abdominal hemorrhage in man. Surgery. 1954;36(1):65–8.
64. Hesse FG, Kletschka HD. Rupture of abdominal aortic aneurysm. Ann Surg. 1962;155(2):320–2. https://doi.org/10.1097/00000658-196200000-00025.
65. Bath J, Leite JO, Rahimi M, Giglia J, Jain A, Shelton K, Meier GH. Contemporary outcomes for ruptured abdominal aortic aneurysms using endovascular balloon control for hypotension. J Vasc Surg. 2018;67(5):1389–96. https://doi.org/10.1016/j.jvs.2017.09.031.
66. Berland TL, Veith FJ, Cayne NS, Mehta M, Mayer D, Lachat M. Technique of supraceliac balloon control of the aorta during endovascular repair of ruptured abdominal aortic aneurysms. In: Ruptured abdominal aortic aneurysm; 2017. p. 403–8. https://doi.org/10.1007/978-3-319-23844-9_21.
67. Desgranges P, Kobeiter H, Katsahian S, Bouffi M, Gouny P, Favre J-P, Alsac JM, Sobocinski J, Julia P, Alimi Y, Steinmetz E, Haulon S, Alric P, Canaud L, Castier Y, Jean-Baptiste E, Hassen-Khodja R, Lermusiaux P, Feugier P, et al. Editor's choice—ecar (endovasculaire ou chirurgie dans les anévrysmes aorto-iliaques rompus): a French randomized controlled trial of endovascular versus open surgical repair of ruptured Aorto-iliac aneurysms. Eur J Vasc Endovasc Surg. 2015;50(3):303–10. https://doi.org/10.1016/j.ejvs.2015.03.028.
68. Reimerink JJ, Hoornweg LL, Vahl AC, Wisselink W, van den Broek TA, Legemate DA, Reekers JA, Balm R. Endovascular repair versus open repair of ruptured abdominal aortic aneurysms. Ann Surg. 2013;258(2):248–56. https://doi.org/10.1097/sla.0b013e31828d4b76.
69. Comparative clinical effectiveness and cost effectiveness of endovascular strategy versus open repair for ruptured abdominal aortic aneurysm: three-year results of the improve randomised trial. BMJ. 2017. https://doi.org/10.1136/bmj.j4859.
70. Shantikumar S, Patel S, Handa A. The role of cell salvage autotransfusion in abdominal aortic aneurysm surgery. J Vasc Surg. 2011;54(5):1538. https://doi.org/10.1016/j.jvs.2011.09.057.
71. Arthurs ZM, Sohn VY, Starnes BW. Ruptured abdominal aortic aneurysms: remote aortic occlusion for the general surgeon. Surg Clin N Am. 2007;87(5):1035–45. https://doi.org/10.1016/j.suc.2007.07.002.
72. Islamoglu F, Apaydın AZ, Posacıoglu H, Çalkavur T, Yagdı T, Atay Y. Effects of thoracic and HIATAL clamping in repair of ruptured abdominal aortic aneurysms. Ann Vasc Surg. 2007;21(4):423–32. https://doi.org/10.1016/j.avsg.2006.12.005.
73. Ohki T, Veith FJ. Endovascular grafts and other image-guided catheter-based adjuncts to improve the treatment of ruptured AORTOILIAC aneurysms. Ann Surg. 2000;232(4):466–79. https://doi.org/10.1097/00000658-200010000-00002.
74. Mulcare RJ, Royster TS, Weiss HJ, Phillips LL. Disseminated Intravascular coagulation as a complication of abdominal aortic aneurysm repair. Ann Surg. 1974;180(3):343–9. https://doi.org/10.1097/00000658-197409000-00015.
75. Graham AP, Fitzgerald O'Connor E, Hinchliffe RJ, Loftus IM, Thompson MM, Black SA. The use of heparin in patients with ruptured abdominal aortic aneurysms. Vascular. 2012;20(2):61–4. https://doi.org/10.1258/vasc.2011.ra0051.
76. Cuen-Ojeda C, Li B, Zhu J, Roche-Nagle G. The effect of heparin on mortality after open ruptured abdominal aortic aneurysm repair: a propensity score-matched analysis. J Vasc Surg. 2021;74(5) https://doi.org/10.1016/j.jvs.2021.08.016.
77. Sicard GA, Allen BT, Munn JS, Anderson CB. Retroperitoneal versus transperitoneal approach for repair of abdominal aortic aneurysms. Surg Clin N Am. 1989;69(4):795–806. https://doi.org/10.1016/s0039-6109(16)44885-1.
78. Shepard AD. Retroperitoneal approach to high-risk abdominal aortic aneurysms. Arch Surg. 1986;121(4):444. https://doi.org/10.1001/archsurg.1986.01400040082013.
79. Mei F, Hu K, Zhao B, Gao Q, Chen F, Zhao L, Wu M, Feng L, Wang Z, Yang J, Zhang W, Ma B. Retroperitoneal versus transperitoneal approach for elective open abdominal

AORTIC ANEURYSM REPAIR. Cochrane Database Syst Rev. 2021;2021(6) https://doi.org/10.1002/14651858.cd010373.pub3.
80. Panthofer AM, Olson SL, Rademacher BL, Grudzinski JK, Chaikof EL, Matsumura JS. Anatomic eligibility for endovascular aneurysm repair preserved over 2 years of surveillance. J Vasc Surg. 2021;74(5) https://doi.org/10.1016/j.jvs.2021.04.044.
81. Mehta M. Technical tips for EVAR for ruptured AAA. Semin Vasc Surg. 2009;22(3):181–6. https://doi.org/10.1053/j.semvascsurg.2009.07.010.
82. Powell JT, Hinchliffe RJ, Thompson MM, Sweeting MJ, Ashleigh R, Bell R, Gomes M, Greenhalgh RM, Grieve RJ, Heatley F, Thompson SG, Ulug P. Observations from the IMPROVE trial concerning the clinical care of patients with ruptured abdominal aortic aneurysm. Br J Surg. 2014;101(3):216–24. https://doi.org/10.1002/bjs.9410.
83. Mouton R, Rogers CA, Harris RA, Hinchliffe RJ. Local anaesthesia for endovascular repair of ruptured abdominal aortic aneurysm. Br J Surg. 2018;106(1):74–81. https://doi.org/10.1002/bjs.10973.
84. Faizer R, Weinhandl E, El Hag S, Le Jeune S, Apostolidou I, Shafii SM, Lee CJ, Rosenberg MS, Reed A, Fanola CL. Decreased mortality with local versus general anesthesia in endovascular aneurysm repair for ruptured abdominal aortic aneurysm in the Vascular Quality Initiative Database. J Vasc Surg. 2019;70(1) https://doi.org/10.1016/j.jvs.2018.10.090.
85. Mayer D, Pfammatter T, Rancic Z, Hechelhammer L, Wilhelm M, Veith FJ, Lachat M. 10 years of emergency endovascular aneurysm repair for ruptured abdominal AORTOILIAC aneurysms: lessons learned. Ann Surg. 2009;249(3):510–5. https://doi.org/10.1097/sla.0b013e31819a8b65.
86. Mehta M, Taggert J, Darling RC, Chang BB, Kreienberg PB, Paty PSK, Roddy SP, Sternbach Y, Ozsvath KJ, Shah DM. Establishing a protocol for endovascular treatment of ruptured abdominal aortic aneurysms: outcomes of a prospective analysis. J Vasc Surg. 2006;44(1):1–8. https://doi.org/10.1016/j.jvs.2006.02.057.
87. Veith FJ, Rockman CB. The recent randomized trials of EVAR versus open repair for ruptured abdominal aortic aneurysms are misleading. Vascular. 2015;23(2):217–9. https://doi.org/10.1177/1708538114568417.
88. Rubenstein C, Bietz G, Davenport DL, Winkler M, Endean ED. Abdominal compartment syndrome associated with endovascular and open repair of ruptured abdominal aortic aneurysms. J Vasc Surg. 2015;61(3):648–54. https://doi.org/10.1016/j.jvs.2014.10.011.
89. Sá P, Oliveira-Pinto J, Mansilha A. Abdominal compartment syndrome after R-EVAR: a systematic review with meta-analysis on incidence and mortality. J Vasc Surg. 2020;72(4):1500–1. https://doi.org/10.1016/j.jvs.2020.07.042.
90. Ersryd S, Djavani Gidlund K, Wanhainen A, Smith L, Björck M. Abdominal compartment syndrome after surgery for ABDOMINAL AORTIC ANEURYSM: subgroups, risk factors, and outcome. J Vasc Surg. 2019;70(6):2102. https://doi.org/10.1016/j.jvs.2019.10.018.
91. Burlew CC. Abdominal compartment syndrome and the open abdomen. In: Management of musculoskeletal injuries in the trauma patient; 2013. p. 321–9. https://doi.org/10.1007/978-1-4614-8551-3_15.
92. De Laet IE, Malbrain ML, De Waele JJ. A clinician's guide to management of intra-abdominal hypertension and abdominal compartment syndrome in critically ill patients. Crit Care. 2020;24(1) https://doi.org/10.1186/s13054-020-2782-1.
93. IMPROVE Trial Investigators. Endovascular or open repair strategy for ruptured abdominal AORTIC ANEURYSM: 30 Day outcomes from improve randomised trial. BMJ. 2014b;348(jan13 2) https://doi.org/10.1136/bmj.f7661.
94. Jones M, Koury H, Faris P, Moore R. Impact of an emergency endovascular Aneurysm Repair Protocol on 30-day ruptured abdominal aortic aneurysm mortality. J Vasc Surg. 2022;76(3) https://doi.org/10.1016/j.jvs.2022.02.050.
95. Guéroult AM, Khan FA, Stather PW, Harrison SC, Boyle JR. Long-term outcomes following endovascular aneurysm repair for ruptured abdominal aortic aneurysms. J Endovasc Ther. 2020;27(3):428–35. https://doi.org/10.1177/1526602820919901.

96. Wang LJ, Locham SS, Dakour-Aridi H, Malas M. Endovascular repair of ruptured abdominal aortic aneurysm is superior to open repair: propensity-matched analysis in the vascular quality initiative. J Am Coll Surg. 2019;229(4) https://doi.org/10.1016/j.jamcollsurg.2019.08.717.
97. Li B, Eisenberg N, Witheford M, Lindsay TF, Forbes TL, Roche-Nagle G. Sex differences in outcomes following ruptured abdominal aortic aneurysm repair. JAMA Netw Open. 2022;5(5) https://doi.org/10.1001/jamanetworkopen.2022.11336.

Chapter 22
Treatment of Mycotic Abdominal Aortic Aneurysms and Infected Aortic Grafts and Endografts

J. Gregory Modrall and Antonio Solano

Introduction

Mycotic aneurysms and infected aortic grafts and endografts are among the most challenging conditions that clinicians who treat aortic disease will face in clinical practice. Without proper treatment, these conditions are often lethal. Despite advances in treatment, the mortality for both conditions remains substantial. The challenges posed by these conditions lie both in their diagnosis and treatment. To aid clinicians in optimizing outcomes for these conditions, this chapter will review the pathogenesis, diagnosis, treatment, and outcomes of these vexing clinical problems. Mycotic aneurysms and aortic graft and endograft infections will be addressed separately, although similar principles guide treatment of both conditions. The diagnosis and management of aortoenteric fistulas are addressed in a separate chapter.

Mycotic Aneurysms

Pathogenesis

The term *mycotic aneurysm* was initially introduced by Osler to denote infected aneurysms associated with endocarditis [1]. Today the term is broadly applied to any infected aneurysm, regardless of etiology. For the purposes of this discussion, mycotic aneurysms will include primary arterial infections causing aneurysm

J. G. Modrall (✉) · A. Solano
Division of Vascular and Endovascular Surgery, University of Texas Southwestern Medical Center, Dallas, TX, USA
e-mail: Greg.Modrall@UTSouthwestern.edu; antonio.solanoavendano@utsouthwestern.edu

G. J. Arnaoutakis et al. (eds.), *Aortic Aneurysms*, Contemporary Cardiology,
https://doi.org/10.1007/978-3-032-13134-8_22

formation, infected arteritis related to contiguous spread of infection, and preexisting aneurysms that become secondarily infected.

Primary arterial infections are believed to result either from hematogenous seeding of the arterial wall during episodes of bacteremia or contiguous spread of local infections. Since the intima of an artery provides a relative barrier to infection, intimal injury related to atherosclerosis is usually required as a cofactor in the development of arteritis [2, 3]. Histopathology of involved sections of artery typically shows transmural acute inflammation with focal microabscesses superimposed on a diffuse intimal atherosclerosis in the wall of mycotic aneurysms [3]. Since wall destruction is a critical element in the pathogenesis of aneurysms related to bacterial arteritis, it should be recognized that many aneurysms related to bacterial arteritis are actually *pseudoaneurysms*.

In the era prior to the introduction of antibiotics, the causative organisms were those associated with endocarditis, including *Streptococcal* species, *Staphylococcal* species, and *Pneumococcus* [4]. A more recent series from the Mayo Clinic [3] found that Gram-positive cocci were responsible for 50% of cases (*Staphylococcus* in 30% and *Streptococcus* in 20%) and Gram-negative bacilli were cultured in 35% (*Salmonella* species in 20% and *Escherichia coli* in 15%). Patients with Gram-negative mycotic aneurysms were far more likely to present with frank rupture, compared to Gram-positive mycotic aneurysms (84% versus 10%) [5]. Fungal species are rare causes of mycotic aneurysms, especially in immunocompromised patients [6].

Bacterial arteritis may also result from contiguous spread from adjacent infected tissues, such as vertebral osteomyelitis, psoas abscess, or suppurative lymphadenitis. Alternatively, preexisting aortic aneurysms may become secondarily infected by hematogenous seeding due to infection of the atherosclerotic intima or mural thrombus within an aneurysm [2, 3].

Clinical Presentation

The clinical presentation of patients with mycotic aortic aneurysms ranges from overt aortic rupture and systemic inflammatory response syndrome (SIRS) to asymptomatic findings on radiological imaging studies. Between 46% and 61% of patients have a history of a recent or ongoing septic illness [7, 8]. Comorbid conditions associated with relative immunosuppression are present in more than two-thirds of patients, including diabetes (33%), chronic renal failure (30%), chronic steroid use (16%), and chronic illnesses (16%) [8]. Ninety-three percent of patients in a series from the Mayo Clinic were symptomatic, and the average duration of symptoms was 38 days [8]. Symptoms may be broadly categorized as septic symptoms, pain syndromes, and hemodynamic symptoms. Fever (77%), chills (51%), and sweats (28%) were typical septic symptoms [8]. Abdominal or back pain was present in 65% of patients [8]. Hemodynamic instability was present in only 7% of patients, despite aortic rupture in 21% of cases [8]. Laboratory abnormalities typically include elevated sedimentation rate (86%) or C-reactive protein (79%) and leukocytosis (54%) [7, 8]. Seventy percent of patients with mycotic aneurysms of the aorta meet the clinical criteria for SIRS syndrome at initial presentation [9, 10].

Diagnosis and Imaging

Imaging tests are often helpful in ascertaining the diagnosis of a mycotic aneurysm. Contrast-enhanced computed tomography (CT) scan is the mainstay of imaging tests for the diagnosis of a mycotic aneurysm. The entire aorta should be imaged since mycotic aneurysms are found throughout the aorta: ascending aorta (6%), descending thoracic aorta (23%), paravisceral aorta (6%), juxtarenal aorta (10%), and infrarenal aorta (32%). A key element in the diagnosis of mycotic aneurysms is the aneurysm morphology. Mycotic aneurysms are characteristically saccular in 93% of cases [11]. Secondary signs of infection on CT scan include the presence of a para-aortic soft tissue mass, stranding, or fluid, which are seen in nearly half of cases (Fig. 22.1) [11]. Thirty percent of patients have CT evidence of aortic rupture [10]. Retroperitoneal gas in the context of a saccular aneurysm is rare (7% of cases), but pathognomonic for a mycotic aneurysm (Fig. 22.1) [11]. Vertebral body destruction with psoas abscess adjacent to an aortic aneurysm is another ominous finding on CT scan [11]. Among patients with serial CT scans available for comparison, periaortic edema and interval development or expansion of an aneurysm are highly suspicious for the presence of an infected aneurysm [11]. Overall, 75% of CT scans

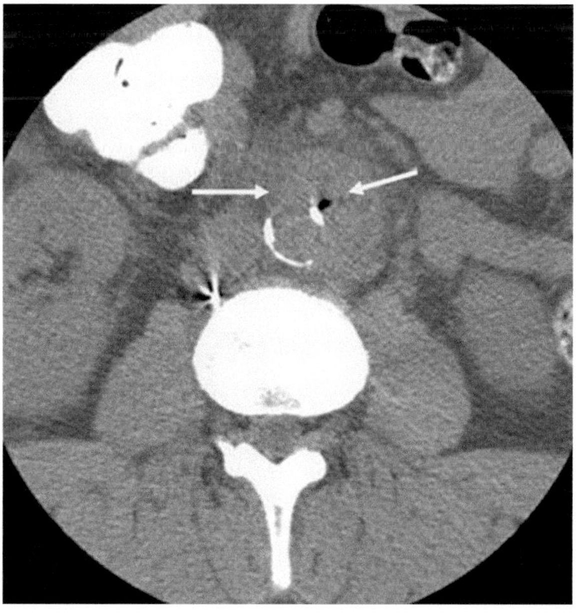

Fig. 22.1 CT of mycotic aneurysm. Periaortic fluid is evident anterior and lateral to the aorta with gas noted within the fluid collection (*arrows*)

will have findings consistent with a mycotic aneurysm in surgically proven cases of mycotic aneurysm [3].

Nuclear imaging often shows increased activity in the vicinity of the aneurysm, consistent with an infection [11]. In recent years, the diagnostic accuracy of contrast-enhanced CT has been augmented by merging CT with radionuclide scanning in the form of positron emission tomography CT with ^{18}F-fluorodeoxyglucose (FDG-PET/CT). A head-to-head comparison of CT with PET/CT showed that PET/CT had a higher diagnostic accuracy than CT [12].

Magnetic resonance imaging (MRI) of mycotic aneurysms may show a saccular aneurysm with high intensity signal on T2-weighted images [11, 13]. Since most cases may be diagnosed by clinical presentation and CT, other imaging studies such as FDG-PET/CT, MRI, and nuclear imaging should be reserved for stable patients in whom the diagnosis remains uncertain. Since the various secondary signs of a mycotic aneurysm discussed above are not be visualized on arteriography, arteriography is rarely helpful, except for answering specific anatomic questions (Fig. 22.2).

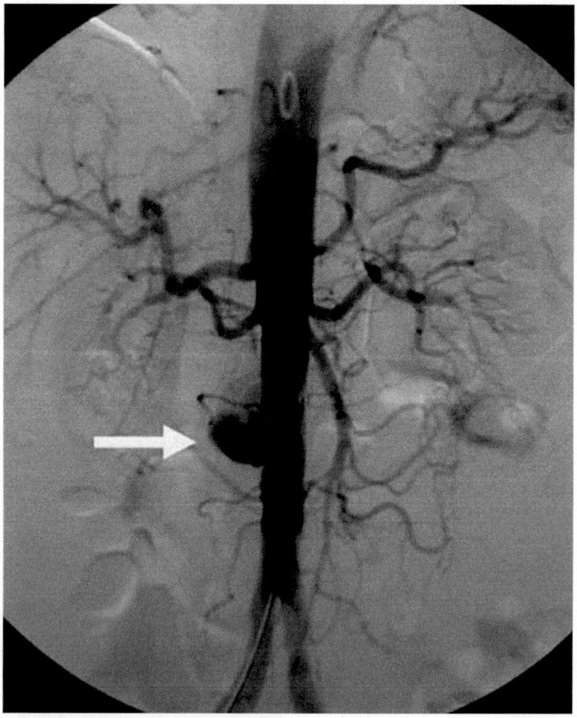

Fig. 22.2 Aortogram of saccular aneurysm. A lobulated saccular aneurysm (*arrow*) typical of a mycotic aneurysm is noted

Treatment

The first priority after the presumptive diagnosis of a mycotic aneurysm is initiation of appropriate antibiotic therapy. A history of recent septic episodes or invasive procedures will guide the choice of antibiotics based on the likely organisms [7, 8]. Without such a history, broad-spectrum antibiotics are appropriate since both Gram-positive cocci and Gram-negative bacilli have been isolated from mycotic aneurysms [3]. The goal of antibiotics is to limit the septic complications until definitive surgical therapy may be undertaken and to lessen the risk of reinfection after surgery.

The guiding principle of surgical treatment of mycotic aneurysms is surgical debridement of the infected aortic tissue and periaortic tissue, followed by revascularization to reestablish distal perfusion. Often a contained aneurysm rupture is identified at surgery [8, 10, 14], so proximal and distal aortic control should be obtained well away from the inflamed segment of aorta (Fig. 22.3) to avoid inadvertent entry into a contained rupture. An important goal of surgical therapy is complete debridement of the grossly infected aorta and surrounding periaortic tissues. The aorta should be debrided back to healthy tissue (Fig. 22.4) which should be ascertained by direct visual inspection rather than intraoperative Gram stain or histopathology.

After debridement, distal flow may be reconstituted by either in situ graft placement or aortic ligation with extra-anatomic bypass. The approach will be dictated by several factors. First, the location of the mycotic aneurysm is a primary determinant. Extra-anatomic bypass of the thoracic or paravisceral aorta is difficult and fraught with problems, so in situ repair is usually necessary for mycotic aneurysms in these segments of the aorta. For the infrarenal aorta, both forms of aortic reconstruction (in situ vs extra-anatomic bypass) have been described. In this location, additional variables may dictate the approach. For instance, hemodynamic instability of the patient may dictate an expeditious in situ repair as the more appropriate strategy. The relative virulence of the organisms may also play a role in the decision-making.

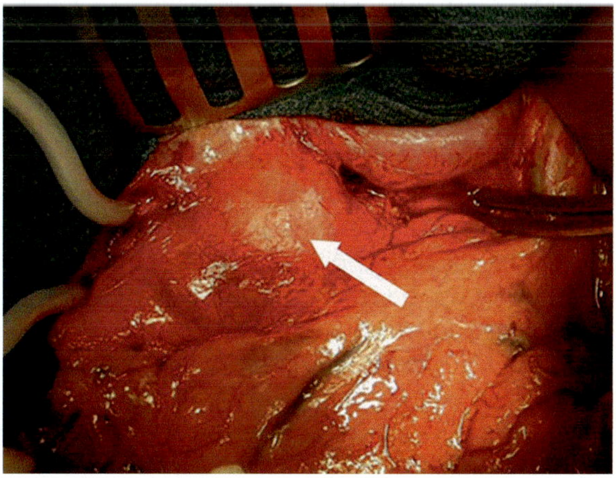

Fig. 22.3 Mycotic aneurysm. A bulge representing a mycotic aneurysm of the aorta is evident in the retroperitoneum (*arrow*). To the right, an aortic cross-clamp is occluding the aorta proximal to the mycotic aneurysm. To the left, tourniquets are occluding the common iliac arteries distal to the infected aneurysm

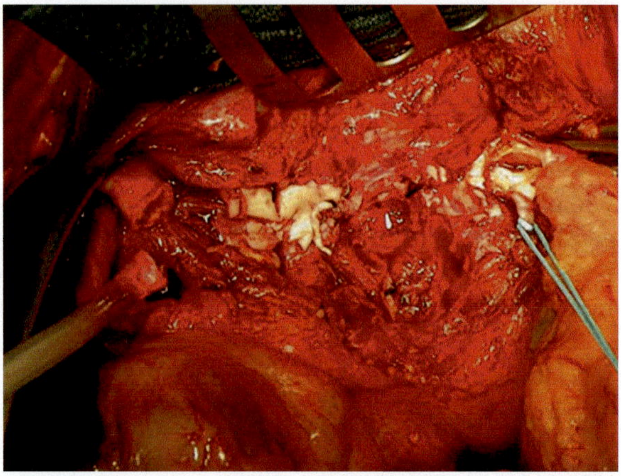

Fig. 22.4 Retroperitoneum after mycotic aneurysm resection. The infected aorta and periaortic tissues from Fig. 22.3 have been debrided, leaving a large defect in the aorta and proximal iliac arteries (*See Color Plates*)

Intraoperative Gram stain of the resected tissue should be performed if an in situ repair is contemplated on a relatively stable patient, as the presence of Gram-negative rods, probable anaerobes, or fungal species may increase the risk of reinfection of an in situ repair, with potentially devastating consequences. Conversely, the presence of Gram-positive cocci consistent with staphylococcal species is suggestive of a relatively low-grade infection that may be amenable to in situ repair. The intraoperative finding of substantial aortic destruction with "tissue-paper" consistency of the adjacent aortic wall is indicative of a high-grade infection with a relatively virulent organism, which would favor an extra-anatomic repair. In the final analysis, neither approach is appropriate for all cases, so the surgeon should be well versed in the technical aspects of both approaches.

The classic approach to treatment of infected aneurysms was aggressive debridement of the infected aortic tissue, followed by closure of the aortic stump in three layers [14]. Aortic stump closure is performed with two layers of nonabsorbable polypropylene suture, followed by reinforcement of the closure with either omentum, ligamentum flavum, or other retroperitoneal tissue. Three-layer closure of the aortic stump is critical to minimizing the risk of stump blowout—a highly lethal complication of this operation. Distal revascularization is then performed using a prosthetic bypass through uninvolved tissue planes (extra-anatomic bypass), such as axillofemoral bypass to the lower extremities. If the diagnosis of a mycotic aneurysm is known preoperatively and the patient is stable, the extra-anatomic bypass should be performed prior to resection of the infected aneurysm. This approach minimizes the risk of cross-contamination of the extra-anatomic bypass graft and lessens the duration of distal ischemia. The results of aortic resection with extra-anatomic bypass are reported below (in section "Outcomes").

Over the past several years, in situ aortic reconstruction has become the favored approach in most centers because of the poor results for extra-anatomic bypass (in section "Outcomes"). In situ aortic reconstruction after resection of a mycotic aneurysm may seem contrary to the traditional principle of performing a bypass in an uncontaminated field whenever possible. However, several modifications to the operative technique have been introduced to minimize the risk of graft infection after in situ aortic reconstruction in an infected or contaminated field. These modifications involve the use of antibiotic-soaked Dacron grafts, cryopreserved human allografts, and autogenous vein as the conduit for in situ repair [8, 10, 15–18]. Another critical adjunct is the use of omental flap coverage of a prosthetic Dacron graft. Each of these techniques of in situ reconstruction merits further discussion.

The use of antibiotic-impregnated grafts was initially described as an approach for the treatment of infected aneurysms of the paravisceral aorta, where it is difficult to perform an extra-anatomic bypass. Popularized by Bandyk and colleagues, this technique entails bonding of rifampin (1200 mg in 20 cc sterile water, >30 min) to a gelatin-impregnated Dacron graft, producing persistent antistaphylococcal activity in vivo [19]. This group described its clinical use in two patients, and both patients survived without evidence of graft infection at 10 months. Other centers have since adopted this approach as an alternative to extra-anatomic bypass [20]. The appeal of in situ reconstruction with a rifampin-soaked Dacron graft is its simplicity. It is also feasible in emergency operations.

The use of cryopreserved allograft was initially described for in situ repair of an infected aneurysm of the infrarenal aorta [21]. The purported advantage of allograft is its relative resistance to reinfection, compared to Dacron grafts. Many centers preferentially use cryopreserved allograft as first-line therapy for elective repair of mycotic aneurysms [7, 16, 17, 22, 23]. A disadvantage of cryopreserved allograft is the need to procure a graft in advance of the operation, which is not always feasible.

Another option for in situ repair is autogenous femoral vein (FV; Fig. 22.5). This approach was based on the experience using FV for in situ aortoiliac reconstruction after excision of infected aortic grafts [24–26]. FV offers resistance to reinfection and excellent long-term patency. The use of FV for in situ repair will be described in greater detail below (see section "Infected aortic grafts and endografts"). Fillmore and Valentine described the use of FV in four patients with infected infrarenal aortic aneurysms with acceptable clinical results [10].

Omental flap coverage is an adjunct that should be employed, whenever feasible, for any in situ aortic reconstruction for infection. Omental flap coverage was described as a means of providing a vascularized pedicle flap to cover a Dacron graft used for in situ repair in an infected operative field [27, 28]. The technique for omental flap coverage involves mobilization of the omentum from the transverse colon to create a long flap that remains attached at its origin on the transverse colon, followed by transposition to the infrarenal retroperitoneal space through an opening of the transverse mesocolon to wrap the prosthetic graft and fill the infected space [27, 28].

Open surgical reconstruction for mycotic aneurysms is associated with a high risk of morbidity and mortality (see section "Outcomes"), especially in older, frail patients. These outcomes have fueled an interest in in situ repair with aortic endografting (endovascular aneurysm repair, EVAR). The advantages of endografting include lessening the magnitude of the operation for patients who are often profoundly ill. In addition, endografting provides an opportunity to temporize, even

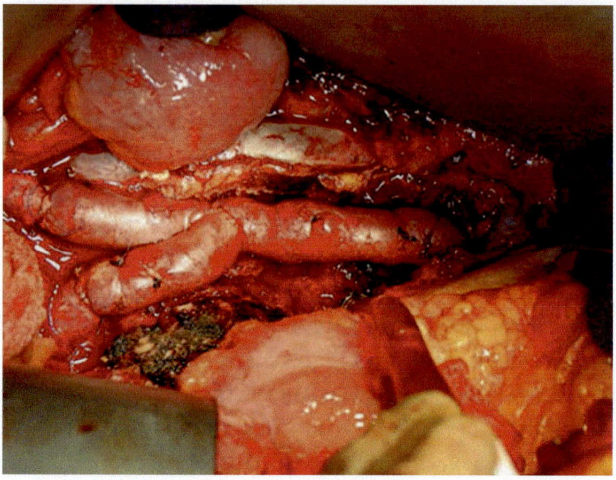

Fig. 22.5 In situ aortic repair with superficial femoral vein (*FV*). The FV has been used to reconstruct the aorta and iliac segments after debridement of the mycotic aneurysm pictured in Figs. 22.3 and 22.4 (*See Color Plates*)

definitively treat, contained ruptures in unstable patients. The results of endografting of mycotic aneurysms are discussed below (see section "Outcomes"). The disadvantage of EVAR is the lack of debridement of infected aorta and periaortic tissue aimed at removing necrotic and infected tissues, with a potential risk of persistent or recurrent infection.

Postoperative management of the treated mycotic aneurysm will entail long-term antibiotic therapy and imaging for recurrent infection. The appropriate duration of antibiotic therapy is not known, although the available data suggests that the first 3 months postoperatively is the highest risk period for infection-related complications and most reinfections occur within the first year. The durations of therapy described in the literature are highly variable, but most series report using 6 weeks of antibiotics or longer. A systematic review of the management of mycotic aortic aneurysms found that antibiotic treatment for more than 6 months postoperatively was associated with better survival [29]. Some authors advocate lifelong suppressive antibiotic therapy [8, 14].

Surveillance of grafts placed into infected fields mandates CT scans for regular intervals. Signs of infection would include a pseudoaneurysm adjacent to a surgical repair, fluid or air persisting around a graft greater than 4 months postoperatively, or inflammatory stranding that persists beyond the perioperative period.

Outcomes

A systematic review of the management of mycotic aortic aneurysms found that open surgical repair predominated prior to 2010, but EVAR has become the more common mode of repair thereafter [29]. While the treatment of mycotic aneurysms of the aorta is associated with significant morbidity and mortality [7, 8, 10, 14, 16, 18], operative mortality rates for aneurysm resection have decreased over the past decade [29]. A comparison of open surgical repair versus EVAR for mycotic aortic aneurysms in Sweden showed significantly higher survival at 3 months postoperatively for EVAR (96%), compared to open surgical repair (74%) [30]. However, the differences in survival were no longer significant at 1 and 5 years postoperatively [30]. A systematic review of 963 mycotic aortic aneurysms found that factors associated with adverse outcomes were increasing age, rupture, suprarenal aortic aneurysm, and non-*Salmonella* positive culture [29].

A number of small series comparing in situ and extra-anatomic reconstructions for mycotic aneurysms failed to show any influence of the type of reconstruction on outcomes [7, 8, 10]. However, data from a large systematic review suggested that in situ reconstruction may be associated with a trend towards fewer complications and lower 30–90 day mortality with no difference in infection-related complications [29].

Infection-related complications after mycotic aneurysm repair include persistent or recurrent infection and sepsis. A large systematic review found that infection-related complications occurred in 21% of cases and many of those infections (46–70%) were fatal. In that series, there were no differences in the rates of infection-related complications between open surgical repair and EVAR [29]. However, a meta-analysis of 14 observational studies with 1203 patients found that the rate of recurrent infection was 2.4 times higher after EVAR than open surgical repair of infected aortic aneurysms [31].

In summary, the available data suggest that both open surgical repair and EVAR have a role in the treatment of mycotic aortic aneurysms. As noted above, the mortality rates for the two treatments are similar, but recurrent infection occurs more commonly after EVAR. Complicating interpretation of the data is the high probability of selection bias impacting treatment decisions. In general, stable patients with a reasonable life expectancy should be considered for open surgical repair. We favor in situ repair, with the conduit dependent on the probable causative organism. In less stable patients and patients with a limited life expectancy, EVAR is a reasonable option. With either treatment, at least 6 months of antibiotic therapy appears to be optimal.

Infected Aortic Grafts and Endografts

Pathogenesis

Graft infection is an uncommon, but not rare, complication after aortic surgery, occurring in 1–5% of cases [32, 33]. The pathogenesis of graft infection is likely multifactorial. Since *Staphylococcal* species is a common offending organism in aortic graft and endograft infections, most authorities have concluded that the majority of graft infections occur through seeding from the patient's skin flora at the time of graft implantation [34]. Operative factors may increase the risk of an aortic graft infection. Aortic operations that require a groin incision, such as aortobifemoral bypass, increase the risk of graft infection severalfold, which probably relates to the bacterial milieu of the groin. The groin is known to harbor high surface concentrations of *Staphylococcus* species [35]. Furthermore, a groin dissection to expose the femoral vessels disrupts the rich network of lymphatics that drain the leg, which may potentially release bacteria draining from the lower leg into the wound. Finally, persistent leakage of lymph fluid in the groin after a groin incision may cause a lymphocutaneous fistula, or lymphorrhea, which provides a ready portal of entry for bacterial influx from the skin and increases the risk of graft infection.

Graft contamination may also occur months or years later due to reoperation or percutaneous access of a graft for an unrelated procedure. Patients with infected aortobifemoral grafts will often relate a history of multiple procedures performed via a graft limb that presents with evidence of infection months or years later. These procedures may inadvertently expose the graft to skin flora despite topical antiseptic preparation of the skin.

For many years Gram-positive organisms, especially *Staphylococcus epidermidis*, were the most common cause of aortic graft infections. *Staphylococcus epidermidis* produces a glycocalyx slime layer, or biofilm, that coats the graft, shielding the organisms from phagocytosis. This biofilm produces the "unincorporated" appearance of a graft that is characteristic of a peri-graft infection at operative exploration. This finding has been associated with positive cultures in 71% of cases [36].

Over the past decade, however, the microbiology of graft infections has evolved from primarily Gram-positive organisms, especially *Staphylococcal* species, to a higher proportion of Gram-negative organisms. A recent study found that 58% of aortic graft infections were caused by Gram-negative organisms and 27% were polymicrobial. In addition, multidrug-resistant bacterial strains are common, causing 72% of early graft infections and 35% of late graft infections [37].

Clinical Presentation

The presentation for aortic graft infections varies according to the time frame after surgery. Bandyk defined *early* graft infections as those occurring within 4 months of surgery, while *late* graft infections presented after 4 months [34]. He further subdivided graft infections based on their presentation as peri-graft infection, graft-enteric erosion, and graft-enteric fistula. The latter two categories will be addressed in a separate chapter. The remainder of this section will be devoted to peri-graft infections. Early perigraft infections usually present as a surgical site infection or wound complication with graft exposure. Purulent drainage and signs of sepsis are the most common findings. Less-frequent manifestations of a perigraft infection are pseudoaneurysm formation or anastomotic disruption with hemorrhage. Early infection of an aortic graft confined to the abdomen usually presents with relatively nonspecific findings such as an ileus, persistent low-grade fever, or leukocytosis.

Late graft infections (>4 months after surgery) may present as a persistent sinus tract, anastomotic pseudoaneurysm or rupture, graft occlusion, or sepsis. A subset of late graft infections are asymptomatic and discovered incidentally during an imaging study for an unrelated indication. Most late graft infections present more than 1 year after graft implantation.

Diagnosis and Imaging

Early graft infections involving aortic grafts confined to the abdomen present a particular challenge for diagnosis. These infections produce nonspecific signs, such as a persistent ileus, fever, or leukocytosis. As will be discussed below, imaging is rarely helpful in the early postoperative period unless a pseudoaneurysm or rupture is visualized. If there is a high index of suspicion, operative exploration and examination of the graft for purulence may be necessary to ascertain the diagnosis. Infections of aortic grafts confined to the abdomen are rare.

The vast majority of *early* graft infections involve aortic grafts that include a groin incision. In this circumstance, an early graft infection usually manifests as a wound infection in the groin overlying the graft. While cellulitis may be treated initially with empiric antibiotics, any significant drainage or partial dehiscence of the postoperative wound overlying a wound mandates operative exploration. The goal of operative exploration is to ascertain the full extent and depth of involvement of the wound in any infectious process. If there is viable, uninfected tissue overlying the graft, the likelihood of graft infection is low. If the infectious process extends to the graft, however, the graft itself is assumed to be infected and definitive therapy should be planned. Any graft that develops an early postoperative pseudoaneurysm or hemorrhage should be considered infected.

Late graft infections are usually more subtle in presentation. Any aortic graft that presents with a persistent wound or sinus tract overlying a graft, anastomotic pseudoaneurysm, or graft thrombosis should be investigated further with an imaging study. Anastomotic pseudoaneurysms may be caused by late degeneration of the artery to which a graft is sutured, but 60% of anastomotic pseudoaneurysms are culture positive [38]. There are several choices for imaging for possible graft infection, including CT, FDG-PET/CT, MRI, radionuclide scanning, ultrasound, and arteriography. The utility of each modality will be discussed.

CT provides excellent visualization of the various secondary signs of a *late* graft infection, including ectopic gas, perigraft fluid, increased perigraft inflammatory changes ("stranding"), anastomotic pseudoaneurysm, and thickening of adjacent bowel (Fig. 22.6) [39–41]. CT scan has a sensitivity of 94% for the diagnosis of late graft infection [42]. In his series of 12 patients, Low et al. found that the presence of perigraft fluid, increased perigraft soft tissue, or ectopic gas identified all cases of graft infections, providing a sensitivity 100% [42]. Ectopic gas is the only single finding that is diagnostic of a late graft infection, but it is present in a minority of cases (Fig. 22.7) [42].

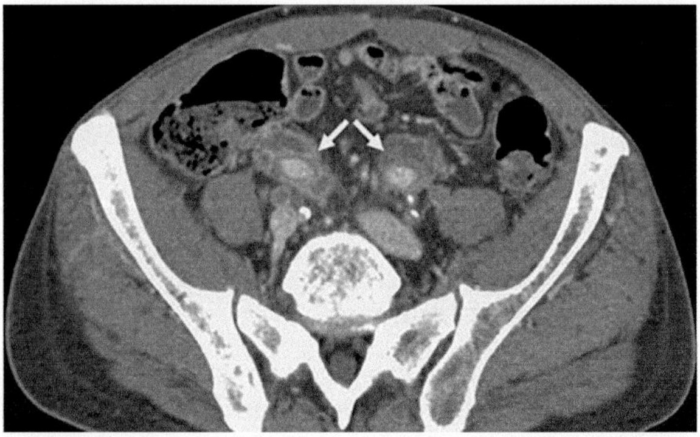

Fig. 22.6 Perigraft fluid. Note the loculated fluid surrounding the two limbs (*arrows*) of an aortobifemoral bypass graft

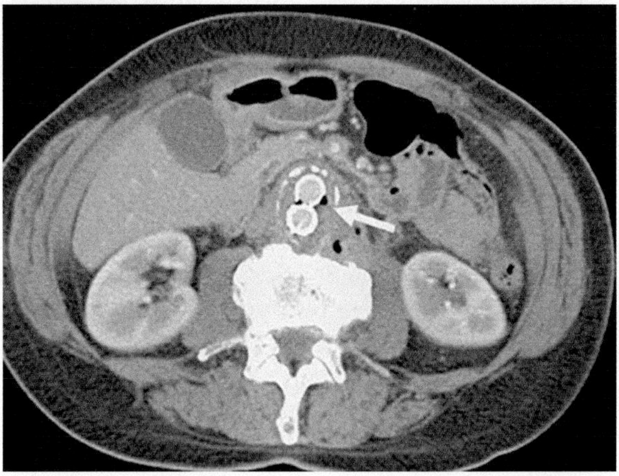

Fig. 22.7 Gas adjacent to aortic endograft. Gas (*arrow*) is observed adjacent to an aortic endograft years after graft implantation

In contrast, CT offers little assistance in the diagnosis of *early* graft infections because perigraft hematoma and retained ambient gas are normal findings in the early postoperative period. Serial scanning of postoperative aortic grafts found that perigraft hematoma should resolve within 3 months, and no ectopic gas should be present beyond 3–4 weeks after surgery [43]. By 3 months after graft implantation, hematoma should resorb, perigraft tissue planes should normalize, and perigraft fluid should be minimal (<5 mm) or absent [39, 42, 43]. After 3 months, CT scanning is considered the diagnostic test of choice in most cases.

FDG-PET/CT may further increase the sensitivity of CT for the detection of *late* graft infections. Increased glucose metabolism in the peri-graft soft tissues may be detected earlier in the infectious process before perigraft soft tissue thickening, gas formation, or pseudoaneurysm formation occurs, allowing for earlier, more accurate detection of graft infections (Fig. 22.8). In a prospective study of 34 patients with suspected graft infections, the diagnostic accuracy of FDG-PET/CT was 94% [44]. An important caveat in interpreting FDG-PET/CT is that inflammation and infection enhance equally in these studies. Furthermore, no systematic study of the time course of postoperative changes on FDG-PET/CT has been performed. Inflammatory

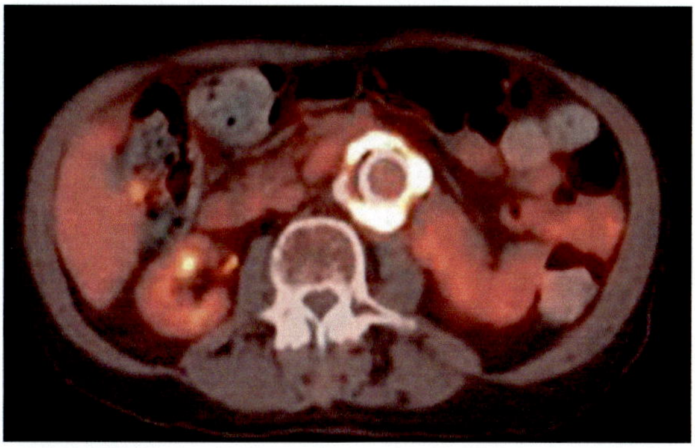

Fig. 22.8 FDG-PET/CT showing enhancement of the peri-graft soft tissues and the abdominal portion of a fenestrated endovascular aneurysm repair

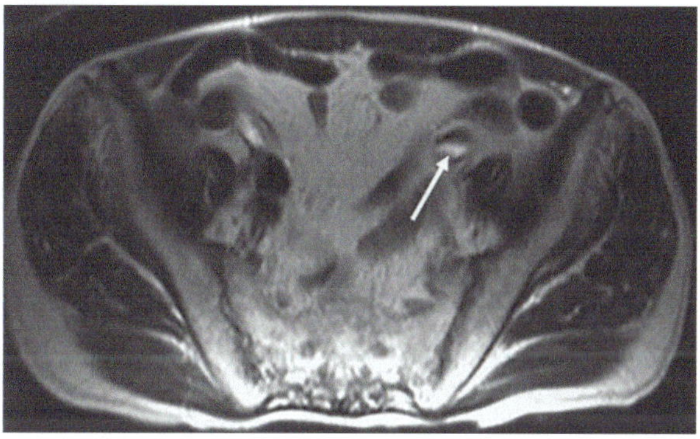

Fig. 22.9 MRI with T2-weighted image. This heavily weighted T2 image shows high-intensity signal (*arrow*) posterior to the left limb of an aortobifemoral bypass graft

changes in the early postoperative period may result in peri-graft enhancement on a FDG-PET/CT scan, so FDG-PET/CT should be considered less reliable in the diagnosis of early postoperative graft infections (Fig. 22.8).

MRI is an alternative modality for imaging-suspected aortic graft infections. On MRI, the perigraft fluid of a graft infection is characterized by a low-to-medium intensity signal on T1-weighted images and high intensity on T2-weighted images (Fig. 22.9) [45]. The characteristic T1- and T2-weighted images will also permit differentiation of perigraft fluid soft tissue inflammation from subacute or chronic hematoma, which is a distinction that is difficult on CT [46]. Using operative exploration as the gold standard for comparison, Auffermann et al. found that MRI had a sensitivity of 85% and a specificity of 100% [45]. A shortcoming of MRI is its inability to distinguish perigraft gas from calcification in the remnant aorta [46]. Because the characteristic high-intensity signal on T2-weighted images permits visualization of even small amounts of fluid, MRI remains a useful modality for imaging of graft infections and may be used when CT findings are equivocal for graft infection.

Radionuclide scanning using ^{111}indium-labeled white blood cells (WBCs; Fig. 22.10) is a favored approach of many infectious disease specialists. The advantage of this approach is its high sensitivity, which approaches 100% in some centers

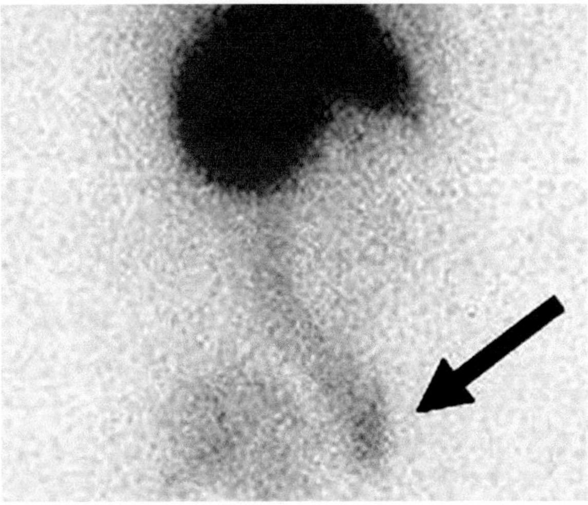

Fig. 22.10 ^{111}Indium-labeled WBC scan. Increased activity (*arrow*) indicative of a possible graft infection is noted on lateral view of an aortobifemoral bypass graft

[47–49]. The primary shortcoming of radionuclide scanning has been a propensity for yielding false-positive results, producing relatively low specificity (80–82%) [47–49]. It has been suggested that inadvertent radiolabeling and inclusion of platelets in the ^{111}indium-labeled WBC preparation may result in nonspecific adherence of the platelets to pseudointima of a vascular grafts, leading to false-positive results. This phenomenon is particularly evident in the early postoperative period when there is active adherence of platelets to prosthetic grafts. Sedwitz et al. found that ^{111}indium-labeled WBC scans are positive in 80% of grafts imaged within 4 months of implantation [50]. Thus, indium scanning is far less accurate in the diagnosis of a suspected *early* graft infection. For the diagnosis of *late* graft infections, radionuclide scanning is a reasonable option. The combination of high sensitivity and specificity for CT, FDG-PET/CT, and MRI has supplanted indium scanning in most centers.

Ultrasonography offers few advantages for the diagnosis of graft infection. The resolution is usually insufficient to provide adequate information. Arteriography plays an equally limited role in the diagnosis of graft infections. While anastomotic pseudoaneurysms are well visualized by arteriography, the majority of extraluminal manifestations of a graft infection will not be imaged by arteriography. The primary role of arteriography is to provide anatomic information for planning definitive therapy after the diagnosis of a graft infection is secure.

Some authors have proposed using CT guidance for percutaneous aspiration of perigraft fluid to confirm the diagnosis of a graft infection [51, 52]. The utility of CT-guided aspiration may be highest in diagnosing aortic endograft infections. A Swedish group was able to obtain a diagnosis of graft infection in 81% of cases with CT-guided aspiration of the aneurysm sac [53]. It is important to recognize, however, that this technique poses a risk of seeding a sterile perigraft fluid collection while performing the aspiration. For that reason, this approach should be reserved for cases in which the diagnosis remains ambiguous.

Belair et al. tested percutaneous drainage as a therapeutic modality for the treatment of confirmed aortic graft infections [52]. In 11 patients, 4 were successfully treated with percutaneous drainage and antibiotics alone. Of the remaining seven patients, six ultimately proceeded to surgery for surgical drainage or graft excision, and one died of procedure-related hemorrhage. Percutaneous drainage should be reserved for patients who cannot survive a more definitive procedure.

Treatment

The guiding principles in the surgical management of infected aortic grafts are analogous to the principles outlined for management of mycotic aneurysms. Surgical dogma has traditionally dictated complete graft excision, ligation of the aorta, and extra-anatomic bypass. Whenever feasible, it is optimal to stage the operations with the extra-anatomic operation performed through uninfected tissue planes first [54]. However, this approach is not without significant potential pitfalls, including a risk of aortic stump blowout, late infection of the prosthetic extra-anatomic bypass, and poor long-term graft patency of extra-anatomic bypasses [32, 54, 55].

In most centers, in situ replacement aortic reconstruction after excision of the infected aortic graft has largely replaced extra-anatomic bypass, except in the most frail patients. The appeal of this approach lies in its direct revascularization of the lower extremities and avoidance of an extra-anatomic bypass with inferior long-term patency. Various conduits have been proposed for in situ repair. Rifampin-soaked prosthetic graft replacement and arterial allografts were discussed previously (see section "Mycotic aneurysms"). The use of FV or femoral-popliteal vein for in situ graft replacement was described by Clagett et al. [24] Clagett described the creation of a neo-aortoiliac system with FV to reconstruct the aortoiliac segments after complete graft excision. The purported advantages of FV are its relative resistance to infection, excellent long-term patency, and avoidance of stump blowout. The technique for harvest is described in detail elsewhere [56]. Harvesting FV for aortic reconstruction may produce an acute compartment syndrome in a minority of patients, although late venous morbidity is surprisingly infrequent in the harvested limbs [57–59]. The primary disadvantage of this approach is the length and magnitude of this operation [32].

Important adjuncts to any in situ reconstruction are aggressive debridement of the retroperitoneum and omental flap coverage of the reconstruction. Debridement of the retroperitoneum is aimed at decreasing the peri-aortic bacterial counts to minimize the risk of reinfection of the new aortic reconstruction. Omental flap coverage of the aortic reconstruction creates a vascularized tissue pedicle for coverage and protection of the new aortic reconstruction, with a goal of preventing reinfection.

Endograft explantation, especially for an endograft with suprarenal fixation, poses a different challenge, compared to excision of a surgically implanted aortic graft. Obtaining proximal control above the site of fixation is key. Some authors believe that retroperitoneal exposure facilitates proximal control in these cases [60].

Removal of the entire endograft and debridement of the aneurysm sac are important adjuncts after endograft explantation to prevent reinfection.

In cases in which the entire graft is not infected, partial graft excision is an option. The advantage of this approach is the ability to minimize the extent of operation in frail patients. The concern with this approach relates to the risk of recurrent infection in the residual graft. The results for each approach to aortic graft infection are described below (see section "Outcomes").

Finally, conservative management is an option in frail patients or those with limited life expectancy. Traditional teaching has been that nonoperative management condemns the patient to an early death due to sepsis or exsanguination. In reality, the frailest patients have a limited life expectancy no matter the treatment and often cannot tolerate a major aortic operation, making conservative treatment an attractive option. A cohort study from Sweden of patients deemed unfit for partial or complete graft excision reported 30-day, 1-year, and 3-year survival rates of 98%, 88%, and 79%, respectively, with conservative management [61]. In that study, conservative management consisted of appropriate antimicrobial therapy. In addition, 1 in 5 patients in that series had adjunctive procedures without graft explantation, including CT- or ultrasound-guided drainage of an abscess in 10% and aneurysm sac resection or repair of an enteric fistula in 10%. Only 12% of deaths with conservative management were deemed related to the graft infection.

Outcomes

The most comprehensive analysis of the outcomes of total graft excision with extra-anatomic bypass was reported by Seeger and colleagues [55]. Seeger reported an 11% operative mortality rate and an aortic stump blowout rate of 2.8% [55]. Seeger found that the long-term patency of the extra-anatomic bypass was dependent on the type of bypass performed. The 5-year primary patency rates were 75% and 64% for axillofemoral—femoral bypass and axillofemoral bypasses, respectively, whereas none of the axillopopliteal bypasses in his series were patent beyond 7 months [55]. In multiple series, reinfection of the extra-anatomic bypass was observed in 10–20% of cases [32, 62, 63].

The operative mortality rate for in situ repair has been reported to vary between 4% and 18% [64, 65]. A nonrandomized cohort study from the Mayo Clinic compared in situ repair with rifampin-soaked grafts to traditional aortic ligation with extra-anatomic bypass [66]. In situ repair provided superior 5-year primary patency (89%), compared to axillofemoral bypass (48%) [66]. Moreover, major morbidity or procedure-related mortality were two-fold higher after graft excision with axillofemoral bypass compared with in situ reconstruction [66]. Operative mortality, limb salvage, and reinfection rates were not statistically different between groups, although the trends favored in situ repair [66]. These data argue strongly that in situ repair with rifampin-soaked grafts and omental flap coverage is superior to extra-anatomic reconstruction.

In situ graft replacement with cryopreserved arterial allograft is the option of choice in many centers. Kieffer et al. reported a series of 179 patients operated for aortic graft infections or secondary aortoenteric fistulas [67]. In Kieffer's series, the operative mortality was 20.1%. Early and late allograft ruptures occurred in 2.8% and 2.1% cases, respectively. Another series of 200 patients with in situ reconstruction with cryopreserved arterial allograft reported a 30-day mortality of 11%. Early revision surgery was required in 29.5% and one-quarter of those were allograft-related. Reinfection within 6 months was identified in 8.5% [68]. A nonrandomized comparison of in situ reconstruction with rifampin-soaked Dacron versus cryopreserved arterial allografts showed a significantly higher rate of reintervention for cryopreserved arterial allograft and a trend toward higher reinfection for rifampin-soaked Dacron [69].

Clagett and colleagues described the use of FV for in situ aortic reconstruction in 179 patients with long-term follow-up [70]. Operative mortality was 10%. Graft reinfection was 5%. All patients with reinfection occurred in patients with polymicrobial infections. Major amputations occurred in 7.4%. Primary patency at 6 years was 81%. Venous morbidity after FV or femoral-popliteal vein harvest included a risk of fasciotomy, but a low incidence (15%) of minor venous insufficiency (CEAP Class C_3, leg edema, or less) [70, 71].

The available options for in situ repair—Rifamin-soaked Dacron, cryopreserved arterial allograft, and FV—have advantages and disadvantages. Rifampin-soaked Dacron is attractive due to its immediate availability and relatively low cost. However, rifampin-soaked Dacron carries a life-long risk of reinfection. Cryopreserved arterial allgraft is intuitively attractive because the conduit is most analogous to the excised aorta. However, arterial allograft is expensive and most centers do not maintain an inventory. And the short-term reintervention and reinfection rate of cryopreserved arterial allograft is significant. Finally, femoral vein is attractive because it is the only autogenous option for aortic replacement. However, femoral vein is time-consuming to harvest and carries a low risk of venous morbidity. No single conduit for in situ reconstruction is ideal for all circumstances. The choice should be dictated by the clinical scenario and the options available at the time.

For grafts in which preoperative imaging suggests that only a portion is infected, such as a femoral limb of aortobifemoral bypass, partial excision is a viable option. A critical prerequisite for this approach is meticulous care to avoid cross-contaminating uninfected portions of the graft. Separate studies by Towne and Calligaro found that 86–92% of grafts will remain free of infection during follow-up using this approach [71, 72]. If partial excision is attempted, long-term antibiotics and careful long-term surveillance with CT is an important component of aftercare for these patients.

Summary

Mycotic aneurysms of the aorta and aortic graft and endograft infections are dreaded complications of aortic disease. A thoughtful plan for treatment that is tailored to each case will minimize the risk of major morbidity or mortality. While both in situ and extra-anatomic approaches are viable options, in situ reconstruction offers significant advantages in patients who can tolerate an open aortic operation. EVAR is a reasonable option in patients who are clinically unstable or frail. For infected aortic grafts and endografts, evidence suggests that in situ aortic reconstruction has significant advantages over traditional extra-anatomic approaches. No single approach to in situ repair is appropriate for all patients, so a thorough understanding of the various options and their utility will permit the clinician to optimize outcomes.

References

1. Osler W. The gulstonian lectures, on malignant endocarditis. Br Med J. 1885;1(1262):467–70.
2. Hankins JR, Yeager GH. Primary mycotic aneurysm. Surgery. 1956;40:747–56.
3. Miller DV, Oderich GS, Aubry M-C, Panneton JM, Edwards JD. Surgical pathology of infection aneurysms of the descending thoracic and abdominal aorta: clinicopathologic correlations in 29 cases (1976 to 1999). Hum Pathol. 2004;35:1112–20.
4. Revell STR Jr. Primary mycotic aneurysms. Ann Intern Med. 1945;22:431–40.
5. Jarrett F, Darling RC, Mundth ED, Austen WG. Experience with infected aneurysms of the abdominal aorta. Arch Surg. 1975;110:1281–6.
6. Brunner S, Engelmann MG, Nabauer M. Thoracic mycotic pseudoaneurysm from *Candida albicans* infection. Eur Heart J. 2008;29:1515.
7. Muller BT, Wegener OR, Grabitz K, Phillny M, Thomas L, Sandmann W. Mycotic aneurysms of the thoracic and abdominal aorta and iliac arteries: experience with anatomic and extra-anatomic repair in 33 cases. J Vasc Surg. 2001;33:106–13.
8. Oderich GS, Panneton JM, Bower TC, Cherry KJ Jr, Rowland CM, Noel AA, Hallett JW Jr. Infected aortic aneurysms: aggressive presentation, complicated early outcomes, but durable results. J Vasc Surg. 2001;34:900–9008.
9. Muchart DJ, Bhagwanjee S. American College of Chest Physicians/Society of Critical Care Medicine Consensus Conference definitions of systemic inflammatory response syndrome and allied disorders in relation to critically injured patients. Crit Care Med. 1997;25:1281–6.
10. Fillmore AJ, Valentine RJ. Surgical mortality in patients with infected aortic aneurysms. J Am Coll Surg. 2003;196:435–41.
11. Macedo TA, Stanson AW, Oderich GS, Johnson CM, Panneton JM, Tie ML. Infected aortic aneruysms: imaging findings. Radiology. 2004;231:250–7.
12. Husmann L, Huellner MW, Ledergerber B, Eberhard N, Kaelin MB, Anagnostopoulos A, Kudura K, Burger IA, Mestres CA, Rancic Z, Hasse B. Diagnostic accuracy of PET/CT and contrast enhanced CT in patients with suspected infected aortic aneurysms. Eur J Vasc Endovasc Surg. 2020;59:972–81.
13. Wang TKM, Griffin B, Cremer P, Shrestha N, Gordon S, Pettersson G, Desai M. Diagnostic utility of CT and MRI for mycotic aneurysms: a meta-analysis. Am J Roentgen. 2020;215:1257–66.
14. Moneta GL, Taylor LM Jr, Yeager RA, Edwards JM, Nicoloff AD, McConnell DB, Porter JM. Surgical treatment of infected aortic aneurysm. Am J Surg. 1998;175:396–9.

15. Fichelle JM, Tabet G, Cormier P, Farkas JC, Laurian C, Gigou F, Marzelle J, Acar J, Cormier JM. Infected infrarenal aortic aneurysms: when is in situ reconstruction safe? J Vasc Surg. 1993;17:635–45.
16. Arbatli H, DeGeest R, Demirsoy E, Wellens F, Degrieck I, VanPraet F, Korkut AK, Vanermen H. Management of infected grafts and myctoic aneurysms of the aorta using cryopreserved homografts. Cardiovasc Surg. 2003;11:257–63.
17. Vogt PR, Brunner-LaRocca H-P, Lachat M, Ruef C, Turina MI. Technical details with the use of cryopreserved arterial homografts for aortic infection: influence on early and midterm mortality. J Vasc Surg. 2002;35:80–6.
18. Ihaya A, Chiba Y, Kimura T, Morioka K, Uesaka T. Surgical outcome of infectious aneurysm of the abdominal aorta with or without SIRS. Cardiovasc Surg. 2001;9:436–40.
19. Gupta AK, Bandyk DF, Johnson BL. In situ repair of mycotic abdominal aortic aneurysms with rifampin-bonded gelatin-impregnated Dacron grafts: a preliminary case report. J Vasc Surg. 1996;24:472–6.
20. Uchida N, Katayama A, Tamura K, Miwa S, Masatsugu K, Sueda T. In situ replacement of mycotic aneurysms on the thoracic and abdominal aorta using rifampin-bonded grafting and omental pedicle grafting. Ann Thoracic Surg. 2012;93:438–42.
21. Alonso M, Caeiro S, Cachaldora J, Segura R. Infected abdominal aortic aneurysm: in situ replacement with cryopreserved arterial homograft. J Cardiovasc Surg. 1997;38:371–5.
22. Kerzmann A, Caeiro S, Daenen G, Linder JL. Infected abdominal aortic aneurysm treated by in situ replacement with cryopreserved arterial homograft. Acta Chir Belg. 2006;106:447–9.
23. Couture T, Gaudric J, Davaine JM, Jayet J, Chiche L, Jarraya M, Koskas F. Results of cryopreserved arterial allograft replacement for thoracic and abdominal aortic infections. J Vasc Surg. 2021;73:626–34.
24. Clagett GP, Bowers BL, Lopez-Viego MA, et al. Creation of a neo-aortoiliac system from lower extremity deep and superficial veins. Ann Surg. 1993;218:239–48.
25. Clagett GP, Valentine RJ, Hagino RT. Autogenous aortoiliac/femoral reconstruction from superficial femoral-popliteal veins: feasibility and durability. J Vasc Surg. 1997;25:255–66.
26. Gordon LL, Hagino RT, Jackson MR, Modrall JG, Valentine RJ, Clagett GP. Complex aortofemoral prosthetic infections: the role of autogenous superficial femoropopliteal vein reconstruction. Arch Surg. 1999;134:615–21.
27. Yokoyama H, Maida K, Takahashi S, Tanaka S. Purulently infected abdominal aortic aneurysm: in situ reconstruction with transmesocolic omental transposition technique. Cardiovasc Surg. 1994;2:78–80.
28. Oderich GS, Bower TC, Hofer J, Kalra M, Duncan A, Wilson JW, Cha S, Gloviczki P. Rifampin-soaked grafts with omental coverage and antibiotic suppression are durable with low infection rates in patients with aortic graft enteric erosion or fistula. J Vasc Surg. 2011;53:99–106.
29. Sorelius K, Budtz-Lilly J, Mani K, Wanhainen A. Systematic review of the management of mycotic aneurysms. Eur J Vasc Endovasc Surg. 2019;58:426–35.
30. Sorelius K, Wanhainen A, Furebring M, Bjorck M, Gillgren P, Mani K. Nationwide study of the treatment of mycotic aortic aneurysms comparing open and endovascular repair. Circulation. 2016;134:1822–32.
31. Shirasu T, Kuno T, Yasuhara J, Yokoyama Y, Takagi H, Cullen MJ, Kent CK, Clouse WD. Meta-analysis finds recurrent infection is more common after endovascular than open repair of infected abdominal aortic aneurysm. J Vasc Surg. 2022;75:348–55.
32. Valentine RJ. Diagnosis and management of aortic graft infection. Sem Vasc Surg. 2001;14:292–301.
33. Hallett JW Jr, Marshall DM, Petterson TM, Gray DT, Bower TC, Cherry KJ Jr, Gloviczki P, Pairolero PC. Graft-related complications after abdominal aortic aneurysm repair: reassurance from a 36-year population-based experience. J Vasc Surg. 1997;25:277–84.
34. Bandyk DF, Esses GE. Aortic graft infection. Surg Clin North Am. 1994;74:571–90.
35. Seabrook GR. Pathobiology of graft infections. Sem Vasc Surg. 1990;3:77–80.

36. Padberg FT Jr, Smith SM, Eng RH. Accuracy of disincorporation for identification of vascular graft infection. Arch Surg. 1995;130:183–7.
37. Melo RG, Martins B, Pedro DM, Santos CM, Duarte A, Fernandes RF, Garrido P, Pedro LM. Microbial evolution of vascular graft infections in a tertiary hospital based on positive graft cultures. J Vasc Surg. 2021;74:276–84.
38. Seabrook GR, Schmitt DD, Bandyk DF, Edmiston CE, Krepel CJ, Towne JB. Anastomotic femoral pseudoaneurysm: an investigation of occult infection as an etiologic factor. J Vasc Surg. 1990;11:629–34.
39. Hilton S, Megibow AJ, Naidich DP, Bosniak MA. Computed tomography of the postoperative abdominal aorta. Radiology. 1982;145:403–7.
40. Mark A, Moss AA, Lusby R, Kaiser JA. CT evaluation of complications of abdominal aortic surgery. Radiology. 1982;145:409–14.
41. Mark AS, Moss AA, McCarthy S, McCowin M. CT of aortoenteric fistulas. Investig Radiol. 1985;20:272–5.
42. Low RN, Wall SD, Jeffrey RB Jr, Sollitto RA, Reilly LM, Tierney LM Jr. Aortoenteric fistula and perigraft infection: evaluation with CT. Radiology. 1990;175:157–62.
43. Qvarfordt PG, Reilly LM, Mark AS, Goldstone J, Wall SD, Ehrenheld WK, Stoney RJ. Computerized tomographic assessment of graft incorporation after aortic reconstruction. Am J Surg. 1985;150:227–31.
44. Sah BR, Husmann L, Mayer D, Scherrer A, Rancic Z, Puippe G, Weber R, Hasse B. Diagnostic performance of 18F-FDG-PET/CT in vascular graft infections. Eur J Vasc Endovasc Surg. 2015;49:455–64.
45. Auffermann W, Olofsson PA, Rabahie GN, Tavares NJ, Stoney RJ, Higgins CB. Incorporation versus infection of retroperitoneal aortic grafts: MR imaging features. Radiology. 1989;172:359–62.
46. Orton DF, LeVeen RF, Saigh JA, Culp WC, Fidler JL, Lynch TJ, Goertzen TC, McCowan TC. Aortic prosthetic graft infections: radiologic manifestations and implications for management. Radiographics. 2000;20:977–93.
47. Brunner MC, Mitchell RS, Baldwin JC, James DR, Olcott C 4th, Mehigan JT, McDougall IR, Miller DC. Prosthetic graft infection: limitations of indium white blood cell scanning. J Vasc Surg. 1986;3:42–8.
48. Lawrence PF, Dries DJ, Alazraki N, Albo D Jr. Indium 111-labeled leukocyte scanning for detection of prosthetic vascular graft infection. J Vasc Surg. 1985;2:165–73.
49. Reilly DT, Grigg MJ, Cunningham DA, Thomas EJ, Mansfield AO. Vascular graft infection: the role of indium scanning. Eur J Vasc Surg. 1989;3:393–7.
50. Sedwitz MM, Davies RJ, Pretorius HT, Vasquez TE. Indium 111-labeled white blood cell scans after vascular prosthetic reconstruction. J Vasc Surg. 1987;6:476–81.
51. Harris KA, Kozak R, Carroll SE, Meads GE, Sweeney JP. Confirmation of infection of an aortic graft. J Cardiovasc Surg. 1989;30:230–2.
52. Bélair M, Soulez G, Oliva VL, Laperriere J, Gianfelice D, Blair JF, Sarrazin J, Therasse E. Aortic graft infection: the value of percutaneous drainage. Am J Roentgenol. 1998;171:119–24.
53. Ljungquist O, Dias N, Haidl S, Sonesson B, Sorelius K, Ahl J. Guided aspiratoin for determining the microbial aetiology of aortic vascular graft and endograft infections. Eur J Vasc Endovasc Surg. 2021;62:935–43.
54. Reilly LM, Stoney RJ, Goldstone J, Ehrenfeld WK. Improved management of aortic graft infection: the influence of operation sequence and staging. J Vasc Surg. 1987;5:421–31.
55. Seeger JM, Pretus HA, Welborn MB, Ozaki CK, Flynn TC, Huber TS. Long-term outcome after treatment of aortic graft infection with staged extra-anatomic bypass grafting aortic graft removal. J Vasc Surg. 2000;32:451–9.
56. Valentine RJ. Harvesting the superficial femoral vein as an autograft. Semin Vasc Surg. 2000;13:27–31.

57. Wells JK, Hagino RT, Bargmann KM, Jackson MR, Valentine RJ, Kakish HB, Clagett GP. Venous morbidity after superficial femoral-popliteal vein harvest. J Vasc Surg. 1999;29:282–9.
58. Modrall JG, Sadjadi J, Ali AT, Anthony T, Welborn MB III, Valentine RJ, Hynan LS, Clagett GP. Deep vein harvesting: predicting the need for fasciotomy. J Vasc Surg. 2004;39:387–94.
59. Modrall JG, Hocking JA, Rosero E, Timaran CH, Arko FA III, Valentine RJ, Clagett GP. Late incidence of chronic venous insufficiency after deep vein harvest. J Vasc Surg. 2007;46:520–5.
60. Lyden S, McNamara JAM, Sternbach Y, Illig K, Woldman DL, Green DM. Technical considerations for late removal of aortic endografts. J Vasc Surg. 2002;36:674–8.
61. Ljungquist O, Haidl S, Dias N, Sonesson B, Sorelius K, Tragardh E, Ahl J. Conservative management first strategy in aortic vascular graft and endograft infections. Eur J Vasc Endovasc Surg. 2023;65:896–904.
62. Yeager RA, Taylor LM Jr, Moneta GL, Edwards JM, Nicoloff AD, McConnell DB, Porter JM. Improved results with conventional management of infrarenal aortic infection. J Vasc Surg. 1999;30:76–83.
63. Reilly LM, Altman H, Lusby RJ, Kersh RA, Ehrenfeld WK, Stoney RJ. Late results following surgical management of vascular graft infection. J Vasc Surg. 1984;1:36–44.
64. Bandyk DF, Novotney ML, Back MR, Johnson BL, Schmacht DC. Expanded application of in situ replacement for prosthetic graft infection. J Vasc Surg. 2001;34:411–9.
65. Hayes PD, Nasim A, London NJ, Sayers RD, Barrie WW, Bell PR, Naylor AR. In situ replacement of infected aortic grafts with rifampicin-bonded prostheses: the Leicester experience (1992 to 1998). J Vasc Surg. 1999;30:92–8.
66. Oderich GS, Bower TC, Cherry KJ Jr, Panneton JM, Sullivan TM, Noel AA, Carmo M, Cha S, Kalra M, Gloviczki P. Evolution from axillofemoral to in situ prosthetic reconstruction for the treatment of aortic graft infections at a single center. J Vasc Surg. 2006;43:1166–74.
67. Kieffer E, Gomes D, Chiche L, Fleron MH, Koskas F, Bahnini A. Allograft replacement for infrarenal aortic graft infection: early and late results in 179 patients. J Vasc Surg. 2004;39:1009–17.
68. Couture T, Gaudric J, Du Montzel ST, Jayet J, Verscheure D, Davaine JM, Jarraya M, Chiche L, Koskas F. Short and mid-term outcomes of aortic allografts used as a substitute for infected prosthetic grafts in 200 patients. Eur J Vasc Endovasc Surg. 2021;62:89–97.
69. Tabiei A, Cifuentes S, Glasgow AE, Colglazier JJ, Kalra M, Mendes C, Rasmussen TE, Shuja F, DeMartino RR. Cryopreserved arterial allografts vs rifampin-soaked Dacron for the treatment of infected aortic and iliac grafts. J Vasc Surg. 2023;78:1064–73.
70. Ali AT, Modrall JG, Hocking J, Valentine RJ, Spencer H, Eidt JF, Clagett GP. Long-term results of the treatment of aortic graft infection by in situ replacement with femoral popliteal vein grafts. J Vasc Surg. 2009;50:30–9.
71. Towne JB, Seabrook GR, Bandyk D, Freischlag JA, Edmiston CE. In situ replacement of arterial prosthesis infected by bacterial biofilms: long-term follow-up. J Vasc Surg. 1994;19:226–33.
72. Calligaro KD, Veith FJ, Valladares JA, McKay J, Schindler N, Dougherty MJ. Prosthetic patch remnants to treat infected arterial grafts. J Vasc Surg. 2000;31:245–52.

Chapter 23
Evaluation and Management of Aortoenteric Fistula

Salvatore T. Scali and Scott T. Robinson

Introduction

Historical Perspectives and Definitions The earliest known description of an aorto-enteric fistula (AEF) was by Sir Astley Cooper in 1829 [1] when he documented a primary aortic infection resulting in an enteric erosion that precipitated exsanguinating hemorrhage in a patient with an abdominal aortic aneurysm (AAA). It was in this publication that the classic triad of abdominal pain, pulsatile abdominal mass, and gastrointestinal (GI) hemorrhage was first described. The post-mortem identification of the communication between the AAA and 3rd portion of the duodenum ushered in the modern era of AEF management. Despite documentation of primary AEF in the early 1800s, due to limitations in anesthesia and surgical techniques of the time, it was not until 1954 that Zenker performed the first surgical repair. Interestingly, the operation featured an account of a "pigeon-egg-sized" AAA that perforated into the duodenum. Subtotal resection of the eccentrically shaped aneurysm was performed with primary closure of the aorta and lateral sutures were applied to the defect in the duodenum. Remarkably, the patient survived for over 2 years after this index operation.

In contrast to a primary AEF that features the aforementioned *de novo* communication between the native aorta and GI tract, the first depiction of a secondary AEF, which occurs when there is a false communication between a previous aortic graft (or endograft) and an enteric structure, was by Brock in 1953 [2]. The patient was a 44-year-old woman with disabling claudication and an infrarenal aortic occlusion who underwent native aortic excision and in-situ reconstruction (ISR) with an

S. T. Scali (✉) · S. T. Robinson
Division of Vascular Surgery and Endovascular Therapy, University of Florida College of Medicine, Florida, USA
e-mail: salvatore.scali@surgery.ufl.edu; Scott.Robinson@surgery.ufl.edu

G. J. Arnaoutakis et al. (eds.), *Aortic Aneurysms*, Contemporary Cardiology,
https://doi.org/10.1007/978-3-032-13134-8_23

aortic homograft using an aorto-bi-iliac configuration. The patient received an arteriogram before hospital discharge, and a small peri-anastomotic pseudoaneurysm between the left limb of the homograft and native common iliac artery was identified but was not remediated. Unfortunately, 3 months postoperatively, the patient died suddenly due to exsanguinating GI hemorrhage. The autopsy revealed a direct communication between the third portion of the duodenum and the false aneurysm arising from the left homograft-common iliac artery anastomosis. Subsequently, in 1958, McKenzie and associates reported the first successful repair of a secondary AEF due to an aortic homograft that was originally used for an AAA resection [3]. Notably, it was during this era that providers started to increasingly use prosthetic graft materials so not surprisingly, by 1959, Gryska and colleagues reported the first repair of an AEF secondary to a Dacron graft that was originally implanted to repair an AAA [4]. The authors described redundancy in the main body of the prosthetic graft so they resected and primarily repaired the conduit, as well as simultaneously performing a lateral duodenorrhaphy but the patient ultimately died due to sepsis.

Incidence and Nomenclature The incidence of AEF is estimated to be 0.04–0.07% among patients who die from massive GI hemorrhage; however, this frequency is reported to be higher (e.g., 0.69–2.36%) among subjects with an AAA [5, 6]. In fact, the occurrence of an AEF after an open AAA repair has been estimated to be as high as 1–2% and usually occurs at a median time of 4–5 years postoperatively. It is worth noting that these historical estimates may be significantly overestimated since they are likely influenced by both ascertainment and referral bias that is common for this highly complex and rare entity, since the overall reported incidence of any aortic graft infection (AGI) within clinical trials is only 0.19–2.0% [7–9]. In the modern era, endovascular aortic stent repair (e.g., EVAR) is thought to have a lower long-term risk of secondary AEF compared to open aortic reconstructions (e.g., 0.02–0.46%) [10, 11]; however, the continued adoption of EVAR and its dominant position as the first-line therapy for the spectrum of aortic pathologies is likely to lead to a higher observed incidence in the future. Interestingly, mean time from index EVAR to presentation with secondary AEF has been reported to be around 32–36 months which is significantly shorter than time to presentation after open aortic operations.

Patients with secondary AEF are the most common subtype (comprising >80–90% of most cases in modern series) but it is worthwhile to further delineate anatomical differences that may exist with their presentations. Specifically, some patients present with graft-enteric erosion (GEE) without direct fistulization but others may have “true” AEF. The typical feature that distinguishes this difference is for subjects harboring GEE, there is an abnormal communication between the prosthetic graft and the mucosa of the GI tract; however, there is no direct involvement of the anastomosis between the graft and the aorta. In this scenario, bleeding is usually attributed to GI mucosal irritation and friability which is commonly less catastrophic when compared to a true secondary AEF. Although this distinction exists in the literature, the management principles governing either entity remain the same.

Presentation

Signs and Symptoms Patients with AEF may present with a variety of different complaints and symptoms which in many ways are influenced by the underlying type of fistula, associated microbiology, and host immunological response. An important teaching point is that any provider managing a GI bleed in a patient with prior aortic surgery should strongly consider the possibility of an underlying AEF until the work-up identifies an alternative diagnosis. In general, hematemesis, hematochezia, and melena are the most common presenting signs but abdominal pain (~50%) and shock (~33%) may also occur. For example, in a historical review of the literature surrounding management of AEF, 94% of patients presented with a history of a herald bleed, which is defined as a brisk GI bleeding episode that subsequently resolves by the time the patient is evaluated by a vascular surgeon [12]. These events can foreshadow massive GI hemorrhage by hours to months which provokes a significant amount of anxiety for patients and surgeons alike.

It has been our institutional experience that more subtle presentations of AEF are actually more common including unintentional weight loss, malaise, anemia, and/or abdominal pain. Additionally, some patients are assumed to only have an AGI but at the time of graft removal, the GI communication is identified. Due to the complexity of the problem and variable nature of the presentation, a high index of suspicion is always needed whenever an AGI is being evaluated since AEF can be present in up to 20–30% of cases [13]. Accordingly, these patients are probably best managed in centers that can offer the full spectrum of vascular, GI surgical, critical care, and ancillary consultation services that are frequently needed to treat this complex and highly morbid problem.

Pathophysiology and Demographics The underlying pathophysiology that drives development of a primary AEF is poorly understood. Either primary aortic infection or remote infection with secondary seeding of the aortic wall has been described that ultimately leads to aortic wall degeneration and fistulous communication with an adjacent enteric structure. Further, it is thought that aortic pulsatility plays a role since repetitive mechanical trauma from the native aortic wall and adjacent bowel (e.g., overlying duodenum) can theoretically occur. This anatomical relationship is somewhat supported by the observation that over 80% of patients who present with a primary AEF have an AAA. Among patients with primary AEF, the clinical phenotype tends to include older male patients usually in their 6th decade of life. A previous history of foreign body ingestion, penetrating aortic ulceration, remote infection (e.g., dental abscess, endocarditis), chronic infection (e.g., tuberculosis, syphilis), cancer, and radiation have all been reported as possible contributing factors.

Correspondingly, patients with secondary AEF are also more likely to be male; however, the age profile is somewhat older (e.g., seventh decade) than primary AEF subjects. These similarities and differences in patient demographics are related to the higher prevalence of AAA and peripheral arterial occlusive disease among men compared to women. Moreover, a patient would have to have undergone a previous aortic reconstruction that then requires a certain "dwell time" before re-presentation with the AEF. The current proposed pathophysiologic mechanism that leads to secondary AEF is from AGI that generates retro-peritoneal inflammation which, when combined with mechanical stress from aortic pulsatility, causes enteric erosion and/or fistula formation.

This concept has been supported by animal model studies involving *S. aureus* [14] and further underscores the critical need to avoid primary graft seeding with the index aortic operation through stringent adherence to aseptic surgical technique, routine use of prophylactic perioperative antibiotics and meticulous handling of retroperitoneal and peri-duodenal tissues both during peri-aortic dissection and when closing. It is for this reason that a commonly espoused principle of aortic surgery is to ensure that during closure of the retroperitoneum, the duodenum (or any enteric structure) should not remain in direct contact with the aortic graft and if needed, liberal use of omental pedicle flaps and/or non-autogenous biologic materials can be interposed between the new aortic graft and overlying bowel.

Microbiology It is common for AEF patients to receive variable exposure to parenteral antibiotics either at a referring hospital or the primary destination center that definitively manages the problem. Accordingly, the diagnostic yield of blood cultures reported in most series can be low (e.g., 30–40%), and some providers may assume that there is a non-infectious etiology responsible for the clinical presentation. In fact, only 50–60% of intra-operative cultures taken at the time of the AEF extirpation yield a positive Gram stain. Most commonly, positive operative cultures contain polymicrobial organisms (40–50%), including Gram-positive cocci (*Staphylococcus* and *Streptococcus* species [30–40%]), *Escherichia coli* (10–15%), *Klebsiella* (1–2%), Enterobacter (0.5–2%), and *Candida* species (1–2%) [15–17]. Due to the prevalence of these organisms, the authors generally empirically prescribe broad-spectrum IV antimicrobial therapy to cover gram-positive, gram-negative, anaerobic, and fungal organisms (e.g., Vancomycin, Cefepime, Metronidazole, Fluconazole) which is then refined postoperatively in coordination with the infectious disease consulting service.

Preoperative Preparation

General Principles and Diagnostic Evaluation Patients with AEF can present in a variety of different physiologic states which dramatically influences the expediency of the work-up and implementation of the operative plan. As previously described, some patients can have more occult signs and symptoms that may lead to delays in diagnosis which can be catastrophic. A high-resolution, thin-cut (e.g., 1 mm or less) computed tomographic arteriogram (CTA) is the most common imaging modality that is employed during the diagnostic evaluation (Fig. 23.1). The reported sensitivity and specificity of CTA to detect AEF are 94% and 84%, respectively [18]. It is rare to see the direct connection of a fistula between the aorta and the enteric structure with contrast extravasation on CTA but this finding would be considered pathognomonic for the diagnosis (Fig. 23.2). More frequently, there is effacement of the retroperitoneal fat plane that is normally interposed between the aorta and 3rd/4th portion of the duodenum (or other enteric structure). Additional CT findings are synonymous with AGI and may include peri-aorta/graft phlegmon, abscess, and/or ectopic air. This is especially relevant for patients with an infected EVAR since presence of air within the excluded AAA sac should raise suspicion for an enteric communication.

Many centers have reported on the use of various adjunctive imaging modalities including esophagogastroduodenoscopy (EGD), magnetic resonance imaging (MRI), PET-CT with fluorodeoxyglucose, catheter-based angiography, as well as nuclear medicine scanning (e.g., Gallium 67 or Indium 111-labelled WBC scan). Although these specific tests may be helpful in unique clinical scenarios, they generally have limited practical application in most patients with AEF (especially if they are unstable). For example, the ability for an EGD to reliably detect a secondary AEF is only about 25–50% and even worse for primary AEF [19, 20]. While it is common for patients with less dramatic GI bleeding presentations from an AEF to have undergone an EGD, it has been our center's experience that identification of the GEE or presence of clot/bleeding at the fistulous connection is infrequent. If an EGD is performed, the endoscopy team needs to be experienced and the patient should have appropriate intravenous access. A complete evaluation of the duodenum is needed including the 3rd and 4th portions since most (e.g., 60–70%) of AEFs are located in this region. If the fistula is not identified it certainly does not rule out a missed communication with the duodenum or localization of the fistula in another segment of the GI tract (e.g., jejunum [10–15%], ileum [15–18%], cecum [5–10%] [21]).

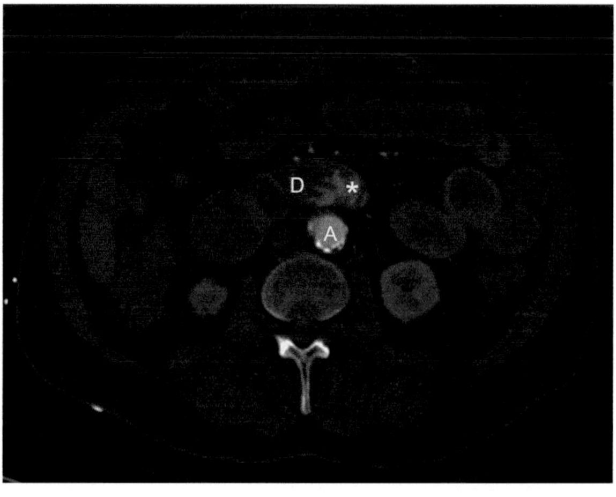

Fig. 23.1 CT arteriogram of a patient who presented with an acute GI bleed that demonstrated a blush of contrast (*) in the lumen of the duodenum consistent with AEF. *D* duodenum, *A* Aorta

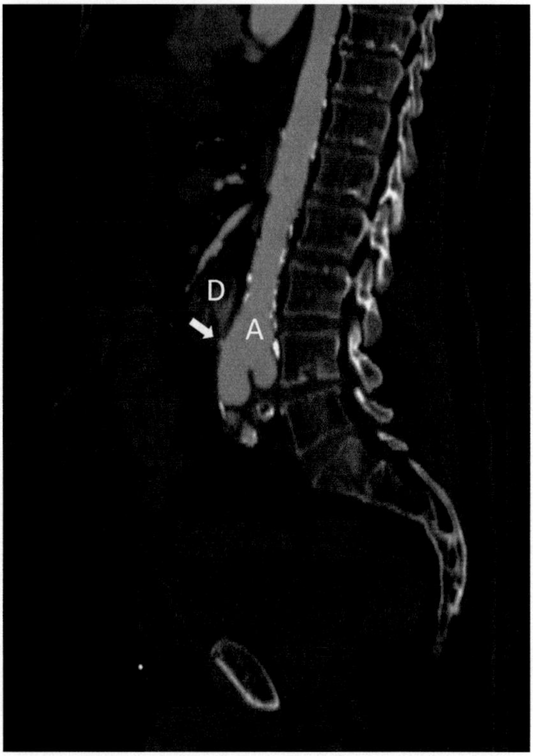

Fig. 23.2 CT arteriogram of a patient presenting with AEF showing a rare finding of the fistulous connection (arrow) between the aorta (A) and duodenum (D) on a sagittal view. *D* duodenum, *A* Aorta

Preoperative Planning and Preparation Patients presenting with suspected AEF require rapid and judicious resuscitation, early initiation of broad-spectrum parenteral antibiotics that cover gram-positive, gram-negative, and anaerobic bacteria, as well as fungal organisms (due to the frequency of foregut involvement). The authors strongly recommend preoperative monitoring of the patient in a critical care setting even when "stable"' given the proclivity for decompensation and hemodynamic instability. For stable patients, evaluation includes testing to identify pre-existing acute or chronic azotemia, cardiac dysfunction and pulmonary mechanics which commonly involves ascertainment of blood cultures (before exposure to antibiotics), arterial blood gas profiles, complete blood count with differential, coagulation parameters, comprehensive metabolic panel with liver function testing (including albumin and pre-albumin), femoral vein mapping (e.g., if considering neo-aortoiliac system, NAIS) and trans-thoracic echocardiography.

If an AEF patient presents with either hemorrhagic and/or septic shock, the management follows that of a ruptured mycotic aneurysm. The resuscitation strategy is usually one that prescribes a permissive hypotension philosophy (e.g., SBP 70–100 mmHg) since over-resuscitation can exacerbate bleeding. This is especially true in patients who have a herald bleed followed by an intervening period of relative clinical stability since aggressive isotonic crystalloid infusion can lead to dislodgement of the temporary clot that may have formed at the site of the AEF. In these scenarios, control of hemorrhage is paramount. Therefore, we have favored selective use of temporizing endovascular stent-graft exclusion to convert an unstable bleeding presentation into a more stable infected problem. Moreover, these types of maneuvers (e.g., transfemoral or trans-axillary aortic balloon control or temporizing aortic endograft cuff placement) can provide a bridge to the definitive therapy that is ultimately selected after the patient has had an interval period of resuscitation.

For more stable patients, the previously described clinical testing scheme can be undertaken which provides anatomic and physiologic information that informs perioperative decision-making. Importantly, during this phase of the expedited work-up, the value of a goals of care discussion among all the stakeholders cannot be overstated. Patients, healthcare surrogates, critical care, vascular, and general surgical team members should have a very transparent and blunt discussion about the significant morbidity, mortality, and protracted convalescence that usually is associated with AEF management. The sobering reality is that 30-day mortality rates of 30–50% are commonplace in the literature and complications occur in up to 70% of patients [17, 22]. Also, these results are probably optimistic since the publication bias that exists includes outcomes from higher-volume centers. Lastly, there are no functional or patient-reported outcome data after recovery from AEF surgery so discussions about anticipated quality of life for the patient are exceedingly difficult to predict and largely unknown.

Pitfalls and Danger Points

The complex nature of AEF is underscored by the myriad of potential pitfalls that can contribute to poor outcomes. Further, a number of danger points must be confronted and managed by the surgical team in order to obtain a successful repair. First, a classic pitfall is a false reassurance that the lack of contrast extravasation from the aorta into the bowel on CTA eliminates the possibility of an AEF. As previously mentioned, any GI bleed in a patient with previous aortic surgery history should be assumed to have an AEF until proven otherwise. Also, despite the preponderance of presentations that include a GI bleed history, many AEF do not have any enteric tract bleeding so this should not rule out the possibility of this highly lethal condition. Another common problem that befalls patients and their care teams alike are delays in definitive operative treatment due to over-ordering tests, especially advanced diagnostic imaging beyond the preoperative CTA. The sensitivity for a CTA to detect an AEF is high as already stated (sensitivity—94%, specificity—84%) so MRI and/or PET-CT (or even nuclear medicine scans) are not likely to add substantially to the diagnostic yield. An analog to this issue is the over-dependence on EGD to "rule out" an AEF. The poor sensitivity (~25–50%) should not reassure the surgical team so contingency plans still need to be generated for what will be done if an AEF is discovered intraoperatively.

Danger points that can be encountered may occur along the entire spectrum of care for the AEF patient and an exhaustive accounting exceeds the scope of this chapter. However, the authors would highlight hazards with the intraoperative management of these problems. More contemporaneously, we have taken a more flexible approach to our surgical management philosophy and selectively employed different staged vs. non-staged and ISR vs. extra-anatomic revascularization strategies. This management algorithm is similar to our experience with AGIs (Fig. 23.3) [13]. Indeed, use of this philosophy has led to improved mortality outcomes after surgical management of AEF at our center over the past 20 years [22].

Intraoperatively, when performing the peri-aortic and duodenal dissection, we routinely obtain both a suitable proximal aortic cross-clamp location (e.g., transperitoneal, supraceliac aortic access) and distal iliac artery control before attempting fistula resection. The rationale being that the infra- or para-renal aorta may have dense adhesions and inflammatory changes that make attempts at obtaining proximal control in this location dangerous. Some authors have expressed enthusiasm for endoluminal aortic balloon control but we have not employed this strategy in stable subjects. Similarly, the mobilization of the small bowel (e.g., duodenum) should be conducted in a deliberate manor trying to balance the risk of exacerbating the enteric defect while reducing operative time. A pitfall of the repair is not sufficiently mobilizing the Ligament or Treitz and elevating the transverse mesocolon to facilitate the subsequent aortic reconstruction and bowel repair. Aggressive extirpation of all offending prosthetic material with wide excisional debridement of native aortic and retroperitoneal tissues is necessary to reduce residual contamination that can compromise the repair.

Intraoperative consultation with the acute care surgery (ACS) team is crucial and for patients in physiologic duress, definitive management of the enteric defect can occur with second look operations after stapling the bowel if needed. Judgments about the type of duodenal repair are challenging and require good communication with the general surgeons. Smaller duodenal injuries can be repaired primarily but larger defects may require enteric exclusion and/or bypass. If aortic ligation is undertaken, a pitfall and danger are not resecting all compromised tissues back to healthy appearing aorta before double ligation with non-pledgeted 2–0 polypropylene suture. Independent of which strategy is ultimately employed for revascularization and restoration of bowel continuity, omental pedicle flaps have been shown to be associated with reduced recurrent fistula formation and/or anastomotic dehiscence in the perioperative period.

Operative Strategy and Technique

Fistula Resection and Peri-Aortic Debridement As outlined previously, our strategy has included application of multiple different operative approaches in the management of AEF. We contend that despite multiple descriptions in the published literature of various reconstruction techniques, there is a paucity of evidence

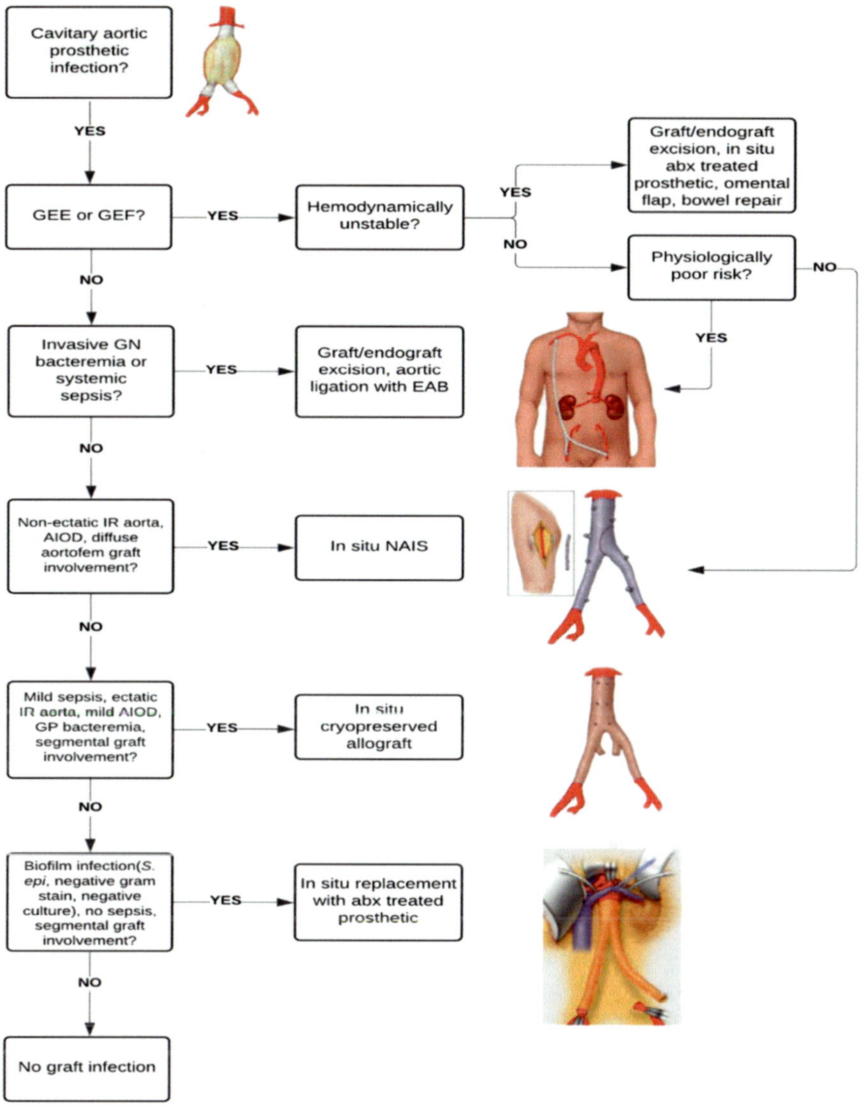

Fig. 23.3 A proposed decision algorithm for surgical management of aortic graft infection. *Abx* antibiotic, *AIOD* aortoiliac disease, *EAB* extra-anatomic bypass, *GEE* graft enteric erosion, *GEF* graft enteric fistula, *GN* gram-negative, *GP* gram-positive, *IR* infrarental, *NAIS* neo-aortoiliac system, *S. epi* Staphylococcus epidermidis. (Reprinted from Annals of Vascular Surgery, Vol 76, Oct 2021, Filiberto et al., Treatment and Outcomes of Aortic Graft Infections Using a Decision Algorithm, 2021, with permission from Elsevier)

describing comparative effectiveness of the different management strategies. For stable patients that are selected for staged extra-anatomic (e.g., bilateral axillo-femoral prosthetic bypass) bypass followed by subsequent midline laparotomy with extirpation of infected tissues/graft and repair of the enterotomy with aortic ligation, usually a period of 48–72 h is used between operations. This decision is predominantly impacted by judgments about adequacy of the patient's recovery from the initial procedure. Alternatively, some AGI patients are identified intraoperatively to have GEE and/or AEF. In these scenarios, if an ISR strategy were selected, conduit choice of antibiotic-impregnated Dacron graft vs. cryopreserved allograft vs. NAIS is impacted by availability, physiologic status of the patient, size of the proximal aorta, and degree of retroperitoneal contamination. More contemporarily, we have not used cryopreserved allograft for AEF due to several early failures including lethal arterial anastomotic dehiscence.

Once proximal and distal control are obtained, the removal of infected tissues and dissection of the tethered bowel off the aorta/aortic graft ensues. Some authors recommend removing a portion of native aortic wall (or graft) *en bloc* with the small bowel mobilization to reduce contamination (Fig. 23.4). It has generally been our approach to separate the bowel from the aorta/aortic graft and temporarily over-sew (or staple) the defect until definitive management occurs with the ACS service. Once the bowel is freed, the peri-aortic dissection is conducted and if healthy peri-renal aortic tissue is identified, the cross-clamp can be moved down to this position. If a primary AEF is present, usually there is a relatively small communication between the bowel and the aorta but debridement needs to persist until healthy appearing tissue is identified. In the scenario of a secondary AEF, removal of all prosthetic material is undertaken ensuring no residual elements remain in situ.

The safe removal of an infected EVAR merits additional description due to the additional complexity. Specifically, if the endograft has supra-renal fixation elements, removal can lead to further injury of attenuated aortic tissues that are friable and may compromise the ability to construct a new anastomosis or ligate safely. Significant judgment and some intraoperative techniques can be applied to try and safely compress and recapture the bare stent elements. The authors' approach has included use of umbilical tapes that are applied sequentially to constrain the endograft (similar to constraining an endograft during physician-modified EVAR) or to attempt placement of a modified 20 cc syringe cephalad along the axis of the graft and intussuscept the bare stent elements into the syringe. However, occasionally these elements may prove too difficult to remove and need to remain in the patient to avoid disruption of the proximal aorta. Management of the excluded AAA sac including wide excisional debridement and over-sewing of lumbar collaterals (which may be quite robust) should occur expeditiously.

Axillo-Bi-Femoral Bypass with Aortic Stump Ligation A conventional approach to AEF management is the use of single vs. multi-staged extra-anatomic reconstruction including bilateral axillo-femoral bypass, infected tissue/graft removal, enteric repair, and double-layer aortic stump ligation with omental pedicle flap placement. The advantage to this approach is that most vascular surgeons are familiar with all

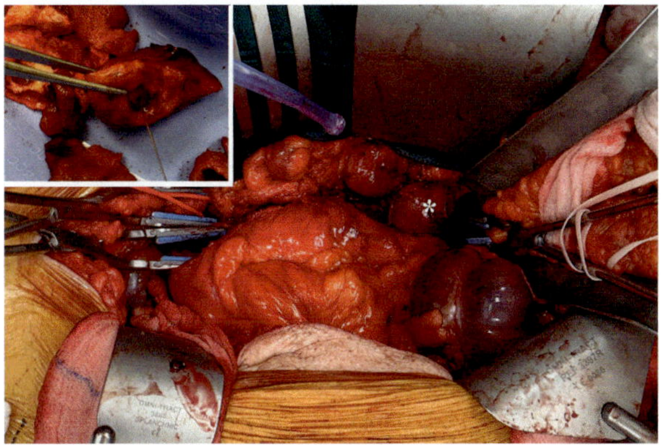

Fig. 23.4 Aorto-enteric fistula after prior aorto-bi-femoral bypass. Here a segment of adherent duodenum was excluded and left *in situ* at the site of the AEF (*) while the proximal aorta and distal aortic graft were dissected and exposed. The specimen was then removed *en bloc* with aortic wall and adjacent graft material (insert) where the fistulous connection was identified with a vessel dilator

the steps of the procedure and has been shown to be effective in the management of AEF. The optimal interval between staging is unknown; however, due to risks of competitive flow and interval graft thrombosis, some authors advocate ligation of the native femoral arteries proximal to the newly placed extra-anatomic bypass or alternatively, use of low-intensity heparin anticoagulation until the second stage procedure. Historical literature surrounding patency of axillo-bi-femoral bypass for AEF (or AGI) has been suboptimal (e.g., 60–80% @5-years) and reported to be associated with both high re-infection (e.g., 20–22%) and major limb amputation rates (10–20%). The most dreaded and catastrophic complication is an aortic stump dehiscence that can occur between 2 weeks and 3 months postoperatively in up to 30% of cases [23–25].

In-Situ Reconstruction Due to the sobering results of extra-anatomic reconstruction in the management of AEF, over the past 20 years, there has been renewed enthusiasm to advocate for a variety of various ISR techniques. Indeed, individual centers each espouse advantages of different conduit choices; however, the data remain confounded due to the publication bias, ascertainment bias, referral bias, and small sample sizes [26]. Interestingly, the studies comparing extra-anatomic to ISR of AEF demonstrated equipoise between approaches [19], unlike management of secondary AGI without enteric involvement [27] where in-situ bypass has been shown to be associated with superior infection-free survival [27]. Notwithstanding limitations of the current data in the field, taken together, the overriding perspective within the peer-reviewed literature is that ISR is preferred to extra-anatomic bypass with aortic stump ligation (Table 23.1). Interestingly, despite impassioned debate about conduit choice, no clear “best” option exists, so surgeon/institutional preference and availability generally inform operative strategy.

Table 23.1 Comparison of outcomes between extra-anatomic and in-situ reconstruction for aorto-enteric fistula repair

Procedure type	30-day mortality	Overall survival	Bypass patency	Amputation rate	Persistent/ recurrent infection
Bilateral axillo-femoral bypass + aortic stump ligation	15–45%	57–60% @5-years	60–80% @5-years	15–20% @5-years	5–20%
Rifampin-soaked Dacron graft + omental wrapping	10–15%	60% @5-years	80–90% @5-years	0–10% @5-years	5%
Silver-impregnated Dacron graft	22%	55% @1-year	60% @1-year	28% @1-year	22%
Cryopreserved aorto-iliac allograft	25–30%	66% @5-years	80–90% @5-years	5–10%	10–15%
Neo-aorto iliac surgery (NAIS)	25%	55% @60-days 20% @5-years	80% @5-years	10–15%	5%

In patients with AEF and hemodynamic instability, we favor an ISR using rifampin-soaked Dacron graft and use of an omental pedicle to wrap the reconstruction similar to the technique described by Oderich and colleagues [20]. Alternatively, in more stable patients who are judged to be good physiologic candidates with no evidence of infrainguinal occlusive disease and more limited infection (aortic tube graft or aorto-bi-iliac) with suitable proximal aortic diameters, NAIS procedures are selectively employed [13].

Postoperative Management

The postoperative management of AEF patients follows similar patterns to AGI patients and includes admission to a dedicated cardiovascular intensive care unit. Postoperative antibiotic choice and schedule are usually determined based upon microbiology data in coordination with infectious disease consultants. In our practice, patients usually receive a minimum of 6–8 weeks of culture-directed postoperative parenteral antibiotics individual providers at our institution ultimately had the 'final say' about whether or not patients were

placed on lifelong oral suppresion therapy after repair of AEF (e.g., ISR with prosthetic or non-autologous biologic grafts frequently receive indefinite antimicrobial prophylaxis). Transitions in care and patient disposition are usually determined by the vascular surgery team with direct feedback from the consulting intensive care and GI surgical teams. Similarly, re-introduction of enteral feeding has been in direct coordination with the ACS service and selective use of upper GI studies (depending on the type of GI surgical procedure performed to address the enteral defect associated with the AEF) has occurred to rule out evidence of leak before resuming oral intake. Follow-up includes surveillance CTA and ABIs, generally at some time between 1 and 3 months postoperatively and then annually, thereafter.

Complications

Similar to other large-magnitude extirpative procedures, the risk of complications is exceedingly high after surgical management of AEF. Morbidity events are catalogued in up to 70% of cases and include the entire spectrum of adverse events that may occur among complex aortic procedures. Unique to AEF procedures are the constellation of re-infection, sepsis, arterial anastomotic dehiscence, GI tract, limb amputation, and mortality events that can occur. Causes of death after AEF operations are most commonly linked to hemorrhagic shock (either at the index repair or postoperatively from the new arterial reconstruction such as aortic stump blow-out), sepsis or multi-organ failure, as well as major adverse cardiac events (e.g., myocardial infarction, ventricular arrhythmia) [28].

The impact of a GI tract complication on overall AEF outcomes deserves additional discussion. Larger institutional series have previously identified enteric complications to be associated with a two to threefold increased risk of morbidity and mortality [17]. Although this seems like a potentially modifiable risk factor, a significant amount of judgment is required by the attending ACS team member who must adhere to the principles of reapproximating well-vascularized, tension-free bowel edges after wide excisional debridement has occurred.

Outcomes

Aggregated outcomes of the different repair strategies, as well as the largest published institutional series featuring results after surgical management of AEF are depicted in Tables 23.1 and 23.2. The historical approach of using bilateral axillo-femoral bypass has been plagued by poor patency, high major amputation rates, and high reinfection rates. Mortality ranges between 15% and 45%, with the lower rates cited in the staged procedures. Aortic stump dehiscence can occur in up to 30% of patients at 3 months. Notably, aortic stump ligation requires two layers of 2-0 monofilament closure, which may not be feasible depending on the proximity of the fistula communication relative to the renal arteries. Patency ranges between 60% and 80% at 5 years, with reinfection rates as high as 20%.

Compared to extra-anatomic reconstruction, other ISR options such as NAIS and rifampin-soaked Dacron graft appear to have more favorable outcomes. However, the authors would caution interpretation of these data due to the limitations that exist with single-center retrospective experiences with small sample sizes. For example, Clagett and colleagues [29] were able to demonstrate a reduction in mortality from ~17% to 38% with alternative strategies down to 10% with the NAIS

Table 23.2 Complication incidence and 30-day mortality outcomes among contemporary series highlighting results after surgical management of aorto-enteric fistula

Series (year)	No.	Complication rate	30-day mortality
Bartley, A., (2021) [22]	57	70%	35%
Chopra, A., (2017) [17]	50	72%	24%
Delva, J. C., (2012) [31]	18	66%	22%
Oderich, G. S., (2011) [20]	54	52%	9%
Batt, M., (2011) [19]	37	59%	43%
Bíró, G., (2011) [32]	48	NA	45.8%
Valentine, R. J., (2008) [33]	38	61%	38%
Baril, D. T., (2006) [34]	16	50%	18.8%
Armstrong, P. A., (2005) [35]	29	NA	21%
Menawat, S. S., (1997) [36]	52	48%	27%
Kuestner, L. M., (1995) [37]	33	NA	18.2%

procedure. There was a 12–15% compartment syndrome rate related to the femoral vein procurement but overall amputation rates were 5%. Durability of the NAIS is well-described with 5-year primary patency exceeding 80% (secondary patency >90%). Similar to the NAIS procedure, different authors report on the utility of antibiotic impregnated prosthetic and cadaveric allograft conduits. We embrace most of these strategies and selectively apply them based on our decision algorithm [13].

Lastly, use of a temporizing endovascular implant (e.g., aortic cuff) to provide a bridge to the final destination therapy has been used, especially in hemodynamically unstable patients. Unfortunately, there are no large series highlighting the role of this therapy; however, a pooled analysis revealed that recurrent/persistent infection or hemorrhage occurs in >40% of patients at a median time of 13 months [30]. If EVAR with suppressive antibiotics is used as the definitive therapy, it is likely for compassionate reasons since the EVAR neither removes the infectious nidus nor does it correct the enteric defect.

References

1. Cooper A. The lectures of Sir Astley Cooper on the principles and practice of surgery. Haswell, Barrington, and Haswell; 1839.
2. Brock RC. Aortic homografting; a report of six successful cases. Guys Hosp Rep. 1953;102:204–28.
3. MacKenzie RJ, Buell AH, Pearson SC. Aneurysm of aortic homograft with rupture into the duodenum. AMA Arch Surg [Internet]. American Medical Association; 1958 [cited 2022 Oct 2];77:965–9. Available from: https://jamanetwork.com/journals/jamasurgery/fullarticle/557341

4. CASE records of the Massachusetts General Hospital. Case 45522. N Engl J Med. 1959;261:1339–42.
5. Skourtis G, Gerasimos P, Sotirios M, Fotios K, Georgios K, Sotirios G, et al. Primary aorto-enteric fistula due to septic aortitis. Ann Vasc Surg [Internet]. Elsevier Inc.; 2010 [cited 2022 Oct 2];24:825.e7–825.e11. Available from: http://www.annalsofvascularsurgery.com/article/S0890509610001019/fulltext
6. Duncan JR, Renwick AA, Mackenzie I, Gilmour DG. Primary aortoenteric fistula: pitfalls in the diagnosis of a rare condition. Ann Vasc Surg. Elsevier; 2002;16:242–5.
7. Hallett J, Marshall DM, Petterson TM, Gray DT, Bower TC, Cherry J, et al. Graft-related complications after abdominal aortic aneurysm repair: reassurance from a 36-year population-based experience. J Vasc Surg [Internet]. J Vasc Surg; 1997 [cited 2022 Oct 2];25:277–86. Available from: https://pubmed.ncbi.nlm.nih.gov/9052562/
8. Participants TUKSAT. Long-term outcomes of immediate repair compared with surveillance of small abdominal aortic aneurysms. https://doi.org/101056/NEJMoa013527 [Internet]. Massachusetts Medical Society; 2002 [cited 2022 Oct 2];346:1445–52. Available from: https://www.nejm.org/doi/10.1056/NEJMoa013527
9. Vogel TR, Symons R, Flum DR. The incidence and factors associated with graft infection after aortic aneurysm repair. J Vasc Surg [Internet]. J Vasc Surg; 2008 [cited 2022 Oct 2];47:264–9. Available from: https://pubmed.ncbi.nlm.nih.gov/18241747/
10. Kahlberg A, Rinaldi E, Piffaretti G, Speziale F, Trimarchi S, Bonardelli S, et al. Results from the multicenter study on aortoenteric fistulization after stent grafting of the abdominal aorta (MAEFISTO). J Vasc Surg [Internet]. J Vasc Surg; 2016 [cited 2022 Oct 2];64:313–320.e1. Available from: https://pubmed.ncbi.nlm.nih.gov/27289529/
11. Capoccia L, Speziale F, Menna D, Esposito A, Sirignano P, Rizzo AR, et al. Preliminary results from a national enquiry of infection in abdominal aortic endovascular repair (Registry of Infection in EVAR—R.I.EVAR). Ann Vasc Surg. Elsevier; 2016;30:198–204.
12. Reilly LM, Ehrenfeld WK, Goldstone J, Stoney RJ. Gastrointestinal tract involvement by prosthetic graft infection. The significance of gastrointestinal hemorrhage. Ann Surg [Internet]. Lippincott, Williams, and Wilkins; 1985 [cited 2022 Oct 2];202:342. Available from: https://pubmed.ncbi.nlm.nih.gov/3876083/
13. Filiberto AC, Scali ST, Patterson S, Neal D, Elder CT, Shah SK, et al. Treatment and outcomes of aortic graft infections using a decision algorithm. Ann Vasc Surg. 2021;76:254–68.
14. Busuttil RW, Rees W, Baker JD, Wilson SE. Pathogenesis of aortoduodenal fistula: experimental and clinical correlates. Surgery. 1979;85:1–13.
15. Dossa CD, Pipinos II, Shepard AD, Ernst CB. Primary aortoenteric fistula: part I. Ann Vasc Surg. Elsevier; 1994;8:113–20.
16. Kakkos SK, Bicknell CD, Tsolakis IA, Bergqvist D. Editor's choice management of secondary aorto-enteric and other abdominal arterio-enteric fistulas: a review and pooled data analysis. Eur J Vasc Endovasc Surg [Internet]. Eur J Vasc Endovasc Surg; 2016 [cited 2022 Oct 2];52:770–86. Available from: https://pubmed.ncbi.nlm.nih.gov/27838156/
17. Chopra A, Cieciura L, Modrall JG, Valentine RJ, Chung J. Twenty-year experience with aorto-enteric fistula repair: gastrointestinal complications predict mortality. J Am Coll Surg. Elsevier Inc.; 2017;225:9–18.
18. Low RN, Wall SD, Jeffrey RB, Sollitto RA, Reilly LM, Tierney LM. Aortoenteric fistula and perigraft infection: evaluation with CT. https://doi.org/101148/radiology17512315475 [Internet]. 1990 [cited 2022 Oct 2];175:157–62. Available from: https://pubs.rsna.org/doi/10.1148/radiology.175.1.2315475
19. Batt M, Jean-Baptiste E, O'Connor S, Saint-Lebes B, Feugier P, Patra P, et al. Early and late results of contemporary management of 37 secondary aortoenteric fistulae. Eur J Vasc Endovasc Surg [Internet]. Eur J Vasc Endovasc Surg; 2011 [cited 2022 Oct 2];41:748–57. Available from: https://pubmed.ncbi.nlm.nih.gov/21414817/
20. Oderich GS, Bower TC, Hofer J, Kalra M, Duncan AA, Wilson JW, et al. In situ rifampin-soaked grafts with omental coverage and antibiotic suppression are durable with low reinfection rates

in patients with aortic graft enteric erosion or fistula. J Vasc Surg [Internet]. J Vasc Surg; 2011 [cited 2022 Oct 2];53. Available from: https://pubmed.ncbi.nlm.nih.gov/21184932/
21. Pipinos II, Carr JA, Haithcock BE, Anagnostopoulos PV, Dossa CD, Reddy DJ. Secondary aortoenteric fistula. Ann Vasc Surg. 2000;14:688–96.
22. Bartley A, Scali ST, Patterson S, Rosenthal MD, Croft C, Arnaoutakis DJ, et al. Improved perioperative mortality after secondary aortoenteric fistula repair and lessons learned from a 20-year experience. J Vasc Surg [Internet]. J Vasc Surg; 2022 [cited 2022 Oct 2];75:287–295.e3. Available from: https://pubmed.ncbi.nlm.nih.gov/34303801/
23. Reilly LM, Stoney RJ, Goldstone J, Ehrenfeld WK. Improved management of aortic graft infection: the influence of operation sequence and staging. J Vasc Surg. 1987;5:421–31.
24. Seeger JM, Pretus HA, Welborn MB, Ozaki CK, Flynn TC, Huber TS. Long-term outcome after treatment of aortic graft infection with staged extra-anatomic bypass grafting and aortic graft removal. J Vasc Surg. 2000;32:451–9; discussion 460-1.
25. Yeager RA, Taylor LM, Moneta GL, Edwards JM, Nicoloff AD, McConnell DB, et al. Improved results with conventional management of infrarenal aortic infection. J Vasc Surg. 1999;30:76–83.
26. Chung J. Management of aortoenteric fistula. Adv Surg [Internet]. Academic Press Inc.; 2018 [cited 2022 Oct 2];52:155–77. Available from: http://www.advancessurgery.com/article/S0065341118300071/fulltext
27. Janko MR, Hubbard G, Back M, Shah SK, Pomozi E, Szeberin Z, et al. In-situ bypass is associated with superior infection-free survival compared with extra-anatomic bypass for the management of secondary aortic graft infections without enteric involvement. J Vasc Surg. Mosby; 2022;76:546–555.e3.
28. Bergqvist D, Björck M. Secondary arterioenteric fistulation—a systematic literature analysis. Eur J Vasc Endovasc Surg [Internet]. Eur J Vasc Endovasc Surg; 2009 [cited 2022 Oct 2];37:31–42. Available from: https://pubmed.ncbi.nlm.nih.gov/19004648/
29. Clagett GP, Bowers BL, Lopez-Viego MA, Rossi MB, Valentine RJ, Myers SI, et al. Creation of a neo-aortoiliac system from lower extremity deep and superficial veins. Ann Surg [Internet]. Lippincott, Williams, and Wilkins; 1993 [cited 2022 Oct 2];218:239. Available from: https://pubmed.ncbi.nlm.nih.gov/8373267/
30. Antoniou GA, Koutsias S, Antoniou SA, Georgiakakis A, Lazarides MK, Giannoukas AD. Outcome after endovascular stent graft repair of aortoenteric fistula: a systematic review. J Vasc Surg [Internet]. J Vasc Surg; 2009 [cited 2022 Oct 2];49:782–9. Available from: https://pubmed.ncbi.nlm.nih.gov/19028054/
31. Delva JC, Déglise S, Bérard X, Dubuisson V, Delva F, Stecken L, et al. In-situ revascularisation for secondary aorto-enteric fistulae: the success of silver-coated dacron is closely linked to a suitable bowel repair. Eur J Vasc Endovasc Surg. W.B. Saunders; 2012;44:417–24.
32. Bíró G, Szabó G, Fehérvári M, Münch Z, Szeberin Z, Acsády G, et al. Late outcome following open surgical management of secondary aortoenteric fistula. Langenbeck's Arch Surg. 2011;396:1221–9.
33. Valentine RJ, Timaran CH, Modrall GJ, Smith ST, Arko FR, Clagett GP. Secondary aortoenteric fistulas versus paraprosthetic erosions: is bleeding associated with a worse outcome? J Am Coll Surg. Elsevier; 2008;207:922–7.
34. Baril DT, Carroccio A, Ellozy SH, Palchik E, Sachdev U, Jacobs TS, et al. Evolving strategies for the treatment of aortoenteric fistulas. J Vasc Surg [Internet]. J Vasc Surg; 2006 [cited 2022 Oct 2];44:250–7. Available from: https://pubmed.ncbi.nlm.nih.gov/16890849/
35. Armstrong PA, Back MR, Wilson JS, Shames ML, Johnson BL, Bandyk DF. Improved outcomes in the recent management of secondary aortoenteric fistula. J Vasc Surg [Internet]. J Vasc Surg; 2005 [cited 2022 Oct 2];42:660–6. Available from: https://pubmed.ncbi.nlm.nih.gov/16242551/
36. Menawat SS, Gloviczki P, Serry RD, Cherry KJ, Bower TC, Hallett JW. Management of aortic graft-enteric fistulae. Eur J Vasc Endovasc Surg. 1997;14(Suppl A):74–81.

37. Kuestner LM, Reilly LM, Jicha DL, Ehrenfeld WK, Goldstone J, Stoney RJ. Secondary aortoenteric fistula: contemporary outcome with use of extraanatomic bypass and infected graft excision. J Vasc Surg [Internet]. J Vasc Surg; 1995 [cited 2022 Oct 2];21:184–96. Available from: https://pubmed.ncbi.nlm.nih.gov/7853593/

Chapter 24
Management of Abdominal Aortic Aneurysm in the Setting of Coexistent Renal and Splanchnic Disease

Fernando Motta, F. Ezequiel Parodi, and Mark A. Farber

Introduction

Aortic aneurysms are characterized by localized or diffuse enlargement of the aorta. The aorta is considered aneurysmal when the aortic diameter is 50% greater than the "normal" vessel diameter [1]. Aneurysms have a predilection for the abdominal component of the aorta, occurring 3.7 times more frequently in the infrarenal segment compared with the thoracic segment [2]. By definition, an infrarenal abdominal aortic aneurysm (AAA) is located in the distal portion of the abdominal aorta, inferior to the renal arteries. The segment of aorta between the renal arteries and an infrarenal aneurysm is commonly referred to as the "neck" of the aneurysm. The anatomic characteristics of this area are of critical importance when considering therapeutic strategies for both open and endoluminal interventions. Juxtarenal aneurysms encroach on the renal arteries but do not involve the renal artery ostia, whereas suprarenal AAAs involve one or more renal vessels but spare the superior mesenteric artery (SMA). Aneurysmal aortic degeneration in the region of the mesenteric vessels may occur as a localized process or may occur in conjunction with aneurysmal changes in other portions of the aorta. In these circumstances, the most familiar classification system described by Crawford allows stratification of thoraco-AAAs into Types I, II, III, IV, and V.

When aneurysmal aortic disease involves the visceral portion of the aorta, the complexity of potential therapeutic options increases exponentially. A treacherous

This chapter is an update of the first edition.

F. Motta · F. E. Parodi · M. A. Farber (✉)
Department of Surgery, Division of Vascular Surgery, University of North Carolina at Chapel Hill School of Medicine, Chapel Hill, NC, USA
e-mail: fernando_motta@med.unc.edu; ezequiel_parodi@med.unc.edu; mark_farber@med.unc.edu

G. J. Arnaoutakis et al. (eds.), *Aortic Aneurysms*, Contemporary Cardiology,
https://doi.org/10.1007/978-3-032-13134-8_24

combination of limited end-organ redundancy and variable collateral communication between visceral vessels increases the clinical imperative of appropriate assessment and management. Furthermore, the presence of divergent pathological processes, such as branch-vessel ostial stenosis occurring in proximity to aortic aneurysmal disease, can compound the complexity of management algorithms.

Prior to the endovascular era, optimal management of coexistent aortic aneurysmal disease and visceral pathology was somewhat controversial. While some centers advocated open endarterectomy for stenotic ostial lesions of the renal and visceral vessels at the time of aneurysm repair, others preferred reimplantation or bypass for similar lesions. The choice of intervention was often individualized and based somewhat upon surgeon preference.

With the advent and the widespread uptake and utilization of endovascular techniques, it is readily evident that many infrarenal and thoracic aortic aneurysms can be repaired using intraluminal stent-graft devices. Furthermore, the successful deployment of fenestrated or branched stent-graft have expanded the limits of endoluminal aneurysm repair.

The first challenge when dealing with the presence of an aortic aneurysm and coexisting branch-vessel stenosis is to accurately define the anatomic features of the aneurysmal process. This involves defining the size of the aneurysm, its location within the aorta, and proximity of the aneurysm to the renal or visceral vessels. Factors that influence candidacy for endovascular repair are specifically sought. Identification of appropriate "landing-zones" or "seal-zones" both proximal and distal to the aneurysm are fundamental considerations. Defining an appropriate proximal landing zone for an aortic stent-graft device is a somewhat complex undertaking. The process requires device-specific consideration of landing-zone diameter, length, angulation, and geometry. This process also requires identification of mural thrombus or calcification within the landing zone that may compromise integrity of the seal or fixation of the device. Further considerations include caliber and patency of access vessels in the iliofemoral segment. In situations of small-caliber iliofemoral vessels, the possible requirement for placement of an iliac conduit to facilitate insertion of the endoluminal device may need to be considered.

If the patient is considered a candidate for endovascular intervention, the next challenge is to accurately identify and define the functional significance of any proximate branch-vessel pathology. This process incorporates conceptual stratification of lesions into those that meet requirement for intervention and those that may be managed conservatively. All these patients should be evaluated carefully with preoperative duplex scanning of the visceral vessels and mandatory high-resolution cross-sectional imaging, preferably CT angiography with at least 2.0 mm cuts augmented with reconstructions. At our institution, we use CT angiography with sagittal and coronal cuts and augment this with three-dimensional reconstruction using the TeraRecon software package. This has allowed us to detail the exact relationships between the AAA and the visceral vessels. Only with this information at hand can a clear plan be formulated. The final conceptual challenge involves determination of whether the branch-vessel stenosis is best treated in a synchronous, metachronous, or independent manner to the aneurysmal process. In some situations,

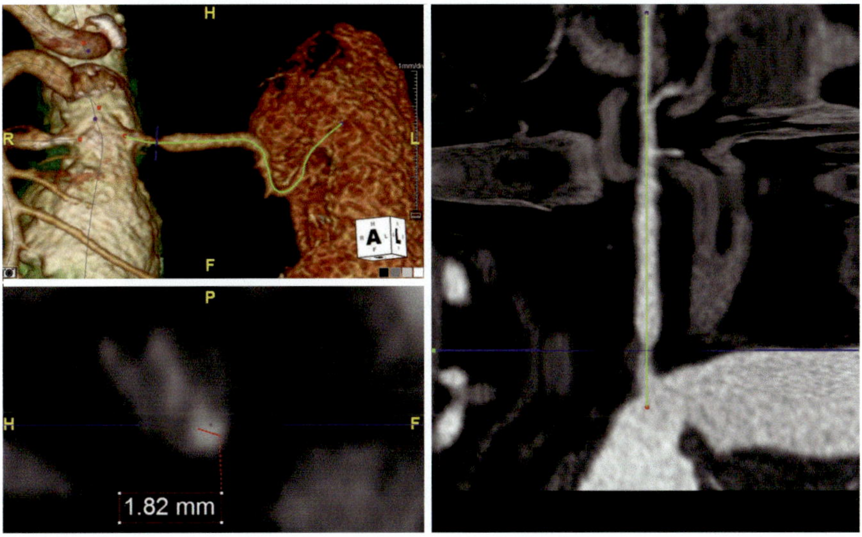

Fig. 24.1 A patient with TAAA and bilateral renal artery stenosis who underwent a F-BEVAR

there will be an absolute requirement for simultaneous intervention on the branch-vessel stenosis, whereas in other situations, a staged approach may be preferable. In a setting of fenestrated-branched endovascular aneurysm repair (F-BEVAR), 3D reconstruction and evaluation of each vessel with centerline of flow allows to identify and diagnosis the degree of stenosis (Fig. 24.1).

Optimal management of aortic aneurysm and coexisting arterial branch-vessel occlusive disease is predicated on a thorough knowledge of the anatomy, pathophysiology, clinical picture, natural history, and therapeutic options that are available for each of the underlying disease processes. A logical platform from which to commence evaluating these processes is to review the current understanding of stenotic lesions affecting the renal arteries, SMA, and the celiac artery.

Renal Artery Stenosis and Aneurysms

History

Richard Bright of Guy's Hospital, London, called attention to the association between hypertension and renal disease in 1836. It was not until 1934 that Goldblatt's dog experiment demonstrated that constriction of a renal artery resulted in systemic hypertension and renal parenchymal atrophy [3]. These findings prompted further investigation and stimulated successful performance of nephrectomy for uncontrolled hypertension. It was not until 1954 that Freeman et al. performed aortorenal endarterectomy on a patient resulting in successful resolution of refractory hypertension [4]. Presently, renal artery stenosis (RAS) may be treated via endovascular or open surgical techniques.

Prevalence

RAS refers to narrowing of the renal artery. Variant pathological processes ranging from fibromuscular dysplasia to atherosclerosis may result in narrowing of the renal arteries, thereby providing partial explanation for the predilection of RAS to occur at the extremes of age [5]. Regardless of the underlying etiology, activation of the renin—angiotensin system results in systemic hypertension. Hypertension has an estimated prevalence of 40–50 million in the United States and RAS is thought to be the underlying stimulus in 5–10% of these patients [6].

It is generally accepted that atherosclerosis is a systemic disease. Patients who have atherosclerotic disease of their coronary arteries have a high incidence of atherosclerotic disease in remote arterial beds. In one study, 47% of hypertensive patients referred for coronary angiography for suspected ischemic heart disease had some degree of atherosclerotic renovascular disease when screened with abdominal aortography at the time of cardiac catheterization [7]. This population demonstrated greater than 50% unilateral RAS in 19.2% of patients, high-grade stenosis (>70%) was identified in 7%, and bilateral RAS in 3.7%.

The prevalence of renovascular disease is even greater in patients with aortoiliac disease. In one retrospective review, some degree of RAS was detected in 96 of 201 patients (48%) who underwent abdominal aortography for aortoiliac disease. In this study, 26% of the patients had a greater than 50% RAS, and 22% had greater than 70% stenosis. In this cohort, 40 patients (20%) had bilateral stenoses, including four with greater than 70% stenosis bilaterally [8]. Hansen et al. found a 50% incidence of RAS in patients older than 60 years of age and with diastolic blood pressure higher than 110 mmHg [9]. When severe hypertension and elevated serum creatinine exist in the elderly, approximately 70% of patients were found to have RAS, with half of these cases involving bilateral renal arteries.

There is also an established association between renovascular disease and infrarenal aortic aneurysms. Cher et al. [10] looked at the incidence of RAS in their surgically revascularized population and found 26% of their patients had a concomitant AAA. In a retrospective review of cases, Olin et al. [11] showed that RAS greater than 50% was present in nearly 40% of patients with AAA. They also found that bilateral RAS was present in approximately 13% of patients with AAA and totally occluded renal arteries occurred in 5% of the patients in this population. Valentine et al. [12] also found a 22% incidence of significant RAS (>50%) in a retrospective review of AAA patients. Interestingly, they also discovered a high correlation between the presence of RAS and mesenteric artery stenosis (MAS). Brewster et al. [13] in 1975 looked at the utility of angiography for planning of AAA repair and they noted a 20% incidence of RAS and 9% incidence of celiac or SMA stenosis.

The relatively high incidence of concomitant RAS and AAA (20–40%) mandates a clear understanding of management options, technical pitfalls, and a candid review of how each strategy affects clinical outcome measures.

Intervention on Renovascular Disease

Interventional management of renovascular occlusive disease remains a controversial topic. Initial data were derived from observational studies. Hunt and Strong evaluated the progression of chronic kidney disease in patients who received medical or drug therapy and compared them with those receiving operative treatment for renovascular hypertension (RVH). Outcomes were followed for 14 years [14]. The results identified a significant difference in survival rates, with 84% survival noted in the patient group receiving operative therapy while 66% survived medical treatment (100 patients operative, 114 medical). They also showed that 93% of the patients in the operative group were cured or had improvement and 21% of the patients in the medical therapy group required crossover to surgical intervention for treatment of their RVH.

Dean et al. reported on 41 patients treated nonoperatively for RVH over a mean follow-up of 28 months. They found 19 patients had a decline in their serum creatinine clearance by 25–50%, glomerular filtration rates decreased 25–50% in 12 patients, a 10% reduction in renal parenchymal length occurred in 14 patients, progression to renal artery occlusion occurred in 4 patients, and a total of 17 patients had worsening of renal function that led to operation. Dean et al. also showed that in patients with hypertension, RAS progressed in the ipsilateral renal artery in 44% of the time, with a 12% rate of progression to renal artery occlusion. Of these occlusions, 3% had loss of revascularization options [15].

Wollenweber et al. [16] and Schreiber et al. [17] have also shown a similar deteriorating relationship of RAS and renal function. They report an ipsilateral progression of RAS in 44% of patients with 16% progressing to occlusion. Renal artery revascularization has been demonstrated to result in significant improvement in renal function and hypertension control, especially when revascularization is performed after rapid decline in renal excretory function.

Hallett et al. make a distinction between prophylactic (no presence of hypertension or renal insufficiency) and empirical RAS repair (presence of hypertension or renal insufficiency) [18]. They conclude that only 5% of patients with known RAS, and without hypertension, would benefit from prophylactic renal artery revascularization. They recently reported from the Cardiovascular Health Study cohort that only 4% of diseased renal arteries progressed to significant stenosis and concluded that progression of RAS is rare.

In order to provide a guide for planning endovascular therapies, endovascular treatment of RAS will have to be evaluated. Primary percutaneous angioplasty (PTA) has not been shown to be a durable therapy. Many reports have indicated that PTA enjoys only a 24–25% success rate and restenosis occurs in 15–42% [19].

Leertouwer et al. [20] have published a meta-analysis of renal artery stenting versus angioplasty. They accumulated data from 14 articles resulting in 678 patients receiving renal artery stents and 10 articles resulting in 644 patients published before 1998. They showed that renal stenting was technically successful in 98% of cases with an overall hypertension cure rate of 20% and clinical improvement in 49% of patients. In terms of renal function, they found a serum creatinine and glomerular filtration rate improvement in 30% of patients and stabilized function in 38% of the patients. They concluded based on statistical significance that the stent group had a higher technical success rate (98% vs 77%) and lower restenosis rate (17% vs 26%) than PTA.

Although the superior technical success rate and lower re-stenosis of renal artery stenting versus PTA, there is a lack of evidence based from clinical trials supporting widespread intervention over medical treatment for renovascular hypertension or ischemic nephropathy. To date, there are two clinical trials conducted in Europe and one in the United States that compared the medical treatment and stenting of renal arteries for RVH and ischemic nephropathy [21–23]. It is important to mention that none of the studies have specifically address RAS and its impact in patients undergoing aortic aneurysm repair.

Management Options for Aortic Aneurysm with Associated RAS

Open Surgical Options for Management of Aortic Aneurysm and Associated RAS

The approach to open surgical repair of an aortic aneurysm is influenced by several factors, including the anatomic location of the aneurysm, presence or absence of a hostile peritoneal cavity, and the requirement for exposure of the renal or visceral vessels. Common surgical approaches include midline celiotomy, retroperitoneal incision, and thoracoabdominal incision.

Infrarenal AAAs are typically repaired with prosthetic material such as Dacron, utilizing a tubular conduit or a bifurcated graft based upon the distal extent of the aneurysmal process. If significant RAS is present in the setting of an infrarenal AAA, and concomitant open surgical intervention is felt to be indicated, options can be broadly divided into aortorenal endarterectomy, renal artery bypass, and renal artery reimplantation.

Open aortorenal endarterectomy directly removes atherosclerotic plaque from the aorta and the ostia of the renal artery but requires suprarenal application of an aortic cross-clamp. An important concept to remember is that aorto-renal endarterectomy should only be contemplated in a nonaneurysmal portion of the aorta. This concept significantly influences open surgical options in the management of suprarenal AAA.

Different techniques have been described for performing renal artery endarterectomy. Stoney et al. [24] described the transaortic technique in 1989. They performed aortic replacement surgery with renal artery endarterectomy in 44 patients with aortic disease and concomitant RAS in symptomatic [35] and asymptomatic [9] patients. To effectively treat the combined aortic and renal disease in these patients, a supraceliac aortic cross-clamp was necessary in three patients, supramesenteric clamp was applied in 20 patients, and a suprarenal clamp was applied in 21 patients. They reported a mean renal ischemic time of 30 min (range 17–81 min). Follow-up of 33 patients demonstrated that 79% had improved or stable renal function and 69% with preoperative hypertension had improved blood pressure control. Stoney et al. claim adequate visualization of the distal intimal flap and stand behind this technique for patients with combined aortic disease and RAS. However, most would agree that the major contraindication to the use of this technique is aneurysmal degeneration of the perirenal aorta or extensive distal renal artery atherosclerosis past the ostia. Hansen et al. [25] advocate a transaortic longitudinal aortotomy and endarterectomy when both renal arteries are diseased. They recommend a transrenal approach for unilateral disease or when the renal arteries potentially need ostial expansion with the use of a patch. Mainly, the techniques are surgeon-dependent.

Renal artery bypass is an alternative option which includes constructing a bypass that circumvents the stenotic renal artery lesion. This procedure has been successfully performed utilizing a variety of inflow sources (e.g., aortorenal, splenorenal, hepatorenal, ileorenal) and a variety of conduits ranging from autogenous material (vein) to prosthetic material (Daron, PTFE). Another frequently utilized technique involves mobilization of the renal artery and reimplantation onto the aorta or aortic graft.

Cherr et al. [10] retrospectively studied 500 patients who underwent both unilateral and bilateral surgical procedures. Techniques used for renal artery revascularization included aortorenal bypass graft (384, Vein 204, PTFE 159, Dacron 21), splanchnorenal bypass graft [13], reimplantation (56), and endarterectomy (267). Of note, 200 patients (41%) had renal revascularization combined with aortic or mesenteric reconstruction. Seventy-six patients underwent combined repair of clinically significant aortic occlusive disease, and 57 patients underwent concomitant repair of AAA. The authors stressed the increased complexity of the combined procedure indicating that renal artery revascularization in conjunction with aortic reconstruction resulted in all but one of their 23 perioperative deaths. Mortality rates after isolated renal artery repair (0.8%) differed significantly from the rates for combined aortic and bilateral repair (6.9%). Therefore, Cherr et al. conclude that caution should be used when considering concomitant renal artery and aortic aneurysm repair.

Juxtarenal AAA by definition encroaches upon at least one of the renal arteries. When open repair is undertaken, positioning of the proximal cross-clamp tends to be guided by individual patient anatomy. In situations where the renal arteries originate from the aorta at different levels, the proximal clamp can occasionally be applied at an oblique orientation preserving perfusion to the more cephalad renal artery at the time of clamp application. In many regards, the therapeutic options and considerations for open renal revascularization for RAS associated with juxtarenal AAA overlap the therapeutic considerations of RAS and infrarenal AAA.

If an AAA has a proximal extension that involves the bilateral renal arteries then the aneurysm may be classified as a suprarenal AAA. Although conceptually simplistic, it is technically challenging to repair a suprarenal AAA from a transabdominal approach. The principal challenge in this circumstance arises from obtaining safe suprarenal control in the retroperitoneum without injuring the pancreas or compromising arterial flow to the SMA. A left retroperitoneal approach provides appropriate exposure and control of the proximal aorta; however, repair of the right renal artery becomes somewhat challenging. These factors raise the specter of performing initial revascularization of the right renal artery (e.g., right hepatorenal bypass), followed by retroperitoneal or thoracoabdominal approach to repair the aneurysm and revascularize the left renal artery (Fig. 24.2).

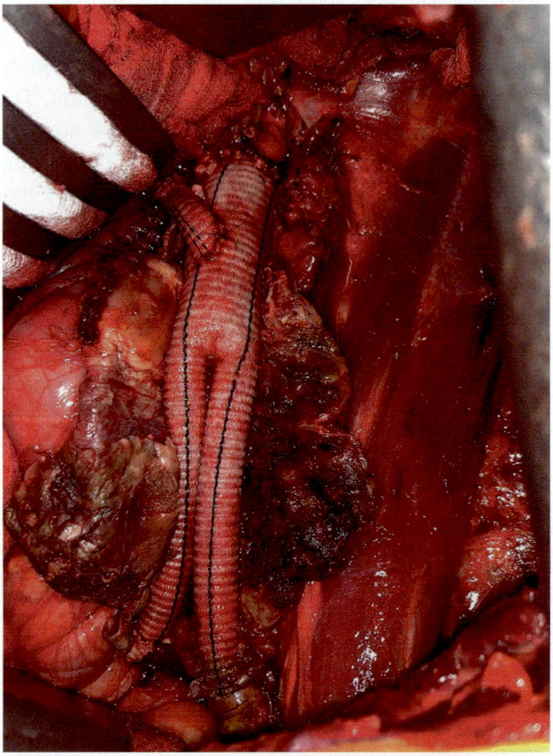

Fig. 24.2 Open suprarenal AAA repair through a retroperitoneal approach in which left renal artery was revascularized with a sidegraft bypass

Endovascular Options for Management of Aortic Aneurysm and Associated RAS

The first endovascular aneurysm repair (EVAR) was performed by Parodi in 1991. This procedure utilized a handmade device consisting of a balloon expandable Palmaz stent surrounded by (and sutured to) Dacron [26] Since that time, significant advancements have been made in device design and the FDA has approved several devices for endovascular repair of infrarenal AAAs. Each device has its own unique "pros and cons." For patients with AAA and concomitant splanchnic artery disease, thoughtful consideration of device selection is required because proximally located suprarenal fixation stents may theoretically complicate or compromise options for endovascular intervention.

When evaluating a patient who meets criteria for EVAR, a couple of key concepts need to be addressed. First, the location of the aneurysm in relation to the renal arteries is critical (infrarenal, juxtarenal, and suprarenal). For all FDA-approved devices, at least a 10 mm neck is required for adequate proximal fixation depending on what device is used.

If this criterion is not met, then the planning for repair of coexistent RAS becomes more complex and involves either planning for a hybrid approach or a branched or fenestrated stent-graft approach. In addition, severe neck angulations (>60°), reverse tapering, and presence of intramural thrombus in the neck provide for challenging proximal seal zones. Although FDA has approved the Medtronic Endurant device with Endoanchors for short neck AAA (4 mm length), some surgeons would favor to incorporate the renal arteries using fenestrated device for short neck aneurysms. In 2012, the FDA approved the Cook Zenith Fenestrated device for juxta-renal AAA and this device remains the only commercially available in the United States [27]. Although long-term results have been published with excellent results [28], the trial designs excluded patients with pre-existing renal artery stenosis.

Once the anatomical considerations have been worked out, timing of renal artery stenting is of the next importance. Three scenarios can be categorized: (1) RAS before EVAR, (2) RAS during EVAR, and (3) RAS after EVAR.

Renal artery stent deployment followed by staged performance of EVAR can be a consideration in patients with significant renal insufficiency who need maximal protection from contrast nephropathy by staging the contrast loads. With this theory, patients who are at high risk for postoperative contrast nephropathy could potentially benefit from improved blood flow to the renal parenchyma. In patients with renovascular disease-induced nephropathy, further benefit may be achieved secondary to reduction of antihypertensive medicines resulting in improved renal artery perfusion, and more stable blood pressure control. The major concern involves the placement of the EVAR device after renal stent placement. An appropriately placed renal stent protrudes 2–3 mm into the aorta, and can be displaced or kinked during the placement of the aortic stent-graft. To avoid this complication, during the EVAR, the left renal artery and stent can be cannulated before inserting the main EVAR component. Then, a balloon is inflated and the main body is inserted with the renal artery stent protected. Effort should be made using endografts with infra-renal fixation, therefore minimizing the renal stents to be compressed by the bare metal stent present in devices with supra-renal fixation. Both the Zenith and Endurant devices involve manipulation above the renal arteries. Both have high risk of renal stent displacement or kinking if the stent is placed prior to EVAR. To avoid this potential hazard, the authors prefer to angioplasty an RAS rather than stent placement. After repair of the AAA, a stent can be placed in the renal artery if or when restenosis occurs.

EVAR followed by staged placement of renal artery stent would likely be the sequence of choice in patients who have mild clinical indicators for treatment such as marginally controlled RVH or slowly declining renal function. In this scenario, the surgeon delays the repair of significant RAS to repair a clinically significant AAA. Multiple factors may influence this decision-making process. Complex aneurysm anatomy will increase operative time and increase contrast load, especially when coupled with renal stenting. The choice of EVAR device has not been found to inhibit future cannulation and stenting of a diseased renal artery. Whenever possible, the authors prefer to stage the procedure in this order.

Simultaneous renal artery stent deployment at time of EVAR would likely be the planning of choice in a patient with an uncomplicated infrarenal AAA who also has clinically significant RAS. While these procedures are performed in the same setting, the authors place the EVAR device prior to placing the renal artery stent to avoid the unwanted renal stent complications discussed above. In renal vessels with severe disease, brachial artery access with placement of a 0.014″ wire into the affected vessel prior to EVAR device deployment will potentially simplify the renal stent placement after EVAR (Figs. 24.3 and 24.4). Although initial experience with bare metal stents in treating RAS, currently the authors have moved to use covered stents instead (iCAST or VBX).

In the current era of complex aortic aneurysm being treated with fenestrated-branched endografts, excellent outcomes have been published, not only demonstrating low mortality and morbidity at the perioperative period, but also excellent long-term branched patency [29–33]. However, incorporating visceral vessels with pre-existing stenosis makes the repair more challenging and with potential

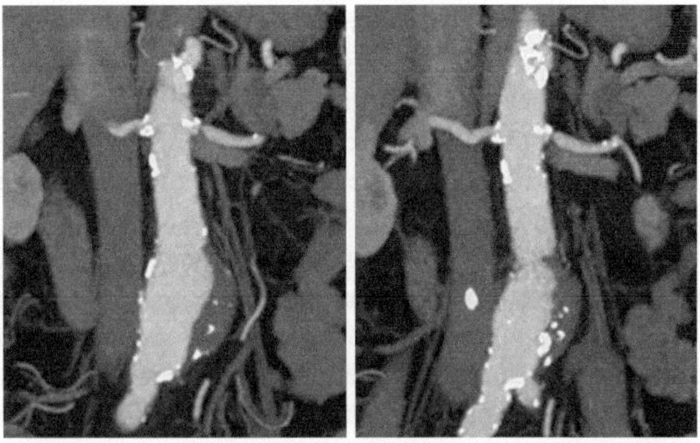

Fig. 24.3 Preoperative computed tomography angiogram (*CTA*) of a 76-year-old male with symptomatic abdominal aortic aneurysm (*AAA*) and severe left renal artery stenosis (*RAS*) and renal insufficiency

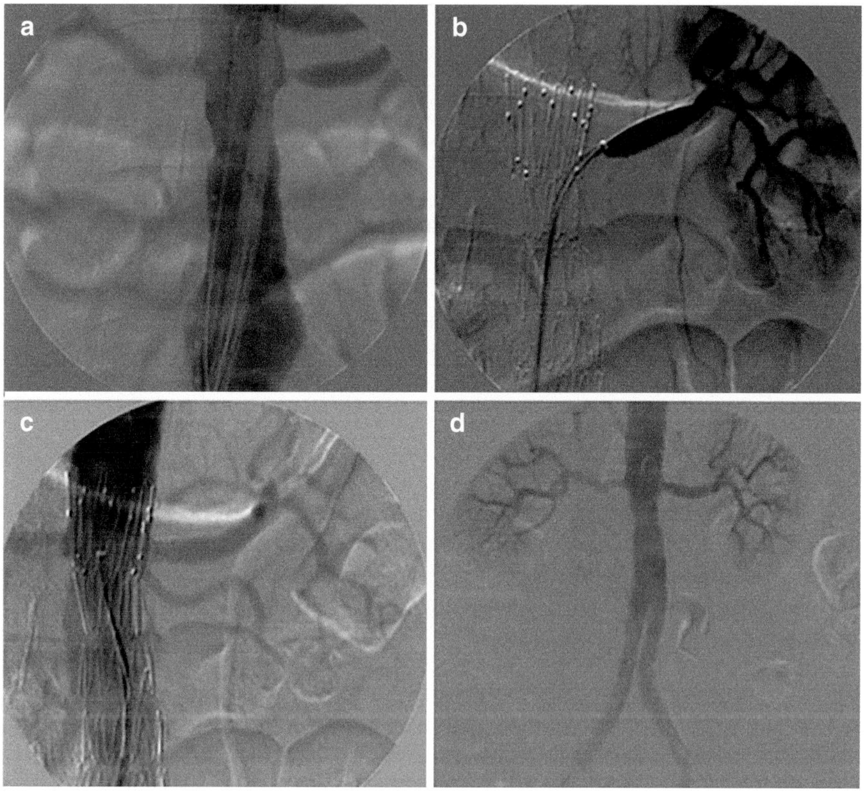

Fig. 24.4 (**a**) Intraoperative aortogram showing the severe left renal artery (*RA*) stenosis from the patient above. (**b**) Cook Zenith endovascular repair with suprarenal fixation allowing access to the left RA with a 6 French sheath and 014 Spartacore wire. (**c**) Balloon expandable Herculink 7-mm stent deployed with complete resolution of stenosis. (**d**) Completion aortogram after Cook Zenith abdominal aortic aneurysm (*AAA*) repair with iliac extensions and left RA stent

increasing risks when manipulating these vessels. Adjunctive designs help to overcome with the challenges of cannulation of visceral vessels during complex aneurysm repair. Oderich described the benefits of using preloaded wires during aortic repair with physician-modified endografts (PMEG) [34]. This concept expanded and is currently used more often during complex AAA treated with manufactured custom modified grafts (CMD). Timaran et al. also published the advantage of preloaded wires and catheters to facilitate catheterization of visceral branches [35]. Data from six PS-IDE trial centers were analyzed. A total of 2157 arteries were incorporated in 564 patients (preloaded systems were used in 387 (68.6%) patients). The overall technical success was 98.8% (preloaded and standard grafts) (99.5% vs. 97.2%; p = .022, respectively). The 30-day mortality rate was 1.9%, and low for both preloaded grafts and standard grafts (0.8% vs. 4.5%; p = .003).

Combination Approaches for Management of Aortic Aneurysm and Associated RAS

Hybrid approach: Renal BPG followed by EVAR repair is generally applied in patients who are poor candidates for traditional open juxtarenal AAA repair secondary to the likely complications from aortic cross-clamping in the supra-renal aorta. These patients are generally elderly and have increased baseline creatinine making them especially high risk for open AAA repair. Multiple extra-anatomical approaches can be applied to this patient population. Restoration of perfusion to the renal arteries using hepatorenal, splenorenal, or ileorenal conduits negates the need for manipulation and cross-clamping of a badly diseased aorta and offers the advantage of extending the proximal landing zone for a stent-graft device (Fig. 24.5). The results from these conduits have generally been exceptionally good. An analysis of 222 patients treated more than 10 years earlier indicates that these procedures were performed with low mortality (2.2%) and low rates of restenosis (7.3%) and good long-term survival. The predictors of late mortality were age above 60 years, coronary disease, and previous vascular surgery [36, 37]. Also, for patients undergoing F-BEVAR for complex aortic repair, renal bypass can be used to rescue these vessels from an occlusion when minimally invasive techniques are not successful (Fig. 24.6).

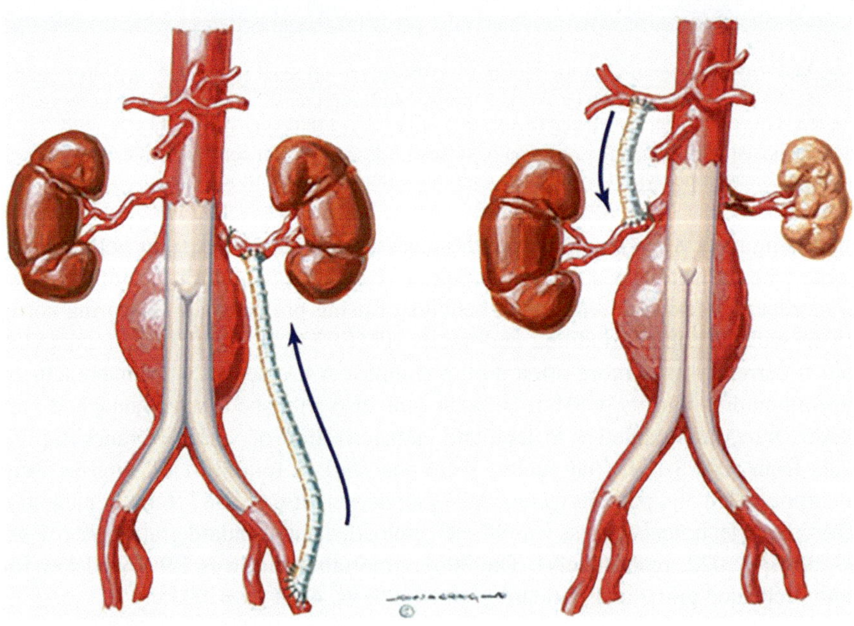

Fig. 24.5 Examples of iliorenal and hepatorenal bypass graft

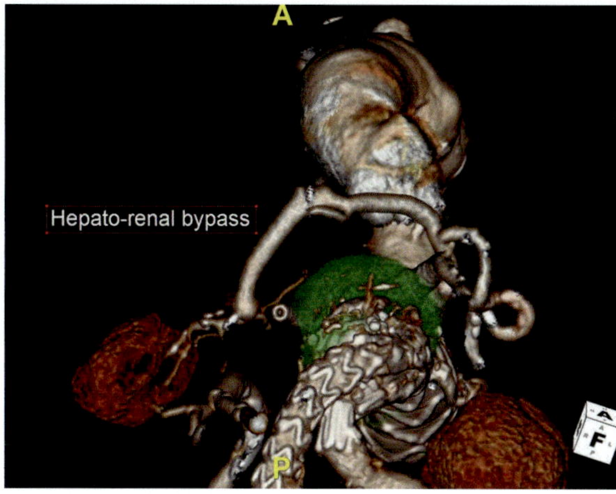

Fig. 24.6 Example of a patient with a right renal artery branch occlusion after F-BEVAR. The patient underwent hepato-renal bypass, with improvement of renal function

MAS and Aortic Aneurysms

Prevalence

The prevalence of MAS has not been as frequently reported in association with AAA. Likely, there is a similar association to aortic aneurysms as there is between RAS and AAA. Valentine et al. [12] retrospectively evaluated the incidence of MAS in patients with AAA. They found in their series that 55% of patients with AAA had celiac artery stenosis. Twenty-two percent had mild stenosis (0–49%), 29% had moderate or severe stenosis, and 4% were occluded. In this same group, the SMA was mildly occluded in 7% and only 4% had moderate stenosis. Four percent were found to have an occluded SMA. All of the patients with occluded or moderate SMA stenosis had moderate or greater celiac artery stenosis. They also pointed out that there was a significant correlation with hypertension and MAS.

As discussed earlier, Valentine et al. evaluated RAS rates in the AAA population and found that 22% of those patients had more than 50% stenosis. It was also reported that 50% of the severe RAS patients had concomitant celiac artery stenosis, suggesting that MAS is more prevalent in patients with known RAS [12, 15].

It is important to understand the time course of clinically relevant disease progression of MAS in the patient with aortic aneurysmal disease. AAAs frequently have intramural thrombus that can adversely affect the mesenteric blood supply by occluding the inferior mesenteric artery. Thomas et al. [38] reported the progression of asymptomatic mesenteric stenosis on approximately 1000 patients over a 6-year course. Eighty-two of these patients had SMA stenosis and 60 of these patients had significant stenosis (>50% diameter reducing). Fifteen of these patients had three-vessel disease. Four (27%) patients of the 15 developed acute mesenteric ischemia during follow-up and 1 (7%) died. Each of these four patients had significant (>50%) stenosis or occlusion of the celiac artery, SMA, and inferior mesenteric artery. Four additional patients of the 15 died from coronary disease. Therefore, 8 of 15 patients with three-vessel disease died or developed MI in a 2.6-year follow-up. They concluded that patients with significant three-vessel mesenteric arterial stenosis should be considered for prophylactic mesenteric arterial reconstruction.

For the general vascular patient with or without aortic disease, an occluded IMA is well tolerated and rarely if ever causes clinical manifestations of ischemia. This is not true for celiac or SMA stenosis or occlusion. For these patients, the risk of ischemia is high. Thomas et al. [38] showed that nearly 40% of patients with more than 50% mesenteric stenosis on abdominal angiogram died in 3 years and of the patients with three-vessel disease, about 30% developed symptomatic ischemia.

Intervention on Mesenteric Artery Disease

One fundamental question in mesenteric revascularization is the number of vessels to revascularize. In reports from the Mayo Clinic, it was first suggested that complete revascularization resulted in decreased symptomatic recurrence [39] and later that graft patency and survival in patients with three-vessel revascularization were improved compared with single-vessel revascularization [40]. Proponents of both celiac and SMA revascularization maintain that it may result in decreased symptomatic recurrence even if reocclusion of one of the grafts occurs [39, 40].

However, Foley et al. [41] demonstrated comparable durability with primary assisted 9-year patency rate of 79% in a series of 49 patients undergoing SMA reconstruction alone, and they concluded that multiple bypass grafts to other splanchnic vessels are unnecessary when adequate SMA reconstruction has been accomplished.

Farber et al. [42] provided a report on 18 patients with chronic mesenteric ischemia of which all had weight loss and chronic abdominal pain. Two of these patients had acute on chronic exacerbation of symptoms requiring urgent revascularization. Fourteen (78%) patients had both celiac and SMA disease, whereas three (17%) had only SMA involvement. All bypasses were performed from the descending thoracic aorta with PTFE grafts. Their results showed only one (6%) perioperative death from multisystem organ failure and three (17%) major complications (two myocardial infarctions and one reintubation). Graft durability was measured by survival rates and symptom relief, which were found to be 89%, 89%, and 76% at 1, 3, and 5 years, respectively. All grafts were found to be patent at 35-month follow-up.

Endovascular treatment of mesenteric ischemia has also been shown to be a safe and effective option. Kasirajan et al. in 2001 [43] reported prospective data comparing endovascular treatment on CMI on patients from 1995 to 1998 with open repair on patients from 1977 to 1997. Twenty-eight patients received an endovascular treatment while 85 patients had a surgical bypass. Endovascular therapies included balloon expandable stents in 23 arteries, 3 self-expanding stents, and 6 angioplasties. Whereas surgical intervention included bypass grafting in 71% (retrograde 40%, antegrade 28%, reimplantation 30%) of the patients, eversion endarterectomy in 22%, and patch repair in 7%. No significant reduced length of stay could be appreciated in the endovascular group and the 3-year cumulative recurrent stenosis and mortality rates did not differ. However, patients receiving an endovascular therapy had a higher incidence of recurrent symptoms. Initially, the utility of endovascular revascularization of mesenteric vessels was reserved for patients unfit for surgery and as a bridge to more definitive and durable open revascularization [44]. With the advent of covered stents, the patency rates have improved compared to the use of bare metal stents [45].

Management Options for Aortic Aneurysm Repair with Associated MAS

Evaluation of Aortic Aneurysm and Associated MAS

Aside from the complex nature of AAA with concomitant RAS, MAS further adds to the complexity of the procedural and timing of visceral artery repair. For the vascular surgeon, it is imperative to identify patients who are at risk for mesenteric ischemia before and after AAA repair. The three abdominal aortic vessels and the internal iliac vessels become the focus of attention for open, endovascular, or a hybrid repair. Classically, the open repair of infrarenal AAA has the mandatory intraoperative evaluation of the inferior mesenteric artery. When the celiac and SMAs are without disease and the IMA has no back bleeding, there is no need to revascularize the IMA. Likewise, brisk back bleeding from the IMA with knowledge of widely patent celiac and SMAs does not require reimplantation of the IMA. However, the algorithm becomes immediately more complex in patients with stenotic celiac, SMA, or even diseased hypogastric arteries. It is in this population of patients that the vascular surgeon needs to heighten the awareness for mesenteric ischemia before and after AAA repair.

It becomes an important intraoperative decision to reimplant the IMA when the vessel has poor to moderate back bleeding, likely provided by mesenteric collaterals such as the Arc of Riolan, Marginal Artery of Drummond, or from branches of the hypogastric vessels. This potentially indicates poor collateral perfusion to the distal bowel, specifically, distal to the splenic flexure. Mesenteric stenosis is well tolerated in patients who have stenosis in one of the three vessels supplying the intestines. However, the risk of acute bowel ischemia increases as the number of stenotic vessels increases, and it is greatest if the SMA is critically stenosed and the hypogastric vessels are heavily diseased.

Therefore, it is our practice to address the issue of mesenteric perfusion before any AAA repair. Each patient gets a thorough workup for clinical signs and symptoms of mesenteric ischemia and this is complemented with a thin-cut CT angiogram to evaluate the morphology of the AAA and, in symptomatic patients, noninvasive duplex scanning to obtain hemodynamic information-associated visceral stenosis. Since the notion of prophylactic repair of radiographic or duplex-identified significant (50%) stenosis is controversial, the algorithm for intervention is dependent on the extent of urgency for AAA repair and the extent of visceral disease.

In an asymptomatic patient with concomitant AAA and >50% diameter stenosis of the SMA or celiac, the authors prefer to evaluate the mesenteric vessels with an arteriogram. Selective injection of the three vessels gives an indication of dominant collateral blood supply and hints to the dominant vessel supplying the viscera. If the IMA is a large vessel, and selective injection with contrast shows reconstitution of the SMA, then the IMA is a critical vessel for blood supply. If there is competitive flow from the SMA, minimal filling of the Arc of Riolan, or Marginal Artery of Drummond, then collateral flow from the SMA is usually adequate.

Open Surgical Options for Management of Aortic Aneurysm and Associated MAS

It is very rare to consider an open approach to repair both mesenteric disease and AAAs simultaneously. However, if necessary, the authors prefer a thoraco-mesenteric bypass via a thoracoabdominal approach and subsequent retroperitoneal repair of the AAA. Other institutions may use a retrograde bypass from the iliac vessels or the aortic graft, while others describe an antegrade approach from the supraceliac aorta to supply the mesenteric vessels prior to a transabdominal repair of the aortic aneurysm. Simultaneous repair places significant stress on the patient and staging of the procedure would always be preferred.

Endovascular Options for Management of Aortic Aneurysm and Associated MAS

An endovascular approach has become the preferred method of AAA repair for patients with adequate anatomy, especially for the patient that is unable to tolerate an open procedure. The procedures are usually staged by first stenting the mesenteric vessels followed by EVAR of the aneurysm. This theoretically reduces the potential ischemic time of the viscera as an EVAR typically occludes inflow from the IMA.

Care must be taken when selecting the EVAR device. Whenever possible, the authors prefer using device with infra-renal fixation to avoid potential encroachment of the SMA stent by the endograft bare metal stent of devices with supra-renal fixation. The Zenith (Cook), Endurant (Medtronic), Trio (Terumo), and Alto (Endologix) devices have bare suprarenal fixation that may potentially extend to, or above, the SMA. This may cause a kink or even create a dislodgement of the SMA stent. Detailed preoperative planning avoids critical mistakes.

The Zenith Fenestrated endograft has the option to include the SMA during the repair for juxta-renal AAA. The visceral vessels can be incorporated using a small fenestration, a large fenestration, or an scallop. The SMA is usually incorporated with scallop, allowing to stent the SMA according to the surgeon's preference. Per instructions for use of the device, stenting the scallop is optional and the manufacture recommends not stent the large fenestrations because there are struts across the fenestration. The role of stenting the SMA during fenestrated aoric repair has been published and varies regarding preference. Lala et al. from UTSW group recommended routinely stenting the SMA [46]. The author's preference has been selective stenting the SMA. Situation that SMA ais routinely stents are: native vessel stenosis, endograft design with only one renal fenestration and one scallop (to avoid axial rotation of the device and future shuttering of the SMA) or when, using a balloon test at the end, the scallop is not perfectly aligned to the SMA origin [47].

Combination Approaches for Management of Aortic Aneurysm and Associated MAS

Hybrid Approach: Mesenteric BPG followed by EVAR repair is generally applied in patients who are poor candidates for traditional open AAA repair secondary to the likely complications from aortic cross-clamping. These patients are generally elderly and have poor cardiac function, making them especially high risk for open AAA repair. Multiple extra-anatomical approaches can be applied to this patient population. Reconstruction of perfusion to the mesenteric arteries using thoraco-mesenteric, aortomesenteric (supraceliac origination), or ileomesenteric conduits negates the need for manipulation and cross-clamping of a diseased aorta in a high-risk patient.

The procedure is usually staged to reduce patient stress that is imposed with prolonged operative times. The endovascular repair of the aneurysm is performed several days later. Care must be taken to avoid coverage of the inflow source of the mesenteric bypass if an ileomesenteric bypass was performed. With current data leaning toward surgical bypass for treatment of mesenteric disease, due to lower recurrence of symptoms, the authors prefer this approach to the treatment of concomitant AAA and symptomatic mesenteric disease.

Conclusion

Management of AAA in the current era of open, endovascular, and hybrid procedures is a complex undertaking. Development of modern generation endovascular devices has opened the door for many high-risk patients who would otherwise have limited therapeutic options. Depending on neck length, size, angulation, and iliac anatomy, most of the available devices can be applied to complex aneurysm anatomy. In the population of AAA, those with concomitant visceral artery stenosis possess an even more complex treatment algorithm, due to simultaneous advances in endoluminal therapy for the management of diverse pathological processes affecting the renal and mesenteric vessels.

The historical paradigm of "hitting two birds with one stone" using open surgical techniques in patients with concomitant AAA and visceral vessel pathology has led to increased end-organ morbidity and patient mortality. An augmented understanding of the underlying data has leaned the pendulum toward an increased frequency of performing staged interventions. The planning of aortic aneurysm repair in patients with visceral vessel disease needs to be highly individualized based on the thorough understanding of visceral and aortic pathology, anatomy, and accessibility. The availability of fenestrated repair incorporating the visceral vessels created an important opportunity to treat these complex aortic aneurysm and splanchnic vessels disease minimally invasive, especially for patients unfit for open repair.

References

1. Johnston KW, Rutherford RB, vascular MTJO. Suggested standards for reporting on arterial aneurysms. Elsevier; 1991.
2. Bickerstaff LK, Hollier LH, Van Peenen Journal of vascular HJ. Abdominal aortic aneurysms: the changing natural history. Elsevier; 1984.
3. Goldblatt H, Lynch J, Ramon F, Ward WS. Studies on experimental hypertension I. The production of persistent elevation of systolic blood pressure by means of renal ischemia. J Exp Med. 1934;59(3):347–79.
4. Freeman NE, Leeds FH, Association WEM. Thromboendarterectomy for hypertension due to renal artery occlusion. jamanetworkcom; 1954.
5. Lawson JD, Boerth R, Foster JH, Surgery RDAO. Diagnosis and management of renovascular hypertension in children. jamanetworkcom; 1977.
6. Burt VL, Whelton P, Roccella EJ, Brown C, Cutler JA. Prevalence of hypertension in the US adult population: results from the Third National Health and Nutrition Examination Survey, 1988–1991. Am Heart Assoc; 1995.
7. Rihal CS, Textor SC, Breen JF, Clinic MMM. Incidental renal artery stenosis among a prospective cohort of hypertensive patients undergoing coronary angiography. Elsevier; 2002.
8. Iglesias JI, Hamburger RJ. The natural history of incidental renal artery stenosis in patients with aortoiliac vascular disease, of LFTAJ. Elsevier; 2000.
9. Benjamin ME, Hansen KJ. Renovascular disease. In: Sidawy AN, Perler BA, editors. Rutherfords vascular surgery and endovascular therapy, Open surgical treatment; volume 2. 9th ed. Philadelphia.
10. Cherr GS, Hansen KJ, Craven TE, vascular MEJO. Surgical management of atherosclerotic renovascular disease. Elsevier; 2002.
11. Olin JW, Melia M, Young JR, of RGTAJ. Prevalence of atherosclerotic renal artery stenosis in patients with atherosclerosis elsewhere. europepmcorg; 1990.
12. Valentine RJ, Martin JD, Myers SI, vascular MRJO. Asymptomatic celiac and superior mesenteric artery stenoses are more prevalent among patients with unsuspected renal artery stenoses. Elsevier; 1991.
13. Brewster DC, Retana A, Journal AWNE. Angiography in the management of aneurysms of the abdominal aorta: its value and safety. Mass Medical Soc; 1975.

14. Hunt JC, Cardiology CSTAJO. Renovascular hypertension: mechanisms, natural history and treatment. Elsevier; 1973.
15. Dean RH, Kieffer RW, Smith BM, of JOA. Renovascular hypertension: anatomic and renal function changes during drug therapy. jamanetworkcom; 1981.
16. Wollenweber J, Sheps SG, cardiology GDTAJO. Clinical course of atherosclerotic renovascular disease*. Elsevier; 1968.
17. Schreiber MJ, Novick AC, Urology MPWJO. The natural history of atherosclerotic and fibrous renal artery disease. Springer; 1989.
18. Hallett JW Jr, Mills JL, Earnshaw J, Reekers JA, Rooke T. Comprehensive vascular and endovascular surgery. Elsevier Health Sciences; 2009. p. 1.
19. Blum U, Krumme B, of PFEJ. Treatment of ostial renal-artery stenoses with vascular endoprostheses after unsuccessful balloon angioplasty. Mass Medical Soc; 1997.
20. Leertouwer TC, Gussenhoven EJ, Radiology JB. Stent placement for renal arterial stenosis: where do we stand? A meta-analysis. pubsrsnaorg; 2000.
21. Investigators ASTRAL, Wheatley K, Ives N, Gray R, Kalra PA, Moss JG, et al. Revascularization versus medical therapy for renal-artery stenosis. N Engl J Med. 2009;361(20):1953–62.
22. Bax L, Woittiez A-JJ, Kouwenberg HJ, Mali WPTM, Buskens E, Beek FJA, et al. Stent placement in patients with atherosclerotic renal artery stenosis and impaired renal function: a randomized trial. Ann Intern Med. 2009;150(12):840–8–W150–1.
23. Cooper CJ, Murphy TP, Cutlip DE, Jamerson K, Henrich W, Reid DM, et al. Stenting and medical therapy for atherosclerotic renal-artery stenosis. N Engl J Med. 2014;370(1):13–22.
24. Stoney RJ, Messina LM, vascular JGJO. Renal endarterectomy through the transected aorta: a new technique for combined aortorenal atherosclerosis—a preliminary report. Elsevier; 1989.
25. MEB and KJH. Open surgical repair of renovascular diseases. In: F RBRM, editor. Rutherford, 10th edition. 2023.
26. Parodi JC, Palmaz JC, surgery HBAOV. Transfemoral intraluminal graft implantation for abdominal aortic aneurysms. Elsevier; 1991.
27. Oderich GS, Correa MP, Mendes BC. Technical aspects of repair of juxtarenal abdominal aortic aneurysms using the Zenith fenestrated endovascular stent graft. J Vasc Surg. 2014;59(5):1456–61.
28. Oderich GS, Farber MA, Schneider D, Makaroun M, Sanchez LA, Schanzer A, et al. Final 5-year results of the United States Zenith Fenestrated prospective multicenter study for juxtarenal abdominal aortic aneurysms. J Vasc Surg. 2020;73(4):1128–1138.e2.
29. Oderich GS, Ribeiro M, Hofer J, Wigham J, Cha S, Chini J, et al. Prospective, nonrandomized study to evaluate endovascular repair of pararenal and thoracoabdominal aortic aneurysms using fenestrated-branched endografts based on supraceliac sealing zones. J Vasc Surg. 2017;65(5):1249–1259.e10.
30. Mastracci TM, Greenberg RK, Eagleton MJ, Hernandez AV. Durability of branches in branched and fenestrated endografts. J Vasc Surg. 2013;57(4):926–33; discussion 933.
31. Eagleton MJ, Follansbee M, Wolski K, Mastracci TM, Kuramochi Y. Fenestrated and branched endovascular aneurysm repair outcomes for type II and III thoracoabdominal aortic aneurysms. J Vasc Surg. 2016;63(4):930–42.
32. Motta F, Crowner JR, Kalbaugh CA, Marston WA, Pascarella L, McGinigle KL, et al. Outcomes and complications after fenestrated-branched endovascular aortic repair. J Vasc Surg. 2019;70(1):15–22.
33. Verhoeven ELG, Vourliotakis G, Bos WTGJ, Tielliu IFJ, Zeebregts CJ, Prins TR, et al. Fenestrated stent grafting for short-necked and Juxtarenal abdominal aortic aneurysm: an 8-year single-centre experience. Eur J Vasc Endovasc Surg. Elsevier Ltd. 2010;39(5):529–36.
34. Oderich GS, Mendes BC, Correa MP. Preloaded guidewires to facilitate endovascular repair of thoracoabdominal aortic aneurysm using a physician-modified branched stent graft. J Vasc Surg. 2014;59(4):1168–73.

35. Timaran CH, Oderich GS, Tenorio ER, Farber MA, Schneider DB, Schanzer A, et al. Expanded use of preloaded branched and fenestrated endografts for endovascular repair of complex aortic aneurysms. Eur J Vasc Endovasc Surg. 2021;61(2):219–26.
36. Novick AC, Ziegelbaum M, Vidt DG, JAMA RG. Trends in surgical revascularization for renal artery disease: ten years' experience. jamanetworkcom; 1987.
37. Steinbach F, Novick AC, Campbell S, Dykstra D. Long-term survival after surgical revascularization for atherosclerotic renal artery disease. J Urol. 1997;158(1):38–41.
38. Thomas JH, Blake K, Pierce GE, vascular AHJO. The clinical course of asymptomatic mesenteric arterial stenosis. Elsevier; 1998.
39. Hollier LH, Bernatz PE, Pairolero PC, Surgery WP. Surgical management of chronic intestinal ischemia: a reappraisal. surgjournalcom; 1981.
40. McAfee MK, Cherry KJ Jr, of JNTAJ. Influence of complete revascularization on chronic mesenteric ischemia. Elsevier; 1992.
41. Foley MI, Moneta GL, vascular AA-ZJJO. Revascularization of the superior mesenteric artery alone for treatment of intestinal ischemia. Elsevier; 2000.
42. Farber MA, Carlin RE, Marston WA, Owens LV, Burnham SJ, Keagy BA. Distal thoracic aorta as inflow for the treatment of chronic mesenteric ischemia. YMVA Mosby. 2001;33(2):281–8.
43. Kasirajan K, O'Hara PJ, Gray BH, vascular NHJO. Chronic mesenteric ischemia: open surgery versus percutaneous angioplasty and stenting. Elsevier; 2001.
44. Biebl M, Oldenburg WA, Paz-Fumagalli R, McKinney JM, Hakaim AG. Endovascular treatment as a bridge to successful surgical revascularization for chronic mesenteric ischemia. Am Surg. 2004;70(11):994–8.
45. Oderich GS, Erdoes LS, LeSar C, vascular BMJO. Comparison of covered stents versus bare metal stents for treatment of chronic atherosclerotic mesenteric arterial disease. Elsevier; 2013.
46. Lala S, Knowles M, Timaran D, Baig MS, Valentine J, Timaran C. Superior mesenteric artery outcomes after fenestrated endovascular aortic aneurysm repair. J Vasc Surg. 2016;64(3):692–7.
47. Motta F, Crowner JR, Kalbaugh CA, Knowles M, Pascarella L, McGinigle KL, et al. Stenting of superior mesenteric and celiac arteries does not increase complication rates after fenestrated-branched endovascular aneurysm repair. J Vasc Surg. 2019;70(3):691–701.

Chapter 25
Management of Abdominal Aortic Aneurysms in Patients with Renal Ectopia and Renal Fusion

Jonathan R. Krebs and Michol A. Cooper

Introduction

In contrast to aberrant renal arteries, which are present in 25–40% of kidneys and usually easily handled by the experienced vascular surgeon, congenital renal anomalies are present in <1% of patients and can pose substantial technical challenges [1]. Congenital anomalies of the upper urinary tract are generally categorized as those involving variations in number, ascent, and rotation [2]. The most common congenital renal anomaly is horseshoe kidney, present in 0.25% of the general population, followed by renal ectopia, present in 1 in 500 to 1 in 1200 of the general population in autopsy studies [2]. Coexisting aberrancies of renal vasculature and the collecting system affect 75% of these patients and warrant careful consideration in the preoperative setting [2].

Based on the previous edition chapter "Management of Abdominal Aortic Aneurysms in Patients with Renal Ectopia and Renal Fusion" by Patrick J O'Hara.

J. R. Krebs · M. A. Cooper (✉)
Department of Surgery, Division of Vascular Surgery, University of Florida, Gainesville, FL, USA
e-mail: Jonathan.krebs@surgery.ufl.edu; Michol.cooper@surgery.ufl.edu

G. J. Arnaoutakis et al. (eds.), *Aortic Aneurysms*, Contemporary Cardiology,
https://doi.org/10.1007/978-3-032-13134-8_25

Embryology

An understanding of the congenital renal anomalies encountered during aortic surgery is predicated on a basic understanding of normal embryological development of the urinary system. During embryonic development, three primitive nephritic systems called the pronephros, mesonephros, and metanephros form from the intermediate mesoderm. Formation of the pronephros initiates a developmental cascade resulting in development of the metanephros, the definitive fetal kidney, in the sacral region by the fourth week of gestation. From this single structure, paired ureteric buds develop from the mesonephric ducts and interact with metanephric mesenchyme to form a pair of fetal kidneys. A series of ureteric bud bifurcations results in formation of the renal pelvis and calyces of the renal collecting system. Between the sixth and ninth weeks, the kidneys ascend from the sacral region to a lumbar site on either side of the dorsal aorta. The relocating kidney is progressively revascularized by a series of arterial sprouts from the aorta and the original renal artery in the sacral region regresses. Occasionally, one or more of the inferior renal arteries fail to regress resulting in accessory renal arteries. The final result is usually a single pair of renal arteries, one for each kidney [3].

Classification

Congenital renal anomalies are categorized as variations in number, form, ascent, and rotation. All can be associated with accessory or aberrant renal arteries and abnormalities in the collecting system [2]. Anomalies associated with accessory or aberrant renal arteries only rarely complicate aneurysm repair (Table 25.1), while

Table 25.1 Renal anomalies infrequently complicating aortic aneurysm repair [2]

Agenesis
Unilateral
Bilateral
Ascent
Simple ectopia
Cephalad renal ectopia
Thoracic kidney
Rotation
Ventral
Dorsal
Lateral

those involving problems with renal form and ascent can have significant ramifications for the vascular surgeon during aortic aneurysm repair (Table 25.2) [2].

Pelvic and ectopic kidneys arise from problems with ascent. If the kidney fails to ascend and remains in the pelvis, it is known as a pelvic kidney. If the kidneys only partially ascend, the resulting kidney is known as an ectopic kidney. Pelvic and ectopic kidneys are typically associated with some degree of malrotation [4]. If the metanephric bud fails to separate following ureteric bud development, a variety of fusion abnormalities including discoid or lump kidney may result [4]. Crossed fused renal ectopia is fusion anomaly that arises when one kidney fuses to the contralateral kidney and the fused kidneys ascend to the contralateral side.

Horseshoe kidney may result if the inferior poles of the two metanephroi make contact and fuse during relocation (Fig. 25.1). A longstanding theory is that the

Table 25.2 Renal anomalies frequently complicating aortic aneurysm repair [2]

Crossed renal ectopia without fusion
Solitary
Bilateral
Crossed renal ectopia with fusion
Inferior ectopic kidney
S-shaped (sigmoid) kidney
Lump kidney
L-shaped kidney
Disc kidney
Superior ectopic kidney
Horseshoe kidney

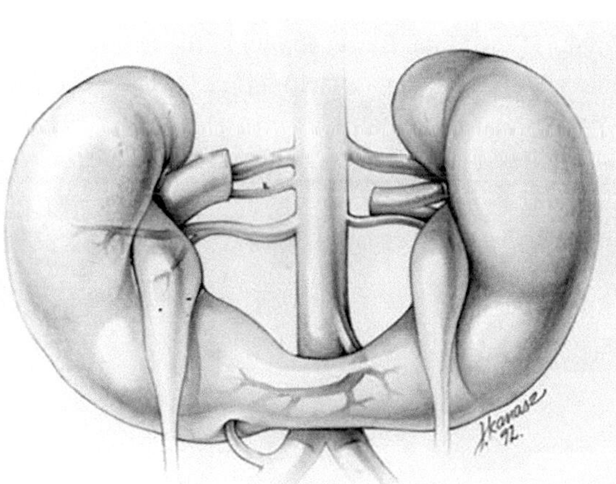

Fig. 25.1 Diagrammatic representation of horseshoe kidney anomaly and its relationship to the abdominal aorta. (Reprinted with permission from O'Hara et al. [5])

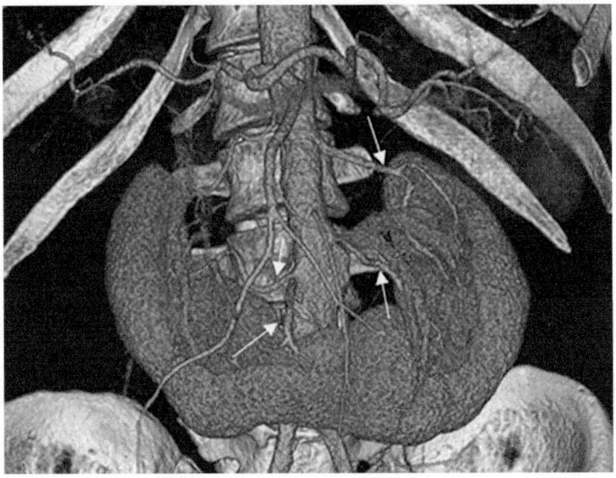

Fig. 25.2 3-Dimensional reconstruction of a CT image of an abdominal aortic aneurysm and coexistent horseshoe kidney. Note the multiple aberrant renal arteries (*arrows*)

fused kidney becomes caught under the inferior mesenteric artery during its ascent resulting in a more caudad location [3]. Multiple, abnormally located renal arteries are a common feature of horseshoe kidney likely as a result of disturbances in the normal ascent and rotation of the developing horseshoe kidney (Fig. 25.2) [5, 6]. Only one-third of horseshoe kidneys have renal arteries located in the usual anatomic position, while the remaining two-thirds can have either single or multiple arteries (Fig. 25.3) [7–10]. Horseshoe kidney and other forms of ectopia alter the medial rotation of the primitive renal unit and are associated with collecting system abnormalities including presence of multiple ureters, a common renal pelvis lying just anterior to the abdominal aorta, or in the case of horseshoe kidney, ureters lying anterior to the renal isthmus. The isthmus itself may occasionally be a fibrous band amenable to division, but more often is composed of a thick segment of renal parenchyma (Fig. 25.4). Blood supply to the isthmus may be asymmetric and unpredictable with poor collateralization [5, 11]. These variations can make abdominal aortic exposure hazardous [5, 11].

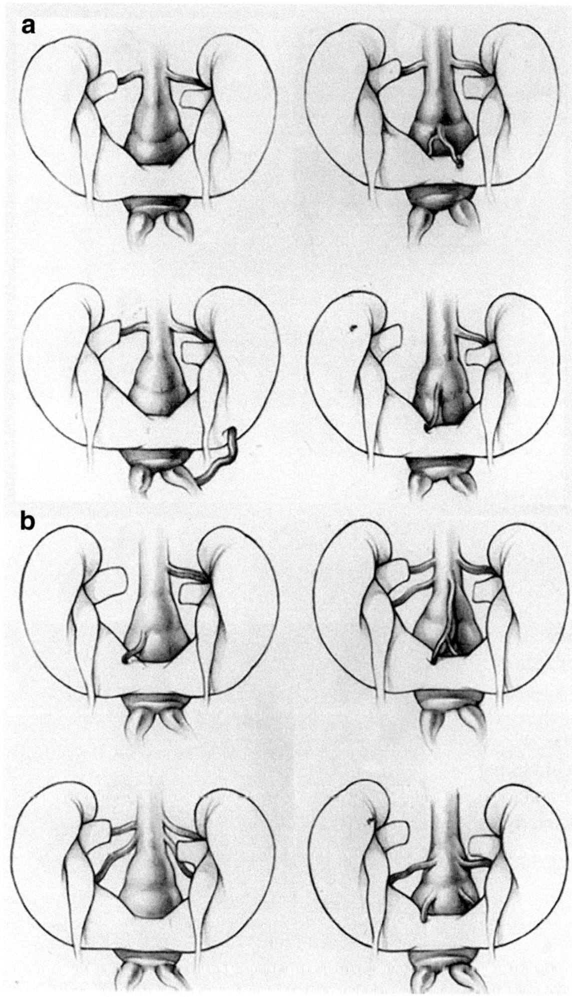

Fig. 25.3 Diagram of renal arterial patterns found in 19 patients with aortic aneurysms and coexistent horseshoe kidneys. (**a**) Four common patterns each found in more than one patient. (**b**, **c**) Seven uncommon patterns each found in a single patient. (Reprinted with permission from O'Hara et al. [5])

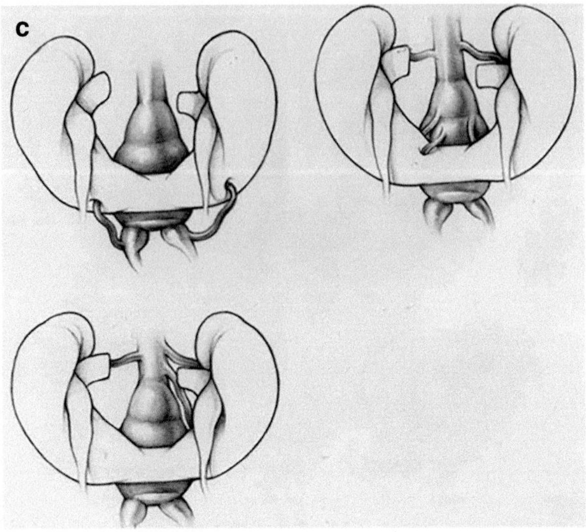

Fig. 25.3 (continued)

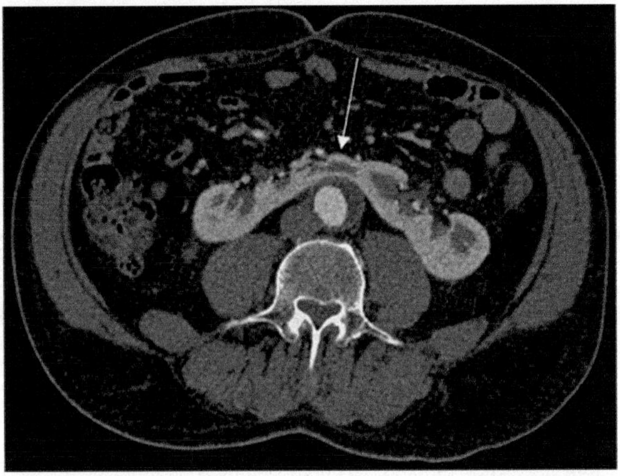

Fig. 25.4 CT scan demonstrating horseshoe kidney overlying a small abdominal aortic aneurysm. Note the isthmus (*arrow*) containing renal parenchyma and collecting system overlying the aorta

Diagnosis and Imaging

On physical exam, aneurysm diameter may be overestimated due to overlying renal parenchyma, but the diagnosis of horseshoe kidney or renal ectopia is readily apparent with several imaging modalities. Ultrasonography is usually able to correctly estimate size of aneurysm, but has a reduced sensitivity in obese patients or air-filled intestines and historically has been able to identify horseshoe kidney in a minority of patients (Fig. 25.5) [5, 12]. Routine preoperative computed tomography angiography (CTA) in abdominal aortic aneurysm surgery has greatly facilitated the identification of renal anomalies and can accurately identify the number and

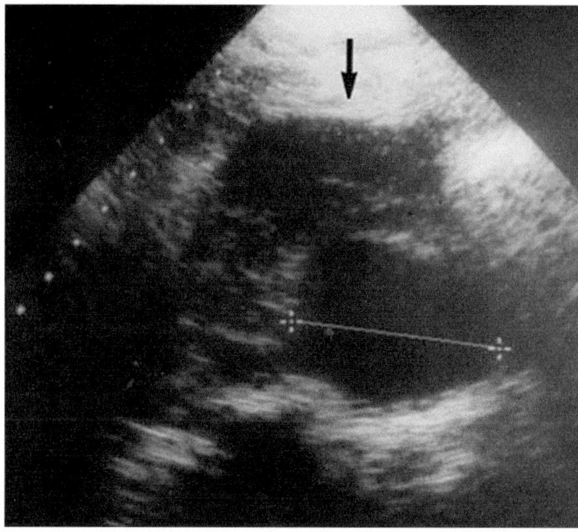

Fig. 25.5 Ultrasound examination of the abdominal aorta with horseshoe kidney (*arrow*) anterior to the aortic aneurysm. (Reprinted with permission from O'Hara et al. [5])

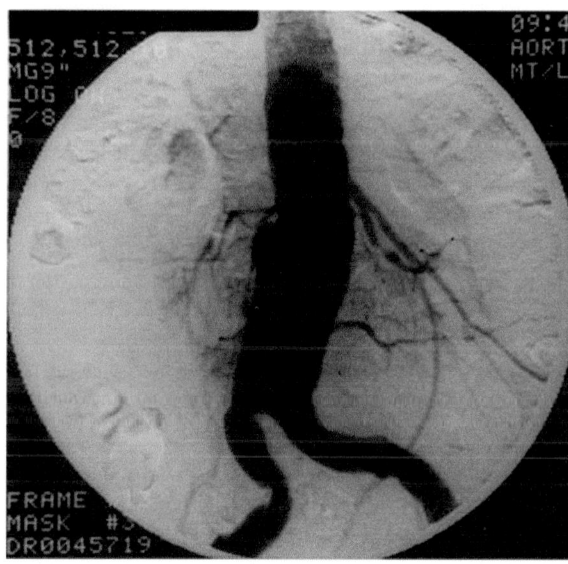

Fig. 25.6 Transfemoral aortogram of a patient with an abdominal aortic aneurysm and coexistent horseshoe kidney. (Reprinted with permission from O'Hara et al. [5])

location of accessory renal arteries (Fig. 25.4) [7, 13]. If ureteral anatomy is unclear, intravenous pyelography can be used to clarify the course and number of ureters [14]. Digital angiography may further define renal perfusion patterns, but as an invasive procedure should be reserved for endovascular interventions in which accessory arteries would be covered (Fig. 25.6). CTA with three-dimensional image reconstruction is the most useful diagnostic tool for detection of horseshoe kidney or renal ectopia and preoperative planning for either an open or endovascular intervention (Fig. 25.7) [7].

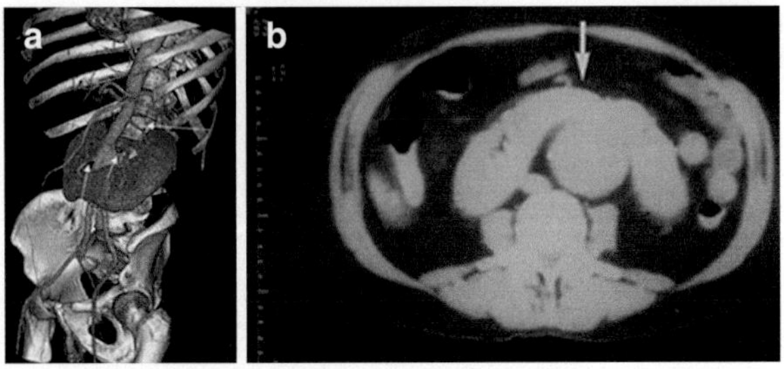

Fig. 25.7 (**a**) 3-Dimensional reconstruction of a CT image of an abdominal aortic aneurysm and coexistent horseshoe kidney. Note the multiple aberrant renal arteries (*arrows*). (**b**) CT scan demonstrating horseshoe kidney overlying an abdominal aortic aneurysm. Note the isthmus (*arrow*) containing renal parenchyma overlying the aorta

Therapy

Open Repair

Preservation of renal blood supply, collecting system, and renal mass in the setting of horseshoe kidney or other renal anomalies should virtually always be feasible during open abdominal aortic aneurysm repair in an acceptable operative risk candidate. For horseshoe kidney, three technical considerations should be carefully considered in the preoperative setting: transperitoneal versus retroperitoneal approach, management of the renal isthmus, and ligation or salvage of renal arteries [7].

Both transperitoneal and retroperitoneal approaches to abdominal aortic aneurysm repair in patients with coexistent renal fusion have been described with technical success, the first of which was performed at Mayo Clinic in 1956 via a transperitoneal approach [5, 13, 15, 16]. During this case, in which the horseshoe kidney was discovered incidentally on exploration, no aberrant vascular anomalies were encountered and an aortic homograft was tunneled posterior to the undivided isthmus of the horseshoe kidney [15]. Historically, the transperitoneal approach was often chosen as the presence of horseshoe kidney was not appreciated preoperatively. While the transperitoneal approach does offer rapid access to the aneurysm sac and better access to both iliac arteries, reconstruction with reimplantation or bypass of anomalous renal arteries is often less than ideal (Fig. 25.8). This is particularly true in cases where aberrant arteries arise from the aorta or iliac arteries directly posterior to the horseshoe kidney. Furthermore, if the length of the renal artery is inadequate to reach the graft after aneurysm decompression, the renal bypass grafts are often difficult to construct and position without kinking [5, 11]. For these reasons, some advocate for routine use of the left retroperitoneal approach as it provides optimal exposure for reimplantation of short aberrant renal arteries and minimizes iatrogenic injury to the urinary tract and renal isthmus [5, 7, 9, 11].

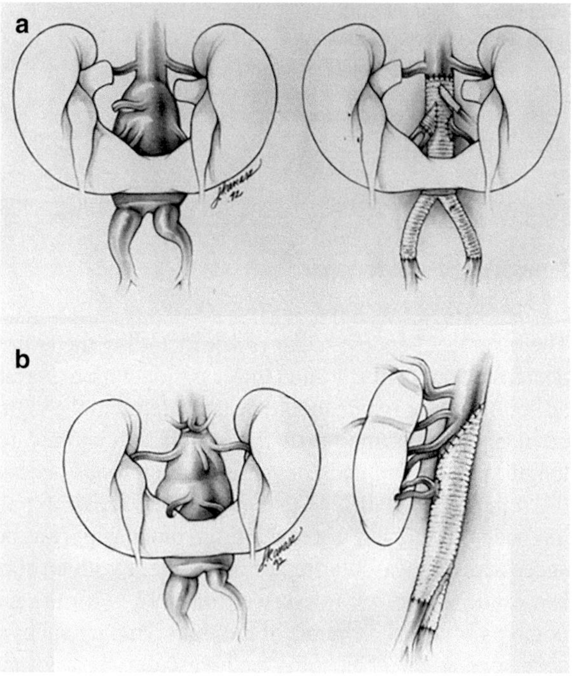

Fig. 25.8 Diagram of surgical exposure and reconstruction options. (**a**) Transperitoneal exposure through a midline abdominal incision with Dacron graft placed beneath renal isthmus and renal branches reconstructed by implantation or bypass grafting. (**b**) Retroperitoneal exposure through a low left thoracoabdominal incision. Dacron graft placed within the aneurysm sac and renal arterial branches reconstructed by implantation. (Reprinted with permission from O'Hara et al. [5])

Due to significant variations in renal isthmus anatomy ranging from a thin fibrous sheath to a significant volume of renal parenchyma, management of the renal isthmus should be considered on an individual basis. Exposure and division of the isthmus can carry a significant risk of infarction, hydronephrosis, and urine leak as the ureters are often positioned more medially and cross the isthmus anteriorly [5]. As approximately 13% of patients with horseshoe kidney have chronic urinary infection, urine leak may carry a significant risk of subsequent graft infection [6]. If the decision to divide the isthmus has been undertaken, it should only be performed in cases of a thin fibrous band of tissue [17]. It is again for these reasons that the retroperitoneal approach may be favorable for many patients as it provides adequate exposure without needing to directly encounter the renal isthmus.

The third consideration involves the management of aberrant and multiple renal arteries. Small arteries <2 mm may be selectively ligated without significant risk of renal dysfunction [18]. Attempts to preserve arteries with diameter >2 mm should be undertaken to prevent postoperative renal infarction and dysfunction [5, 18]. Reimplantation can be performed directly to the prosthetic graft material or using Carrel patch. Some form of renal protection is recommended particularly if the period of warm ischemia time is expected to be lengthy. Several methods of renal protection have been described including renal shunting, temporary bypass, in situ cold perfusion, and extracorporeal pump oxygenation [19–21]. A representative renal perfusate solution is shown in Table 25.3. In this solution, a total of 600 mL is infused into the renal mass to provide 30–45 min of relative renal protection [5, 11].

Table 25.3 Example cold renal perfusate composition

1000 cc Ringer's lactate
1 ampoule (18 g) mannitol
500 mg methylprednisolone
2000 units heparin
Chill to 3 °C

Endovascular Repair

The benefits of endovascular repair including the reduced morbidity of laparotomy, decreased length of stay, and lower perioperative mortality are well documented and an endovascular repair should be considered in the higher risk patient with favorable renal anatomy. Other than the standard anatomic requirements including neck length, angulation, and adequate landing zones necessary for endovascular repair, the principle impediment to endovascular repair in patients with horseshoe kidney has been the anomalous renal arterial blood supply as described previously. The first successful endovascular repair of a patient with an abdominal aortic aneurysm and horseshoe kidney was described in 1997, with the patient's postoperative course notable for partial ischemia of the right renal parenchyma after graft exclusion of an accessory artery [22]. Early endovascular repairs suggested that small accessory renal branches (<3 mm) could be safely sacrificed provided preoperative renal function was normal, although small renal infarcts were identified in 20–50% of those patients with renal branches that were covered [1, 23, 24]. There is also a theoretical risk of type II endoleak with coverage of accessory renal arteries, but back-bleeding is typically minimal and low pressure so the clinical significance of this is unknown [23, 25].

Due to the limitations of traditional endovascular repair, several strategies have been successfully used to preserve the accessory renal arteries in horseshoe kidney. In cases where accessory arteries arise from the proximal iliac artery, deployment of a unilateral aortoiliac endograft with femorofemoral bypass can exclude the aneurysm while preserving renal flow [7]. Advances in customized fenestrated endografts have allowed for selective catheterization of anomalous arteries although there remain outstanding concerns regarding long-term patency [26]. Another group published a case whereby chimney graft was performed to preserve flow to a large inferior mesenteric artery during endovascular aneurysm repair [27]. Shirakawa et al. reported on their use of a hybrid approach, whereby endovascular repair was combined with open revascularization of aberrant left renal arteries with satisfactory outcome [28].

Advances in endovascular technology have provided the vascular surgeon with a range of endovascular, open, and hybrid approaches to abdominal aortic aneurysm repair with coexistent renal fusion or ectopia. Endovascular repair should be considered in patients with favorable anatomy and normal baseline renal function.

Regardless of approach, with a thorough assessment of the patient's baseline operative fitness and anatomy safe aneurysm repair with renal preservation is a realistic goal.

Complications and Results

Few large published series on the results of open or endovascular treatment of aortic aneurysm and horseshoe kidney or other form of renal ectopia exist due to its rare occurrence in clinical practice. Most published information regarding perioperative results and complications consists of case reports, case series, and literature reviews. Results of the largest series of open management are summarized in Table 25.4.

Among all open case series, mortality is low. This is true even when considering earlier case series that included both emergency and elective cases in addition to cases performed prior to widespread availability and use of computed tomography. It is well known that abnormal preoperative renal function is associated with increased perioperative morbidity and mortality regardless of operative approach [9, 20, 21, 29]. In the largest open series to date from O'Hara et al., preoperative renal failure was the strongest indicator of poor outcome following open aneurysm repair in the presence of horseshoe kidney [5]. Fifty percent (3/6) of patients with preoperative renal insufficiency required postoperative hemodialysis. Conversely, none of the 13 patients with normal baseline renal function required postoperative hemodialysis, a difference that was statistically significant ($p = 0.02$). The early mortality rate for the entire series was 16% (3/19), 6% (1/16) for those patients not requiring postoperative dialysis, and 67% (2/3) for those patients who did require postoperative hemodialysis ($p = 0.05$) [5]. No large case series exist for endovascular repair. A systemic review analyzing 50 patients who had undergone endovascular repair for horseshoe kidney demonstrates the safety of this approach, with no early postoperative deaths and a complication rate of 14% (7/50) [30]. Complications included

Table 25.4 Outcomes following open repair of coexistent abdominal aortic aneurysms and horseshoe kidney or renal ectopia in selected series

	Abdominal aortic aneurysm and coexistent horseshoe kidney or renal ectopia				
Author	Year	Approach	Patients	Early postoperative deaths	Complications
de Virgilio et al. [29]	1995	Open	16	0	29% (includes dialysis)
Shortell et al. [31]	1995	Open	8	0	Dialysis 13% (1/8)
O'Hara et al. [5]	1993	Open	19	16% (3/19)	Dialysis 16% (3/19)
Crawford et al. [9]	1988	Open	13	15% (2/13)	Not specified

four endoleaks (all type II), one wound infection, one late iliac limb occlusion, and one graft stenosis [30]. Renal infarction was observed in 14% of patients (7/50) and associated with preoperative chronic kidney disease [30]. The number of patients requiring hemodialysis postoperatively was not specified although it was suggested that long-term renal impairment appeared low [30].

References

1. Kaplan DB, Kwon CC, Marin ML. Endovascular repair of abdominal aortic aneurysms in patients with congenital renal vascular anomalies. J Vasc Surg. 1999;30 https://doi.org/10.1016/S0741-5214(99)70067-4.
2. Bauer SB. Anomalies of the upper urinary tract. In: Wein AJ, editor. Campbell-Walsh urology. WB Saunders Co; 2007.
3. Schoenwolf GC, et al. Larsen's human embryology. 5th ed. Elsevier; 2014.
4. Park JM. Normal development of the urogenital system. In: Wein AJ, editor. Campbell-Walsh urology. WB Saunders Co; 2007.
5. O'Hara PJ, Hakaim AG, Hertzer NR, Krajewski LP, Cox GS, Beven EG. Surgical management of aortic aneurysm and coexistent horseshoe kidney: review of 31-year experience. J Vasc Surg. 1993;17 https://doi.org/10.1067/mva.1993.44344.
6. Glenn JF. Analysis of 51 patients with horseshoe kidney. N Engl J Med. 1959;261 https://doi.org/10.1056/NEJM195910012611402.
7. Sachsamanis G, Charisis N, Maltezos K, et al. Management and therapeutic options for abdominal aortic aneurysm coexistent with horseshoe kidney. J Vasc Surg. 2019;69(4):1257–67. https://doi.org/10.1016/j.jvs.2018.10.009.
8. Boatman DL, Cornell SH, Kolln CP. The arterial supply of horseshoe kidneys. Am J Roentgenol. 1971;113(3):447–51. https://doi.org/10.2214/ajr.113.3.447.
9. Crawford ES, Coselli JS, Safi HJ, Martin TD, Pool JL. The impact of renal fusion and ectopia on aortic surgery. J Vasc Surg. 1988;8(4):375–83. https://doi.org/10.1016/0741-5214(88)90098-5.
10. Eisendrath DN, Phifer FM, Culver HB. Horseshoe kidney. Ann Surg. 1925;82(5):735.
11. Kasirajan K, O'Hara PJ. Renal ectopia and renal fusion in patients requiring abdominal aortic operations. In: Ernst CB, Stanley JC, editors. Current therapy in vascular surgery. Mosby; 2001.
12. Taylor DC, Sladen JG, Maxwell T. Aortic surgery and horseshoe kidney: a challenging surgical problem. Can J Surg. 1987;30(6):431–3.
13. Göksel O, Çınar B, Kömürcü G, Ahin S, Eren T. Surgical treatment of abdominal aortic aneurysms associated with horseshoe kidney. Vascular. 2006;14(1):27–31. https://doi.org/10.2310/6670.2006.00002.
14. Kawanishi Y, Tanaka H, Nakagiri K, Yamashita T, Okada K, Okita Y. Abdominal aortic aneurysm associated with horseshoe kidney. Asian Cardiovasc Thorac Ann. 2008;16(3):e28–9. https://doi.org/10.1177/021849230801600325.
15. Phelan JT, Bernatz PE, DeWeerd JH. Abdominal aortic aneurysm associated with a horseshoe kidney: report of a case. Mayo Clin Proc. 1957;32(4):77–81.
16. Davidović LB, Kostić DM, Jakovljević NS, et al. Abdominal aortic surgery and horseshoe kidney. Ann Vasc Surg. 2004;18(6):725–8. https://doi.org/10.1007/s10016-004-0076-8.
17. Connelly TL, McKinnon W, Smith RB III, Perdue GD. Abdominal aortic surgery and horseshoe kidney: report of six cases and a review. Arch Surg. 1980;115(12):1459–63. https://doi.org/10.1001/archsurg.1980.01380120031008.
18. Canova G, Masini R, Santoro E, et al. Surgical treatment of abdominal aortic aneurysm in association with horseshoe kidney. Three case reports and a review of technique. Tex Heart Inst J. 1998;25(3):206. https://pmc.ncbi.nlm.nih.gov/articles/PMC325551/. Accessed 19 July 2022.

19. Schneider JR, Cronenwett JL. Temporary perfusion of a congenital pelvic kidney during abdominal aortic aneurysm repair. J Vasc Surg. 1993;17 https://doi.org/10.1067/mva.1993.38803.
20. Hollis HW, Rutherford RB, Crawford GJ, Cleland BP, Marx WH, Clark JR. Abdominal aortic aneurysm repair in patients with pelvic kidney. Technical considerations and literature review. J Vasc Surg. 1989;9 https://doi.org/10.1067/mva.1989.vs0090404.
21. Hollis HW, Rutherford RB. Abdominal aortic aneurysms associated with horseshoe or ectopic kidneys: techniques of renal preservation. Semin Vasc Surg. 1988;1:148–59.
22. Ferko A, Krajina A, Jon B, Leško M, Vobořil Z. Juxtarenal aortic aneurysm associated with a horseshoe kidney: transfemoral endoluminal repair. Arch Surg. 1997;132(3):316–7. https://doi.org/10.1001/archsurg.1997.01430270102021.
23. Ruppert V, Umscheid T, Rieger J. Endovascular aneurysm repair: treatment of choice for abdominal aortic aneurysm coincident with horseshoe kidney? Three case reports and review of literature. J Vasc Surg. 2004;40 https://doi.org/10.1016/j.jvs.2004.04.014.
24. Aquino RV, Rhee RY, Muluk SC. Exclusion of accessory renal arteries during endovascular repair of abdominal aortic aneurysms. J Vasc Surg. 2001;34 https://doi.org/10.1067/mva.2001.118814.
25. Frego M, Bianchera G, Angriman I. Abdominal aortic aneurysm with coexistent horseshoe kidney. Surg Today. 2007;37 https://doi.org/10.1007/s00595-006-3451-y.
26. Brown K, Robinson D, Bray A. Customized fenestrated endovascular graft repair of abdominal aortic aneurysm with concomitant horseshoe kidney. Vascular. 2013;22(3):193–7. https://doi.org/10.1177/1708538113480577.
27. Kfoury E, Almanfi A, Dougherty KG, Krajcer Z. Endovascular abdominal aortic aneurysm repair by means of the chimney technique in a patient with crossed fused renal ectopia. Tex Heart Inst J. 2016;43(3):232–5. https://doi.org/10.14503/THIJ-15-5025.
28. Kin K, Takano H, Nakagawa T, Shirakawa Y. Hybrid repair of an abdominal aortic aneurysm: debranching with endovascular aneurysm repair in a patient with horseshoe kidney. Ann Vasc Dis. 2017;10(1):41. https://doi.org/10.3400/AVD.CR.16-00107.
29. Virgilio C, Gloviczki P, Cherry KJ. Renal artery anomalies in patients with horseshoe or ectopic kidneys: the challenge of aortic reconstruction. Cardiovasc Surg. 1995;3 https://doi.org/10.1016/0967-2109(95)94161-O.
30. Gonzalez-Urquijo M, Padilla-Armendariz DP, Hinojosa-Gonzalez DE, Lozano-Balderas G, Flores-Villalba E, Fabiani MA. EVAR in patients with abdominal aortic aneurysm and horseshoe kidney: a systematic review. J Endovasc Ther. 2021;29(4):637–45. https://doi.org/10.1177/15266028211059447.
31. Shortell CK, Welch EL, Ouriel K, Green RM, DeWesse JA. Operative management of coexistent aortic disease and horseshoe kidney. Ann Vasc Surg. 1995;9 https://doi.org/10.1007/BF02015326.

Chapter 26
Aortocaval Fistula

David Strosberg and Alan Dardik

Introduction

A fistula between the inferior vena cava and aorta is a rare finding, occurring in 0.2–1.3% of abdominal aortic aneurysms (AAA). The incidence is 1% in asymptomatic and 3–4% in symptomatic aneurysms. Most fistulae occur as a complication of AAA, but 5–10% can occur because of mycotic aneurysms. Ehlers-Danlos and Marfan's syndromes or Takayasu's arteritis can also cause fistulae. Rarely, low-velocity penetrating trauma, such as a stab wound, can result in an aortocaval fistula. However, the majority of penetrating injuries to the aorta result in either death or hemodynamic instability necessitating surgical exploration, such that a fistula does not have the opportunity to form. Nevertheless, congestive heart failure in a young patient with a history of trauma should alert the physician to a possible aortocaval fistula.

The simultaneous presentation of an aneurysm and congestive heart failure (CHF) usually represents unrelated processes, and thus typically the CHF should be treated prior to elective AAA repair. However, the persistence of CHF despite treatment suggests a fistula or some other ominous finding.

Patients may complain of back or abdominal pain. On physical examination, there may be a pulsatile abdominal mass, 75% will have an audible continuous bruit and 25% a palpable thrill. In a study performed at the Mayo Clinic, 94% of patients

---

D. Strosberg (✉)
Division of Vascular Surgery and Endovascular Therapy, Department of Surgery, Yale School of Medicine, New Haven, CT, USA
e-mail: david.strosberg@yale.edu

A. Dardik (✉)
Department of Surgery, Icahn School of Medicine at Mount Sinai, New York, NY, USA
e-mail: alan.dardik@mountsinai.org

G. J. Arnaoutakis et al. (eds.), *Aortic Aneurysms*, Contemporary Cardiology,
https://doi.org/10.1007/978-3-032-13134-8_26

with aortocaval fistulae were symptomatic at presentation, but only 17% had a triad of pain, pulsatile mass, and abdominal bruit [1].

CHF associated with an aortocaval fistula is a hyperdynamic, high-output state. Therefore, patients may present with tachycardia, hypertension, decreased diastolic blood pressure, cardiac dilation with an associated murmur, jugular venous distension, hepatomegaly, swollen legs, or venous stasis disease. There have also been reports of saphenous vein bruit [2]. Previously undiagnosed congenital abnormalities such as patent foramen ovale or central malignancies, may contribute to circulatory overload and heart failure. Renal failure is often present. Rarely, patients may present with lower gastrointestinal bleeding in cases with visceral ischemia or hematuria if venous engorgement of the bladder is present. Lower extremity claudication may also be present.

Diagnosis

The initial test suggesting the presence of an AAA is frequently an ultrasound, but this is not the best imaging option for a fistula. Occasionally, a fistula may be discovered with color flow on the duplex ultrasound, but this is rare, and preoperative planning is not routinely performed with ultrasound. In the past, aortocaval fistulae were more often discovered unexpectedly in the operating room, during the course of open repair of an aneurysm.

Aortography is the gold standard for diagnosis, but now, more commonly, computed tomography (CT) and magnetic resonance (MR) angiograms are used to assess AAA and an associated fistula. CT is more commonly used, especially as patients are routinely evaluated with CT to determine candidacy for endovascular repair (EVAR). Routine imaging has led to increased preoperative detection of fistulae, and early filling of the inferior vena cava (IVC) after intra-aortic contrast

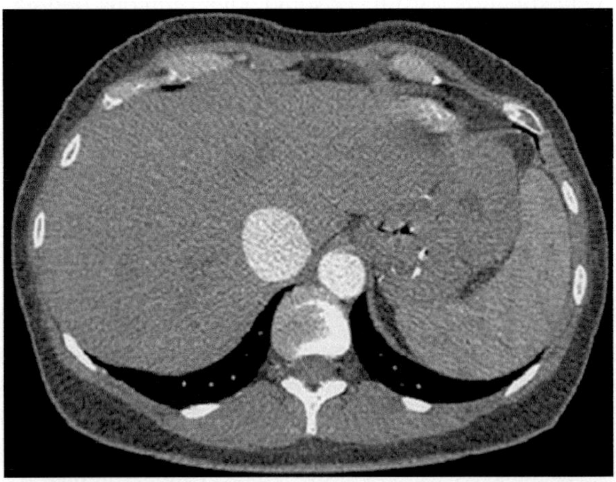

Fig. 26.1 Arterial phase computed tomography (*CT*) demonstrating an aortocaval fistula. In addition to contrast in the aorta, contrast is also simultaneously present in the inferior vena cava (*IVC*)

injection is indicative of a fistula (Fig. 26.1). MR angiography can demonstrate this finding as well, but is less commonly used.

Treatment

The natural history of an aortocaval fistula is progressive CHF leading to death, and therefore, the fistula and associated AAA should be immediately repaired. However, even with successful open surgical repair, there is an associated 22–51% mortality largely due to blood loss, cardiac decompensation, and pulmonary embolus. Survival rates are generally higher for elective repairs and lower for emergency repairs of ruptured AAA or elective repairs of AAA in which the fistula was not preoperatively diagnosed. Today, with routine preoperative imaging studies, it is increasingly rare for a fistula to go undiagnosed and encountered unexpectedly during open aneurysm repair.

Preoperatively, all patients with suspected aortocaval fistula should receive a transesophageal echocardiogram to evaluate cardiac performance and hemodynamics as well as to assess alternative sites of, or potential additional, fistulae, including those due to a previously undiagnosed patent foramen ovale. The central venous pressure is usually elevated and patients may have varying degrees of renal failure. Therefore, in patients with severe symptoms requiring therapy, a pulmonary artery catheter should be used to evaluate left-to-right shunt or high-output cardiac failure, and it can also be used to guide fluid management. In most cases, renal function will return to normal after a successful repair.

The hemodynamic consequences of AAA-IVC fistula repair should be anticipated intraoperatively. Both the cardiac output and the mixed venous oxygen content should fall to normal values. Continued fall in cardiac output to low values likely reflects low filling pressures that will be responsive to fluids. Mild acidosis may be present after repair as well.

Operative Repair

Traditional open repair is performed either from the transperitoneal or from the retroperitoneal approach, depending on aneurysm configuration and surgeon preference. Although successful operation is expected with comprehensive preoperative diagnosis and planning, potential complications include bleeding, infection, hemodynamic instability, impotence, colon ischemia, cardiac failure, prolonged ventilator dependence, stroke, air embolism, pulmonary embolism, acute limb ischemia, and death.

Repair should proceed in standard fashion including dissection, vessel control, and heparinization. Acute fistulas are easily entered, whereas chronic fistulae can be encased in fibrous tissue or an inflammatory mass. Chronic fistulae may also have thinned, large arteries and bulging veins, adding to the difficulty of vascular isolation. Patients must be adequately positioned and draped so that major bleeding can be controlled. For high abdominal fistulae, the chest should be included in the field. The fistula and IVC do not need to be isolated or dissected individually. After aneurysm exclusion and opening of the sac, back bleeding from the fistula is characteristically quite large. Sponge sticks are typically used to compress the IVC for hemostasis (Fig. 26.2). Venous control may also be achieved by intermittent clamping of the fistula from the arterial side, but Fogarty and Foley catheters may also be used. Control of the IVC may diminish venous return to the heart, and should be performed cautiously. Massive venous bleeding upon opening the aneurysm sac should alert the surgeon to an undiagnosed fistula, but can be generally easily controlled (Fig. 26.2).

Once control of the aorta has been achieved, repair of the fistula should be performed from within the aneurysm sac. Care should be taken not to manipulate the aneurysm as clot may be dislodged into the fistula and lead to a pulmonary embolus. The vein should be repaired first, usually by primary closure, but Teflon pledgets may be helpful. Next, the aortic aneurysm should be repaired with a standard aortic graft.

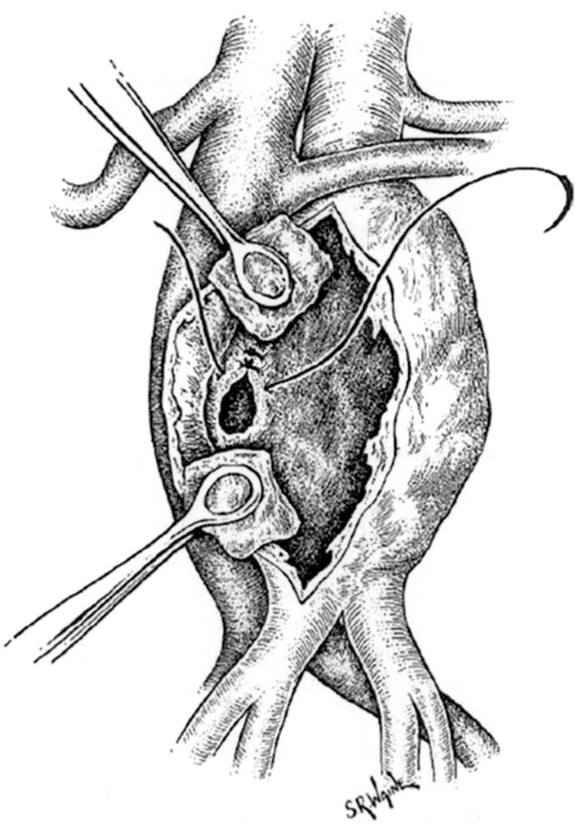

Fig. 26.2 Technique for controlling bleeding from an aortocaval fistula and fistula repair via an intra-aortic suture closure. (From Dardik et al. [3])

Rarely, aortocaval fistula is a complication of aortitis. If the surgical field is contaminated due to severe aortic infection, routine principles of vascular surgery are followed and the septic tissue should be debrided. The fistula is oversewn, the artery closed proximally and distally, and extra-anatomic arterial bypass performed. Once the abdomen is closed, a subcutaneous bypass can be placed in a clean surgical field to allow adequate perfusion of the legs. Alternatively, a prosthetic graft can be placed into the contaminated field after the aorta has been debrided and thoroughly irrigated with saline or antibiotic solution. An antibiotic-coated graft can be used, if available. Once the graft has been placed, an omental pedicle should be used to cover the graft.

Endovascular Repair

In patients who are suitable candidates for EVAR, preoperative diagnosis of an aortocaval fistula suggests consideration for simultaneous endovascular repair of the fistula. Given the relatively high operative mortality and morbidity of open repair, the EVAR option offers the potential benefits of decreased blood loss, virtually no chance for air embolus, decreased hospital stay, and a more rapid return to normal activities. Once anatomical suitability has been determined, typically by the presence of adequate proximal and distal sealing zones, then EVAR may be an acceptable approach for repair of an aneurysm with an IVC fistula [4, 5].

As with all aortic stent grafts, careful follow-up must be maintained to evaluate for endoleaks, as endoleaks can cause fistula reoccurrence [6–8]. However, isolated non-aneurysmal aortocaval fistulae represent a different disease process than AAA; the purpose of treatment in AAA is to prevent rupture, whereas in aortocaval fistulae, the primary measurement of success is restoration of normal physiology via the treatment of a large arteriovenous shunt [9]. This has implications for follow-up. In EVAR for AAA, the purpose of surveillance is to eliminate any endoleak that presents a risk for late rupture. Conversely, in aortocaval fistulae, a small, hemodynamically insignificant endoleak likely needs no treatment at all. It has been proposed that nonaneurysmal, aortocaval fistulae treated via EVAR can be followed adequately by yearly IVC duplex scanning; if elevated arterial velocities are not encountered, then the radiation and contrast of a CT can be eliminated, whereas abnormal duplex examinations should prompt a contrast CT or MR angiogram for additional study.

There have been reports of aortocaval fistula treatment with coil embolization, with coils placed into the midfistula tract [10]. This method is likely suitable only for very small fistulae with long fistula tracks. Large, short fistulae are high-flow phenomena. Endovascular coils placed in these high-flow communications carry a high risk of coil embolization to the lungs. Future endovascular solutions may involve occlusion devices, similar to the Amplatzer septal occluder or the Helex septal occluder device (W.L. Gore) used to treat intracardiac septal defects with large shunts; however, this is off-label and not currently considered to be standard of care; the potential for embolization of the device is unclear. Another endovascular repair option is placement of a covered stent across the inferior vena cava and iliac venous system; however, extensive iliocaval deep venous thrombosis remains a potential complication.

The endovascular treatment of aortocaval fistulae lacks long-term data to evaluate the outcome of this treatment modality. Most case reports have only a 1-year follow-up [8, 11], and randomized, controlled trials or multicenter studies are unlikely to ever be reported given the rarity of this condition. Nevertheless, endovascular options appear promising and deserve additional study.

A hybrid approach to aortocaval fistulae may be optimal in select patients. In patients with decompensated heart failure or cardiogenic shock, an aortic endograft may be placed first to allow for cardiac optimization, followed by an open repair of the fistula and endoleaks. Alternatively, endovascular balloon tamponade of the inferior vena cava from a transfemoral approach may also be utilized during open repair to decrease blood loss after opening the aneurysm sac.

Aortocaval fistula repair is traditionally associated with high mortality, approaching 50%. In the presence of persistent renal failure, the results are dismal. Aortocaval fistulae should be repaired as soon as possible after diagnosis in order to minimize end-organ damage from sustained high cardiac output. EVAR is a new approach to repair an aortocaval fistula and the associated aortic aneurysm, and will be considered more often as CT is used preoperatively to identify aortocaval fistulae. However, long-term data must be obtained to determine the durability of this technique.

References

1. Davis PM, Gloviczki P, Cherry KJ. Aorto-caval and ilio-iliac ateriovenous fistulae: rare and challenging problems. Am J Surg. 1998;176:115.
2. Phillips AW, Chaudhuri A, Meyer FJ. Bilateral long saphenous bruits: a marker of aortocaval fistula. Eur J Vasc Endovasc Surg. 2006;32:529–31.
3. Dardik H, Dardik I, Strom MG, Attai L, Carnevale N, Veith FJ. Intravenous rupture of arteriosclerotic aneurysms of the abdominal aorta. Surgery. 1976;80:647–51.
4. Orion K, et al. Aortocaval fistula: is endovascular repair the preferred solution? Ann Vasc Surg. 2016;31:221–8.
5. Esmat HA, Naseri MW. Endovascular management of aortocaval fistula complicating abdominal aortic aneurysm presenting as an acute renal failure. Ann Med Surg. 2021;62:477–80.
6. Maeda H, et al. Surgery for ruptured abdominal aortic aneurysm with an aortocaval and iliac vein fistula. Surg Today. 2007;37:445–8.
7. Pathak S, et al. Endovascular repair of a recurrent aortocaval fistula and anastamotic false aneurysm. Br J Radiol. 2006;79:e62–3.
8. Vetrhus M, et al. Endovascular repair of abdominal aortic aneurysms with aortocaval fistula. Eur J Vasc Endovasc Surg. 2005;30:640–3.
9. Dabbouseh NM, et al. Endovascular repair of delayed traumatic aortocaval fistula. J Vasc Surg Cases Innov Tech. 2019;5(4):467–71.
10. Kashyap VS, et al. Aortocaval fistula. J Am Coll Surg. 2006;203(5):780.
11. Waldrop JL Jr, Dart BW, Barker DE. Endovascular stent graft treatment of a traumatic aortocaval fistula. Ann Vasc Surg. 2005;19:562–5.

Chapter 27
Mesenteric Ischemia Following Abdominal Aortic Aneurysm Repair

Amanda C. Filiberto, Gilbert R. Upchurch Jr., and Michol Cooper

Introduction

Intestinal ischemia following abdominal aortic aneurysm (AAA) repair is a rare but highly morbid complication. It has been shown that increased attentiveness to prevent, detect, and intervene early on intestinal ischemia in the setting of AAA repair can decrease the incidence and mortality of this frequently lethal disease [1].

Definition

The term intestinal ischemia refers to a spectrum of disease. The common endoscopic grading system includes Grade I ischemia, which affects the mucosa and may lead to sloughing; Grade II ischemia, which penetrates the muscularis layer; and Grade III, or transmural ischemia, which includes gross bowel infarction.

Incidence

The reported incidence of postoperative intestinal ischemia varies from 0.5% to 4% for elective AAA (non-ruptured) repairs and from 4% to 23% for urgent/emergent AAA repairs [2]. The incidence of intestinal ischemia is higher with open repair as

A. C. Filiberto · G. R. Upchurch Jr. · M. Cooper (✉)
Department of Surgery, Division of Vascular Surgery and Endovascular Therapy, University of Florida College of Medicine, Gainesville, FL, USA
e-mail: Michol.cooper@surgery.ufl.edu

G. J. Arnaoutakis et al. (eds.), *Aortic Aneurysms*, Contemporary Cardiology, https://doi.org/10.1007/978-3-032-13134-8_27

compared with endovascular repair for both elective and emergent repairs [3, 4]. Open repair, emergency repair, perioperative hypotension, abdominal compartment syndrome, and female sex are known risk factors for developing intestinal ischemia after AAA repair [3–6].

Patients who undergo open repair of ruptured AAAs are at highest risk for intestinal ischemia, with an incidence of 10–36%, depending on whether the diagnosis is made based on clinical or endoscopic findings [3]. In a prospective study of 100 patients undergoing open AAA repair, Bast et al. found some degree of ischemia on routine postoperative colonoscopy in 4.5% patients who underwent elective repair as compared with 17.6% of patients who underwent emergent repair [7]. In a large series of 2196 patients who underwent both elective and emergent open AAA repair, Ultee et al. found that patients who developed intestinal ischemia were more likely to have longer operative time, blood loss greater than one liter, a suprarenal clamp, and reimplantation of the IMA [6].

For patients who undergo endovascular repair, a recent systematic review that included over 150,000 patients in 11 studies demonstrated a reduced incidence of intestinal ischemia in patients undergoing elective EVAR as compared with open repair (0.5–1% vs 2.1–3.6%, $p = .007$) [8]. Similar to open repair, Ultee et al. found that patients who underwent elective EVAR that developed intestinal ischemia were more likely to have a longer operative time, extensive blood loss, and intraoperative blood transfusion. Additionally, arterial injury (unspecified) and type III endoleak at completion occurred more often in those with bowel ischemia [6].

As with open repair for ruptured AAA, endovascular repair of ruptured AAA results in higher rates of intestinal ischemia compared to elective repair. In a study by Champagne et al. in which patients with ruptured AAA treated with endovascular repair underwent routine postoperative endoscopy, 23% showed evidence of intestinal ischemia, of which 8% required surgical intervention [9].

Mesenteric Arterial Anatomy

The mesenteric arterial system involves extensive collateralization (Fig. 27.1), such that chronic intestinal ischemia rarely occurs unless at least two of the three main mesenteric arteries are compromised. The celiac and the superior mesenteric artery (SMA) exchange collaterals via the pancreaticoduodenal and gastroduodenal arteries (Fig. 27.2). The SMA and the inferior mesenteric artery (IMA) collateralize via the marginal artery of Drummond, which joins the left branch of the SMA's middle colic artery to the ascending branch of the IMA's left colic artery (Figs. 27.3 and 27.4). In addition, the meandering mesenteric artery, also known as the central anastomotic artery, provides a route of direct collateralization between the trunks of the

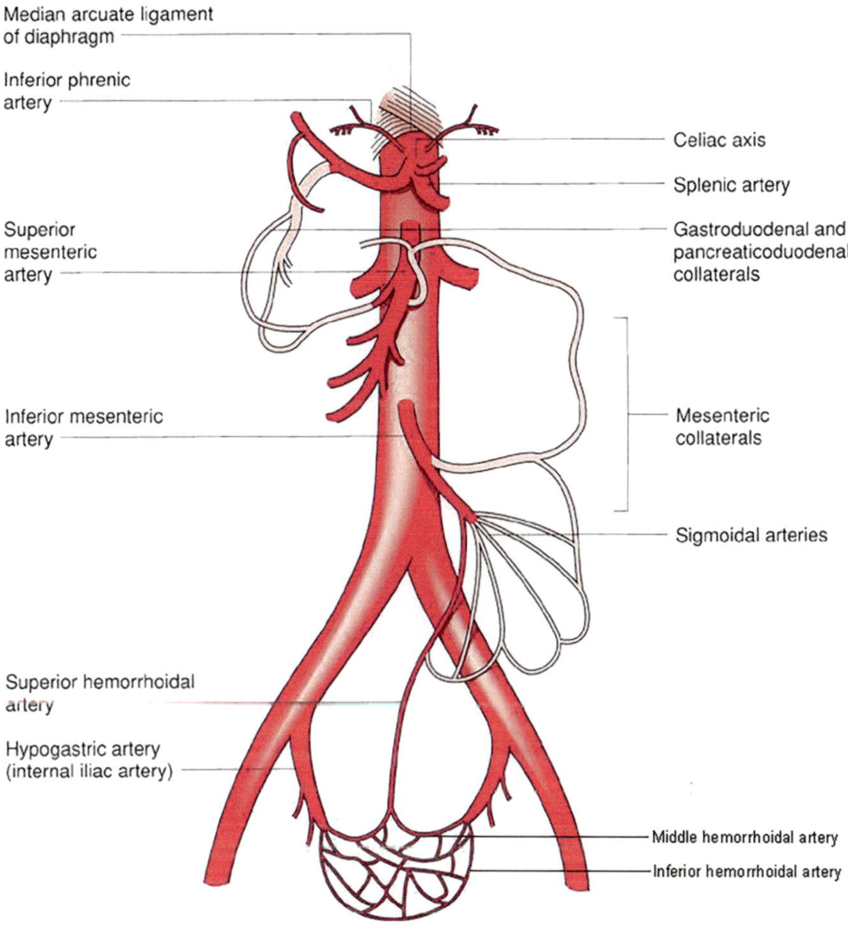

Fig. 27.1 Mesenteric collateral vessels. (Reproduced with permission from: Figure 94.4A. Greenfield's Surgery: Scientific Principles & Practice. Ed. Michael W. Mulholland, MD, PhD, et al. 4th ed. Philadelphia, PA: Lippincott Williams & Wilkins, 2006. http://thegreenfieldsolution.com)

SMA and IMA (Fig. 27.5). The IMA also collateralizes with the iliac system via the capillary network in the rectal wall, through which the IMA's superior hemorrhoidal artery exchanges with the middle and inferior hemorrhoidal branches of the internal iliac, or hypogastric, arteries (Figs. 27.1, 27.3 and 27.4). The internal iliac arteries receive collaterals from the external iliac, lumbar, and femoral arteries.

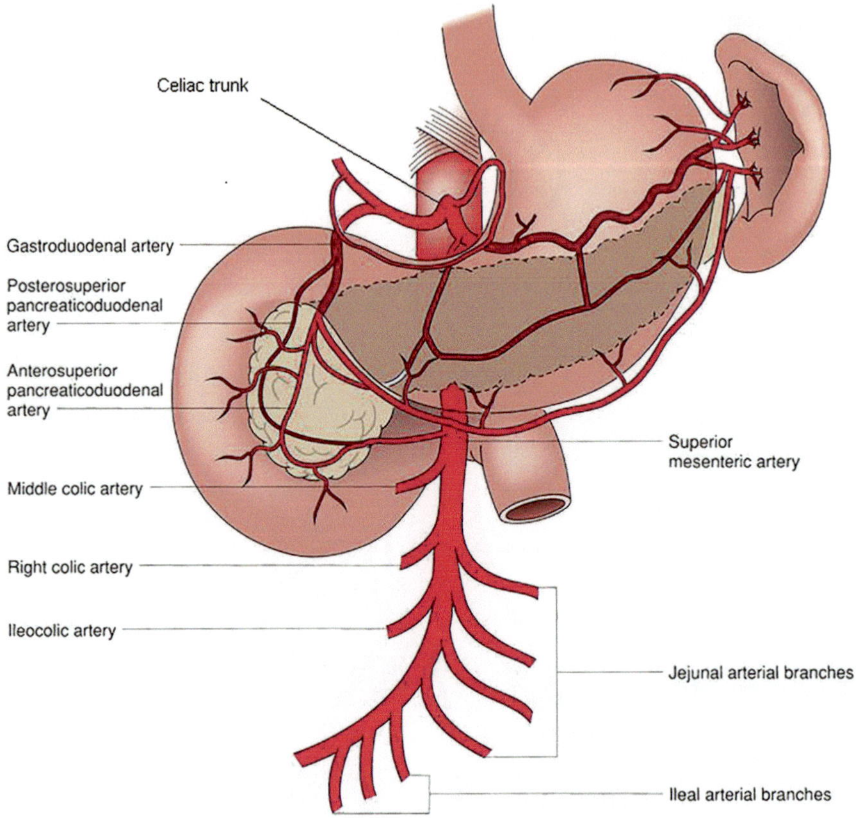

Fig. 27.2 Distribution of the celiac artery and SMA. (Reproduced with permission from: Figure 94.1. Greenfield's Surgery: Scientific Principles & Practice. Ed. Michael W. Mulholland, MD, PhD, et al. 4th ed. Philadelphia, PA: Lippincott Williams & Wilkins, 2006. http://thegreenfieldsolution.com)

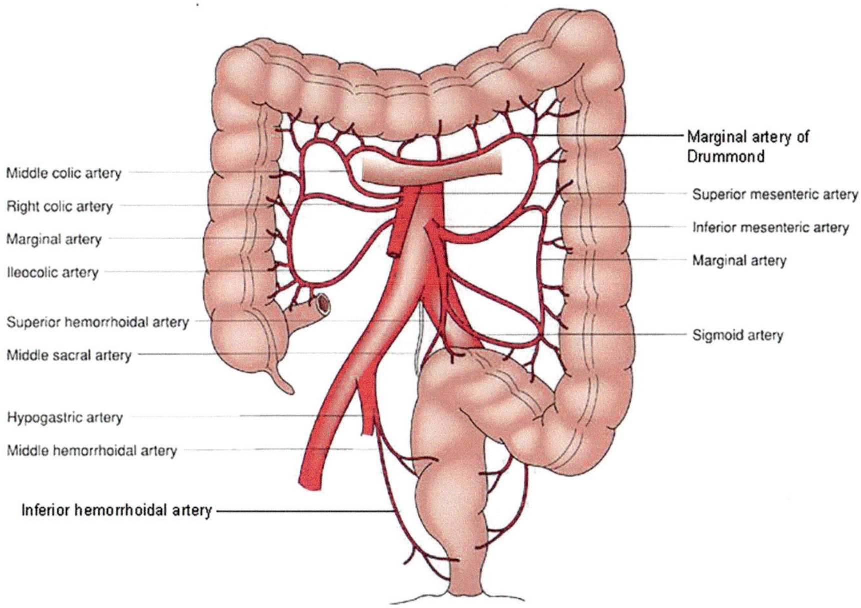

Fig. 27.3 Distribution of the SMA and IMA. (Reproduced with permission from: Figure 94.2. Greenfield's Surgery: Scientific Principles & Practice. Ed. Michael W. Mulholland, MD, PhD, et al. 4th ed. Philadelphia, PA: Lippincott Williams & Wilkins, 2006. http://thegreenfieldsolution.com)

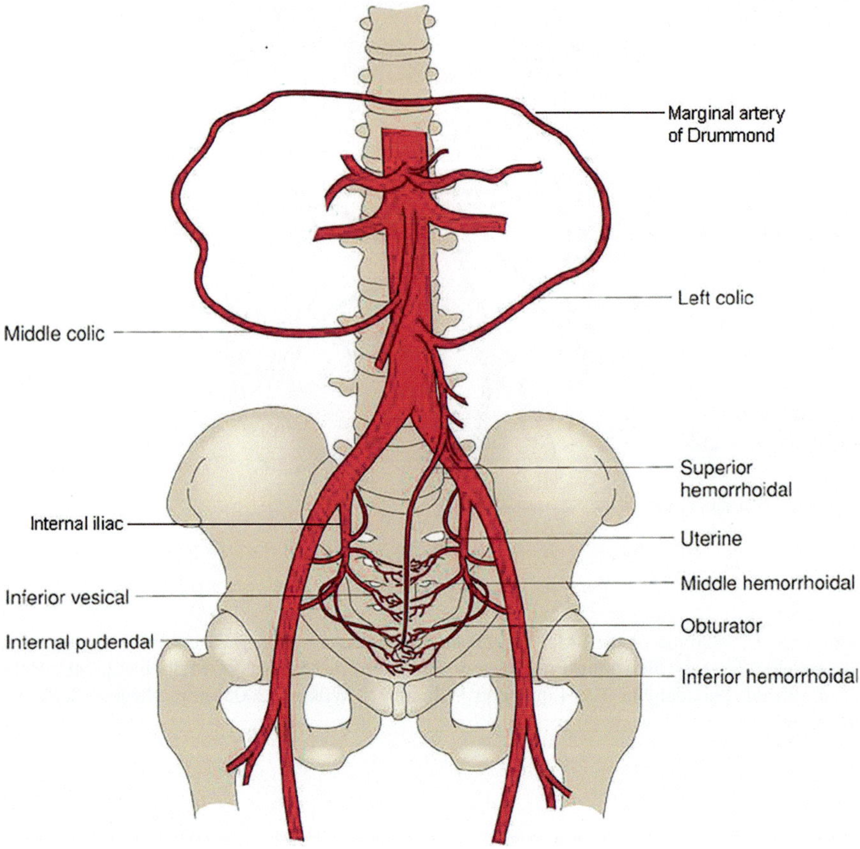

Fig. 27.4 Marginal artery of Drummond. (Reproduced with permission from: Figure 95.3. Greenfield's Surgery: Scientific Principles & Practice. Ed. Michael W. Mulholland, MD, PhD, et al. 4th ed. Philadelphia, PA: Lippincott Williams & Wilkins, 2006. http://thegreenfieldsolution.com)

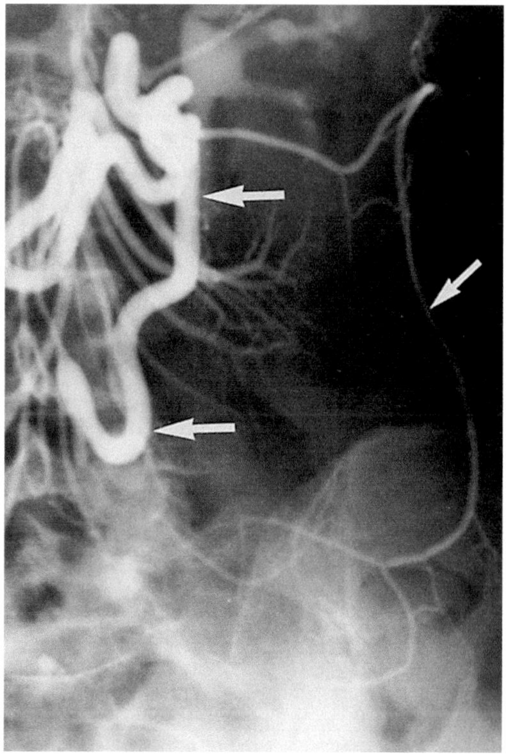

Fig. 27.5 Angiography demonstrates an enlarged IMA (black arrow) and meandering mesenteric artery (white arrow) in the setting of celiac and SMA occlusion. (Reproduced with permission from: Figure 94.16B. Greenfield's Surgery: Scientific Principles & Practice. Ed. Michael W. Mulholland, MD, PhD, et al. 4th ed. Philadelphia, PA: Lippincott Williams & Wilkins, 2006. http://thegreenfieldsolution.com)

Etiology

The etiologies of intestinal ischemia in the setting of AAA repair can be divided into anatomic, embolic and mechanical, and physiologic causes.

Anatomic

Given the collateral flow within the mesenteric arterial system, ligation or exclusion of the IMA, as often performed during AAA repair, should not compromise intestinal blood flow in the setting of otherwise non-diseased vessels. Patients with AAAs, however, often have coexistent atherosclerotic disease and, in the setting of diseased mesenteric vessels, ligation or exclusion of the IMA could be the critical event that precipitates overt bowel ischemia. In the setting of celiac stenosis, in which the SMA is the main source of blood flow to the stomach and duodenum via the pancreaticoduodenal collaterals, ligation or exclusion of the IMA, leaving the SMA as the primary source of blood supply to the entire gastrointestinal tract may be detrimental. In the setting of SMA stenosis, on the other hand, the role of the internal iliac arteries as collateral flow to the left colon gains importance if the IMA is ligated. During an endovascular AAA repair, an internal iliac artery and sometimes bilateral internal iliac arteries are sacrificed, which may put patients at risk for bowel ischemia if conscious steps are not taken to maintain flow to the left colon. In the setting of atherosclerosis of the IMA, the left colon receives most of its blood supply from other sources, including collaterals from the SMA or from the internal iliac arteries. Therefore, theoretically, ligation at the root of the IMA should not affect that supply to any great extent, provided that the collateral sources are left intact. Finally, in the setting of a previous right hemicolectomy where the collateral pathways from the SMA have been disrupted and the IMA is then covered/ligated during AAA repair, the patient is at risk for descending and sigmoid colonic ischemia.

Embolic and Mechanical

Embolization of atherosclerotic plaque during aortic clamping in open AAA repair, or during intraluminal stent manipulation in endovascular repair, is another factor that may play an important role in intestinal ischemia. This has been evidenced by histologic review of the pathology specimens of patients who underwent surgical intervention for bowel ischemia in the setting of endovascular AAA repair [9]. In the case of open AAA repair, compression of or damage to mesenteric vessels by retractors is also a potential cause of bowel ischemia.

Physiologic and Intraoperative

Physiologic factors alone, including intra- or perioperative hypotension, hypovolemia, or use of pressors, might be sufficient to precipitate intestinal ischemia. Piotrowski et al. published findings suggesting that preoperative shock was the most important risk factor for colon ischemia following open repair of ruptured AAA, while large intraoperative blood loss was also predictive [10]. In contrast, a study by Meissner et al. found no correlation between intestinal ischemia following ruptured AAA repair and either perioperative shock or volume administration, but documented that low perioperative cardiac output and use of alpha adrenergic pressors were predictive [11]. Additionally, during open surgery aortic cross-clamping has been shown to cause ischemia and reperfusion injury. This was demonstrated in one study that found a threefold increase in colonic mucosal apoptosis in biopsies obtained immediately after open AAA repair as compared to those who underwent EVAR [12].

Diagnosis and Management

Diagnosis

For intraoperative detection of inadequate intestinal perfusion during AAA repair, several methods have been proposed. Other than in cases of gross ischemia or infarction, visual inspection of the bowel is generally inadequate to recognize malperfusion. Management of the IMA appears critical. Relatively simple adjuncts to determine the safety of IMA ligation versus the need for implantation into the aortic graft include Doppler ultrasound of the relevant mesenteric vessels [13], endoluminal pulse oximetry of the bowel wall [14], or laser Doppler monitoring of serosal blood flow [15, 16] following IMA occlusion. Each of these methods has demonstrated good sensitivity in small, non-randomized studies, but has not been universally adopted. Intravenous fluorescein injection followed by Wood's lamp examination of the bowel wall [17], intraperitoneal xenon injection followed by gamma-activity monitoring [18], and measurement of intraluminal pH [19] are other methods that have been proposed. However, none of these methods have been universally implemented due to need for specialized equipment and lack of validation in the literature.

The classic presenting sign of intestinal ischemia following AAA repair is hematochezia. Common symptoms, such as abdominal pain out of proportion to physical examination, may be masked by the use of epidural anesthesia or intravenous narcotics; while fever, leukocytosis, lactic acidosis, or general sepsis are less specific signs that may be confounded by the physiologic changes associated with the operation itself. Postoperative diarrhea, whether bloody or not, is uncommon following AAA repair, and should lead to a high index for suspicion of colon ischemia with urgent consideration of sigmoidoscopy. Liberal use of endoscopy has been suggested to avoid the catastrophic event of intestinal infarction. In the setting of ruptured AAA repair, several authors have advocated for the routine use of postoperative endoscopy in the first 24–48 h following surgery. Vascular surgeons at Case Medical Center instituted routine colonoscopy following open ruptured AAA repair, with improved mortality rates for ischemic colitis that they attributed to earlier diagnosis and treatment [20]. In a second study, these authors instituted the same mandate for endovascular repair of ruptured AAA [9]. While an effect on mortality was not documented due to the lack of a comparison group, it is notable that among the patients in the study found to have any degree of intestinal ischemia, not a single death occurred during the 30-day follow-up. The effects on outcome of routine endoscopy

Table 27.1 Management of intestinal ischemia

Grade I	Grade II	Grade III
Supportive management: optimization of fluid status, bowel rest, empiric antibiotics, serial abdominal examinations, consideration of follow-up endoscopy	Supportive management: lower threshold for follow-up endoscopy; contrast enema to evaluate for intestinal strictures after the acute phase of ischemia has resolved	Urgent exploratory laparotomy

after ruptured AAA repair await more rigorous examination to determine whether this strategy should become common practice.

Of note, flexible sigmoidoscopy, as opposed to full colonoscopy, is usually sufficient to diagnose intestinal ischemia, as the rectosigmoid colon is involved in 95% of cases in which intestinal ischemia occurs [21].

Management

Management of intestinal ischemia varies with endoscopic findings (Table 27.1). Mucosal ischemia alone (i.e., grade I), associated with a near-zero mortality rate, generally warrants only supportive management, including optimization of fluid status, bowel rest, empiric antibiotics, serial abdominal examinations, and repeat endoscopy to confirm resolution or evaluate for progression that may warrant more aggressive management. With more advanced ischemia that penetrates the muscularis propria (grade II), recovery also commonly occurs with conservative management alone. Patients with grade II ischemia, however, are at risk of developing strictures as the bowel wall heals, and therefore they should undergo contrast enema once the acute phase of ischemia has resolved. Finally, transmural involvement of the bowel (grade III) requires urgent laparotomy. Even in the setting of prompt operation, mortality rates are as high as 90%, generally due to sepsis and multisystem organ failure.

Recommendations

Preoperative Planning

Preoperative assessment of the patency and dominance of the celiac, SMA, IMA, and internal iliac arteries is essential prior to AAA repair. A complete history and physical examination should be obtained to detect any history of symptoms suggesting mesenteric ischemia, such as post-prandial pain, unintentional weight loss, or food fear. In most cases, CT angiography (CTA) is adequate to assess the characteristics and measurements of the aortic aneurysm and the relationship to visceral and renal arteries, as well as the patency of the visceral vessels themselves. Compromise of any one or combination of the mesenteric arteries may require a more unique operative plan, varying from IMA implantation into the aortic graft, to internal iliac artery bypass, to a more complex reconstruction involving the celiac or SMA or SMA stenting.

Treatment of the IMA

A study from Massachusetts General Hospital of 2137 patients undergoing infrarenal abdominal aortic reconstruction cited ligation of a patent IMA as the most common factor found to be present, at a rate of 74%, in patients who developed colon ischemia following open abdominal aortic surgery [22]. Implantation of the IMA into the aortic graft, therefore, has been proposed to lessen the risk of intestinal ischemia. This, however, remains theoretical and there are few studies to support implantation of the IMA. Senekowitsch et al. performed a study in which 128 patients were prospectively, randomly assigned to undergo IMA ligation or implantation during infrarenal aortic aneurysm repair [23]. There were no significant differences in rates of ischemic colitis as diagnosed by routine postoperative colonoscopy and biopsy sampling. In a recent retrospective study of 700 patients undergoing open elective infrarenal AAA repair, IMA reimplantation was actually found to be a significant predictor of ischemic colitis and wound complications on multivariable analysis [24]. Therefore, the role of IMA reimplantation remains to be identified, but should be considered in certain subsets of patients, such as in the patient with an SMA stenosis and a large IMA supplying the majority of intestinal blood flow (Fig. 27.5). For purposes of assessing benefit in more subtle cases, measurement of IMA stump pressure has been proposed, with a pressure of at least 40 mm Hg thought to be sufficient to allow for safe ligation [25]. In practice, however, simple visual inspection of IMA backflow is usually employed. When the IMA must be ligated without implantation, it is recommended that ligation be performed at the wall of the aorta in order to avoid interruption of any proximal collateral vessels.

Treatment of the Internal Iliac Arteries

In a study of 2196 patients undergoing open repair for ruptured AAA, hypogastric ligation was found to be associated with a higher rate of intestinal ischemia [6]. Therefore, it has been hypothesized that maintaining patency of one or both internal iliac arteries lessens the risk of bowel compromise. Multiple retrospective studies, however, have demonstrated that unilateral or bilateral internal iliac artery interruption can be performed during either endovascular or open AAA repair without inducing buttock necrosis or colon ischemia requiring operation [26, 27]. However, for this to be successful the following must occur: [1] the internal iliac arteries are

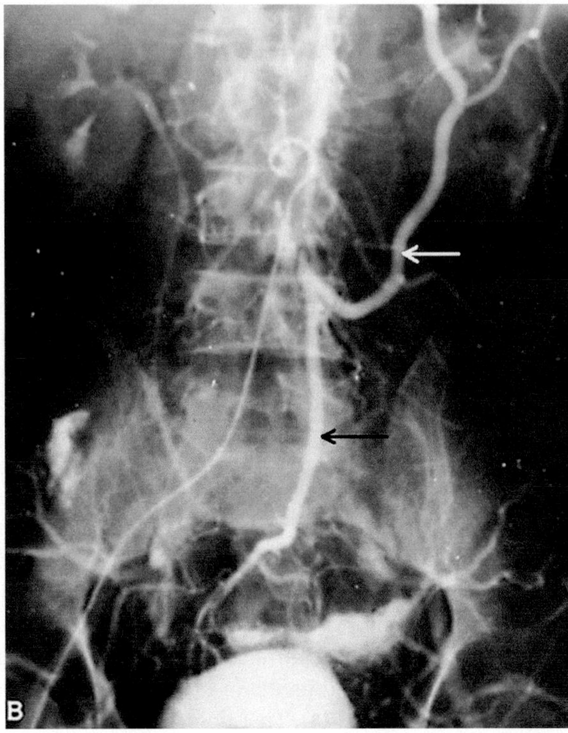

Fig. 27.6 Selective inferior mesenteric artery angiography demonstrates the marginal artery of Drummond (single arrow, image right) and the larger meandering mesenteric artery, or central anastomotic artery (paired arrows, image left). (Reproduced with permission from: Figure 94.3. Greenfield's Surgery: Scientific Principles & Practice. Ed. Michael W. Mulholland, MD, PhD, et al. 4th ed. Philadelphia, PA: Lippincott Williams & Wilkins, 2006. http://thegreenfieldsolution.com)

interrupted as proximally as possible, ideally at their origin, in order to maintain distal collateral flow from the external iliac and femoral arteries; [2] distal embolization is avoided; and [3] ligation, when bilateral, is performed in a staged fashion (Fig. 27.6).

Conclusion

Intestinal ischemia following AAA repair is a highly morbid, but potentially preventable complication in the elective setting. Vigilance on the part of the surgeon and perioperative team is essential. Appropriate preoperative planning, procedural execution, and postoperative monitoring are critical to allow for timely diagnosis and intervention in order to decrease the incidence and mortality of this otherwise deadly complication.

References

1. Zelenock GB, Strodel WE, Knol JA, Messina LM, Wakefield TW, Lindenauer SM, et al. A prospective study of clinically and endoscopically documented colonic ischemia in 100 patients undergoing aortic reconstructive surgery with aggressive colonic and direct pelvic revascularization, compared with historic controls. Surgery. 1989;106(4):771–9; discussion 9–80.
2. Behrendt CA, Riess HC, Schwaneberg T, Larena-Avellaneda A, Kolbel T, Tsilimparis N, et al. Incidence, predictors, and outcomes of colonic ischaemia in abdominal aortic aneurysm repair. Eur J Vasc Endovasc Surg. 2018;56(4):507–13.
3. Becquemin JP, Majewski M, Fermani N, Marzelle J, Desgrandes P, Allaire E, et al. Colon ischemia following abdominal aortic aneurysm repair in the era of endovascular abdominal aortic repair. J Vasc Surg. 2008;47(2):258–63; discussion 63.
4. Willemsen SI, Ten Berge MG, Statius van Eps RG, Veger HTC, van Overhagen H, van Dijk LC, et al. Nationwide study to predict colonic ischemia after abdominal aortic aneurysm repair in the Netherlands. Ann Vasc Surg. 2021;73:407–16.
5. Lee MJ, Daniels SL, Drake TM, Adam IJ. Risk factors for ischaemic colitis after surgery for abdominal aortic aneurysm: a systematic review and observational meta-analysis. Int J Color Dis. 2016;31(7):1273–81.
6. Ultee KH, Zettervall SL, Soden PA, Darling J, Bertges DJ, Verhagen HJ, et al. Incidence of and risk factors for bowel ischemia after abdominal aortic aneurysm repair. J Vasc Surg. 2016;64(5):1384–91.
7. Bast TJ, van der Biezen JJ, Scherpenisse J, Eikelboom BC. Ischaemic disease of the colon and rectum after surgery for abdominal aortic aneurysm: a prospective study of the incidence and risk factors. Eur J Vasc Surg. 1990;4(3):253–7.
8. Williamson JS, Ambler GK, Twine CP, Williams IM, Williams GL. Elective repair of abdominal aortic aneurysm and the risk of colonic ischaemia: systematic review and meta-analysis. Eur J Vasc Endovasc Surg. 2018;56(1):31–9.
9. Champagne BJ, Lee EC, Valerian B, Mulhotra N, Mehta M. Incidence of colonic ischemia after repair of ruptured abdominal aortic aneurysm with endograft. J Am Coll Surg. 2007;204(4):597–602.
10. Piotrowski JJ, Ripepi AJ, Yuhas JP, Alexander JJ, Brandt CP. Colonic ischemia: the Achilles heel of ruptured aortic aneurysm repair. Am Surg. 1996;62(7):557–60; discussion 60–1.
11. Meissner MH, Johansen KH. Colon infarction after ruptured abdominal aortic aneurysm. Arch Surg. 1992;127(8):979–85.
12. Ghosh J, Khwaja N, Howarth V, Murray D, Murphy MO, Byers R, et al. Colonic epithelial apoptosis during conventional and endoluminal aortic surgery. Br J Surg. 2005;92(1):113–8.
13. Hobson RW 2nd, Wright CB, Rich NM, Collins GJ Jr. Assessment of colonic ischemia during aortic surgery by Doppler ultrasound. J Surg Res. 1976;20(3):231–5.
14. Yilmaz EN, Vahl AC, van Rij G, Nauta SH, Brom HL, Rauwerda JA. Endoluminal pulse oximetry of the sigmoid colon and the monitoring of the colonic circulation. Cardiovasc Surg. 1999;7(7):704–9.
15. Krohg-Sorensen K, Kvernebo K. Laser Doppler flowmetry in evaluation of colonic blood flow during aortic reconstruction. Eur J Vasc Surg. 1989;3(1):37–41.
16. Sakakibara Y, Jikuya T, Saito EM, Mitsui T, Ijima H. Does laser Doppler flowmetry aid the prevention of ischemic colitis in abdominal aortic aneurysm surgery? Thorac Cardiovasc Surg. 1997;45(1):32–4.

17. Bergman RT, Gloviczki P, Welch TJ, Naessens JM, Bower TC, Hallett JW Jr, et al. The role of intravenous fluorescein in the detection of colon ischemia during aortic reconstruction. Ann Vasc Surg. 1992;6(1):74–9.
18. Gharagozloo F, Bulkley GB, Zuidema GD, O'Mara CS, Alderson PO. The use of intraperitoneal xenon for early diagnosis of acute mesenteric ischemia. Surgery. 1984;95(4):404–11.
19. Fiddian-Green RG, Amelin PM, Herrmann JB, Arous E, Cutler BS, Schiedler M, et al. Prediction of the development of sigmoid ischemia on the day of aortic operations. Indirect measurements of intramural pH in the colon. Arch Surg. 1986;121(6):654–60.
20. Champagne BJ, Darling RC 3rd, Daneshmand M, Kreienberg PB, Lee EC, Mehta M, et al. Outcome of aggressive surveillance colonoscopy in ruptured abdominal aortic aneurysm. J Vasc Surg. 2004;39(4):792–6.
21. Bjorck M, Bergqvist D, Troeng T. Incidence and clinical presentation of bowel ischaemia after aortoiliac surgery—2930 operations from a population-based registry in Sweden. Eur J Vasc Endovasc Surg. 1996;12(2):139–44.
22. Brewster DC, Franklin DP, Cambria RP, Darling RC, Moncure AC, Lamuraglia GM, et al. Intestinal ischemia complicating abdominal aortic surgery. Surgery. 1991;109(4):447–54.
23. Senekowitsch C, Assadian A, Assadian O, Hartleb H, Ptakovsky H, Hagmuller GW. Replanting the inferior mesentery artery during infrarenal aortic aneurysm repair: influence on postoperative colon ischemia. J Vasc Surg. 2006;43(4):689–94.
24. Lee KB, Lu J, Macsata RA, Patel D, Yang A, Ricotta JJ, et al. Inferior mesenteric artery replantation does not decrease the risk of ischemic colitis after open infrarenal abdominal aortic aneurysm repair. J Vasc Surg. 2019;69(6):1825–30.
25. Ernst CB, Hagihara PF, Daugherty ME, Griffen WO Jr. Inferior mesenteric artery stump pressure: a reliable index for safe IMA ligation during abdominal aortic aneurysmectomy. Ann Surg. 1978;187(6):641–6.
26. Dadian N, Ohki T, Veith FJ, Edelman M, Mehta M, Lipsitz EC, et al. Overt colon ischemia after endovascular aneurysm repair: the importance of microembolization as an etiology. J Vasc Surg. 2001;34(6):986–96.
27. Mehta M, Veith FJ, Ohki T, Cynamon J, Goldstein K, Suggs WD, et al. Unilateral and bilateral hypogastric artery interruption during aortoiliac aneurysm repair in 154 patients: a relatively innocuous procedure. J Vasc Surg. 2001;33(2 Suppl):S27–32.

Chapter 28
Evaluation and Treatment of Isolated Common Iliac Artery Aneurysms

Karthik Bhat and Guillermo A. Escobar

Introduction

The majority of iliac artery aneurysms are associated with abdominal aortic aneurysms (AAAs), whereas isolated common (or internal) iliac artery aneurysms are uncommon whereas primary external iliac arteries are very rare. Common and external iliac arteries greater than 1.8 cm in diameter and hypogastric arteries greater that 0.8 cm are aneurysms [1]. Isolated iliac artery aneurysms are very uncommon with an estimated prevalence of ≤2% [2, 3] and usually consist of the common or internal iliac artery. Approximately 10% of AAAs will have a coexisting iliac artery aneurysm most often involving the common iliac artery [4, 5].

Iliac artery aneurysms are found unilateral or bilateral with equal frequency and are more common in older males. Frequency of isolated iliac aneurysms is 70% common iliac (Fig. 28.1) and 20% internal iliac (rarely in the external iliac) [6]. The risk factors and pathogenesis of common and internal iliac artery aneurysms are degenerative, similar to that of AAA, and most are diagnosed incidentally in asymptomatic patients [4, 6]. However, true aneurysms of the external iliac artery are extremely rare and nearly all cases will be in patients with either an underlying genetic disorder affecting the walls of the vessel (see below) or are infected (mycotic). A syndrome seen primarily in competitive cyclists is endofibrosis where the external (and common) iliac artery can develop fibrosis and stenosis and/or "post-stenotic" aneurysms which all require open reconstruction. Aneurysms of the external iliac artery that followed trauma, intervention (especially percutaneous access), or surgery (often reported after urology, orthopedic, oncologic, or transplant surgeries) are usually pseudoaneurysms where the vessel wall is disrupted

K. Bhat · G. A. Escobar (✉)
Division of Vascular Surgery and Endovascular Therapy, Emory University, Atlanta, GA, USA
e-mail: karthik.r.bhat@emory.edu; guillermo.escobar@emory.edu

G. J. Arnaoutakis et al. (eds.), *Aortic Aneurysms*, Contemporary Cardiology, https://doi.org/10.1007/978-3-032-13134-8_28

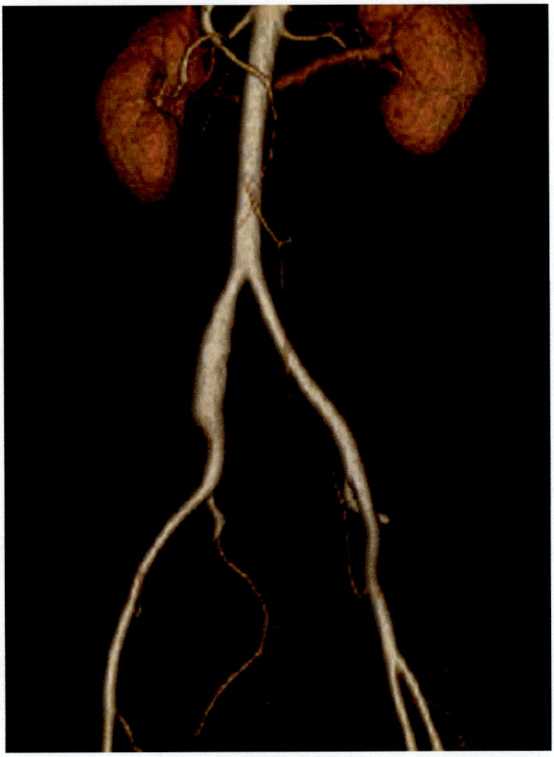

Fig. 28.1 Isolated right-sided common iliac artery aneurysm

with blood outside the vessel walls, but somewhat contained by the surrounding retroperitoneal tissue.

Other etiologies of iliac artery aneurysms include blunt trauma, multiparous-related, and autoimmune diseases. The latter include Behçet's disease, Kawasaki syndrome, Takayasu's arteritis, and Hughes-Stovin syndrome. Post-stenotic iliac artery dilatations secondary to occlusive disease (or endofibrosis) may also acquire aneurysmal dimensions, but these are usually not very large and tend to have a more benign growth rate. Genetic disorders affecting vessel wall, particularly Ehlers-Danlos syndrome type IV (Vascular-type) and Marfan's syndrome, can have isolated (primary or secondary to dissection) iliac artery aneurysms of all three iliacs [1, 4, 7, 8]. Anastomotic pseudoaneurysms of the iliac arteries are not uncommon at the site of a graft anastomosis after aortoiliac reconstruction or iliac-to-femoral bypasses.

Natural History and Risk of Rupture

The natural history of primary iliac artery aneurysms is to progressively enlarge and rupture. Untreated, small (<3 cm) isolated iliac artery aneurysms are estimated to grow at a rate of about 0.5–1.1 mm/year, but may expand at a faster pace (over

2.6 mm/year) when larger than 3 cm [3, 9]. The risk of rupture of iliac artery aneurysm can approach 75% when they reach 5 cm in diameter [9, 10]. Elective repair generally offers a good operative outcome with a low morbidity and mortality. On the other hand, ruptured iliac artery aneurysms carry a high mortality rate similar to that of ruptured AAA (~40%) [4, 6, 10]. Atherosclerotic internal iliac artery aneurysms are thought to present with rupture 40% of the time and have an overall mortality of 31% [6, 11]. The highest risk of iliac aneurysm rupture is in patients with connective tissue diseases such as vascular-type Ehlers-Danlos syndrome type IV (Sack-Barabas syndrome). In addition, operative or endovascular repair of these aneurysms can be very challenging due to their vessels' fragility and often require multiple interventions during their hospitalization [12, 13].

Diagnostic Evaluation

At the time of diagnosis, over half of iliac artery aneurysms are asymptomatic. Internal iliac artery aneurysms tend to be larger at the time of diagnosis and historically were more likely to have clinical manifestations such as pelvic pain, ureteral obstruction (including ipsilateral hydronephrosis), rectal discomfort, arterioenteric fistulae with hematochezia, and aneurysm rupture. Most modern series show that all iliac artery aneurysms are most often found to be asymptomatic and serendipitously found on imaging for other causes. Common and external iliac artery aneurysms are mostly asymptomatic but rarely present with pain, claudication, palpable pulsatile masses, distal embolization, fistulization into the iliac veins, and spontaneous rupture. Iliac artery aneurysms occasionally present with lower limb swelling or deep vein thrombosis secondary to a mass-effect compression of the iliac and pelvic veins [4, 7, 11, 14]. Physical examination of thin patients with iliac aneurysms may reveal a pulsatile mass or bruit in the lower abdomen or abnormal pulsation during a rectal examination (with large internal iliac aneurysms).

Ultrasonography, computed tomography angiography (CTA), digital subtraction angiography, and MRA are useful in the diagnosis of iliac aneurysms, while CTA is the most commonly used for preoperative case planning.

Ultrasound is the screening test of choice, albeit limited by bowel gas and/or severe obesity which makes imaging the pelvic vessels difficult, if not impossible [15, 16]. Nevertheless, when ultrasound is technically feasible, it is very accurate in sizing iliac aneurysms when compared to CTA [9]. CTA is perhaps the optimal imaging modality for evaluating iliac aneurysms, and certainly the test of choice in preparation for surgical or endovascular repair. There is an exponential growth in the technology of this imaging modality. Angiography is in general inadequate to size iliac aneurysms because of the presence of mural thrombus, but may be helpful in some cases to delineate the arterial anatomy in patients with very tortuous vessels.

Repair of Iliac Artery Aneurysms

Iliac artery aneurysms noted at the time of repair of an AAA should be repaired simultaneously if they are >2.5 cm in diameter to prevent aneurysmal growth if left untreated [9, 17, 18]. Isolated iliac artery aneurysms without an associated aortic aneurysm should be repaired when they reach 3–3.5 cm in diameter or if they become symptomatic [9]. Symptoms are an important indication as most iliac aneurysms that rupture are preceded by pain [9, 10].

The first recorded surgical treatment of an iliac artery aneurysm was in 1827 by Valentine Mott. It consisted in the successful blind ligation of the common iliac artery in an awake patient [19]. While much experience has been accumulated with the open surgical repair of iliac aneurysms, there is a paucity of long-term data on endovascular approaches. For this reason, open repair offers the greatest assurance of a lasting repair and is ideal in patients who are at low risk and/or young although the short-term morbidity may be greater.

Patients who are at high risk for open repair, technically difficult to access (obese or reoperations), and/or relatively older are best served with an endovascular approach. Technical considerations that may exclude patients from endovascular therapy include lack of adequate vascular access and absence of landing zones in the arterial segments proximal or distal to the aneurysm. In addition, extreme tortuosity or angulation of the iliac anatomy may also preclude endovascular intervention.

Special consideration must be taken for patients with Ehlers-Danlos syndrome type IV (Sack-Barabas syndrome) who may require both open and endovascular approaches due to the high risk of rupture and reintervention [12, 13].

Endovascular has become the procedure of choice for most AAAs and concurrent IAAs, allowing treatment of both, even in cases with bilateral iliac artery aneurysms (Fig. 28.2). Advances in endovascular technique through the development of iliac branched devices (IBD), pioneered by the Cook Zenith Platform and subsequently by WL Gore and Jotech, have shown excellent technical success in early and midterm patency [20].

Open Surgical Repair

Bilateral iliac aneurysms are best approached by a midline transperitoneal approach. Bilateral common iliac arteries are typically treated with a bifurcated graft from the distal infrarenal aorta to the distal, non-aneurysmal vessel. A decision must be made if the internal iliac artery is to be ligated or included in the reconstruction. If the aneurysm includes the common or internal iliac, then, the first graft is anastomosed from the aorta to the deeper, internal iliac artery in an end-to-end fashion. A "jump" graft is then sewn off the anterior portion of that graft to the external iliac artery to complete reconstruction of the iliac arteries. Care must be taken to identify and spare the ureters and iliac veins, especially in cases of inflammatory aneurysms or

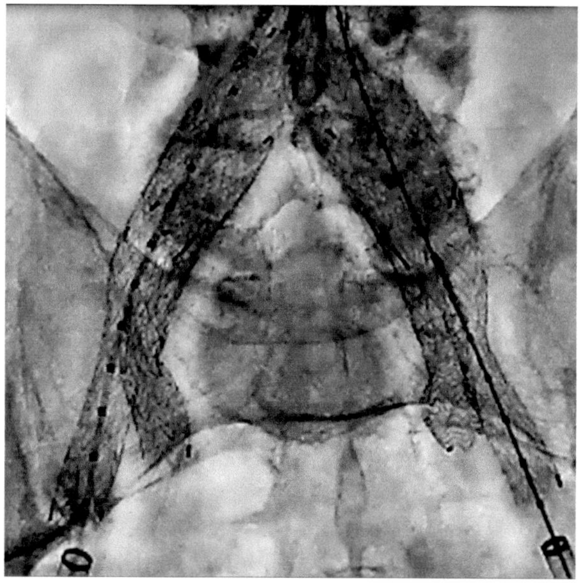

Fig. 28.2 Treatment of bilateral iliac aneurysms using bilateral iliac branch devices, docked into an aortic endograft

re-explorations. Preoperative placement of ureteral stents may be helpful in identifying, preventing (and treating) ureteral injuries.

Unilateral iliac aneurysms are ideally repaired via an ipsilateral retroperitoneal approach and are also replaced with a prosthetic graft as above. The aneurysm can usually be replaced with an end-to-end anastomosis from the proximal (normal) iliac or aorta. If the aneurysm includes the origin of the internal iliac artery, then the latter can be ligated as proximally as possible as long as the contralateral one is widely patent. In younger, physically and sexually active patients, revascularization of the hypogastric artery is advisable (if technically feasible) to prevent the above-mentioned complications. In addition, care to minimize dissection of the common iliac artery and minimal division of the splanchnic nerves that envelop it will minimize sexual dysfunction in males.

Endovascular Repair

Experience with endovascular treatment of iliac artery aneurysms has expanded dramatically in the last decade. Patients who can undergo endovascular reconstruction (especially if they have significant open operative risk) are ideal candidates because it offers a less invasive approach, lower periprocedural morbidity, and much faster recovery [21]. Commercially available bifurcated grafts are available for this repair, and are referred to as "iliac branch devices" (IBD). However, they are not designed to treat isolated iliac artery aneurysms, rather they were created to compliment treating AAA with associated iliac aneurysms and thus, the IBD are designed to anchor inside an AAA endograft. Device options in the world include Cook medical Iliac branched device (straight, helical, or bifurcated configurations) (Bloomington, Indiana), Gore Excluder Iliac Branch Endoprosthesis (IBE) (Flagstaff, Arizona), and the Jotec E-liac stent system (Hechingen, Germany) although only the first two are available in the United States [20]. IBD have been used in patients without an aortic endograft in special cases where the anatomy allows for a good seal (Fig. 28.3) and/or other endovascular options are possible when an IBD are not a possibility. Important considerations and factors leading to technical failure include concomitant aneurysms, diameters and distance of iliac arteries, internal iliac ostial disease, presence of internal iliac aneurysm, landing zones, angulation, tortuosity, and presence of calcification [20]. Immediate technical success has been reported between 86% and 100% and early outcomes show IBD have limited perioperative morbidity. The main reason for technical failure was complex anatomy. Factors resulting in perioperative morbidity in the immediate to early period were iliac artery occlusion, rupture, and medical complications. 30-day mortality was 0–1% [20].

Other endovascular approaches to treat common and internal iliac artery aneurysms without an IBD include [22]:

Internal iliac occlusion/embolization with intentional stent graft from the common iliac to the external iliac (excluding flow to the internal iliac).

Placement of 2 parallel stent grafts starting in the common iliac artery and one sealing in the internal and the other in the external iliac artery.

A hybrid open/endo option which includes occluding flow into the common iliac artery on the affected side, followed by a femoral-femoral bypass and retrograde stenting from the external iliac artery into the ipsilateral internal iliac artery.

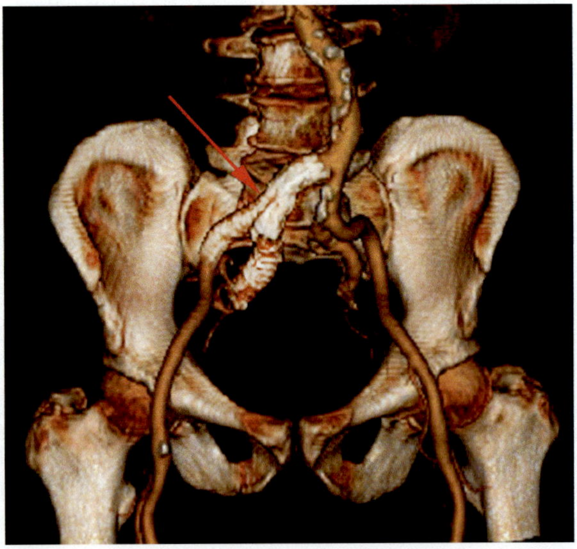

Fig. 28.3 Off-label use of an Iliac branch device as a stand-alone treatment for common iliac and/or internal iliac artery aneurysms when the aorta is normal and the iliac anatomy is favorable

Occlusion of one or both internal iliac arteries is associated with complications secondary to pelvic flow disruption resulting in buttock claudication, thigh claudication, erectile dysfunction, or less commonly in gluteal necrosis, perineal necrosis, ischemic colitis, and even spinal cord ischemia. At least one of these complications is found in 50% of people with unilateral internal iliac occlusion, and up to 80% in bilateral occlusion [2, 20]. Complications cited for endograft exclusion of iliac artery aneurysms include endograft thrombosis, migration of the graft, and continued aneurysm expansion; all of which may require subsequent operative repair [23–25].

Midterm results of the first commercially available IBD show that in 196 patients treated with the Cook device success was 85–100% with no aneurysm-related mortality. However, 24/196 patients had branch occlusions and half with buttock claudication when they used their Cook-made iliac stent [26]. Parlani et al. reviewed their own long-term experience in 100 patients using the Zenith Cook device and found internal iliac branch patency of 91.4% at 5 years, and freedom from any reintervention rate was 81.4% at 5 years. Physician-modified IBDs reported by Oderich et al. had a technical success and patency of 100% in their small series [27]. In the United States, there is only access to the IBD made by Gore (released in 2016) and Cook (released in 2025), but a propensity-matched comparison of outcomes between the original Cook and the Gore endografts in 190 IBD showed no difference and nearly 100% success, patency and freedom of aneurysm-related rupture [28]. Since Cook's original experience was marred with complications from their home-grown internal iliac bridging stentgraft, Cook partnered with a different balloon-expandible stent-graft for their latest release (iCast/Advanta V12; GETINGE Göteborg Sweden) and has published a 90% primary patency during their 5-year PRESERVE II study [29].

Knowledge of endovascular repair of iliac artery aneurysms has improved greatly over the past decade. Mid-term and long-term results are encouraging but device complications, including endoleaks and occlusions, are still present. Meticulous preoperative planning with cross-sectional imaging (CTA) and software with centerline of flow and careful patient selection are of utmost importance of minimize risk of technical failure. Purely endovascular options for isolated common iliac or internal iliac artery aneurysms remain limited, so open or hybrid approaches remain important tools in their management.

References

1. Johnston KW, Rutherford RB, Tilson MD, Shah DM, Hollier L, Stanley JC. Suggested standards for reporting on arterial aneurysms. Subcommittee on Reporting Standards for Arterial Aneurysms, Ad Hoc Committee on Reporting Standards, Society for Vascular Surgery and North American Chapter, International Society for Cardiovascular Surgery. J Vasc Surg. 1991;13(3):452–8.
2. Levi N, Schroeder TV. Isolated iliac artery aneurysms. Eur J Vasc Endovasc Surg. 1998;16(4):342–4.
3. Brunkwall J, Hauksson H, Bengtsson H, Bergqvist D, Takolander R, Bergentz SE. Solitary aneurysms of the iliac arterial system: an estimate of their frequency of occurrence. J Vasc Surg. 1989;10(4):381–4.

4. Krupski WC, Selzman CH, Floridia R, Strecker PK, Nehler MR, Whitehill TA. Contemporary management of isolated iliac aneurysms. J Vasc Surg. 1998;28(1):1–11; discussion 11–13.
5. Gliedman ML, Ayers WB, Vestal BL. Aneurysms of the abdominal aorta and its branches: a study of untreated patients. Ann Surg. 1957;146(2):207–14.
6. Richardson JW, Greenfield LJ. Natural history and management of iliac aneurysms. J Vasc Surg. 1988;8(2):165–71.
7. Markowitz AM, Norman JC. Aneurysms of the iliac artery. Ann Surg. 1961;154:777–87.
8. Kalko Y, Basaran M, Aydin U, Kafa U, Basaranoglu G, Yasar T. The surgical treatment of arterial aneurysms in Behcet disease: a report of 16 patients. J Vasc Surg. 2005;42(4):673–7.
9. Santilli SM, Wernsing SE, Lee ES. Expansion rates and outcomes for iliac artery aneurysms. J Vasc Surg. 2000;31(1 Pt 1):114–21.
10. Lowry SF, Kraft RO. Isolated aneurysms of the iliac artery. Arch Surg. 1978;113(11):1289–93.
11. Dix FP, Titi M, Al-Khaffaf H. The isolated internal iliac artery aneurysm—a review. Eur J Vasc Endovasc Surg. 2005;30(2):119–29.
12. Pepin M, Schwarze U, Superti-Furga A, Byers PH. Clinical and genetic features of Ehlers-Danlos syndrome type IV, the vascular type. N Engl J Med. 2000;342(10):673–80.
13. Oderich GS, Panneton JM, Bower TC, et al. The spectrum, management and clinical outcome of Ehlers-Danlos syndrome type IV: a 30-year experience. J Vasc Surg. 2005;42(1):98–106.
14. Bollinger A. The death of Thomas Mann: consequence of erroneous angiologic diagnosis? Wien Med Wochenschr. 1999;149(2–4):30–2.
15. Spittell PC, Ehrsam JE, Anderson L, Seward JB. Screening for abdominal aortic aneurysm during transthoracic echocardiography in a hypertensive patient population. J Am Soc Echocardiogr. 1997;10(7):722–7.
16. Luke B, Rea K. Studies of aneurysm. JAMA J Am Med Assoc. 1921;72:935–6.
17. Sala F, Hassen-Khodja R, Branchereau P, et al. Outcome of common iliac arteries after aortoaortic graft placement during elective repair of infrarenal abdominal aortic aneurysms. J Vasc Surg. 2002;36(5):982–7.
18. Hassen-Khodja R, Feugier P, Favre JP, Nevelsteen A, Ferreira J. Outcome of common iliac arteries after straight aortic tube-graft placement during elective repair of infrarenal abdominal aortic aneurysms. J Vasc Surg. 2006;44(5):943–8.
19. Mott V. Successful ligature of the common iliac artery. Am J Med Sci. 1827;1:156.
20. Factor D, Oderich GS. Endovascular aortic repair current techniques with fenestrated, branched and parallel stent-grafts. Springer; 2018. p. 579–639.
21. Criado E, Marston WA, Ligush J, Mauro MA, Keagy BA. Endovascular repair of peripheral aneurysms, pseudoaneurysms, and arteriovenous fistulas. Ann Vasc Surg. 1997;11(3):256–63.
22. Giosdekos A, Antonopoulos CN, Sfyroeras GS, et al. The use of iliac branch devices for preservation of flow in internal iliac artery during endovascular aortic aneurysm repair. J Vasc Surg. 2020;71(6):2133–44.
23. Sahgal A, Veith FJ, Lipsitz E, et al. Diameter changes in isolated iliac artery aneurysms 1 to 6 years after endovascular graft repair. J Vasc Surg. 2001;33(2):289–4; discussion 294–285.
24. Boules TN, Selzer F, Stanziale SF, et al. Endovascular management of isolated iliac artery aneurysms. J Vasc Surg. 2006;44(1):29–37.
25. Henry M, Amor M, Henry I, et al. Percutaneous endovascular treatment of peripheral aneurysms. J Cardiovasc Surg. 2000;41(6):871–83.
26. Karthikesalingam A, Hinchliffe RJ, Holt PJ, et al. Endovascular aneurysm repair with preservation of the internal iliac artery using the iliac branch graft device. Eur J Vasc Endovasc Surg. 2010;39(3):285–94.
27. Parlani G, Verzini F, De Rango P, et al. Long-term results of iliac aneurysm repair with iliac branched endograft: a 5-year experience on 100 consecutive cases. Eur J Vasc Endovasc Surg. 2012;43(3):287–92.
28. Masciello F, Fargion AT, Pratesi G, et al. A propensity score-matched comparison of two commercially available iliac branch devices in patients with similar clinical and anatomic preoperative features. J Vasc Surg. 2020;71(4):1207–14.
29. Lee WA, Mantese V, Lee JT, Long G, Cable D, Hu M. Five-year outcomes of the PRESERVE II Zenith iliac branch pivotal clinical study. J Vasc Surg. 2025:S0741–5214(25)01786–0

Chapter 29
Diagnosis, Evaluation, and Management of Isolated Hypogastric Artery Aneurysms

Diego V. S. Rodrigues, Bernardo C. Mendes, and Todd E. Rasmussen

Introduction

Aneurysms of the iliac arteries, which include the common, internal (hypogastric), and external iliac arteries, often present in conjunction with other aneurysms, mainly abdominal aortic aneurysms (AAA), coexisting in around 10–20% of cases [1]. The presence of iliac artery aneurysms in the absence of AAA is rare, accounting for only 2–7% of all intra-abdominal aneurysms. In this cohort of patients, isolated/solitary hypogastric artery aneurysms are even more uncommon representing a range of 0.03–0.4% of all abdominal aneurysms or 20% of all iliac artery aneurysms [2, 3]. External iliac artery aneurysms are the least common corresponding to 10% of the iliac artery aneurysms. These differences may be in part due to the differences in embryological origin and resistance to atherosclerotic degeneration [4, 5]. Isolated/solitary hypogastric artery aneurysms are often followed by contralateral artery disease which manifests as aneurysmal degeneration in 11.4% of cases and occlusion in 11.6% [6].

The pathogenesis behind iliac artery aneurysms is believed to be like that of aorto-iliac aneurysm development, and 80% of hypogastric artery aneurysms are considered degenerative, prevailing in men with a 6:1 male to female sex ratio. Other less common etiological factors are iatrogenic injury, such as traumatic childbirth (forceps use or caesarean section) and hysterectomy, penetrating/blunt trauma, connective tissue disorder, and infection leading to mycotic aneurysms, including cases in the neonatal population related to umbilical artery catheterization once umbilical arteries originate in the hypogastric arteries [1, 7].

D. V. S. Rodrigues · B. C. Mendes · T. E. Rasmussen (✉)
Division of Vascular and Endovascular Surgery, Department of Surgery, Mayo Clinic, Rochester, MN, USA
e-mail: rodrigues.diego@mayo.edu; mendes.bernardo@mayo.edu; rasmussen.todd@mayo.edu

G. J. Arnaoutakis et al. (eds.), *Aortic Aneurysms*, Contemporary Cardiology,
https://doi.org/10.1007/978-3-032-13134-8_29

The Subcommittee on Reporting Standards for Arterial Aneurysms of The Society for Vascular Surgery defines an iliac artery aneurysm as an increase in the diameter of the iliac artery >1.5 times the expected normal diameter of the vessel and, for the hypogastric arteries, a diameter ≥8 mm is considered aneurysmal [8]. The natural history of these aneurysms is enlargement and eventual rupture. Expansion rates for hypogastric artery aneurysms are between 1 and 4 mm per year. However, larger aneurysms (3–5 cm) may have a higher rate of expansion and most reports of rupture have been in hypogastric arteries 5 cm or larger [9, 10]. Because of its rarity and localization within the pelvis, hypogastric artery aneurysms most commonly expand without symptoms, becoming symptomatic only when they reach significant size. Symptoms may arise from stenosis or embolization of outflow vessels causing hip and buttock claudication, or from pain or discomfort associated with the aneurysm's mass effect. Large hypogastric artery aneurysms can also compress or fistulize into surrounding structures in the pelvis such as bowel or ureter [11–13]. Rupture of hypogastric artery aneurysms is associated with mortality rates as high as 60% [14].

The 2019 European Society of Vascular Surgery (ESVS) guidelines recommend elective repair of common, hypogastric, and external iliac artery aneurysms when the diameter exceeds 3.5 cm, although they do not make a distinction among these anatomically distinct arteries. Because the internal iliac is smaller than the common at baseline, an aneurysm of the hypogastric may have a slightly higher risk of rupture compared to a similar-sized aneurysm of the common [15]. Some experts recommend elective repair when any iliac artery aneurysm, common, internal, or external, reaches 3 cm and urgent repair for any patient whose aneurysm is 5 cm or larger or who is experiencing symptoms. In patients with limited functional capacity, cardiopulmonary reserve, and or those of higher operative risk, surveillance with periodic CT imaging should continue until the aneurysm reaches at least 4 cm in diameter, keeping in mind most reported ruptures are in aneurysms 5 cm or larger [14, 15].

Diagnosis and Evaluation

The deep pelvic localization of isolated/solitary hypogastric artery aneurysms makes its diagnosis difficult, thus a negative abdominal physical examination does not rule out its presence. Historically, most of these aneurysms presented as symptomatic due to mass effect on the surrounding compromised pelvic structure. However, increasingly, they have been detected as incidental findings from imaging performed for other purposes [16].

Signs and symptoms, when present, may be dull lower abdominal and flank pain, deep vein thrombosis, hydronephrosis, pyelonephritis, and sepsis from ureteral obstruction, which can turn into renal failure. Others such as pain on defecation from rectal compression, hip pain, lumbosacral pain, sciatic neuralgia, and lower-limb paresis from compression of the pelvic nerves may occur [2, 17]. Intermittent

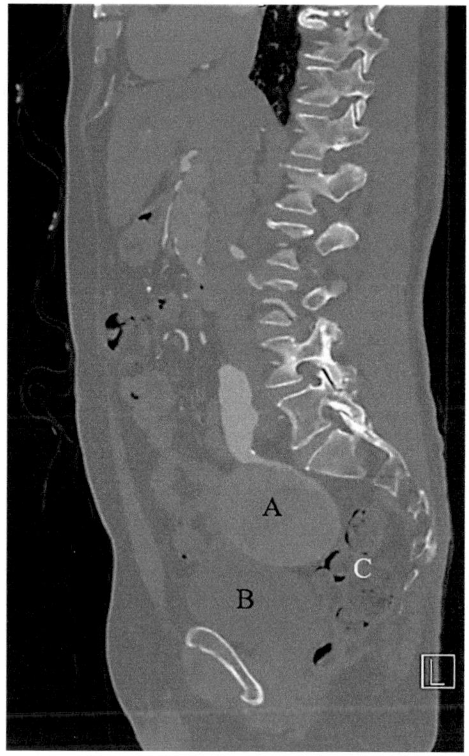

Fig. 29.1 CTA image in sagittal view demonstrates a right internal (hypogastric) iliac artery aneurysm (**a**) slightly compressing the fundus of the bladder (**b**) and in close contact with the sigmoid-rectum transition (**c**)

hematuria and rupture into the bladder, ureter, and scrotal ecchymosis have also been described [16, 18, 19].

Diagnostic imaging modalities used for hypogastric artery aneurysms are the same as used for AAA. Computed tomography angiography (CTA) is well stablished for this purpose and highly accurate, providing details on the aneurysm, the relationship with other organs, presence of retroperitoneal hematoma, as well as aorto-iliac anatomy and contralateral vessels. Currently, CTA is considered essential for pretreatment planning [20] (Fig. 29.1). Doppler ultrasound might be a good non-invasive option to identify the presence of the aneurysm and rule out other differential diagnoses of pelvic masses; however, it is operator dependent and has limited reach due to overlying bowel gas, the deep location, and tortuosity of the vessels. Transanal ultrasonography may be of use for the diagnosis [21].

Magnetic resonance angiography imaging can also be an alternative to the CTA, although not typically used given its higher expense and lower availability [22]. Standard arteriography is invasive and less accurate for determining the true diameter of the vessels; nevertheless, there is general agreement of its possible use as complement to assess the pelvic circulation and for preoperative planning [4].

Treatment Modalities

Early diagnosis, careful surveillance, and timely repair of iliac artery aneurysms are crucial to avoid emergent situations which impose higher morbidity and mortality. In the elective approach, surgery can be planned properly, and challenges can be predicted with reliable anatomic study and identification of potential pitfalls. A systematic review made by Dix et al. highlighted the difference in perioperative mortality between elective and emergent repair of hypogastric artery aneurysms, showing a reduction of nearly 40% in complications with the elective repair (50% to 11%) [22]. Multiple modalities of treatment for iliac artery aneurysms have been described with both open and endovascular techniques being used in isolation or combined [23].

Traditionally, iliac artery aneurysms have been repaired using open surgical techniques; however, similarly to AAA, their treatment has evolved over time and open surgical repair has been superseded by endovascular treatment [24]. The best course of action for treatment relies on careful consideration of critical factors. These factors include the patient's current health status, renal function, the specific segment of the iliac tree affected, coexistent AAA or contralateral disease, as well as the availability of healthy proximal and distal segments of the artery (landing zones), and associated risks with hypogastric artery occlusion [25].

Open Surgical Repair

MacLaren, in 1913, first reported his attempt of correction of a hypogastric artery aneurysm with proximal ligation achieving a partial cure [26]. Other techniques were developed over time and remain in the arsenal of the vascular surgeon like aneurysmectomy (resection of the aneurysmal segment and graft interposition), endoaneurysmorrhaphy (opening the aneurysm sac, sewing collateral vessels from inside, and placing a graft), or proximal and distal hypogastric artery ligation [22, 27].

Resection of the aneurysm imposes higher area of dissection and, due to the presence of pelvic congestion and the deep field, may favor major bleeding. In the open repair of more extensive aneurysms, back bleeding control from the outflow arteries can be attained using balloon catheters once the aneurysm sac is open, facilitating the exposure [14]. Interposition grafting maintains antegrade pelvic flow and should be used whenever possible, primarily in the setting of bilateral aneurysms when one side will require ligation, avoiding the risk of ischemic complications as suggested by recent guidelines [15].

Proximal and distal ligation offers an approach with minimum pelvic dissection especially in small and localized proximal aneurysms; however, despite proximal and distal hypogastric ligation, collateral branches may keep feeding the aneurysm sac, particularly in those extending deeply in the pelvis. In contemporary practice, isolated proximal ligation is no longer considered a valid treatment option [27].

Open surgical repair of hypogastric artery aneurysms has proven to have an up to 7–11% higher mortality than endovascular therapies, primarily owing to hemorrhage during the surgery; however, open surgery may be preferred if preserving the hypogastric artery is critical to pelvic flow and patient is unsuitable for an endovascular approach. Hybrid procedures have been reported with coil or plug embolization of the distal branches of the hypogastric artery and, in a second stage, open approach with only proximal artery control and aneurysm excision [28].

Endovascular Repair

Endovascular techniques have surpassed the open repair treatment of aortoiliac and isolated iliac aneurysms, including isolated hypogastric artery aneurysms, because of better short-to mid-term results, less invasiveness, and low early mortality [3]. A study from our group comparing outcomes of open versus endovascular repair of internal iliac aneurysms in 97 patients observed a significantly lower major adverse events (43% vs 8%, $p < 0.001$) and length of hospitalization (9 days vs 1 day, $p < 0.001$) following endovascular repair, albeit a higher chance of sacrificing the ipsilateral pelvic perfusion [14].

Historically, the most described endovascular treatments for hypogastric artery aneurysms are embolization of the distal branches and the aneurysmal sac, followed by coverage of the origin of the hypogastric artery by a stent-graft from the common to the external iliac, or placement of a plug in the proximal hypogastric artery if the anatomy allows (Fig. 29.2). However, the sacrifice of internal iliac artery brought attention over acute and chronic pelvic ischemic syndromes [29]. A systematic

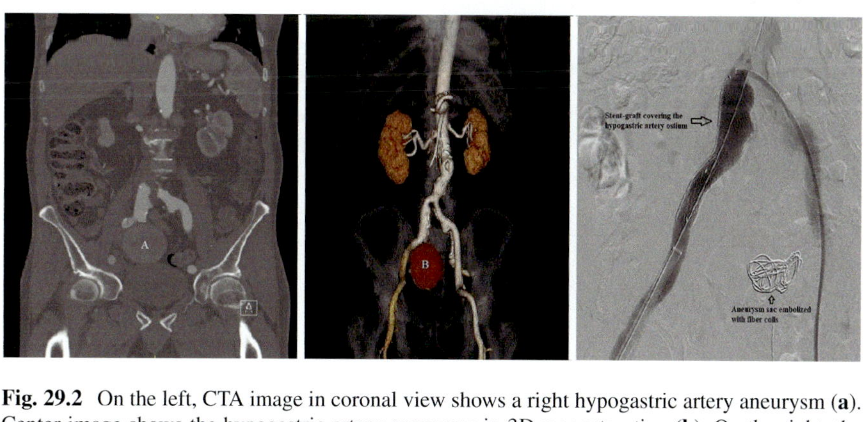

Fig. 29.2 On the left, CTA image in coronal view shows a right hypogastric artery aneurysm (**a**). Center image shows the hypogastric artery aneurysm in 3D reconstruction (**b**). On the right, the completion angiography after endovascular repair with coil embolization of the aneurysm sac and stent-graft coverage from common to external iliac artery

review compared the effects of hypogastric artery occlusion with hypogastric artery revascularization in the context of endovascular treatment for aortoiliac aneurysms. The incidence of buttock claudication was 36.5% in the occlusion group and 4.1% in the revascularization group [30].

Most aneurysms of the hypogastric artery terminate at its bifurcation into the anterior and posterior divisions, with rare involvement of these branches. Furthermore, less extensive aneurysms that end proximal to the bifurcation leave a healthy segment of the primary vessel that can be utilized as a target for endovascular reconstruction. In the context of preserving internal iliac flow, the largest distal branch can be used as a revascularization target with embolization of smaller branches that might be present [6, 14]. Moreover, use of different materials for embolization, such as outer parts of guidewires, acrylic glue, thrombin, autologous blood clot, and gelatin sponge, has been reported. Their use can be in combination with coils or in isolation, inducing thrombosis of the aneurysm sac [31]. When bilateral embolization is necessary, a staged approach has become a common practice to allow collateral development; nevertheless, some recent small nonrandomized studies have not shown obvious benefits from this approach [32] (Fig. 29.3).

Multiple strategies have been used to preserve pelvic flow in the setting of iliac artery aneurysm repair, such as hybrid or parallel stent-graft techniques that include snorkel/sandwich procedures. Even though these procedures have an important place in the surgical arsenal, they have shown suboptimal results [10, 24]. Use of physician-modified devices with branches or fenestrations has also been described, although they require time for modification and should only be used by highly trained physicians in patients without other options [33].

Currently, development of iliac branch devices has allowed totally endovascular incorporation of one or both internal iliac arteries. In 2016, the WL Gore Excluder iliac branch endoprosthesis (IBE; WL Gore, Flagstaff, AZ), designed to preserve

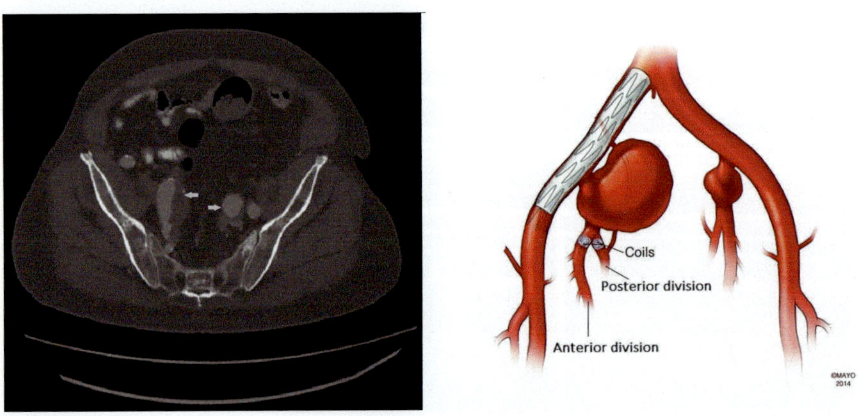

Fig. 29.3 On the left, CTA image in axial view demonstrates partially thrombosed bilateral internal (hypogastric) iliac artery aneurysms (arrows). On the right, depiction of the endovascular repair using coils for embolization of the hypogastric artery distal branches and stent-graft coverage of its origin

hypogastric artery flow during repair of common iliac artery and aortoiliac aneurysms, was approved in the United States by the Food and Drug Administration (FDA) [34]. Various studies have demonstrated better outcomes with endovascular repair using iliac branch endoprosthesis when compared with open surgical repair, including shorter length of hospitalization, lower estimated blood loss, and need for transfusions [24, 33]. Over time, its use has been expanded and described as safe and effective for endovascular reconstruction of isolated iliac aneurysms (Fig. 29.4) [24, 33].

Benefits of the endovascular approach are associated with the inherent minimally invasive nature, which allows percutaneous access, possibility of local or regional anesthesia, minimal blood loss, minimized surgical trauma, and lower cardiovascular demand. Some of the limitations of this technique are the impossibility of decompression of pelvic structures which could be attained with an open fashion, and the risk of ongoing or new onset endoleak within the aneurysm sac, which might require further open or percutaneous reintervention.

In emergent situations with ruptured aneurysm, transient hemostasis can be reached with embolization of side-branches of HA combined with the placement of balloon catheters in the CIA and EIA crossing the ostium of the HA. This strategy offers a period for patient stabilization before proceeding with the definitive

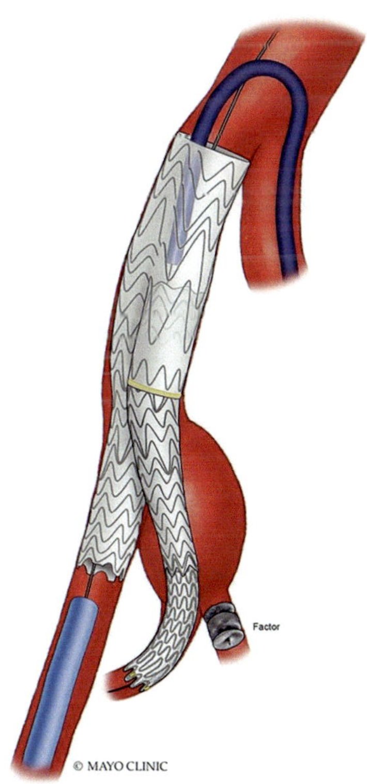

Fig. 29.4 Illustration of the iliac branch endoprosthesis (IBE) Gore graft. The main body of the endograft is inserted from the right common femoral artery and the iliac branch is positioned into the hypogastric artery. From a contralateral access the anterior division of the right hypogastric artery was catheterized and embolized with a plug. From brachial access, a covered stent is then introduced and deployed in the posterior division of the hypogastric artery followed by a bridging stent

treatment of the HAA employing either an open surgical approach or covered stent-graft.

Conclusion

Isolated or solitary hypogastric artery aneurysms are uncommon and often go unnoticed as they expand silently, often to significant dimension. Aneurysm rupture is rare but poses a life-threatening situation leading to high rates of death and disability regardless of how it is managed. It is important to diagnose and closely monitor hypogastric artery aneurysms with CT imaging and intervene when they reach significant size. In patients with few medical comorbidities and who are of low operative risk, repair should be considered when the aneurysm reaches 3–3.5 cm in diameter. Treatment can be deferred until the aneurysm reaches 4–5 cm in patients who are deconditioned or of higher operative risk. Endovascular repair is less invasive and associated with fewer complications than open repair and when feasible it is the preferred treatment approach. Catheter-based treatment is based on the premise of depressurizing the aneurysm by occluding inflow and outflow with or without thrombosing the aneurysm sac. When possible, priority should be given to preserving the contralateral internal iliac artery and as much distal pelvic circulation as possible to reduce the risk of ischemic complications. Early detection, surveillance, and appropriate intervention can improve survival and functional outcomes of patients with solitary hypogastric artery aneurysms.

References

1. Parry DJ, Kessel D, Scott DJ. Simplifying the internal iliac artery aneurysm. Ann R Coll Surg Engl. 2001;83(5):302–8.
2. Uberoi R, Tsetis D, Shrivastava V, Morgan R, Belli AM. Subcommittee on Reporting Standards for Arterial Aneurysms of The Society for Vascular S. Standard of practice for the interventional management of isolated iliac artery aneurysms. Cardiovasc Intervent Radiol. 2011;34(1):3–13.
3. Perini P, Mariani E, Fanelli M, Ucci A, Rossi G, Massoni CB, et al. Surgical and endovascular management of isolated internal iliac artery aneurysms: a systematic review and meta-analysis. Vasc Endovasc Surg. 2021;55(3):254–64.
4. Sandhu RS, Pipinos II. Isolated iliac artery aneurysms. Semin Vasc Surg. 2005;18(4):209–15.
5. Boules TN, Selzer F, Stanziale SF, Chomic A, Marone LK, Dillavou ED, et al. Endovascular management of isolated iliac artery aneurysms. J Vasc Surg. 2006;44(1):29–37.
6. Ciofani L, Massi I, Acciarri P. A rare case of bilateral isolated internal iliac artery aneurysms excluded with VBX covered stents. Vascular. 2023;2023:17085381231155939.
7. Khandanpour N, Chaudhuri A, Roebuck DJ, Armon MP. Neonatal mycotic internal iliac aneurysm due to methicillin-resistant Staphylococcus aureus (MRSA) septicaemia successfully treated by coil embolisation. Eur J Vasc Endovasc Surg. 2007;33(6):687–9.
8. Johnston KW, Rutherford RB, Tilson MD, Shah DM, Hollier L, Stanley JC. Suggested standards for reporting on arterial aneurysms. Subcommittee on Reporting Standards for Arterial

Aneurysms, Ad Hoc Committee on Reporting Standards, Society for Vascular Surgery and North American Chapter, International Society for Cardiovascular Surgery. J Vasc Surg. 1991;13(3):452–8.
9. Santilli SM, Wernsing SE, Lee ES. Expansion rates and outcomes for iliac artery aneurysms. J Vasc Surg. 2000;31(1 Pt 1):114–21.
10. Huang Y, Gloviczki P, Duncan AA, Kalra M, Hoskin TL, Oderich GS, et al. Common iliac artery aneurysm: expansion rate and results of open surgical and endovascular repair. J Vasc Surg. 2008;47(6):1203–10; discussion 10-1.
11. Guille F, Ridoux G, Leguerrier A, Lobel B. Compression of the pelvic ureter by a hypogastric aneurysm. J Urol (Paris). 1983;89(9):635–7.
12. Ito T, Kurita Y, Tamura K, Shinbo H, Ushiyama T. An isolated internal artery aneurysm with complete thrombotic occlusion for which preoperative diagnosis was difficult: a case report. Nihon Hinyokika Gakkai Zasshi. 2015;106(1):49–52.
13. Mineta K, Nomura M, Fujimoto N, Takahashi K, Matsumoto T. Ureteral obstruction due to retroperitoneal fibrosis secondary to a solitary internal iliac aneurysm. Int J Urol. 2004;11(11):1024–7.
14. Rana MA, Kalra M, Oderich GS, de Grandis E, Gloviczki P, Duncan AA, et al. Outcomes of open and endovascular repair for ruptured and nonruptured internal iliac artery aneurysms. J Vasc Surg. 2014;59(3):634–44.
15. Wanhainen A, Verzini F, Van Herzeele I, Allaire E, Bown M, Cohnert T, et al. Editor's choice—European Society for Vascular Surgery (ESVS) 2019 clinical practice guidelines on the management of abdominal aorto-iliac artery aneurysms. Eur J Vasc Endovasc Surg. 2019;57(1):8–93.
16. Zeren G, Can F, Avci II, Sungur MA, Yilmaz MF, Karabay CY. Endovascular management of giant isolated iliac artery aneurysms: a case series. Anatol J Cardiol. 2022;26(9):733–6.
17. Singh R, Moores T, Maddox M, Horton A. Internal iliac aneurysm presenting with lower back pain, sciatica and foot drop. J Surg Case Rep. 2013;2013(2):rjs032.
18. Sangey T, Moledina S. Internal iliac aneurysm causing hydroureteronephrosis. Case Rep Radiol. 2020;2020:8857729.
19. Pirvu A. Uretero-arterial fistula due to a hypogastric aneurysm. Arab J Urol. 2018;16(2):257–9.
20. Rozenblit AM, Cynamon J, Maddineni S, Marin ML, Sanchez LA, Yuan J, et al. Value of CT angiography for postoperative assessment of patients with iliac artery aneurysms who have received endovascular grafts. AJR Am J Roentgenol. 1998;170(4):913–7.
21. Krupski WC, Selzman CH, Floridia R, Strecker PK, Nehler MR, Whitehill TA. Contemporary management of isolated iliac aneurysms. J Vasc Surg. 1998;28(1):1–11; discussion -3.
22. Dix FP, Titi M, Al-Khaffaf H. The isolated internal iliac artery aneurysm—a review. Eur J Vasc Endovasc Surg. 2005;30(2):119–29.
23. Soury P, Brisset D, Gigou F, Saliou C, Angel F, Laurian C. Aneurysms of the internal iliac artery: management strategy. Ann Vasc Surg. 2001;15(3):321–5.
24. Mendes BC, Oderich GS, Sandri GA, Johnstone JK, Shuja F, Kalra M, et al. Comparison of perioperative outcomes of patients with iliac aneurysms treated by open surgery or endovascular repair with iliac branch endoprosthesis. Ann Vasc Surg. 2019;60:76–84.e1.
25. Chaikof EL, Dalman RL, Eskandari MK, Jackson BM, Lee WA, Mansour MA, et al. The Society for Vascular Surgery practice guidelines on the care of patients with an abdominal aortic aneurysm. J Vasc Surg. 2018;67(1):2–77 e2.
26. Maclaren AXIV. Aneurism of the internal iliac: probably immediately following a severe instrumental delivery: operation and partial cure. Ann Surg. 1913;58(2):269–70.
27. Nakajima T, Kawazoe K, Komoda K, Sasaki T, Kin H, Kamada T, et al. Failure of exclusion of internal iliac artery aneurysms. J Vasc Surg. 2001;33(3):476–80.
28. Kawatani Y, Oguri A. Hybrid repair of isolated internal iliac artery aneurysm. J Surg Case Rep. 2020;2020(2):rjz409.

29. Hollis HW Jr, Luethke JM, Yakes WF, Beitler AL. Percutaneous embolization of an internal iliac artery aneurysm: technical considerations and literature review. J Vasc Interv Radiol. 1994;5(3):449–51.
30. Kouvelos GN, Katsargyris A, Antoniou GA, Oikonomou K, Verhoeven EL. Outcome after interruption or preservation of internal iliac artery flow during endovascular repair of abdominal aorto-iliac aneurysms. Eur J Vasc Endovasc Surg. 2016;52(5):621–34.
31. Antoniou GA, Nassef AH, Antoniou SA, Loh CY, Turner DR, Beard JD. Endovascular treatment of isolated internal iliac artery aneurysms. Vascular. 2011;19(6):291–300.
32. Bratby MJ, Munneke GM, Belli AM, Loosemore TM, Loftus I, Thompson MM, et al. How safe is bilateral internal iliac artery embolization prior to EVAR? Cardiovasc Intervent Radiol. 2008;31(2):246–53.
33. D'Oria M, Mastrorilli D, DeMartino R, Lepidi S. Current status of endovascular preservation of the internal iliac artery with iliac branch devices (IBD). Cardiovasc Intervent Radiol. 2019;42(7):935–48.
34. Millon A, Della Schiava N, Arsicot M, De Lambert A, Feugier P, Magne JL, et al. Preliminary experience with the GORE((R)) EXCLUDER((R)) iliac branch endoprosthesis for common iliac aneurysm endovascular treatment. Ann Vasc Surg. 2016;33:11–7.

Chapter 30
True Femoral and Popliteal Artery Aneurysms: Clinical Features and Treatment

Elizabeth Andraska and Rabih Chaer

Introduction

Popliteal artery aneurysms (PAAs) are relatively rare, occurring in an estimated 0.1–1% of the population [1]. Nevertheless, they represent the most common form of peripheral AA, accounting for 70–80% of peripheral aneurysms [2]. True common femoral artery aneurysms (CFAAs) remain relatively uncommon as compared with PAA. Overall, few large series have been published, in part because the evaluation and treatment is straightforward, safe, and durable. Further, the location is not as amendable for endovascular therapies. The benefit from an endovascular repair of an isolated CFAA is unlikely to be achieved, given the branching of the profunda and the fact that these can be repaired under local anesthesia (if need be) with excellent long-term results. The increased number of abdominal aortic aneurysms (AAAs) repaired via an endovascular approach, which mandates femoral artery exposure in many cases, allows the CFAA to be repaired in the same setting.

E. Andraska (✉)
UPMC Department of Surgery, Division of Vascular Surgery, Heart and Vascular Institute, Pittsburgh, PA, USA
e-mail: andraskaea@upmc.edu

R. Chaer
Department of Surgery, Division of Vascular and Endovascular Surgery, Stony Brook University, NY, USA
e-mail: chaerra@upmc.edu

G. J. Arnaoutakis et al. (eds.), *Aortic Aneurysms*, Contemporary Cardiology,
https://doi.org/10.1007/978-3-032-13134-8_30

Demographics

Peripheral AAs predominantly occur in men, which make up nearly 96% of this population. Other risk factors for these aneurysms include: hypertension, smoking, the presence of coronary artery disease, hyperlipidemia, and chronic obstructive pulmonary disease. Other factors which are known to be associated with peripheral AA include abdominal aortic and iliac aneurysms.

More than 60% of PAA patients have concomitant AAAs, and almost 40% have femoral aneurysms [3]. Nearly 65% of patients with PAA disease have bilateral involvement [4–6]. Patients with CFAA have the highest concordance with proximal AA, up to 85% incidence, and associated PAAs are found in 40–50% [7]. Conversely, those with AAA have up to 14% peripheral AA incidence [8].

Pathogenesis

Peripheral AAs have historically been linked to degenerative changes that accumulate as a result of atherosclerosis. Atherosclerotic changes are present in the histological analysis of human peripheral AA tissue, similar to those observed with aortic atherosclerosis and AAA. Further studies, however, have suggested a more specific association with inflammatory changes in the vessel wall, primarily defined from PAA specimens.

Disruption of elastic lamellae and active proteolysis have been shown in excised aneurysmal tissue [4]. Additionally, the expression of molecules linked to apoptosis is increased. Bax, CPP-32, and Fas are significantly elevated in PAA specimens, particularly within vascular smooth muscle cells [4].

Another study found increased expression of CPP-32 in T cells located within the PAA wall itself [5]. The suggested mechanism is that T-cell-induced apoptosis leads to a degradation of the arterial wall matrix. It is unclear, however, whether the apoptotic pathway has a causative role in AA formation, or whether it is merely associated with the degenerative changes that occur.

Anatomic factors may also play a role. The popliteal artery arises from the superficial femoral artery as it passes through the adductor (Hunter's) canal, and continues into the popliteal fossa. Unique structural stresses on the popliteal artery that may contribute to PAA formation include turbulent blood flow associated with branching points and wall fatigue secondary to repeated knee flexion. This may also be a factor in the groin with flexion of the CFA and the branching of profunda femoris artery (PFA) and superficial femoral artery (SFA).

Diagnosis

Diagnosis of a peripheral AA is fairly straightforward, even in the case of an asymptomatic lesion, but due to obesity or other patient features, may be missed on physical examination [8]. A prominent femoral or popliteal pulse or pulsatile mass in the inguinal or popliteal fossa in a patient should arouse suspicion, particularly if the patient is male, older than 50 years of age, has used tobacco, and/or has risk factors for coronary artery disease. Although the CFA is usually not difficult to palpate, it is a different situation with the popliteal artery. Because the popliteal pulse is rarely easily palpable, some practitioners recommend screening for all persons with an easily detectable popliteal pulse. If the aneurysm is thrombosed, a nonpulsatile mass may be present, which should also prompt further diagnostic evaluation [9, 10]. In either scenario, the examination is performed with the knee in a relaxed, flexed position, and the aneurysm itself is defined in relation to the knee joint. A normal popliteal artery measures 5–9 mm in diameter. It is generally considered aneurysmal when the diameter exceeds 15 mm or when it is 1.5 times greater than its normal diameter—either standardized to proximal or distal popliteal artery or contralateral popliteal artery.

The differential diagnosis hinges mainly on whether the lesion detected on physical examination is pulsatile. Hypertrophic or malignant lymph nodes, incarcerated hernias (including femoral hernias), Baker's cysts, deep venous thrombosis, hematoma, lipoma, and sarcoma are all possible differential diagnoses for a mass in the inguinal or popliteal fossa, but are rarely pulsatile. Once the distinction is made, the lesion in question may be further evaluated with duplex ultrasound (DU). For screening, contrast-enhanced computed tomography (CT) and magnetic resonance imaging are rarely indicated. Because of the invasive nature of the procedure, angiography is not an appropriate initial diagnostic test, and the presence of intraluminal thrombus makes it inaccurate for assessing the presence or size of an aneurysm.

Diagnostic DU has several advantages as an initial mode of evaluation. First, it is relatively inexpensive and available in the clinic. Second, DU is accurate in determining the size of the aneurysm and for assessment of intraluminal thrombus [1, 5]. Third, addition of DU measurements can be used postoperatively to detect flow within the aneurysm sac following exclusion [11, 12]. DU can be used to map the availability of the saphenous vein for arterial bypass, as well as to image the proximal and distal arterial tree, sometimes obviating the need for invasive arteriography (Fig. 30.1). DU is also useful as a screening technique for other arterial aneurysms According to the most recent Society of Vascular Surgery (SVS) guidelines, patients found to have a PAA should be screened for contralateral PAA as well as AAA. When considering repair specifically, operative planning is heavily dependent on a pre-operative CTA. This is of critical importance because it can provide anatomical

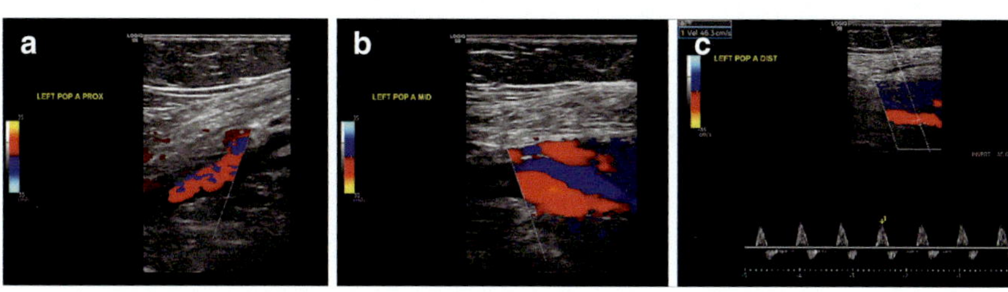

Fig. 30.1 Duplex ultrasound of the popliteal artery aneurysm at the (**a**) proximal popliteal artery, (**b**) mid popliteal artery, and (**c**) distal popliteal artery

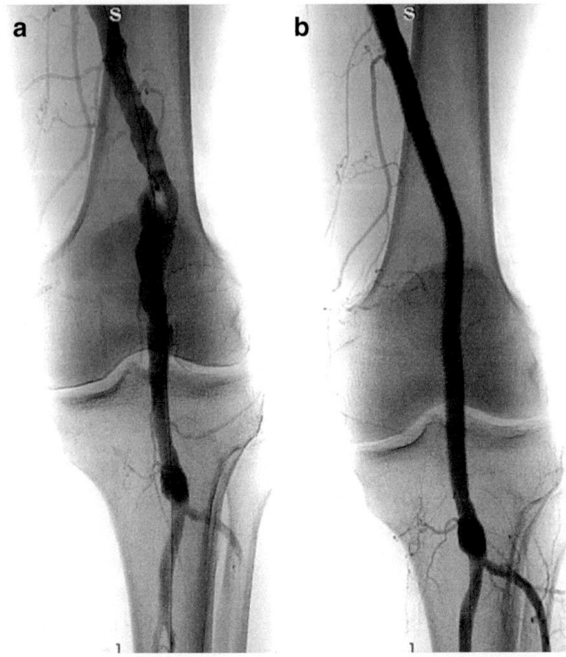

Fig. 30.2 Angiogram demonstrating popliteal artery aneurysm (**a**) prior to stenting and (**b**) after stenting

information that cannot be obtained using an angiogram such as exact location of the aneurysm, the diameter of normal artery proximal and distal to the aneurysm, and whether or not a normal proximal and distal landing zone is available. CTA measurements also help with graft size choice as well as characterizing the patient's runoff score.

Although not appropriate for screening, angiography has an important role in selected preoperative evaluation of PAA, but perhaps less so in CFAA patients. Angiography allows evaluation of arterial inflow, popliteal artery patency, and distal runoff (Fig. 30.2). Although inflow disease does not appear to affect symptoms from the aneurysm, the presence of a proximal stenosis does alter the operative approach, and can increase the complexity of a repair. Knowledge of the lower extremity arterial runoff is important, as the bypass requires a distal target which may be at the level of a tibial artery. Alternatively, CT angiography is sufficiently reliable to base operative decisions in many cases, depending on the surgeon's comfort level and is particularly useful for planning CFAA repair (Fig. 30.3).

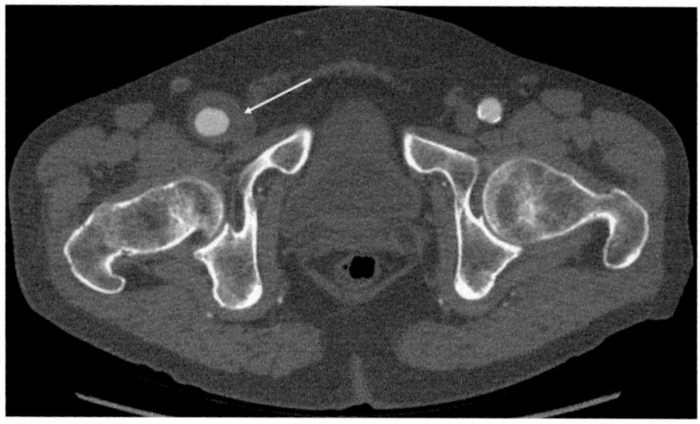

Fig. 30.3 Axial computed tomography (CT) imaging of a right femoral artery aneurysm (white arrow) prior to repair

Medical Management

Given that the pathogenesis of PAA is predominantly atherosclerotic in etiology, optimal medical management should be established at diagnosis. Risk modification strategies such as smoking cessation, and treatment of hypertension, hyperlipidemia, and diabetes, are all essential in this patient population.

Presentation and Indications for Repair

The natural history of peripheral artery aneurysms has been more clearly defined in recent years. For popliteal AA less than 20 mm in diameter, the expected annual growth rate is 0.3–1.5 mm. For aneurysms >20 mm, growth is variable but usually <3 mm per year. Aneurysms that are at baseline larger in diameter are at increased risk of complications including accelerated growth [13]. Between 30% and 50% of patients with peripheral AA are asymptomatic, whereas 50% will present initially with some form of limb ischemia, embolic process, or local pain [4, 6, 14]. Arterial ischemic symptoms include claudication, rest pain, and tissue loss, and these are reported in 20–40% of patients, more commonly associated with PAAs [4, 6]. Apart from complete vascular occlusion, peripheral AA may present with a "blue toe syndrome" resulting from repeated embolization of thrombotic debris to the distal extremity, and may occur in up to 12% of patients presenting with PAA [10, 15, 16]. Local compression from a sizable AA may result in a femoral or tibial nerve neuropathy, or venous obstruction resulting in edema, pain, and potentially deep venous thrombosis.

The complication rate for PAA ranges between 18% and 77%, depending on the definition used and the series reported. Amputation rates in some series are as high as 20%, but more recent studies have demonstrated improved limb salvage rates [10–12]. Even if the aneurysm is asymptomatic at the time of presentation, most patients will require intervention for a complication (such as acute ischemia or embolization) within several years after diagnosis. These patients will frequently require operative intervention to preserve the affected limb [15, 17, 18].

Acute limb ischemia (ALI) is the most common limb-threatening presentation of a peripheral AA, and is distinctly more common with PAA, as compared with CFAA. Between 18% and 30% of PAA will present with some form of ischemic limb [3, 14, 17, 18]. Patients presenting with an ischemic limb in the setting of a PAA usually present with grade IIB ischemia (cool, painful, pulseless limb) as the result of acute thrombosis of the popliteal artery, or a combination of acute thrombosis in the setting of outflow occlusion as the result of chronic embolization [4–6, 19]. Less frequently, patients may present with a ruptured PAA. In either circumstance, immediate intervention is required for limb salvage.

Recent guidelines from the Society of Vascular Surgery (SVS) have advocated for treatment of PAA to reduce the risk of limb ischemia [20]. In patients at low surgical risk, elective repair of PAA when ≥20 mm is recommended to reduce the risk of thromboembolic complications. In a study evaluating 106 patients with asymptomatic PAAs, 18% of patients developed symptoms over a 6-year follow-up. Three risk factors were present for the development of symptoms. This included diameter ≥20 mm, presence of intramural thrombus, and poor tibial runoff. This prompted the SVS to recommend repair when ≥20 mm [21]. In patients who have high surgical risk, a threshold of 30 mm is recommended.

In patients who have higher risk of developing symptoms or complications from the PAA, a lower threshold for repair can be considered. For example, the presence of intramural thrombus or poor tibial runoff can prompt earlier evaluation for repair. This is because aneurysm size has not been consistently associated with complication. For example, Ascher et al. described the risk of thrombotic complications in PAA that were small but were partially thrombosed and poorer outflow vessels [9].

With regard to open versus endovascular repair of PAAs, recommendations are dependent on patient comorbidities and anatomy. For asymptomatic patients with a life expectancy of at least 5 years, open repair of PAA is recommended. There have been recent small center studies comparing open to endovascular repair of PAA which have noted improved patency after open repair. However, this is contingent on the presence of an adequate saphenous vein for conduit [22–24]. Coverage below the knee and single vessel runoff have been described to be predictors of major adverse limb events following endovascular repair of PAAs, therefore in patients with poor runoff or distal extent of aneurysmal dilatation, open repair is preferred [22, 25].Patients presenting with ALI often have compromised tibioperoneal runoff. Degree of ischemia will dictate operative approach. In patients who present with mild or moderate ischemia defined as Rutherford type I or IIA, optimizing runoff is a preferred initial intervention. This can be achieved with thrombolysis or pharmacomechanical interventions to improve the outflow of the ultimate repair. Repair of the PAA can then be staged with either an endovascular or open approach. Patients with Rutherford class IIB ischemia should be promptly repaired in order to avoid further ischemia. The adjunctive use of surgical thromboembolectomy or pharmacomechanical thrombectomy can be used to maximize the tibial runoff. Patients with nonviable limbs, classified as Rutherford type III, require amputation.

Although PAA are clearly associated with other aneurysms, it is not known whether the presence of other aneurysms affects long-term outcome for PAA repair. In one study, when PAA patients had a high rate of either bilateral PAA or extrapopliteal aneurysms, 10-year survival was worse in patients with multiple aneurysms (16% vs. 66%) compared with those who had isolated disease [5]. Mortality in this study, however, was the result of coronary artery disease rather than aneurysmal disease, suggesting a relationship between overall atherosclerotic burden and predisposition to aneurysm formation.

CFAAs are classified as either Type I or Type II. Type I is the most common and isolated to the common femoral artery whereas Type II involves the PFA as well as the common femoral artery. A definitive size criterion for repair has not been defined, but generally those over 2.5–3 cm who are otherwise a good operative candidate should be repaired [7, 26]. Again, CFAA are less often associated with ALI, but whether this is due to a more benign process or less reporting is not clear.

Treatment: Popliteal Artery Aneurysms

Endovascular Treatment

The advent of catheter-based interventions has spurred an increase in the number of centers and surgeons applying endovascular techniques to the management of PAA. This is especially popular in the management of patients, who based on comorbid conditions or lack of conduit would not otherwise be considered ideal operative candidates. Much of the enthusiasm for this technique is based on the success of AAA exclusion with endovascular graft placement.

The most commonly used stent graft is made of a polytetrafluoroethylene-lined nitinol stent with thermal memory (Viabahn, Gore, Tempe, AZ) [19, 27, 29, 30]. The location of the popliteal artery stent grafts requires several considerations not relevant to AAA, including flexibility and graft compliance, given the proximity to the knee joint. The mobility of the joint increases the risk of graft migration and graft kinking. Other potential complications include graft separation following deployment, and endoleaks from incompletely excluded vessels. Neointimal hyperplasia may result in narrowing of the lumen at the proximal and distal endpoints.

In general, the endovascular approach has been shown to be both safe and effective, and a prospective randomized study demonstrated similar patency rates with open repair. Tielliu et al. described a series of 57 endovacular PAA repairs, with 5 treated for acute ischemia [29]. Several retrospective reviews have compared OPAR to EPAR and have found OPAR and EPAR to have similar outcomes (Table 30.1).

When evaluating preoperative imaging, a close examination of proximal and distal landing zones, as well as tibial runoff, is of critical importance. The ideal landing zone length is about 2 cm of nonaneurysmal, nontortuous, healthy artery. If there is a size discrepancy between the proximal and distal landing zones, a tapered configuration is used. With this strategy, if the size discrepancy between the proximal and distal stent is greater than 2–3 mm, a bridging stent is used. If opting for an endovascular approach, the patient should have greater than one tibioperoneal runoff vessel, as this has consistently been correlated to patency [25]. Extent of coverage below the knee should also be considered, as more distal coverage is also associated with worse outcomes [25]. Postoperatively, all EPAR patients should be on dual antiplatelet therapy for at least 6 months as long as this can be tolerated by the patient. Surveillance following EPAR generally consists of a 1-month follow-up with duplex and if normal, the patient will then be followed with a duplex every 6 months.

Surgical Treatment

Open surgical intervention remains the gold standard treatment for PAA in good-risk patients, and includes exclusion of the aneurysm by proximal and distal artery ligation, combined with revascularization (Table 30.1).

Three techniques of PAA exclusion have been described. One method involves proximal and distal ligation of the PAA with short-segment revascularization. This technique is typically employed when there is a focal PAA and when the superficial femoral artery is relatively disease-free so that it can be used as an inflow source. Another technique also involves proximal and distal ligation of the aneurysm but with long segment exclusion (e.g., proximal ligation in upper superficial femoral artery with a common femoral to below-knee popliteal bypass). This procedure is usually performed when an extensive fusiform aneurysm is present, or when there is significant femoral-popliteal artery occlusive disease. A third method involves a

Table 30.1 Selected series of popliteal artery aneurysms treated by endovascular repair compared to open repair

Authors	Year	Approach	Number of aneurysms	Assisted patency (%)	Number with thrombosis	Mean follow-up (months)
Antonello et al. [27]	2005	OPAR	15	100	0	46.1
		EPAR	15	100	1	45.9
Pulli et al. [23]	2012	OPAR	43	81.6	2	22.5
		EPAR	21	78.4	3	
Pulli et al. [28]	2013	OPAR	178	84.7	6	30.6
		EPAR	134	90.8	13	
Serrano Hernando et al. [22]	2015	OPAR	139	79.0	20	49.0
		EPAR	32	79.7	7	

OPAR open popliteal aneurysm repair, *EPAR* endovascular popliteal aneurysm repair, *NA* not available, *PAAs* popliteal artery aneurysms single proximal ligature of the aneurysm and revascularization [31, 32]. Most surgeons agree that full PAA exclusion by proximal and distal ligation is critical for long-term success and this later method has been discounted [31].

Two anatomic approaches can be used for PAA repair. Most repairs are performed using the medial leg approach. Many surgeons prefer this approach due to its familiarity and the greater number of options available in the supine patient. The greater saphenous vein is easily accessible as are the tibial vessels, in the case a more distal arterial bypass is required. Additionally, the superficial or common femoral artery can be used for inflow, which may be necessary if the above-knee popliteal artery is found to be more diseased than expected from the preoperative studies. The posterior approach to PAA repair is typically used when the aneurysm is confined to the popliteal fossa. It is associated with an increased incidence of popliteal vein and tibial nerve injury, as these structures may be adherent to the aneurysm, but the bypass graft is shorter and the incision is smaller.

When selecting the conduit for bypass, autologous vein, specifically the greater saphenous vein, is preferred. Any adequately sized autologous vein, however (including cephalic or lesser saphenous), is associated with good long-term graft patency and limb salvage. Prosthetic grafts may also be employed, but only as a last resort for symptomatic PAA as patency rates are inferior [10].

However, some have reported good success with the posterior approach using a short ePTFE interposition graft [33].

Outcomes for patients undergoing elective repair of their PAA are favorable, especially when in asymptomatic patients with preserved distal vessel runoff. In multiple studies, the range of 5- and 10-year graft patency rates is reported as 90–95% and 64–75%, respectively [4, 5, 10]. Five- and ten-year limb salvage rates are higher. In contrast to these results for asymptomatic aneurysm repair, amputation rates are high for patients presenting with ALI from a PAA. Despite attempts at urgent revascularization and emergent bypass grafting, long-term amputation rates are as high as 25% [3, 6]. Operative mortality for PAA repair is low, with estimates from 0% to 2% overall [1, 34].

Treatment: Common Femoral Artery Aneurysms

Surgical

This aneurysm is approached through a standard groin exposure. Perioperative antibiotics are administered prior to incision and discontinued within 24 h. Isolation and control of the distal external iliac, SFA, and PFA is obtained. Only in rare circumstances it is necessary to obtain separate proximal external iliac artery control through a separate incision. Intravenous heparin is administered to achieve an ACT of more than 250. The AA sac is opened, and an appropriately sized graft is chosen (generally 8–10 mm Dacron or ePTFE). It is essential to preserve the PFA and most of the time the graft is sewn distally at the SFA-PFA junction. Occasionally, a side graft to the PFA is needed, or a transposed PFA patch can be sewn onto the side of the graft. These repairs provide a durable, short segment, modest-sized graft with excellent patency [26].

Profunda femoral aneurysms may actually be more [35] dangerous to the patient as they often grow to a significant size [36] and may present with rupture or ALI in the setting of an occluded SFA. These aneurysms are also more challenging to repair, particularly in a setting of a chronic SFA occlusion. It is important to maintain as many outflow branches with the repair as possible, but occasionally ligation and a femoral to distal bypass may be needed for limb salvage. In brief, a prosthetic graft (6–8 mm) is sewn between the inflow PFA neck and the first- or second-order PFA outflow nonaneurysmal branches. Several series are published on these AA, although the overall number of patients with isolated profunda aneurysms is very rare [35, 36]. Graft patency and limb salvage for CFAA repair is more than 80% at 5 years follow-up [26].

Thrombolysis for Acute Ischemia Related to AA

Peripheral AA may present with ALI resulting from either a thrombosed AA or a chronic embolization, and requires urgent intervention to reestablish flow. This may take the form of open thrombectomy and embolectomy or catheter-directed intra-arterial thrombolysis. As with other forms of ALI, all patients presenting with acute occlusion of a peripheral AA must be given systemic IV Heparin. Unfortunately, for patients who present with critical limb ischemia, the risk of eventual amputation is high, between 9% and 36% [37].

Catheter-directed intra-arterial thrombolysis has replaced open thrombectomy as the primary treatment for PAA, and is less commonly used for acute CFAA occlusions. In addition to avoiding the morbidity of open operation and preserving the options (and conduit) for future bypass, thrombolysis may help improve the patency of the runoff vessels (tibial and peroneal), improving the success of eventual open repair. The newest SVS guidelines recommend thrombolysis or pharmacomechanical intervention as the first step for a patient who presents with ALI. This maximizes tibioperoneal outflow and optimizes patency after repair. This is primarily for patients with mild or moderate ischemia. For patients who present with Rutherford IIB ischemia, thromboembolectomy, pharmacomechanial thrombectomy, or suction thrombectomy should be used as an adjunctive intervention at the time of repair.

Nonoperative Treatment

Several criteria may be used to select patients for nonoperative management, and the patients' general health and suitability for intervention must be considered. Patients with small (≤2 cm) asymptomatic aneurysms without thrombus and thrombosed PAA with stable claudication are reasonable nonoperative candidates. However, this may not apply to thrombosed CFAA which are usually symptomatic. Although no data exist to support the benefit of anticoagulation therapy with Coumadin or a direct oral anticoagulant, it is the author's current practice to use anticoagulation selectively, carefully considering the bleeding risk. Regardless, patients should be followed closely and educated about possible signs/symptoms of emboli or arterial occlusion.

Conclusion

A diagnosis of a peripheral arterial aneurysm mandates evaluation of a more proximal AAA. Imaging is primarily with duplex ultrasonography, and CT angiography has replaced angiography for operative planning. Peripheral arterial aneurysms are more often limb-threatening than life-threatening, and repair is recommended for PAA >2.0 cm and for >2.5 cm CFAA in good-risk patients. Open surgical repair for PAA and CFAA is safe, and durable in properly selected patients. PAA endovascular repair is comparable to surgical repair when anatomically suitable and should be considered depending on the patient's age, co-morbidities, and anatomy.

References

1. GLM. Femoral and popliteal aneurysms. L. W. & W. Publishers; 2001.
2. Dent TL, Lindenauer SM, Ernst CB, Fry WJ. Multiple arteriosclerotic arterial aneurysms. Arch Surg. 1972;105:338–44.
3. Vermilion BD, Kimmins SA, Pace WG, Evans WE. A review of one hundred forty-seven popliteal aneurysms with long-term follow-up. Surgery. 1981;90:1009–14.
4. Jacob T, Ascher E, Hingorani A, Gunduz Y, Kallakuri S. Initial steps in the unifying theory of the pathogenesis of artery aneurysms. J Surg Res. 2001;101:37–43.
5. Dawson I, van Bockel JH, Brand R, Terpstra JL. Popliteal artery aneurysms. Long-term follow-up of aneurysmal disease and results of surgical treatment. J Vasc Surg. 1991;13:398–407.
6. Carpenter JP, Barker CF, Roberts B, Berkowitz HD, Lusk EJ, Perloff LJ. Popliteal artery aneurysms: current management and outcome. J Vasc Surg. 1994;19:63–5.
7. Graham LM, Zelenock GB, Whitehouse WMJ, Erlandson EE, Dent TL, Lindenauer SM, Stanley JC. Clinical significance of arteriosclerotic femoral artery aneurysms. Arch Surg. 1980;115:502–7.
8. Diwan A, Sarkar R, Stanley JC, Zelenock GB, Wakefield TW. Incidence of femoral and popliteal artery aneurysms in patients with abdominal aortic aneurysms. J Vasc Surg. 2000;31:863–9.
9. Ascher E, Markevich N, Schutzer RW, Kallakuri S, Jacob T, Hingorani AP. Small popliteal artery aneurysms: are they clinically significant? J Vasc Surg. 2003;37:755–60.
10. Shortell CK, DeWeese JA, Ouriel K, Green RM. Popliteal artery aneurysms: a 25-year surgical experience. J Vasc Surg. 1991;14:771–9.
11. Ebaugh JL, Morasch MD, Matsumura JS, Eskandari MK, Meadows WS, Pearce WH. Fate of excluded popliteal artery aneurysms. J Vasc Surg. 2003;37:954–9.
12. Kirkpatrick UJ, McWilliams RG, Martin J, Brennan JA, Gilling-Smith GL, Harris PL. Late complications after ligation and bypass for popliteal aneurysm. Br J Surg. 2004;91:174–7.

13. Cousins RS, Dexter DJ, Ahanchi SS, Cain BC, Powell OM, Ongstad SB, Parikh NM, Panneton JM. Determining patient risk factors associated with accelerated growth of popliteal artery aneurysms. J Vasc Surg. 2018;67:838–47.
14. Anton GE, Hertzer NR, Beven EG, O'Hara PJ, Krajewski LP. Surgical management of popliteal aneurysms. Trends in presentation, treatment, and results from 1952 to 1984. J Vasc Surg. 1986;3:125–34.
15. Lowell RC, Gloviczki P, Hallett JWJ, Naessens JM, Maus TP, Cherry KJJ, Bower TC, Pairolero PC, Ascher E, Markevich N, Schutzer RW, Kallakuri S, Jacob T, Hingorani AP. Popliteal artery aneurysms: the risk of nonoperative management. J Vasc Surg. 2003;8:14–23.
16. Batt M, Scotti L, Gagliardi JM, Riberi A, Cassar JP, Porcher G, Le Bas P. Popliteal aneurysms. Our experience apropos of 119 cases. J Chir (Paris). 1985;122:319–25.
17. Stoner MC, Calligaro KD, Chaer RA, Dietzek AM, Farber A, Guzman RJ, Hamdan AD, Landry GJ, Yamaguchi DJ. Reporting standards of the Society for Vascular Surgery for endovascular treatment of chronic lower extremity peripheral artery disease. J Vasc Surg. 2016;64:e1–e21.
18. Puech-Leão P, Kauffman P, Wolosker N, Anacleto AM. Endovascular grafting of a popliteal aneurysm using the saphenous vein. J Endovasc Surg. 1998;5:64–70.
19. Gerasimidis T, Sfyroeras G, Papazoglou K, Trellopoulos G, Ntinas A, Karamanos D. Endovascular treatment of popliteal artery aneurysms. Eur J Vasc Endovasc Surg. 2003;26:506–11.
20. Farber A, Angle N, Avgerinos E, Dubois L, Eslami M, Geraghty P, Haurani M, Jim J, Ketteler E, Pulli R, Siracuse JJ, Murad MH. The Society for Vascular Surgery clinical practice guidelines on popliteal artery aneurysms. J Vasc Surg. 2022;75:109S–20S.
21. Lowell RC, Gloviczki P, Hallett JWJ, Naessens JM, Maus TP, Cherry KJJ, Bower TC, Pairolero PC. Popliteal artery aneurysms: the risk of nonoperative management. Ann Vasc Surg. 1994;8:14–23.
22. Serrano Hernando FJ, Martínez López I, Hernández Mateo MM, Hernando Rydings M, Sánchez Hervás L, Rial Horcajo R, Moñux Ducajú G, Martín Conejero A. Comparison of popliteal artery aneurysm therapies. J Vasc Surg. 2015;61:655–61.
23. Pulli R, Dorigo W, Fargion A, Pratesi G, Innocenti AA, Angiletta D, Pratesi C. Comparison of early and midterm results of open and endovascular treatment of popliteal artery aneurysms. Ann Vasc Surg. 2012;26:809–18.
24. Leake AE, Segal MA, Chaer RA, Eslami MH, Al-Khoury G, Makaroun MS, Avgerinos ED. Meta-analysis of open and endovascular repair of popliteal artery aneurysms. J Vasc Surg. 2017;65:246–256.e2.
25. Zaghloul MS, Andraska EA, Leake A, Chaer R, Avgerinos ED, Hager ES, Makaroun MS, Eslami MH. Poor runoff and distal coverage below the knee are associated with poor long-term outcomes following endovascular popliteal aneurysm repair. J Vasc Surg. 2021;74:153–60.
26. Sapienza P, Mingoli A, Feldhaus RJ, di Marzo L, Cavallari N, Cavallaro A. Femoral artery aneurysms: long-term follow-up and results of surgical treatment. Cardiovasc Surg. 1996;4:181–4.
27. Antonello M, Frigatti P, Battocchio P, Lepidi S, Cognolato D, Dall'Antonia A, Stramanà R, Deriu GP, Grego F. Open repair versus endovascular treatment for asymptomatic popliteal artery aneurysm: results of a prospective randomized study. J Vasc Surg. 2005;42:185–93.
28. Pulli R, Dorigo W, Castelli P, Dorrucci V, Ferilli F, De Blasis G, Monaca V, Vecchiati E, Benincasa A, Pratesi C. A multicentric experience with open surgical repair and endovascular exclusion of popliteal artery aneurysms. Eur J Vasc Endovasc Surg. 2013;45:357–63.
29. Tielliu IFJ, Verhoeven ELG, Zeebregts CJ, Prins TR, Span MM, van den Dungen JJAM. Endovascular treatment of popliteal artery aneurysms: results of a prospective cohort study. J Vasc Surg. 2005;41:561–7.
30. Curi MA, Geraghty PJ, Merino OA, Veeraswamy RK, Rubin BG, Sanchez LA, Choi ET, Sicard GA. Mid-term outcomes of endovascular popliteal artery aneurysm repair. J Vasc Surg. 2007;45:505–10.
31. Mehta M, Champagne B, Darling RC 3rd, Roddy SP, Kreienberg PB, Ozsvath KJ, Paty PSK, Chang BB, Shah DM. Outcome of popliteal artery aneurysms after exclusion and

bypass: significance of residual patent branches mimicking type II endoleaks. J Vasc Surg. 2004;40:886–90.
32. Jones WT 3rd, Hagino RT, Chiou AC, Decaprio JD, Franklin KS, Kashyap VS. Graft patency is not the only clinical predictor of success after exclusion and bypass of popliteal artery aneurysms. J Vasc Surg. 2003;37:392–8.
33. Beseth BD, Moore WS. The posterior approach for repair of popliteal artery aneurysms. J Vasc Surg. 2006;43:940–5.
34. Whitehouse WMJ, Wakefield TW, Graham LM, Kazmers A, Zelenock GB, Cronenwett JL, Dent TL, Lindenauer SM, Stanley JC. Limb-threatening potential of arteriosclerotic popliteal artery aneurysms. Surgery. 1983;93:694–9.
35. Harbuzariu C, Duncan AA, Bower TC, Kalra M, Gloviczki P. Profunda femoris artery aneurysms: association with aneurysmal disease and limb ischemia. J Vasc Surg. 2008;47:31–5.
36. Posner SR, Wilensky J, Dimick J, Henke PK. A true aneurysm of the profunda femoris artery: a case report and review of the English language literature. Ann Vasc Surg. 2004;18:740–6.
37. Ravn H, Björck M. Popliteal artery aneurysm with acute ischemia in 229 patients. Outcome after thrombolytic and surgical therapy. Eur J Vasc Endovasc Surg. 2007;33:690–5.

Index

G. J. Arnaoutakis et al. (eds.), *Aortic Aneurysms*, Contemporary Cardiology,
https://doi.org/10.1007/978-3-032-13134-8

MIX
Papier aus verantwortungsvollen Quellen
Paper from responsible sources
FSC® C105338

If you have any concerns about our products,
you can contact us on
ProductSafety@springernature.com

In case Publisher is established outside the EU,
the EU authorized representative is:
Springer Nature Customer Service Center GmbH
Europaplatz 3, 69115 Heidelberg, Germany

Printed by Libri Plureos GmbH
in Hamburg, Germany